D1258278

In Vitro Methods in Pharmaceutical Research

In Vitro Methods in Pharmaceutical Research

Edited by

José V. Castell

and

María José Gómez-Lechón

University Hospital 'La Fe'
Valencia
Spain

ACADEMIC PRESS

SAN DIEGO LONDON BOSTON NEW YORK
SYDNEY TOKYO TORONTO

This book is printed on acid-free paper

Academic Press, Inc.
525 B Street, Suite 1900, San Diego, California 92101-4495, USA
http://www.apnet.com

Academic Press Limited
24–28 Oval Road, London NW1 7DX, UK
http://www.hbuk.co.uk/ap/

ISBN 0-12-163390-X

Library of Congress Cataloging-in-Publication Data

A catalogue record for this book is available from the British Library

Typeset by Tradespools Ltd, Frome, Somerset
Printed in Great Britain by The University Press, Cambridge

96 97 98 99 00 01 EB 9 8 7 6 5 4 3 2 1

Contents

Contributors vii

Preface xi

Part I: General Aspects of *In Vitro* Testing

1 Replacement Alternative and Complementary *In Vitro* Methods in Pharmaceutical Research 1
Donald W. Straughan, Julia H. Fentem and Michael Balls

2 Integration of QSAR and *In Vitro* Toxicology 15
Martin D. Barratt and Mark Chamberlain

3 Continuous Cell Lines as a Model for Drug Toxicity Assessment 33
Frank A. Barile

Part II: Target Organ Toxicity

4 *In Vitro* Models for Nephrotoxicity Screening and Risk Assessment 55
Peter H. Bach, David K. Obatomi and Stephen Brant

5 Experimental *In Vitro* Models to Evaluate Hepatotoxicity 103
Alison E. M. Vickers

6 Isolation, Culture and Use of Human Hepatocytes in Drug Research. 129
María José Gómez-Lechón, Teresa Donato, Xavier Ponsoda, Ricardo Fabra, Ramón Trullenque and José V. Castell

7 Studies of Neurotoxicity in Cellular Models 155
Elizabeth McFarlane Abdulla and Iain C. Campbell

8 Chondrocyte Culture: A Target System to Evaluate Pharmacotoxicological Effects of Drugs. 181
Monique Adolphe, Sophie Thenet-Gauci and Sylvie Demignot

9 Primary Cultures of Cardiac Myocytes as *In Vitro* Models for Pharmacological and Toxicological Assessments 209
Enrique Chacon, Daniel Acosta and John J. Lemasters

10 Immunotoxicology Testing *In Vitro* 225
Clive Meredith and Klara Miller

Part III: Irritancy Testing

11 Cutaneous Pharmacotoxicology *In Vitro* 241
Roland Roguet

12 Ocular Irritation 265
Horst Spielmann

13 Phototoxicity of Drugs 289
Miguel A. Miranda

Part IV: Genotoxicity and Tetratogenicity Testing

14 *In Vitro* Genotoxicity and Cell Transformation Assessment 317
Ian de G. Mitchell and Robert D. Combes

15 Use of Whole Embryo Cultures in *In Vitro* Teratogenicity Testing 353
Beat Schmid, Rudolf Bechter and Pavel Kucera

Part V: Drug Metabolism and Mechanisms of Toxicity

16 *In Vitro* Investigation of the Molecular Mechanisms of Hepatotoxicity 375
José V. Castell, María José Gómez-Lechón, Xavier Ponsoda and Roque Bort

17 Biotransformation of Drugs by Hepatocytes 411
André Guillouzo

18 Drug Metabolism and Carcinogen Activation Studies with Human Genetically Engineered Cells 433
Katherine Macé, Elizabeth A. Offord and Andrea M. A. Pfeifer

Index 457

Contributors

Daniel Acosta
College of Pharmacy, Department of Pharmacology/Toxicology, University of Texas at Austin, Texas 78712-1074, USA

Monique Adolphe
Laboratoire de Pharmacologie Cellulaire de l'Ecole Pratique des Hautes Etudes, Centre de Recherches Biomédicale des Cordeliers, 15 Rue de l'Ecole de Médecine, 75006 Paris, France

Peter H. Bach
Interdisciplinary Centre for Cell Modulation Studies, Faculty of Science and Health, University of East London, Romford Road, London E15 4LZ, UK

Michael Balls
ECVAM, Joint Research Centre Environment Institute European Commission, I-21020 Ispra (VA), Italy

Frank A. Barile
Department of Natural Sciences, City University of New York at York College, Jamaica, New York 11451, USA

Martin D. Barratt
Unilever Environmental Safety Laboratory, Colworth House, Sharnbrook, Bedford MK44 1LQ, UK

Rudolf Bechter
Sandoz Pharma Ltd, Drug Safety, Toxicology 881, CH-4002 Basle, Switzerland

Roque Bort
Unidad de Hepatología Experimental, Centro de Investigación, Hospital Universitario La Fe, Avda. Campanar 21, E-46009, Valencia, Spain

Stephen Brant
Interdisciplinary Centre for Cell Modulation Studies, Faculty of Science and Health, University of East London, Romford Road, London E15 4LZ, UK

Iain C. Campbell
Department of Neuroscience, Institute of Psychiatry, London SE5 8AF, UK

José V. Castell
Unidad de Hepatología Experimental, Centro de Investigación, Hospital Universitario La Fe, Avda. Campanar 21, E-46009, Valencia, Spain

Enrique Chacon
CEDRA Corporation, 8609 Cross Park Drive, Austin, Texas 78754, USA

Mark Chamberlain
Unilever Environmental Safety Laboratory, Colworth House, Sharnbrook, Bedford MK44 1LQ, UK

Robert D. Combes
FRAME, Russell and Burch House, 96–98 North Sherwood Street, Nottingham NG1 4EE, UK

Sylvie Demignot
Laboratoire de Pharmacologie Cellulaire de l'Ecole Pratique des Hautes Etudes, Centre de Recherches Biomédicale des Cordeliers, 15 Rue de l'Ecole de Médecine, 75006 Paris, France

Teresa Donato
Unidad de Hepatología Experimental, Centro de Investigación, Hospital Universitario La Fe, Avda. Campanar 21, E-46009, Valencia, Spain

Ricardo Fabra
Servicio de Cirugía Digestiva, Hospital General de Valencia, Camino Tres Cruces s/n. E-46014 Valencia, Spain

Julia H. Fentem
ECVAM, TP 580, JRC Environment Institute, I-21020 Ispra (VA), Italy

María José Gómez-Lechón
Unidad de Hepatología Experimental, Centro de Investigación, Hospital Universitario La Fe, Avda. Campanar 21, E-46009, Valencia, Spain

André Guillouzo
Groupe Détoxication et Réparation Tissulaire, Faculté des Sciences Pharmaceutiques et Biologiques, Av. du Professeur Léou Bernard, F-35043 Rennes Cedex, France

Pavel Kucera
Institute of Physiology, University of Lausanne, CH-1005 Lausanne, Switzerland

John J. Lemasters
Department of Cell Biology and Anatomy, Curriculum in Toxicology, School of Medicine, University of North Carolina at Chapel Hill, North Carolina 27599-7090, USA

Katherine Macé
Nestlé Research Centre, Vers chez les Blanc, PO Box 44, CH-1000 Lausanne 26, Switzerland

Elizabeth McFarlane Abdulla
Department of Neuroscience, Institute of Psychiatry, London SE5 8AF, UK

Clive Meredith
Immunotoxicology Department, BIBRA International, Woodmansterne Road, Carshalton, Surrey SM5 4DS, UK

Klara Miller
Immunotoxicology Department, BIBRA International, Woodmansterne Road, Carshalton, Surrey SM5 4DS, UK

Miguel A. Miranda
Departamento de Quimica/Instituto de Tecnología Química UPV-CSIC, Universidad Politécnica de Valencia, Camino de Vera, s/n; Apartado 22012, E-46071 Valencia, Spain

Ian de G. Mitchell
Smith-Kline Beecham Pharmaceuticals, The Frythe, Welwyn, Herts AL6 9AR, UK

David K. Obatomi
Interdisciplinary Centre for Cell Modulation Studies, Faculty of Science and Health, University of East London, Romford Road, London E15 4LZ, UK

Elizabeth A. Offord
Nestlé Research Centre, Vers chez les Blanc, PO Box 44, CH-1000 Lausanne 26, Switzerland

Andrea M. A. Pfeifer
Nestlé Research Centre, Vers chez les Blanc, PO Box 44, CH-1000 Lausanne 26, Switzerland

Xavier Ponsoda
Unidad de Hepatología Experimental, Centro de Investigación, Hospital Universitario La Fe, Avda. Campanar 21, E-46009, Valencia, Spain

Roland Roguet
Life Sciences Research, Advanced Research, L'OREAL, 1 Avenue E. Schueller, Boîte Postale 22, F-93600 Aulnay-sous-Bois, France

Beat Schmid
Zyma SA, Preclinical Development and Drug Safety, CH-1260 Nyon, Switzerland

Horst Spielmann
National Centre for Documentation and Evaluation of Alternatives to Animal Experiments, Federal Institute for Health Protection of Consumers and Veterinary Medicine, Diedersdorfer Weg 1, D-12277 Berlin, Germany

Donald W. Straughan
FRAME, Russell and Burch House, 96–98 North Sherwood Street, Nottingham NG1 4EE, UK

Sophie Thenet-Gauci
Laboratoire de Pharmacologie Cellulaire de l'Ecole Pratique des Hautes Etudes, Centre de Recherches Biomédicale des Cordeliers, 15 Rue de l'Ecole de Médecine, F-75006 Paris, France

Ramón Trullenque
Servicio de Cirugía Digestiva, Hospital General de Valencia, Camino Tres Cruces s/n. E-46014 Valencia, Spain

Alison E. M. Vickers
Drug Safety Assessment, Sandoz Pharma Ltd, CH-4002 Basle, Switzerland

Preface

In the field of pharmaceutical development, researchers face a paradox: they have to search for new active compounds and guarantee consumer safety, but at the same time they are asked to minimize the number of animals used in experimentation. In this context, *in vitro* models are becoming increasingly relevant as they can be used to great advantage, both for screening purposes, and to explore the mechanisms of drug action. Moreover, they require small amounts of the substance to be tested, are relatively simple and fast to perform, and can render valuable scientific information at the very early stages of drug development, at a reasonable cost. *In vitro* models are, however, a simplification of the more complex living animal. This is an intrinsic advantage for researchers as it facilitates the study of complex *in vivo* phenomena, but at the same time, the interpretation of the experimental results is not easy in terms of human risk prediction. To know the limitations of *in vitro* models facilitates understanding of which experiments should be done and which may be meaningless. This is why the correct utilization of such models is of utmost importance. This book is intended to contribute to the wider implementation of *in vitro* techniques by providing a statement of the existing knowledge, models and methods currently being used, practical details of how to carry out the assays, and a discussion of their use and limitation.

The first part of the book is an introduction to the general aspects of *in vitro* screening with future perspectives, and discusses the use of quantitative structure-activity relationships in *in vitro* toxicology. The second part is a pragmatic summary of techniques currently used in *in vitro* toxicology, relating to the most relevant target organs such as the kidneys, liver, central nervous system, heart, cartilagous and immune systems. The book devotes individual chapters to each of these areas, presenting the principal models, their most relevant features and their present use. The third section is focused on irritancy testing, where the optimum utilization of *in vitro* assays for specific groups of compounds is discussed in the light of validation programs in progress. The fourth section of the book addresses the study of drug genotoxicity and teratogenicity. The ability of tests to predict or screen for human toxicity is presented according to the current scientific and regulatory advantages and limitations of human risk assessment. The methods are presented as a starting point and general guide for further investigation, rather than simplified flowcharts for particular procedures. The final section deals with the procedures used to assess *in vitro* hepatic drug metabolism and toxicity due to biotransformation. This section also covers the recent use of genetically engineered cells as a tool in drug metabolism research.

In Vitro Methods in Pharmaceutical Research, although necessarily limited in its scope, is intended to bring pharmaceutical researchers closer to the practical use of *in vitro* approaches. As the contents of this book demonstrate, there are now a broad range of *in vitro* models for use in either identifying or understanding most forms of toxicity. The authors and editors hope that this book will provide a sound basis for broad understanding and practical utilization of these models in drug development.

J. V. Castell
M. J. Gómez-Lechón

1

Replacement Alternative and Complementary *In Vitro* Methods in Pharmaceutical Research

DONALD W. STRAUGHAN, JULIA H. FENTEM AND MICHAEL BALLS

I. Introduction 1
II. Extent of use of *in vivo* and *in vitro* methods by the pharmaceutical industry . 2
A. *In vivo* methods. . . . 2
B. *In vitro* methods 3
III. Drug discovery and development 3
A. *In vitro* screening methods 4
1. Screens for pharmacological activity 4
2. Screens for toxicological activity. . . . 5
3. Limitations of *in vitro* methods. . . . 5
B. *In vivo* screening methods 6
C. Metabolism and pharmacokinetic studies. . . . 7
1. *In vitro* methods for studying biotransformation 7
2. Determination of kinetic parameters 8
3. Other related applications of *in vitro* methods. . . . 8
4. Future needs 8
D. Mechanistic studies 9
IV. Replacement alternative methods 10
V. Reduction and refinement alternatives. . . . 10
A. Antimicrobial agents 10
B. Cancer studies and anticancer drugs 11
VI. Conclusions. . . . 11
References. . . . 12

I. INTRODUCTION

It is now 15 years since the Fund for the Replacement of Animals in Medical Experiments (FRAME) organized a seminal conference on the use of alternatives in drug research,[1] so it is appropriate to look again at this theme. In the light of our experience, we will consider both

IN VITRO METHODS IN PHARMACEUTICAL RESEARCH
ISBN 0-12-163390-X

the general role and varied application of *in vitro* methods in pharmaceutical research, particularly in drug discovery, and then comment more briefly on reduction and refinement alternatives.[2] The size of the pharmaceutical industry makes a discussion of the approaches relevant. The successful record of the industry in relation to basic research and in drug discovery requires such discussion to be positive. The industry provides, and will continue to provide, significant therapeutic, economic and societal benefits.

The pharmaceutical industry is concerned primarily with developing new or better treatments for disease; these medicines are usually administered orally, but may occasionally be administered by inhalation or dermal application. Assurance of efficacy and safety in use is critical. Because many drugs may cause adverse effects, a consideration of the nature of these possible adverse effects and the circumstances in which they might occur is important. Knowledge of mode of action is vital, and information about drug absorption, disposition, metabolism and excretion (ADME), and about the kinetics of these processes, is fundamental. To maximize safety, particular attention is attached to toxicity studies. Depending on the likely duration of treatment, these studies place particular emphasis on the identification of possible target organ toxicity (particularly for the liver, kidney, and haemopoietic and immune systems), reproductive and developmental toxicity, mutagenic and carcinogenic effects, and adverse effects following chronic administration.

Our definition of *in vitro* methods includes the many and varied uses of animal and human tissues and isolated cells, cell lines and cellular components, which are typically maintained in supporting aqueous media outside the living body.[3] In this chapter, we will consider the extent and nature of the use of *in vitro* methods (when, why and how such methods are used, and their role in complementing, as well as in providing replacement alternatives for, *in vivo* methods), and progress in their application in the development and testing of pharmaceuticals in recent years, and the problems encountered. We shall not deal with the plethora of specific applications of *in vitro* methods in drug research, since they have been, and continue to be, covered in a wide range of specialist scientific journals, as well as in several journals dealing primarily with alternative methods (e.g. *ATLA (Alternatives to Laboratory Animals)* and *ALTEX (Alternativen zu Tierexperimenten)*), and in monographs (e.g. reference 4).

II. EXTENT OF USE OF *IN VIVO* AND *IN VITRO* METHODS BY THE PHARMACEUTICAL INDUSTRY

A. *In vivo* methods

In vivo procedures in pharmaceutical research and testing account for a substantial proportion of the numbers of laboratory animals used in many countries. Typically, data are available on the numbers and types of animal procedures conducted by, or for, the pharmaceutical industry in the course of carrying out basic and applied research. Thus, in The Netherlands, medicines research (including toxicity tests) accounted for 25% of the animals used in 1987.[5] In the UK, non-toxicity procedures for the selection of medical, dental and veterinary products comprised 31% of the 2.8 million regulated animal procedures in 1994, while toxicity testing comprised a further 10%.[6]

B. *In vitro* methods

No firm data exist on the extent to which *in vitro* methods are used in pharmaceutical research, but our knowledge of several UK companies suggests that such methods are now widely used, with perhaps more than half the time of biological research staff being taken up with *in vitro* rather than with *in vivo* methods. Zbinden[7] commented that *in vitro* methods are 'widely used whenever a specific type of information is needed', which is often the case during the drug development process. He presented data showing that at least half of the research communications presented by fundamental biomedical scientists at several scientific conferences were based on results obtained by using *in vitro* models.

In the UK, if tissues, cells or subcellular material are obtained fresh by killing otherwise normal animals, the experiment (and its subsequent reporting and enumeration) falls outside the legal controls on animal experiments (i.e. the Animals (Scientific Procedures) Act 1986[8]), but this is not the case in The Netherlands or Sweden. In The Netherlands, the killing of previously untreated animals for organ removal and blood sampling accounted for 12.7% of the animals used in 1994.[9] It seems likely that between one-third and one-half of all the animals supplied to the pharmaceutical industry in the UK could be used as a source of tissues for *in vitro* experiments. The tissues removed from these animals provide for multiple use by several research teams, and can be used in many experiments.

Such broad indicators take no account of the scale of use of previously derived cell lines and biological materials. In the USA, the use of human tumour cell lines in culture has allowed the National Cancer Institute to phase out completely its previous use of six million tumour-bearing animals (mainly mice) per year for screening compounds for antitumour activity.[10] With respect to the numbers of tests rather than staff time, Spink[11] suggested that *in vitro* screens outnumbered *in vivo* screens by three to one at Wellcome Laboratories. This ratio seems likely to have increased considerably in the industry in recent years, both as a consequence of continuing advances in knowledge about target sites and cellular mechanisms, and because of sophisticated technical automation.

III. DRUG DISCOVERY AND DEVELOPMENT

Pharmaceutical research involves three elements: (a) fundamental biological research; (b) method development; and (c) drug discovery and development. The first two of these elements are similar to those undertaken in academic departments and research institutes. Drug discovery and development is the specific objective of the pharmaceutical industry and the reason for its existence.

Essentially, drug discovery involves screening to identify an initial lead compound, which either has a *novel biological activity* in an existing chemical entity, or has a known type of biological activity in a *new chemical entity*. Subsequently, systematic chemical modification and biological testing are undertaken to optimize the perceived useful activity, until one or more potential drug candidates are identified for further research and development. Biological testing includes extensive pharmacological and toxicological evaluation, with a view to administering the new drug to human volunteers and then subjecting it to clinical trials. Because many drugs may cause adverse effects, the nature of these and the circumstances in which they might occur must be determined. Purists might classify these later stages as development, rather than as pharmaceutical research.

A. *In vitro* screening methods

A key consideration in drug discovery is the need for a sound rationale for the initial pharmacological and toxicological screening methods employed during compound selection, whether they be existing compounds or novel entities. Toxicological screening should take place as soon as a group of molecules with a particular pharmacological activity of interest has been identified.[12] The ideal approach is one in which pharmacological and toxicological screening with *in vitro* methods are undertaken concurrently. The findings from these screens can then be used to guide further modification of the compound(s), before any animal tests have to be conducted.[12] In this respect, it is particularly important that the *in vitro* screens are highly predictive of effects known to occur *in vivo*.

In recent years, the purification and identification of macromolecular target sites, combined with powerful physical techniques, or homology modelling, have allowed the molecular structures of the target sites to be determined. This knowledge has provided a better basis for understanding the interaction of drugs with their target sites (DNA, enzymes, membrane receptors, etc.). In turn, through the application of powerful computational techniques, computer-aided drug selection and design (CADD) has become an exciting and important reality.[13] It seems very likely that CADD has rationalized the initial selection of compounds, making it more efficient and successful in several areas. The effect of this is that fewer inactive compounds are being tested, resulting in a corresponding reduction in unsuccessful screening studies and in the associated use of laboratory animals.

In vitro methods are ideal when there is a specific dynamic effect or end-point that can be measured. They provide an environment in which the variables can be controlled carefully and manipulated.[14] The end-points can be pharmacological, biochemical or molecular, immunological, genetic, physiological or pathological. Characteristically, *in vitro* methods are usually easy to set up, yield results quickly, readily permit replication and good quantification, are inexpensive, and are simple to run and automate. These features provide a marked contrast to *in vivo* methods. Orlans[10] put the contrast succinctly: 'Typically, *in vitro* methods can be used to ask certain questions at the cellular or molecular level, whereas whole animals (including humans) are needed to answer questions at the organ and inter-organ level.' As a consequence, *in vitro* methods find particular use in 'high throughput' screening, as well as in basic research and mechanistic studies undertaken during drug discovery. They also play an important role in subsequent drug development and toxicological testing.

Perhaps the greatest advantage of *in vitro* methods is that human cells and tissues can be used,[15,16] thereby obviating the need for extrapolating data from laboratory animals to humans, and making the results obtained of direct relevance to human safety assessments of drugs. Nevertheless, the use of primary cultures of human cells involves a range of ethical, safety, legal and logistical issues, which need to be overcome if the use of human tissues for research and testing is to become more widespread.[17,18]

1. *Screens for pharmacological activity*

When screening for pharmacological activity, an array of *in vitro* methods can be used to provide data on multiple end-points considered likely to confer therapeutic advantage. For example, for antihypertensives the ratio of β-adrenoceptor to α_1-adrenoceptor block can be determined, and for antidepressants the ratio of 5-hydroxytryptamine (5-HT) uptake block, or of α_2-adrenoceptor block, to noradrenaline uptake block can be measured.

Drug concentrations that give effects *in vitro* often correspond very closely to *free* plasma concentrations *in vivo* (i.e. the concentration of drug not bound to plasma proteins). This has been shown for a range of compounds, such as monoamine uptake inhibitors, hormones, ATPase inhibitors, dopamine antagonists and opioid analgesics. It provides the rationale for, and confirms the essential utility of, the *in vitro* approach. Thus, in drug discovery and development, *in vitro* methods (isolated organs, receptor binding studies, etc.) will continue to provide both novel leads from high throughput screens and essential data for the pharmacological classification of receptors, and for establishing structure–activity relationships (SARs).

2. *Screens for toxicological activity*

A multitude of *in vitro* screens for cytotoxicity[7,19] and target organ toxicity[20,21] have been developed. For example, the potential hepatotoxic,[22,23] nephrotoxic[24,25] and neurotoxic[26,27] effects of large numbers of compounds can be readily investigated in relatively simple *in vitro* systems, which employ various end-points and assay procedures. The toxicological end-points determined need to be specific, to avoid the discarding of potentially valuable drugs because of false-positive results.

In terms of toxicological screening during drug discovery and development, the availability of reliable and predictive (i.e. validated) *in vitro* tests for teratogenicity is considered to be a priority. A large number of *in vitro* systems for assessing teratogenic effects has been proposed,[28–31] including whole embryo cultures (e.g. from rat, mouse, chick, fish and frog), organ and micromass limb-bud cultures, micromass cultures of embryonic midbrain, and several cell lines (e.g. measurement of the inhibition of intercellular communication in Chinese hamster V79 cells). By aiding the selection of compounds for subsequent *in vivo* testing, *in vitro* teratogenicity assays could considerably reduce the expense and duration of toxicological studies,[28] in addition to reducing the numbers of animals used. Standard segment II *in vivo* test protocols involve the use of over 100 animals (rats or mice, and rabbits) per test compound, require high levels of technical expertise, and take several weeks to perform.[29,32] It has also been suggested that *in vitro* tests could be more predictive of human teratogenic potential than the current animal procedures, as specific human metabolic systems could be incorporated *in vitro*.[31,32]

3. *Limitations of* in vitro *methods*

In vitro test systems are typically highly simplified models of *in vivo* processes, and thus there are various limitations to the direct extrapolation of *in vitro* data to the *in vivo* situation in both pharmacological and toxicological investigations.

1. The target may be artefactual. For example, in receptor binding assays, binding sites may be created which are not normally functional *in vivo*. Such assays are now used with appropriate targets in a more discriminating fashion, not least because of the potential for information overload. The target may also be artefactual in *in vitro* toxicological screens, due principally to the relatively static nature of most *in vitro* systems and the use of inappropriate drug concentrations, which are markedly higher than those that could ever be achieved *in vivo*.
2. The target may be of low novelty. For example, even if another drug is discovered which inhibits prostaglandin synthetase, blocks β-adrenoceptors or inhibits noradrenaline uptake, there are already many drugs available with such actions. Yet another drug

with these actions seems unlikely to offer obvious therapeutic advantages, although it might have commercial relevance in less discriminating markets.

3. The drug target may be genuine, but its therapeutic utility or advantage may not be known. For example, the pioneering work on β-blockers and 5-HT_3 (M) receptor antagonists necessarily preceded the discovery of their present therapeutic utility. The assumption that a particular pharmacological activity *in vitro* will be useful therapeutically may also be oversimplified, as is the case with the development of cholinomimetics for treating senile dementia. This reflects the current state of knowledge and, in particular, the considerable complexity of the function and pathology of the central nervous system.
4. Compound biokinetics are different *in vitro* and *in vivo*. The biotransformation of a drug often has an important effect on its pharmacological and/or toxicological activities, as can its absorption, distribution and excretion *in vivo*.
5. Drug activity *in vitro* usually relates to the aqueous solubility of the compound. Thus, it is generally necessary to modify the most active, polar, compound *in vitro* (the lead compound), to develop more lipophilic congeners for subsequent oral dosing in *in vivo* studies. This may alter considerably the pharmacological and toxicological properties of the compound, due to effects on its absorption, distribution, metabolism and excretion, and the kinetics of these processes.
6. The concentrations at which the drug is pharmacologically and toxicologically active need to be considered. To be useful, any lead compound should be pharmacologically active *in vitro* at relevant concentrations (i.e. those that are likely to be achieved *in vivo* with realistic dose levels). For example, Na^+K^+-ATPase inhibition with an anti-depressant compound at millimolar (mM) concentrations is irrelevant, because such compounds are active clinically and affect monoamine uptake *in vivo* at submicro-molar (μM) concentrations. The selection of appropriate concentrations for use in *in vitro* toxicological studies is also critical, if the production of non-specific effects is to be avoided (see (1) above). The pharmaceutical industry appreciates concentration relevance, though, on occasion, academic groups do not, and engage in phenomeno-logical studies.

B. *In vivo* screening methods

In vitro methods are frequently undertaken first, as part of a hierarchical testing strategy, and hence complement later investigations conducted *in vivo* to confirm the principal mechanism of drug action, and then to determine the general pharmacology, pharmaco-kinetics and toxicology of selected compounds. If this is an accepted practice, then a fundamental question to be addressed is *whether* and, if so, *when* there is any justification for using *in vivo* rather than *in vitro* tests in the primary screening for new lead compounds. This is an important issue, because of the large numbers of animals (tens of thousands per annum) which may be used, even in a single screen, when trying to identify a new lead compound from the vast 'library' of chemicals available 'in-house' to most pharmaceutical companies.

Any attempt at rational discussion is frustrated by a lack of specific information in the public domain on the numbers of animals used in particular types of *in vivo* screening tests, the circumstances of use, and the absolute justification for such use. In the UK, this information is available only to Home Office inspectors; elsewhere, it should be available to independent review committees in those situations where they inspect protocols for industrial research. Because details of animal use in specific *in vivo* screening tests are not readily accessible, the public is obliged to accept assurances that all such animal use is necessary and justified. At present, even the scientific community does not have the detailed information to know whether *in vitro* methods are, in general, deployed optimally to minimize experimentation on living animals.

In the UK, there has been a marked decrease in the use of *in vivo* tests for initial screening in recent years. This reflects increased knowledge about the mechanisms of action of drugs and about disease processes, and enthusiasm for targeted research where the target can be modelled *in vitro* (e.g. angiotensin-converting enzyme (ACE) inhibitors or angiotensin antagonists). In addition, the introduction of licences for specific research programmes (project licences) under the Animals (Scientific Procedures) Act 1986[8] seems likely to have reduced the extent of *in vivo* screening.

At least some *in vivo* primary screens for several pharmacological activities currently in use can be justified, where it has been argued convincingly that relevant *in vitro* systems are not yet available to model the desired action, or where drugs with anticipated novel mechanisms of action cannot be detected by the use of *in vitro* methods (since it is essential that these involve known mechanisms). Thus, an argument can be made for primary *in vivo* screening of compounds for their effects on spontaneous hypertension in rats (as a model for human idiopathic hypertension), for primary screening in certain inflammatory or immune-based models, and perhaps for the screening of classes of antifungal drugs which are otherwise inactive *in vitro*.

The general proposition that primary screening *in vivo* is always justified to permit oral administration and adequate bioavailability is less satisfactory, given that many lead compounds can be modified chemically to enable their use *in vivo*. The continued primary screening *in vivo* of, for example, antibiotics may reflect habitual practice rather than necessary and best practice. We suspect that *in vivo* screens may be used more extensively in mainland Europe than in the UK, but have no direct information on this. However, if this was the case, then the practice would be difficult to justify, unless it could be shown that mainland Europe had a better record of drug discovery than the UK.

C. Metabolism and pharmacokinetic studies

Another important area of application of *in vitro* methods in pharmaceutical research involves determining how biological systems affect the compound, rather than how the compound affects target sites. Predictions of likely absorption are made routinely, based on physicochemical parameters such as partition coefficients and pK_a values, and are confirmed in artificial (e.g. reconstructed epidermis) or natural (e.g. loops of gut in organ baths) cellular or organotypic preparations.

1. In vitro *methods for studying biotransformation*

A wide range of *in vitro* systems, which employ animal and/or human cells derived from the liver and/or from many extrahepatic tissues, is available for studying the metabolism of compounds. These systems include tissue slices, primary cell cultures, genetically engineered cell lines expressing specific xenobiotic-metabolizing enzymes, and microsomes and other subcellular fractions.[4,16,33] Owing to their high levels of biotransformation enzymes compared with other cell types, isolated hepatocytes are a potentially valuable test system for determining the metabolic profiles of drugs, as well as for measuring the activities and substrate specificities of the various hepatic enzyme systems involved in their biotransformation.[22,34,35]

As mentioned previously, *in vitro* approaches are ideal when many substances have to be compared, as in screening to select lead compounds. They are also very useful for undertaking investigations of species differences in metabolism. For example, the extrapolation of pharmacological and toxicological data between species is often hampered by qualitative and quantitative differences in drug biotransformation, as well as in the intrinsic activities of the compounds and their metabolites. The use of *in vitro* systems derived from different species, including humans, can provide a basis for qualitative and quantitative interspecies comparisons, making it easier to evaluate the relevance of observations made in the species used in pharmacology and/or toxicology studies, and helping to provide confidence in the results of such studies.[22]

2. *Determination of kinetic parameters*

The data obtained in *in vitro* systems are not directly comparable with those on the *in vivo* effects of a chemical, partly because the concentrations used in cell cultures cannot easily be related to the doses administered *in vivo*. For an appropriate *in vitro* to *in vivo* extrapolation, it is therefore necessary to obtain data on the biokinetics of the compound and its metabolites, both *in vivo* and *in vitro*.[22,36]

In vitro data on absorption and drug metabolism can be combined with information, again from *in vitro* studies, on protein binding, transport and drug clearance,[37,38] and with existing data on partitioning, organ blood flow, etc., to make predictions about the distribution, metabolism and excretion of compounds *in vivo*. In some cases, physiologically based pharmacokinetic (PBPK) models may be developed, by using *in vitro* and *in vivo* data, to enable a full understanding of the biological responses resulting from exposure to therapeutic and/or toxic drug concentrations.[39] The integrated use of data from *in vitro* tests and predictive computer modelling approaches (PBPK models; determination of SARs) was the subject of a recent workshop held by the European Centre for the Validation of Alternative Methods (ECVAM).[40]

3. *Other related applications of* in vitro *methods*

In recent years, *in vitro* techniques have facilitated the production, by recombinant DNA techniques, of large quantities of human drug-metabolizing enzymes of known sequences.[41,42] The three-dimensional modelling of the structure of some enzymes (e.g. human cytochrome P450 isozymes) is now being used to predict some drug interactions early in the drug development process. *In vitro* systems have proved particularly valuable for early investigations of possible drug–drug interactions.[43]

4. *Future needs*

There is a need to put more emphasis on the use of *in vitro* models of extrahepatic metabolism, and for more widespread recognition of the importance of drug biotransformation by enzyme systems other than cytochrome P450. Also, it would be valuable if the full functionality (in terms of the maintenance of specific functions associated with the cell/tissue *in vivo*) of tissue slices and isolated cells (particularly those derived from liver) could be maintained in culture for longer periods. In this respect, among 11 specific recommendations[22] about the best ways forward, the participants at a recent ECVAM workshop on hepatocyte culture concluded that:

(a) The relatively poor maintenance of stable biotransformation activities during hepatocyte culture is a major limitation of the current *in vitro* systems. Studies are required to standardize the culture conditions in order to optimize the maintenance of various hepatocyte-specific functions.
(b) The maintenance of hepatocyte-specific functions during long-term culture should be explored further, in particular in co-cultures and in three-dimensional hepatocyte culture systems.

In addition, the workshop participants recognized the critical importance of using human cells and tissues for xenobiotic metabolism and toxicity studies, since these were 'of particular value in bridging the gap between animal and human studies'.

Despite the obvious usefulness of *in vitro* methods in this area, for the time being regulatory authorities will continue to require data on ADME and pharmacokinetics from *in vivo* studies for the further development of lead compounds in the clinic and for the subsequent licensing of new drugs. Vickers *et al.*[44] summarized the current stance of the US Food and Drug Administration (FDA) with respect to the inclusion of *in vitro* metabolism data for investigational new drug (IND) or new drug application (NDA) submissions in this way: 'While *in vitro* information can never replace *in vivo* data, it can often provide insight into questions regarding the human metabolism of a drug prior to the initiation of clinical studies.'

D. Mechanistic studies

In vitro systems are ideally suited to investigations on the molecular, cellular and physiological mechanisms of drug activity (both pharmacological and toxicological effects) which cannot readily be studied *in vivo*.[14,22] Understanding the mechanisms by which drugs cause adverse effects, and the reasons for species differences in biological activity and the increased susceptibility of certain individuals to particular drugs, will markedly improve our ability to undertake human safety assessments. Acquiring an understanding of the mechanism(s) by which a drug acts is often an expensive and time-consuming process, necessitating the use of many different methods (both *in vitro* and *in vivo*).

The literature on the use of *in vitro* methods in toxicological research and testing is vast.[30] In toxicity testing, a few *in vitro* methods, e.g. short-term microbial assays for assessing mutagenesis, are now widely used and accepted by regulatory agencies. Others find particular use as complementary or adjunct methods in investigating mechanisms of toxicity,[23,24] for predicting specific toxic effects (e.g. drug-induced steatosis,[45] peroxisome proliferation[46]), or in selecting compounds with favourable *in vitro* therapeutic ratios.[47]

However, despite our best efforts, many adverse effects *in vivo* cannot be predicted by using *in vitro* systems. Even relatively complex cell aggregates (organotypic and micromass models) cannot mimic the complexity and duration of *in vivo* exposure, with its associated plethora of targets and control mechanisms. For this reason, despite the widespread use of *in vitro* methods, they have not replaced the use of *in vivo* procedures. Ultimately, it is hoped that the application of a suitable battery of mechanistically based *in vitro* tests may permit certain adverse effects of drugs to be predicted, thereby enabling the replacement of some of the acute toxicity tests required by regulatory agencies.

IV. REPLACEMENT ALTERNATIVE METHODS

In vitro methods need to be considered in terms of the Three Rs concept of alternatives pioneered by Russell and Burch,[2] and now enshrined in several national laws, and in Directive 86/609/EEC[48] of the European Union (EU), which regulate animal experimentation. In particular, the *replacement alternative* principle encourages the substitution of insentient material for conscious living animals. Within the EU, the use of replacement alternatives is covered under Article 7 of Directive 86/609/EEC,[48] which requires that: 'An experiment shall not be performed if another scientifically satisfactory method of obtaining the result sought, not entailing the use of an animal, is reasonably and practicably available.'

It will be apparent from the preceding sections of this chapter that *in vitro* methods are being used extensively as adjuncts (i.e. to provide data that can be used in combination with results obtained in *in vivo* studies). In this way, they have contributed to a genuine reduction in the numbers of *in vivo* experiments conducted for drug discovery purposes. However, they have not had as much impact on the number of animal procedures undertaken either for ADME and pharmacokinetic studies, or for toxicity testing.

V. REDUCTION AND REFINEMENT ALTERNATIVES

Where *in vivo* methods are used, it is proper to ask whether animal suffering has been minimized to the greatest extent possible, and whether the smallest practicable number of animals has been (and continue to be) used. Presumably, all responsible scientists accept such objectives, even if they do not have the commitment or the means to achieve them.

In the pharmaceutical industry in the UK, optimal or near-optimal deployment of alternative methods in drug discovery and development should be the general rule, since this is required by the UK project licensing system. In other countries, we expect that much of the industry will have good internal systems for reviewing their research programmes 'in house', but that national attitudes and practices are likely to differ, as is illustrated by the following two examples.

A. Antimicrobial agents

Recently, the UK pharmaceutical industry has devised guidelines for the conduct of infective challenge tests (PD50/rodent protection tests), which are frequently used in early screening to determine the potency of potential antimicrobial agents.[49] This is an important and very welcome first step in self-regulation to encourage the implementation of reduction and refinement alternatives. It is not known whether similar guidelines and principles have been accepted and apply generally in Europe and in the USA, but this is unlikely.

Further progress is still possible in the screening of antimicrobial agents. For example, single threshold doses might be used more frequently to allow a preliminary compound selection (rather than administering the antimicrobial agent at three dose levels to enable a formal potency calculation). Also, it should be possible to revise the end-point to count animals completely protected (i.e. those displaying no adverse symptoms), rather than counting animals which die or have to be killed humanely. There might also be anxieties about whether the minimum numbers of animals suggested by the guidelines are actually used in practice, and the extent to which tests are repeated.

B. Cancer studies and anticancer drugs

The pharmaceutical industry in the UK adheres to the UKCCCR (UK Coordinating Committee for Cancer Research) guidelines when undertaking cancer research, and for the screening and further evaluation of anticancer agents. Similar guidelines have been devised in some other countries, but the extent to which they are applied or can be enforced is not known. Such guidelines are not universal, and it would be useful to attempt to reach agreement on supranational and international guidelines, as a practical and specific means of implementing reduction and refinement alternatives.

VI. CONCLUSIONS

Pharmaceutical research is an area in which many animal experiments are conducted, and so the optimal and consistent implementation of all the Three Rs is clearly a worthwhile objective. We suggest that commitment to this aim will continue to provide scientific, practical and economic benefits to the pharmaceutical industry, as well as enabling it to be seen to be behaving in an ethical manner. The recent furore over the disposal of a North Sea oil rig indicates that a lack of concern for ethical or 'green' environmental issues may also carry an economic penalty. In the case of animal experimentation, good ethics should be good science, and should usually offer economic benefits through preventing unnecessary and unsuccessful *in vivo* experiments from being undertaken.

In our view, progress in further implementing the Three Rs would benefit from the production of clear and detailed European and international guidelines in specific areas of animal use, together with in-depth, expert and, ideally, independent review of all pharmaceutical research projects and protocols. Significant progress has been made in some countries, but further progress internationally requires commitment, the allocation of adequate human and financial resources, and the establishment of appropriate administrative mechanisms. We suggest that ECVAM has a pivotal role to play in the development and introduction of such guidelines, in collaboration with other European institutions and the pharmaceutical industry.[50] Previously, guidelines and ethical concerns have focused mainly on toxicity testing, but basic drug research, during which many animals are used, and in which considerable human and financial resources are invested, is also an important area. Such guidelines should clarify and encourage the optimal use of *in vitro* methods in a hierarchical testing strategy, before undertaking *in vivo* studies considered to be essential.

REFERENCES

1. Rowan, A. N. and Stratman, C. J. (eds) (1980) *The Use of Alternatives in Drug Research.* Macmillan Press, London.
2. Russell, W. M. S. and Burch, R. L. (1959) *The Principles of Humane Experimental Technique.* Methuen, London.
3. Smith, J. A. and Boyd, K. M. (eds) (1991) *Lives in the Balance: The Ethics of Using Animals in Biomedical Research.* Oxford University Press, Oxford.
4. Castell, J. V. and Gómez-Lechón, M. J. (eds) (1992) *In Vitro Alternatives to Animal Pharmaco-toxicology.* Farmaindustria, Madrid.
5. Anonymous (1988) *Animal Experimentation in the Netherlands, 1987.* Veterinary Public Health Inspectorate, Rijswijk, The Netherlands.
6. Anonymous (1995) *Statistics of Scientific Procedures on Living Animals in Great Britain 1994.* Cm 3012. HMSO, London.
7. Zbinden, G. (1992) Development of *in vitro* toxicology. In Jolles, G. and Cordier, A. (eds) *In Vitro Methods in Toxicology*, pp. 3–12. Academic Press, London.
8. Anonymous (1986) *Animals (Scientific Procedures) Act 1986.* HMSO, London.
9. Anonymous (1995) *Animal Experimentation in the Netherlands, 1994.* Veterinary Public Health Inspectorate, Rijswijk, The Netherlands.
10. Orlans, F. B. (1993) *In the Name of Science: Issues in Responsible Animal Experimentation.* Oxford University Press, New York.
11. Spink, J. D. (1977) Drug testing. In *The Welfare of Laboratory Animals: Legal, Scientific and Humane Requirements*, pp. 44–50. UFAW, Potters Bar, UK.
12. Cordier, A. C. (1992) *In vitro* strategy for the safety assessment of drugs. In Jolles, G. and Cordier, A. (eds) *In Vitro Methods in Toxicology*, pp. 21–27. Academic Press, London.
13. Richards, W. G. (1994) Computer-aided drug design. *Pure Appl. Chem.* **66:** 1589–1596.
14. Fentem, J. H. and Balls, M. (1992) *In vitro* alternatives to toxicity testing in animals. *Chemistry and Industry* **6:** 207–211.
15. Hawksworth, G. M. (1994) Advantages and disadvantages of using human cells for pharmacological and toxicological studies. *Hum. Exp. Toxicol.* **13:** 568–573.
16. Rogiers, V., Sonck, W., Shephard, E. and Vercruysse, A. (eds) (1993) *Human Cells in In Vitro Pharmaco-toxicology.* VUB Press, Brussels.
17. Anonymous (1995) *Human Tissue – Ethical and Legal Issues.* Nuffield Council on Bioethics, London.
18. Fentem, J. H. (1994) The use of human tissues in *in vitro* toxicology, Stirling, 28/29 April 1993. Summary of general discussions. *Hum. Exp. Toxicol.* **13:** 445–449.
19. Balls, M. and Fentem, J. H. (1992) The use of basal cytotoxicity and target organ toxicity tests in hazard identification and risk assessment. *ATLA* **20:** 368–388.
20. Frazier, J. M. (ed.) (1992) *In Vitro Toxicity Testing. Applications to Safety Evaluation.* Marcel Dekker, New York.
21. Jolles, G. and Cordier, A. (eds) (1992) *In Vitro Methods in Toxicology.* Academic Press, London.
22. Blaauboer, B. J., Boobis, A. R., Castell, J. V. *et al.* (1994) The practical applicability of hepatocyte cultures in routine testing. The report and recommendations of ECVAM workshop 1. *ATLA* **22:** 231–241.
23. Guillouzo, A. (1992) Hepatotoxicity. In Frazier, J. M. (ed.) *In Vitro Toxicity Testing. Applications to Safety Evaluation*, pp. 45–83. Marcel Dekker, New York.
24. Bach, P. H. and Wilks, M. F. (1992) *In vitro* techniques for nephrotoxicity screening, studying mechanisms of renal injury and novel discoveries about toxic nephropathies. In Jolles, G. and Cordier, A. (eds) *In Vitro Methods in Toxicology*, pp. 59–89. Academic Press, London.
25. Williams, P. D. and Rush, G. F. (1992) An evaluation of *in vitro* models for assessing nephrotoxicity. In Frazier, J. M. (ed.) *In Vitro Toxicity Testing. Applications to Safety Evaluation*, pp. 85–110. Marcel Dekker, New York.
26. Atterwill, C. K., Bruinink, A., Drejer, J. *et al.* (1994) *In vitro* neurotoxicity testing. The report and recommendations of ECVAM workshop 3. *ATLA* **22:** 350–362.
27. Harvey, A. L. (1992) Neurotoxicity. In Frazier, J. M. (ed.) *In Vitro Toxicity Testing. Applications to Safety Evaluation*, pp. 111–129. Marcel Dekker, New York.

28. Bechter, R. (1995) The validation and use of *in vitro* teratogenicity tests. *Arch. Toxicol. Suppl.* **17:** 170–191.
29. Brown, N. A. and Freeman, S. J. (1984) Alternative tests for teratogenicity. *ATLA* **12:** 7–23.
30. Gad, S. C. (1993) Alternatives to *in vivo* studies in toxicology. In Ballantyne, B., Marrs, T. and Turner, P. (eds) *General and Applied Toxicology*, pp. 179–206. Macmillan Press, Basingstoke.
31. Hales, B. F. (1992) Teratogenicity. In Frazier, J. M. (ed.) *In Vitro Toxicity Testing. Applications to Safety Evaluation*, pp. 205–220. Marcel Dekker, New York.
32. Renault, J.-Y. and Cordier, A. (1992) Micromass limb bud cell cultures: a model for the study and detection of teratogens. In Jolles, G. and Cordier, A. (eds) *In Vitro Methods in Toxicology*, pp. 447–460. Academic Press, London.
33. Pacifici, G. M. and Fracchia, G. N. (eds) (1995) *Advances in Drug Metabolism in Man.* Office for Official Publications of the European Communities, Luxemburg.
34. Cholerton, S., Daly, A. K. and Idle, J. R. (1992) The role of individual human cytochromes P450 in drug metabolism and clinical response. *Trends Pharmacol. Sci.* **13:** 434–439.
35. Donato, M. T., Gómez-Lechón, M. J. and Castell, J. V. (1992) Biotransformation of drugs by cultured hepatocytes. In Castell, J. V. and Gómez-Lechón, M. J. (eds) *In Vitro Alternatives to Animal Pharmaco-toxicology*, pp. 149–178. Farmaindustria, Madrid.
36. Frazier, J. M. (1992) Scientific perspectives on the role of *in vitro* toxicity testing in chemical safety evaluation. In Jolles, G. and Cordier, A. (eds) *In Vitro Methods in Toxicology*, pp. 522–529. Academic Press, London.
37. Houston, J. B. (1994) Relevance of *in vitro* kinetic parameters to *in vivo* metabolism of xenobiotics. *Toxicol. In Vitro* **8:** 507–512.
38. Houston, J. B. (1994) Utility of *in vitro* drug metabolism data in predicting *in vivo* metabolic clearance. *Biochem. Pharmacol.* **47:** 1469–1479.
39. Andersen, M. E. (1995) Combining *in vitro* alternatives and physiologically-based computer modeling will improve quantitative health risk assessments. In Goldberg, A. M. and van Zutphen, L. F. M. (eds) *Alternative Methods in Toxicology and the Life Sciences, Vol. 11, The World Congress on Alternatives and Animal Use in the Life Sciences: Education, Research, Testing*, pp. 371–377. Mary Ann Liebert, New York.
40. Barratt, M. D., Castell, J. V., Chamberlain, M. *et al.* (1995) The integrated use of alternative approaches for predicting toxic hazard. The report and recommendations of ECVAM workshop 8. *ATLA* **23:** 410–429.
41. Gonzalez, F. J. (1992) Human cytochromes P450: problems and prospects. *Trends in Pharmacol. Sci.* **13:** 346–352.
42. Langenbach, R., Smith, P. B. and Crespi, C. (1992) Recombinant DNA approaches for the development of metabolic systems used in *in vitro* toxicology. *Mutat. Res.* **277:** 251–275.
43. Boobis, A. R. (1995) Prediction of inhibitory drug–drug interactions by studies *in vitro*. In Pacifici, G. M. and Fracchia, G. N. (eds) *Advances in Drug Metabolism in Man*, pp. 515–539. Office for Official Publications of the European Communities, Luxemburg.
44. Vickers, A., Ferrero, J., Fisher, R. and Brendel, K. (1995) Xenobiotic metabolism in precision-cut dynamic organ cultured human liver slices. In Pacifici, G. M. and Fracchia, G. N. (eds) *Advances in Drug Metabolism in Man*, pp. 683–753. Office for Official Publications of the European Communities, Luxemburg.
45. Ivanov, M. A., Heuillet, E., Vintezou, P., Melcion, C. and Cordier, A. (1992) Primary culture of hepatocytes in the investigation of drug-induced steatosis. In Jolles, G. and Cordier, A. (eds) *In Vitro Methods in Toxicology*, pp. 165–187. Academic Press, London.
46. Lake, B. G., Lewis, D. F. V., Gray, T. J. B. and Beamand, J. A. (1993) Structure-activity relationships for induction of peroxisomal enzyme activities in primary rat hepatocyte cultures. *Toxicol. In Vitro* **7:** 605–614.
47. Parchment, R. E., Huang, M. and Erickson-Miller, C. L. (1993) Roles for *in vitro* myelotoxicity tests in preclinical drug development and clinical trial planning. *Toxicol. Pathol.* **21:** 241–250.
48. Anonymous (1986) Council Directive 86/609/EEC of 24 November 1986 on the approximation of laws, regulations and administrative provisions of the Member States regarding the protection of animals used for experimental and other scientific purposes. *Official Journal of the European Communities* **L358:** 1–29.
49. Acred, P., Hennessey, T. D., MacArthur-Clark, J. A. *et al.* (1994). Guidelines for the welfare of animals in rodent protection tests. *Lab. Anim.* **28:** 13–18.
50. Balls, M. (1994) Replacement of animal procedures: alternatives in research, education and testing. *Lab. Anim.* **28:** 193–211.

2

Integration of QSAR and *In Vitro* Toxicology

MARTIN D. BARRATT AND
MARK CHAMBERLAIN

I. Introduction 15
II. The value of the mechanistic approach 16
III. Development of prediction models 17
IV. Assessment of the mechanistic competence of an *in vitro* assay 19
V. The problem of 'dose' 22
VI. Selection of sets of test chemicals 23
VII. Classification boundaries and biological uncertainty 23
VIII. Validation and acceptance of alternative test methods 24
IX. Integration of QSAR and *in vitro* alternative methods 26
X. Conclusions 29
References 29

I. INTRODUCTION

The properties of achemical are implicit in its chemical structure; this is the principle underlying the development of quantitative structure–activity relationships (QSARs).

A QSAR is a model which relates the magnitude of a particular property of a series of related chemicals to one or more other physicochemical or structural parameters of the chemicals in question. Related chemicals in this context means chemicals for which the dependent property is derived from the parameters by the same mechanism of action. If the mechanistic basis for a particular property of a group of related chemicals can be elucidated and the relevant parameters measured or calculated then, in principle, a structure–activity relationship (SAR) can be established. For a QSAR to be valid and reliable, the dependent property for all of the chemicals covered by the relationship has to be elicited by a mechanism that is both common and relevant. Attempts to derive QSARs for data sets where either the dependent property is derived by more than one mechanism or the mechanism of action is wrongly defined will invariably be unsuccessful.

IN VITRO METHODS IN PHARMACEUTICAL RESEARCH
ISBN 0-12-163390-X

There are several different approaches to the derivation of QSARs. Most of these methods are inductive in that large amounts of information on chemical structure are analysed using correlative methods to determine which molecular parameter or combination of parameters is associated with the toxicity.[1] The major output of such methods is usually a multiparameter equation which provides a mathematical or statistical description of a QSAR. The value of classical QSAR methods such as regression analysis has been demonstrated (e.g. for phenylbenzoates[2]). However, it can be argued that the value of this approach is limited: for example, it is often difficult to interpret the QSAR in terms of a mechanistic model[3] and this could limit its practical application.

For the development of successful *in vitro* alternatives to animal tests, the same principles need to be applied; in many cases, however, they are overlooked. As a result, some alternative tests may predict end-points that are substantially different from those which they are claimed to predict; this is often because the mechanism modelled by the *in vitro* alternative is incomplete compared with the *in vivo* situation, e.g. many *in vitro* skin or eye irritation tests simply model cytotoxicity and may not take partition into the biological system into account adequately. Other tests that are claimed to be applicable to all chemical classes can predict end-points accurately for some classes of chemicals, but not for others. This is because different classes of chemicals may elicit a change in a particular biological end-point via different mechanisms, which would require different parameters to model them.

Within this chapter, we explore ways in which QSARs and *in vitro* toxicology can complement each other in order to assess toxicity as alternatives to live animal experiments. Scientifically based alternatives can be validated with the help of QSAR techniques and, provided their principles can be readily identified, they should be more readily accepted by regulatory authorities. The value of the mechanistic approach to QSAR and *in vitro* methods is examined; different types of predictive models are discussed together with ways in which they might be integrated. Criteria for the selection of sets of chemicals for test development, optimization and validation are put forward; proposals are made for ways in which QSARs might be used to support the use of data from *in vivo* tests which do not meet today's stringent requirements of acceptability. Ways of assessing the mechanistic competence of *in vitro* assays and of improving their design are discussed. Finally, the challenge of achieving the acceptance of alternative methods is discussed in the context of what it is that we are trying to replace.

II. THE VALUE OF THE MECHANISTIC APPROACH

There are sound reasons in favour of the mechanistic approach to the problem of designing alternative methods for the replacement of animal experiments. A mechanistic understanding of the biological process underlying the *in vivo* toxicity assay which is to be replaced can be expected to lead to the identification of the parameters most appropriate to model the toxicity. A 'complete' *in vitro* alternative will be required to respond in terms of all of the relevant chemical parameters with the appropriate weightings. The underlying scientific basis of alternative methods based on these principles should improve their credibility and assist their acceptance by regulatory authorities. It is argued that the fact that regulatory acceptance is not readily forthcoming is based partly on the relatively poor understanding of the scientific (mechanistic) basis of many alternative methods.

In advocating a mechanistic approach to alternative methods, it is pertinent to examine the scope and limitations of such an approach. This is done most easily by considering some requirements and restrictions for the generation and use of QSARs, which are, almost by definition, mechanistic relationships. QSARs in which the parameters are not related mechanistically to the dependent variable in some way can have little or no correlation, except by chance.

The parameters used to construct a QSAR should, where possible, be selected on the basis of an understanding of the mechanism of the process. Where a mechanism is not known in sufficient detail to be used to define appropriate parameters, a QSAR may be derived by computing a large number of parameters and then establishing a statistical relationship with a few of those parameters. In the latter case, the relevance of such a QSAR may be supported if the parameters in question have some mechanistic significance to the process.

The chemicals used to construct a QSAR (the training set) should be selected on the basis of a common mechanism of action (if possible) and should adequately cover the parameter space in terms of dependent and independent variables. It is also important to realize that the predictive domain of the QSAR model is restricted to the same parameter space covered by the training set, i.e. the model can be used for interpolation but not for extrapolation. The same holds for an alternative method.

A further limitation which may apply to QSAR models rather more than to *in vitro* alternatives is that, so far, the successful application of QSAR has been restricted to the modelling of the properties of pure chemicals. As far as *in vitro* alternatives are concerned, it may be possible to construct a complete (i.e. mechanistically competent) *in vitro* model and then to calibrate and validate it using mixtures of chemicals. Provided the constraints described above relating to mechanistic validity and parameter space are taken into account, there appears to be no reason why such a model should not provide useful predictions.

Because many toxicological end-points are effectively colligative properties of chemicals, i.e. a property determined by the dose in terms of the number of molecules present, QSARs relating to these end-points should properly be expressed in molar units. A significant problem is therefore raised by the fact that a large number of regulatory toxicological procedures are conducted using doses expressed in weight units. This point will be amplified later.

III. DEVELOPMENT OF PREDICTION MODELS

Predictions of toxicity can be made with an acceptable degree of certainty only if an appropriate prediction model is used. Prediction models may take several forms. For example, physiologically based pharmacokinetic models (PBPKs) may be used to develop an understanding of the biological responses resulting from exposure to toxic or therapeutic doses of chemicals.[4–8]

The use of rigorously defined prediction models in the validation of *in vitro* tests is being pioneered by the management team of the European Cosmetic, Toiletry and Perfumery Associations (COLIPA) validation study on eye irritation which is currently in progress.[9] Prediction models are algorithms which convert the results from an alternative method into a prediction of toxicity observed *in vivo*. A prediction model must define the relationship between all of the possible results from an *in vitro* test with the *in vivo* end-point, both qualitatively and quantitatively, including confidence limits; it must also define the scope of the alternative test in terms of the physical and chemical properties of the substances for which it is valid, i.e. define the physicochemical parameter space for which it is valid.

A QSAR can be regarded as a prediction model in that, as long as the chemical parameters that are responsible for the toxicity of the chemical in question are within the chemical parameter space of the model, then predictions can be made.[3,10,11]

An example in which a QSAR was used as a prediction model to construct a hypothesis that was subsequently tested is provided by Whittle *et al.*[12] This work was based on a QSAR for the corrosivity of organic acids,[13] with the putative mechanism that corrosivity is a function of the ability of the chemical to permeate the skin together with its cytotoxicity, expressed in this case as acidity (pK_a). The study examined the corrosive potential of a series of fatty acids ranging from propanoic acid (C3) to dodecanoic acid (C12) using the *in vitro* skin corrosivity test (IVSCT).[14] In this series of fatty acids, the cytotoxicity parameter, pK_a remains constant; changes in skin corrosivity potential are therefore determined entirely by the variables that model skin permeability: log(octanol/water partition coefficient) (logP), molecular volume and melting point.[15] Because a number of chemicals have shown significantly different skin corrosivity results when tested on human skin compared with animal skin,[16,17] this series of fatty acids was investigated with the IVSCT using both rat and human skin.

Principal components analysis has been found to be particularly useful for visualizing QSARs. This technique affords a ready understanding of the sometimes conflicting effects of different chemical parameters on the QSAR and has been particularly useful in understanding 'embedded' relationships.[18] In principal components analysis, the original variables are transformed into a new orthogonal set of linear combinants called principal components. The variance from the original descriptors is greatest in the first principal component, less in the second component and so on, allowing multicomponent data sets to be reduced to two- or three-dimensional plots without significant loss of information. The utility of this method has been illustrated in a number of toxicological QSAR studies including teratogenicity,[19] α_2-microglobulin nephropathy,[20] skin corrosivity[13] and eye irritation.[21] A principal components map[12] illustrating the corrosivity of organic acids is shown in Fig. 2.1. The corrosivity/irritation profile of the fatty acids series towards rat skin *in vitro* is identical to that towards rabbit skin *in vivo*.

All of the fatty acids with alkyl chain lengths up to and including C8 were found to be corrosive to rat skin. When human skin was used, the corrosive–non-corrosive threshold was shifted to around the C6 fatty acid. The mechanistic interpretation of these results is consistent with the known greater permeability barrier presented by human skin compared with rat skin. This particular example also serves to illustrate that animals are not necessarily a good model for humans. The power of the QSAR as a predictive model lies in the ability to understand where the rat may not be a good model for humans in terms of chemical parameter space. Although rat skin may be a general model that is useful for predicting corrosivity towards human skin, there are specific chemicals for which the rat would overpredict the corrosive hazard for human skin.

Predictions made in parameter space poorly covered by existing knowledge can be tested by conducting new experiments in an optimum manner and not by incremental expansion or repeated testing over small regions of parameter space.

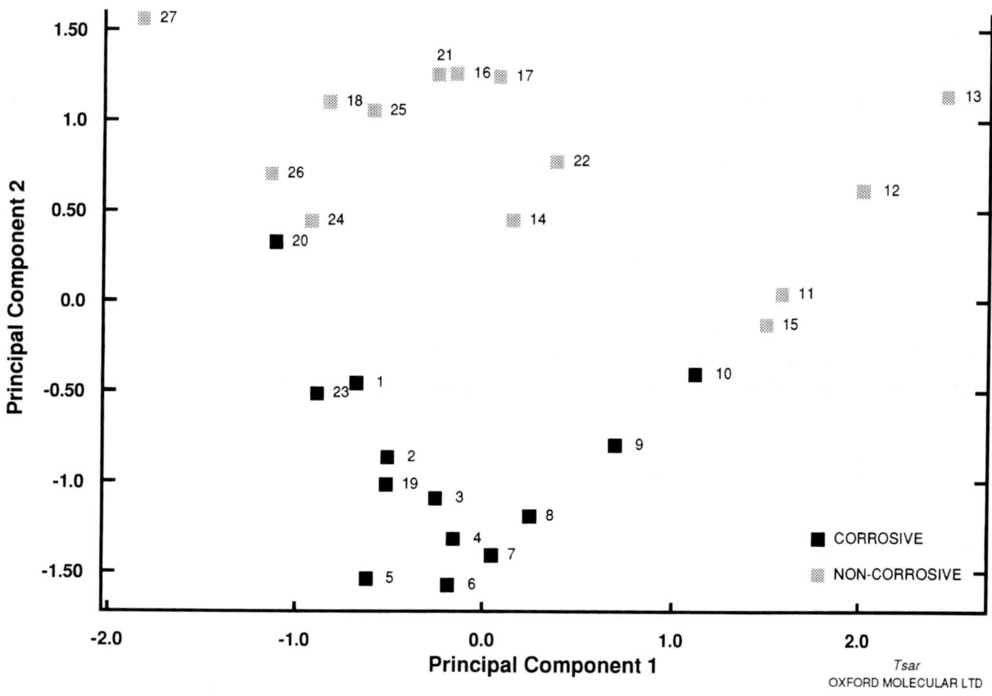

Fig. 2.1 Plot of the first two principal components of logP, molecular volume, melting point and pK_a for 27 organic acids. **Key:** 1, dichloroacetic acid; 2, bromoacetic acid; 3, mercaptoacetic acid; 4, acrylic acid; 5, formic acid; 6, acetic acid; 7, propanoic acid; 8, butanoic acid; 9, hexanoic acid; 10, octanoic acid; 11, decanoic acid; 12, dodecanoic acid; 13, tetradecanoic acid; 14, benzoic acid; 15, 2,4,6-trichlorophenol; 16, 2-bromobenzoic acid; 17, 4-nitrophenylacetic acid; 18, citric acid; 19, lactic acid; 20, oxalic acid; 21, salicylic acid; 22, *trans*-cinnamic acid; 23, cyanoacetic acid; 24, malonic acid; 25, succinic acid; 26, maleic acid; 27, sulphamic acid. (From Whittle *et al.*[12])

IV. ASSESSMENT OF THE MECHANISTIC COMPETENCE OF AN *IN VITRO* ASSAY

The use of mechanistically based QSAR techniques has profound implications for the assessment of the practical utility of *in vitro* tests. Elucidation of the putative mechanism of action of a class of chemicals facilitates evaluation of an *in vitro* method for predicting the *in vivo* toxic potential of an untested chemical. Provided the QSAR is mechanism based, then its independent variables should define the mechanistic requirements of the *in vitro* assay as well as the scope and limitations of its parameter space. Therefore, using this information there is a greater likelihood of being able to determine (or design) an appropriate *in vitro* assay.

For an *in vitro* test reliably to predict *in vivo* toxic potential it should ideally be sensitive to the same parameters that are responsible for the effects *in vivo*. It follows that this test would show a high degree of correlation with the response *in vivo*. However, in the case of an *in vitro* test which is only partially sensitive to the parameters operating *in vivo*, only a partial correlation with the *in vivo* response would be observed. The fewer the number of relevant parameters operating in the *in vitro* assay, the weaker the correlation with the *in vivo* response, and vice versa. Typically, correlation methods have been used to evaluate the performance of *in vitro* methods in predicting the *in vivo* results. Varying degrees of partial correlation have been found with the many *in vitro* methods that have been developed and advocated as alternatives, for example to the Draize rabbit eye irritation test.[22]

The following example serves to illustrate how the mechanistic competence of an *in vitro* assay can be assessed. Recently a QSAR has been developed[21] for a set of neutral organic chemicals consisting of 38 chemicals from the ECETOC database and eight chemicals from the work of Jacobs and Martens.[23] This work proposes that the eye irritation potential of neutral organic chemicals is associated with the following molecular features in a complex way. The mechanistic basis is as follows.

It is proposed that neutral organic chemicals are irritant by virtue of their effects on cell membranes. The putative effect on cell membranes is perturbation of ion transport mechanisms resulting from a change in the electrical properties (e.g. the dielectric properties) of the membrane. This is based on the knowledge that some low molecular weight neutral organic chemicals, e.g. diethyl ether, chloroform and *n*-butanol, can alter the electrical resistance (and thus the ion permeability) of phospholipid membranes.[24,25] It is hypothesized that changes in electrical resistance (and hence ion permeability) in the membranes of the eye might lead to cytotoxicity and result in irritation. The property of the test chemical used to model this change is its dipole moment. For a chemical to affect the electrical resistance properties of a cell membrane it must also be able to partition into the cell membrane and hence must possess the appropriate hydrophobic–hydrophilic properties; the parameter which describes this property is the calculated log(octanol/water partition coefficient) – (clogP). An appropriately small cross-sectional area allowing the chemical to fit easily between lipid components of the membrane also appears to be a requirement; this is modelled by the minor principal inertial axes R_y and R_z which represent the cross-sectional area of the molecule.

The eye irritation data set consisting of these four dependent variables was analysed using principal components analysis and is shown in Fig. 2.2. The vectors for the different molecular features can be mapped on to the plot of the first and second principal components:

1. clogP operates along a vector which is at 28° to the horizontal. The more hydrophobic chemicals are found in the lower right-hand region of the plot, the more hydrophilic in the upper left-hand region.
2. The vectors of the minor principal inertial axes R_y and R_z are virtually contiguous and operate along a vector 35° to the horizontal. Chemicals with larger cross-sectional areas are found in the upper right-hand region, and those with smaller cross-sectional areas are found in the lower left-hand region.
3. The vector of the dipole moment operates at 66° to the horizontal. Chemicals with larger dipole moments are found in the upper left-hand region; molecules with lower dipole moments are found in the lower right-hand region.

Within this data set, irritant chemicals are found in the region of parameter space defined by intermediate hydrophobicity, relatively small cross-sectional area and intermediate dipole moment. Chemicals with zero or low dipole moments are not irritant to the eye (dipole moment is the 'reactivity' parameter: no reactivity = no irritation). To be an eye irritant, a chemical must have a certain dipole and partition easily into the membrane, i.e. it must be reasonably hydrophobic, with not too large a cross-sectional area. Chemicals with a large dipole moment tend to be more polar (low clogP) and vice versa. These two parameters clearly oppose each other. The eye irritation potential of neutral organic chemicals is determined (in part) by the result of these two opposing features.

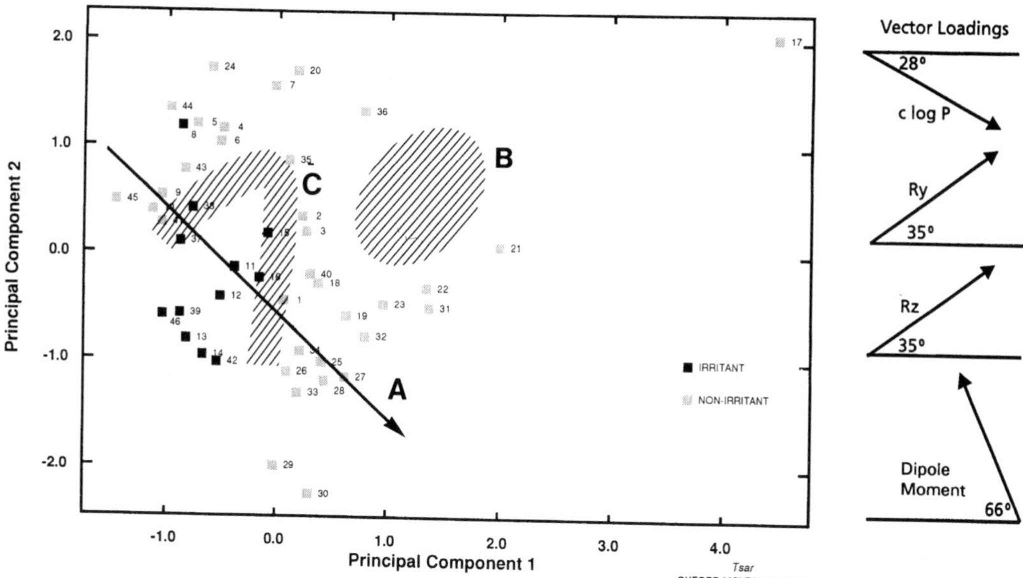

Fig. 2.2 Plot of the first two principal components of clogP, R_y, R_z and dipole moment for 46 neutral organic chemicals showing vector loadings. **Key:** 1, 2-ethyl-hexan-1-ol; 2, methyl trimethyl acetate; 3, ethyl trimethyl acetate; 4, *n*-butyl acetate; 5, ethyl acetate; 6, cellosolve acetate; 7, ethyl 2-methylacetoacetate; 8, methyl acetate (believed to be an eye irritant via a mechanism not covered by this QSAR[21]); 9, propylene glycol; 10, glycerol; 11, *iso*propanol; 12, *iso*butanol; 13, *n*-butanol; 14, *n*-hexanol; 15, butyl cellosolve; 16, cyclohexanol; 17, 4,4-methylene-bis(2,6-di-*t*-butylphenol); 18, 4-bromophenetole; 19, xylene; 20, 3-chloro-4-fluoronitrobenzene; 21, 1,3-di*iso*propylbenzene; 22, 1-methylpropylbenzene; 23, 3-ethyltoluene; 24, 2,4-difluoronitrobenzene; 25, styrene; 26, toluene; 27, 3-methylhexane; 28, 2-methylpentane; 29, 1,9-decadiene; 30, dodecane; 31, 1,5-dimethylcyclo-octadiene; 32, *cis*-cyclooctene; 33, methylcyclopentane; 34, 1,5-hexadiene; 35, methyl *iso*butyl ketone; 36, methyl amyl ketone; 37, methyl ethyl ketone; 38, acetone; 39, allyl alcohol; 40, chloroform; 41, 2-methoxyethanol; 42, octan-1-ol; 43, dimethylformamide; 44, dimethylsulphoxide; 45, formamide; 46, 2(2-ethoxyethoxy)ethanol. (From Chamberlain and Barratt.[11])

Principal components plots and their associated vectors for the different molecular features such as that shown in Fig. 2.2 can also be used to evaluate the performance of *in vitro* assays. Whereas the position of a chemical on the principal components plot is determined solely by its molecular features, assignment of toxicity classification depends entirely on the results from a variable biological assay. Therefore a principal components plot could be compiled for each one of several *in vitro* assays to compare their performance in correctly discriminating between chemicals with different toxicological properties. If an *in vitro* assay correctly predicted the toxicological properties of a set of chemicals, then the principal components plots for both the *in vivo* and *in vitro* assays would be very similar. The similarity would depend on the *in vitro* assay being sensitive to the same molecular parameters that are responsible for the toxicity in the *in vivo* assay. This approach augments the usual correlation methods in that it can provide information on the extent of mechanistic similarity with the *in vivo* assay.

A high degree of mechanistic similarity between the *in vitro* and *in vivo* assays would result in very similar principal components plots. Conversely, a low degree of similarity or the omission of a key dependent variable would result in dissimilar principal components plots. A hypothetical example has been simulated by omitting dipole moment from the principal components analysis of the eye irritation data set and replotting the data (Fig. 2.3). Whilst there is still some discrimination between the irritant and non-irritant substances,

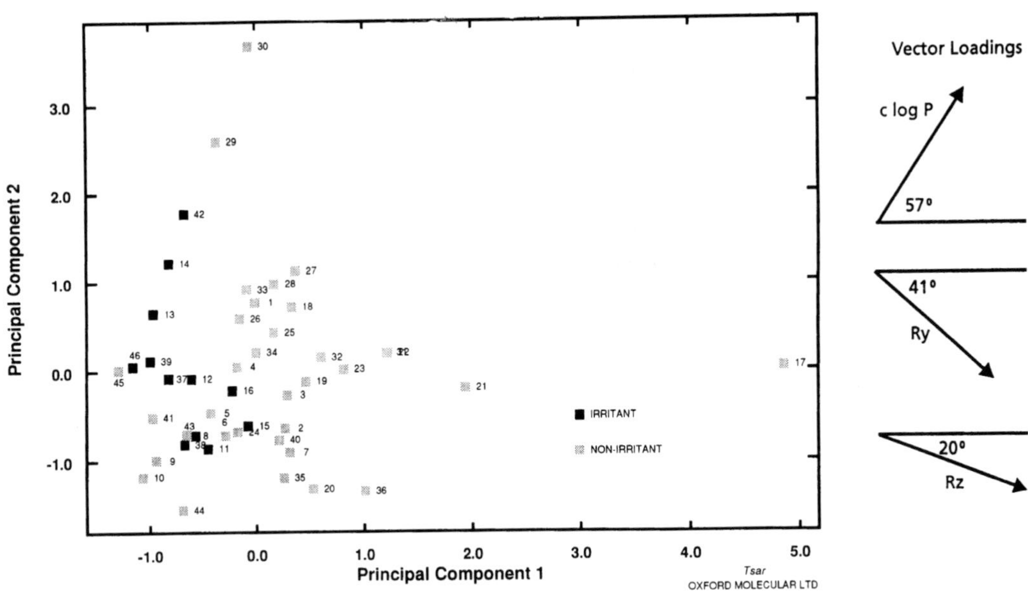

Fig. 2.3 Plot of the first two principal components of clogP, R_y and R_z, i.e. dipole moment omitted, for 46 neutral organic chemicals showing vector loadings. (From Chamberlain and Barratt.[11])

probably because clogP and dipole moment are partially correlated, there is now one area of the plot where irritants and non-irritants show considerable overlap. The molecular parameters that remain in the model are clogP, R_y and R_z: these parameters would determine the ability of a molecule to penetrate into or through a membrane. However, since dipole moment is absent, full assessment of the perturbation of the membrane function cannot be made.

V. THE PROBLEM OF 'DOSE'

A large number of regulatory toxicological procedures are conducted using doses that are expressed in weight or volume units; this is a perfectly reasonable system when assessing hazard to the consumer, but raises a significant problem when attempting to construct a QSAR model. The problem originates from the fact that many toxicological phenomena are colligative properties of chemicals, i.e. determined by the dose in terms of the number of molecules present. In a QSAR, the magnitude of the toxicological response is related quantitatively to the magnitude of certain intrinsic properties of the chemicals within that relationship, i.e. the intrinsic properties of the chemicals are compared with each other. To make an accurate comparison of the potencies of one chemical with another, the toxicological response must therefore be expressed in molar units.

A typical consequence of the 'dose' problem can be seen in eye irritation data, as illustrated by the QSAR in Fig. 2.2. All eye irritation tests are carried out using a standard mass or volume of test chemical. Because eye irritation is a colligative property of a chemical in addition to being a constitutive property, it follows that lower molecular weight chemicals are intrinsically more irritant than higher molecular weight chemicals when tested at constant mass or volume. This QSAR uses a mapping technique which clusters together chemicals with a similar eye irritation potential on the basis of specific physicochemical properties and no specific attempt was made in this QSAR study to model the dose in molar units. The variables R_y and R_z correlate very strongly with molecular volume and molecular weight, which in turn correlate inversely with the number of molecules in a unit weight of chemical, i.e. the dose. In addition to increasing the ability of a molecule to penetrate into a biological membrane, low values of R_y and R_z also reflect a higher molar dose of chemical – both of which lead to increased irritancy.

The 'ideal' solution to the problem of dose would be for all toxicological tests to be repeated using molar doses. As this solution is clearly unacceptable for a large number of reasons, QSAR modellers must either ignore the problem as a first approximation (whilst still bearing it in mind) or accommodate it by the use of an appropriate variable, e.g. reciprocal molecular weight.

VI. SELECTION OF SETS OF TEST CHEMICALS

QSAR affords the ability to select test chemicals for *in vitro* testing in a more scientific way than hitherto.[11] This has been demonstrated using the principal components map for the eye irritation potential of neutral organic chemicals.[21] The use of the principal components map allows the selection of chemicals which cover the widest possible parameter space in terms of both biological activity and physicochemical properties. For example, this may be achieved by selecting a series of chemicals that would start in an area predicted to be non-irritant, pass through the irritant area and out again to the non-irritant area. This is illustrated by track A in Fig. 2.2. The same principal components map can also be used to identify regions of parameter space incompletely covered by the current database, e.g. in the region marked B ($PC1 = 1.5$, $PC2 = 0.5$ in Fig. 2.2). Obtaining biological test data from chemicals in these regions would be essential for the completeness of the non-animal model. Similarly the map can be used to identify regions of parameter space well covered by the current database. In these regions, testing of additional chemicals would add little value and could be a waste of valuable resources. These arguments apply equally well to classical *in vitro* alternatives as well as to QSAR predictive models.

These techniques are currently being used in connection with the selection of test chemicals for a proposed ECVAM-sponsored study on skin corrosivity (see reference 26 and the associated appendix).

VII. CLASSIFICATION BOUNDARIES AND BIOLOGICAL UNCERTAINTY

An important consideration that has stemmed from the above work is that of boundary regions in QSARs. This is a concept that has its origin in the fact that most regulatory schemes operate initially by quantizing continuous biological (toxicological) data into discrete hazard bands which can conveniently be used in the regulatory process. The inherent biological variability in toxicology tests can lead to uncertainty in classification in the boundary regions. An example of a boundary region is illustrated in Fig. 2.2 by the area marked C. In the case of the Draize rabbit eye test the variability is inherent in the design of the test (M. York and L. Bruner, personal communication). This is dependent on several factors, including the number of animals used. The variability could manifest itself as the results of two well-conducted Draize rabbit eye irritation tests on the same chemical leading to a non-irritant classification in one case and an irritant classification in the other. Examples of such variability have been cited previously.[11] QSAR techniques such as principal components analysis afford visualization and hence predictability of regions of chemical parameter space in which ambiguity in *in vivo* results may arise.

Another source of variability in the classification of chemicals can arise from regulatory classification schemes. In the case of the EC classification scheme for skin irritants,[27] two different scoring systems are used, depending on whether the test has been carried out using three or more than three animals. For a three-animal test, the classification is based on two or more animals reaching the threshold score; for more than three animals, the classification is based on the average score calculated over all of the animals tested. The consequence of this scoring system is that a chemical with a skin irritation potential that is on the irritant–non-irritant threshold is less likely to classify as a skin irritant if it is tested in more than three animals, because it is possible for a single animal with a low irritancy score to reduce the average score below the threshold even if the individual scores of all of the other animals are above the threshold. This particular source of biological variability is not insignificant, as examination of individual animal scores show wide variations in response to the same chemical applied at the same dose to different animals.[28] It is common, within the same test, for one or more animals to exhibit a response which is clearly 'irritant', whilst others may show little or no effect.

VIII. VALIDATION AND ACCEPTANCE OF ALTERNATIVE TEST METHODS

It is now accepted that there are several steps in the path from test inception to acceptance by regulatory agencies.[29,30] Broadly, these steps are initial test development, test optimization, chemical database development, validation and acceptance. Relevant sets of chemicals need to be used at each stage. Traditionally in the early stages of test development small sets of test chemicals favoured by the originating laboratory have been used. The set of chemicals probably represents that with which the laboratory is particularly knowledgeable in terms of the *in vivo* response elicited, and possibly the mode of action, and the relevance for the specific *in vitro* assay under development. As test development proceeds, the number of test chemicals is increased and usually collaborations are sought from one or more other laboratories.[31,32] The collaborations can serve several purposes during test development, including exposing the assay to an element of peer review or comment, demonstration of the ability to transfer the technology, and expansion of the set of test chemicals (chemical database development), sometimes outside the domain of knowledge of the originating laboratory.

A validation study has been described as an interlaboratory blind trial in which one or more tests, test batteries or testing strategies are assessed for their relevance and reliability for one or more specific purposes, according to predefined performance criteria.[29]

Typically the performance of an *in vitro* test is assessed by its capability of correctly predicting the *in vivo* response. It is now becoming recognized that the only realistic assessment of the utility of an *in vitro* assay in replacing an animal experiment is that the *in vitro* test should not be expected to predict the result of an *in vivo* test with any more accuracy than would a repeat *in vivo* test. If chemicals for which the *in vivo* responses are unambiguous are included in the test set then, if the *in vitro* responses are a true representation of the *in vivo* responses, it follows that these will also be unambiguous. However, if the test set of chemicals contains a high proportion of chemicals for which there is uncertainty in the *in vivo* data, then consequently the confidence of the *in vitro* predictions will be low.

Following several proposals,[29,33,34] the European Centre for Ecotoxicology and Toxicology of Chemicals (ECETOC) has taken the initiative in establishing acceptance criteria for the quality of the *in vivo* data to be included in reference sets of chemicals for use in development and validation of *in vitro* tests. In the first of these initiatives, an ECETOC Task Force called for, received and reviewed *in vivo* eye irritation data to determine the conformity with the established criteria.[35,36] The criteria were that the experiments had to:

(a) be conducted according to the principles of Good Laboratory Practice (GLP) according to OECD guideline 405;[37]
(b) involve instillation of 0.1 ml or the equivalent weight of undiluted chemical into the conjunctival sac without the use of anaesthetic;
(c) include individual tissue scores for observations at 24, 48 and 72 hours, together with an assessment of reversibility.

The criteria are listed above to illustrate that they were reasonable and not overly stringent since they should be seen only as good scientific practice. Contrary to expectations, it has proved to be difficult to obtain large chemical data sets conforming to such criteria and it may not be possible readily to obtain large data sets in this way. The original exercise was able to include only 55 chemicals. These were from several chemical classes and, although the database is of some utility, the limitations of this data set have been alluded to.[21] A similar exercise for chemicals causing skin irritation and corrosion has been recently completed by the same ECETOC Task Force.[28] This has been somewhat more successful in that more chemicals have been included in the database (176 chemicals in 215 tests).

A major challenge facing researchers developing either *in vitro* models or QSARs is the availability of high-quality data derived from experiments with animals. Ironically, the increasing reluctance to conduct animal experiments may inhibit the development of alternative test methods. However, where there are biological data that do not meet today's stringent requirements of acceptability (see above), particularly historical data generated before the advent of GLP, it is possible that QSARs themselves may be used to 'validate' these data for use in alternative tests. If QSAR techniques can be used to demonstrate that the results of these tests are consistent with the physicochemical attributes of the chemicals, when compared with the results from tests conforming to the current acceptance criteria, they should be deemed to be acceptable for use for the development and validation of *in vitro* alternative methods.

IX. INTEGRATION OF QSAR AND *IN VITRO* ALTERNATIVE METHODS

In vitro tests can be categorized as:

1. Empirical: those for which no mechanistic basis has been identified (e.g. the pollen tube growth inhibition test for eye irritants[38]).
2. Mechanistic: those with a clearly identified mechanistic basis (e.g. *in vitro* photobinding to human serum albumin test for photoallergens[39]).
3. Analogous: those in which the *in vivo* system or part thereof is reproduced; it is implicit that mechanisms relevant to *in vivo* toxicity operate in an analogous assay (e.g. the isolated rabbit eye test,[40] the *in vitro* skin corrosivity test[16]).

In the absence of knowledge of mechanism, QSAR methods may help to elucidate the mechanisms operating in *in vitro* assays. Systematic consideration of multicompartment models, such as is done in PBPK modelling, can help to understand the role of various chemical parameters in influencing toxicity *in vivo*. Similar careful consideration of an *in vitro* test can help to define the role of each parameter and thus assess the mechanistic relevance of the *in vitro* assay.

One of the key recommendations of the European Centre for the Validation of Alternative Methods (ECVAM) workshop held in January 1995 on the integrated use of alternative approaches for predicting toxic hazard,[41] was that there is a need to address the mechanistic basis of currently available *in vitro* tests, in order to: (a) rationalize their predictive power; (b) aid in the design of test batteries and hierarchical testing strategies; and (c) help in the design of new *in vitro* tests.

It has long been recognized that, for a chemical to be biologically active, it must first be transported from its site of administration to its site of action and then it must bind to or react with the receptor or target (as restated in reference 1), i.e. biological activity is a function of partition and reactivity. However, there are many QSAR models, particularly in the area of aquatic toxicity, in which the magnitude of the biological response *appears* to be dependent only on partition parameters. Many non-reactive chemicals exhibit baseline toxicity or non-polar narcosis in aquatic toxicity;[42] for these chemicals, the external lethal concentration is governed simply by the partition coefficient between water and the aquatic organism.[43] Two examples in mammalian toxicology relate to the skin sensitization potential of some haloalkanes[44] and a set of substituted phenyl benzoates.[2] In both of these examples, the biological response is related to parameters that model skin permeability, logP and $(\log P)^2$ in the first case and logP and molecular volume in the second. The reactivity parameters in both cases are implicit in that the predictive power of both QSARs is restricted to other related chemicals working by the same chemical mechanism.

To be effective replacements for animal tests, the alternatives must incorporate all the relevant features pertaining to partition and reactivity; these constraints apply equally to *in vitro* models as they do to QSAR. As has been illustrated above, models that are deficient in key features cannot be expected to reproduce the results of the *in vivo* system. It has been suggested that many *in vitro* alternatives to the Draize rabbit eye test are simple cytotoxicity assays, i.e. they largely omit the partition variable, which perhaps partly explains the poor performance of many *in vitro* alternatives to that test in the recent European Commission/UK Home Office (EC/HO) sponsored validation study.[45]

To design new alternative methods that are mechanistically based, there is clearly a requirement for an improved mechanistic understanding of many toxicological processes. This mechanistic understanding can also be used to determine the mechanistic competence of existing *in vitro* alternative tests, as indicated previously. This will be done for the nine *in vitro* assays included in the EU/HO validation study once the data become available. Because the only QSAR that exists for the chemicals included in that study is for the neutral organic chemicals, the analysis will be limited to those chemicals, but this covers the majority. Simulations can be performed as described previously (see Fig. 2.3) in order to try to understand any mechanistic deficiencies of the *in vitro* assays. In this way it may be possible to recommend modifications to existing assays to improve their predictive performance.

A schema which illustrates how mechanistic understanding of a toxicological phenomenon may be used to develop QSARs or *in vitro* assays is shown in Fig. 2.4. Initially the toxicological phenomenon that is to be modelled has to be defined. The less complex the phenomenon the better. There may be hierarchies of effects that need to be understood before modelling can take place. For example, modelling acute lethal toxicity in mammals is

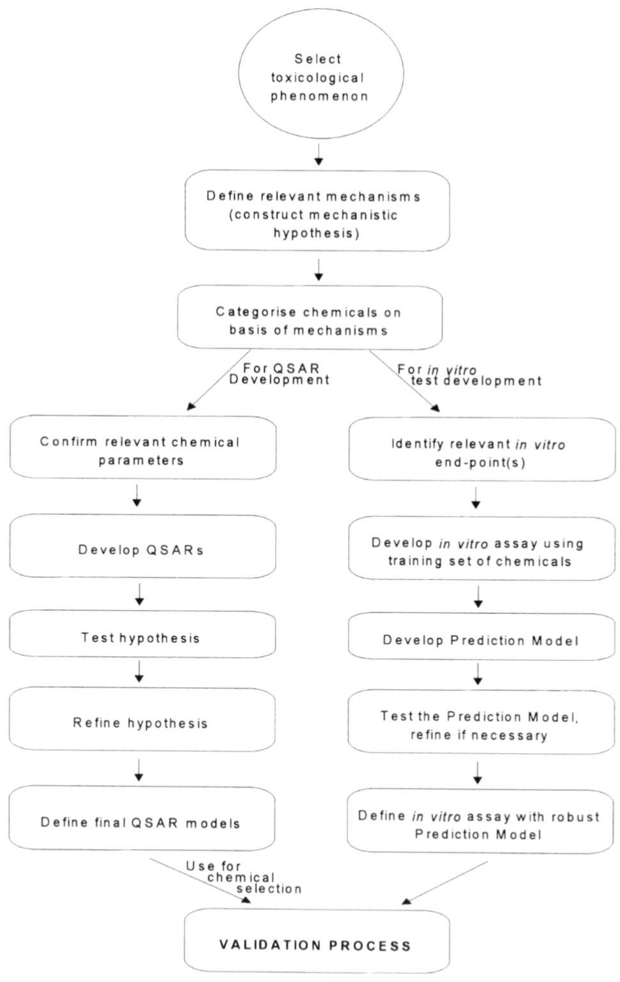

Fig. 2.4 A mechanistic approach to the development of QSARs and *in vitro* assays.

fraught with problems as, clearly, there are many reasons for death. Any one of several organ systems may be targeted with quite different features of the chemicals being responsible for the toxicity. Even within a single toxicological phenomenon, some classes of chemicals may operate by fundamentally different mechanisms but share common features. This is illustrated by an example from a skin corrosivity QSAR.[13] Organic acids and phenols are corrosive by two different reactivity mechanisms which are modelled by the same physicochemical parameter, pK_a, which operates quite differently in the two mechanisms; both classes of chemicals, however, share similar transport parameters which influence their ability to penetrate skin.

Increasingly it is being accepted that the validation of alternative methods should be conducted using sets of chemicals which have common features. This implies that such chemicals operate via common mechanisms of action. Identification of mechanistically relevant chemical parameters affords the development of QSARs and *in vitro* assays. For QSAR development, chemical parameters relevant to the mechanism of action need to be identified. Once developed the QSAR can be used to test the mechanistic hypothesis developed earlier. Significant outliers may indicate that mechanisms outside the existing QSAR are operating and so new QSARs may need to be developed. Eventually a robust QSAR model is developed. The process for development of an *in vitro* assay should similarly start with definition of the toxicological phenomenon to be modelled or replaced, definition of relevant mechanism and categorization of chemicals on the basis of mechanism of action. An end-point in the *in vitro* assay should be selected on the basis of relevance to the *in vivo* toxicity.

The *in vitro* assay is developed using a training set of chemicals, usually one with which the laboratory is knowledgeable. This should lead to the definition of a prediction model (see above) and subsequent testing of the prediction model with an extended set of chemicals. The prediction model may then be refined if necessary. The aim is to define an *in vitro* assay with a robust protocol that can readily be adopted by several laboratories and a prediction model that can readily be interpreted by several laboratories.

Both the *in vitro* assay and its associated prediction model can then enter the validation process.[9] The final QSAR model(s) similarly could enter the validation process either alone as a prediction tool, or could be used to optimize selection of test chemicals for the validation of *in vitro* assays, as is currently in progress for the ECVAM-sponsored validation study on skin corrosivity.

This schema is contrasted with what has actually happened in the development of the majority of alternative assays. There has often been poor identification of the toxicological phenomenon to be modelled. For example, many alternative methods have been developed as replacements for the Draize rabbit eye irritation test. However, scant regard has been paid to which component of the *in vivo* eye response is to be modelled, e.g. corneal opacity or conjunctival erythema. In this case the yardstick that has often been used to assess the performance of the *in vitro* methods is a composite score called the Maximum Average Score (MAS).[22] The validity of the MAS as an adequate descriptor of eye irritation is highly questionable because it treats ordinal numbers as cardinal numbers and introduces subjective weighting factors.[36] Thus, on occasions, a single continuous variable, e.g. neutral red uptake, is expected to predict and correlate with a set of discontinuous variables describing fundamentally different reactions in different tissues. In contrast, some researchers have rationalized their methods in terms of a single end-point change in the eye,[46] but this refinement has not led to any improved predictive power.

There is one further way in which *in vitro* and QSAR techniques may be integrated. We have stated above that biological activity is a function of partition and reactivity. One of the strengths of QSAR is the ease with which it can model partition either directly, e.g. logP, or through the use of a combination of parameters as exemplified by the modelling of skin permeability[15,47] or in PBPK models.[8] On the other hand, one of the major strengths of *in vitro* toxicology is the ease of measurement of cytotoxicity parameters, properties that depend much more on the reactivity properties of the chemical and rather less on partition. Whilst the reactivity parameters of chemicals can be calculated using chemical modelling software or even measured directly, these methods are often comparable only within relatively small areas of chemistry. A practical solution to this problem is to use cytotoxicity data from *in vitro* toxicology techniques as the independent variables for reactivity in QSARs. An example of this approach currently under development is the use of neutral red uptake data to measure the cytotoxicity of electrophilic organic acids. These data, in combination with parameters used in a previous QSAR study of the corrosivity of organic acids,[13] are proving useful in discriminating between chemicals with the EC classifications R34 (corrosive: causes burns) and R35 (corrosive: causes severe burns).[48]

X. CONCLUSIONS

There are excellent opportunities for the integration of QSAR knowledge and *in vitro* method development and evaluation. A major limitation is the mechanistic understanding of many toxicological phenomena. Where such understanding does not already exist we have shown how development of QSARs may help to elucidate and clarify such mechanisms of action. This approach requires careful and systematic consideration of the toxic effects, especially revisiting the descriptors of *in vivo* toxicity. It is admitted that with the current state of our knowledge the more 'simple' toxicities, such as eye and skin irritation and skin sensitization, are more amenable to QSAR analysis but there are already indications that more 'complex' toxicities, e.g. α_2-microglobulin nephropathy[20] and peroxisome proliferation[3] may be similarly amenable to these approaches.

Ultimately QSAR models may be used reliably to predict toxicity of chemicals and thus lead to replacement of animals in some toxicity studies. In the meantime, QSAR methods can help to:

(a) evaluate the mechanistic competence of *in vitro* methods;
(b) help to refine existing *in vitro* methods;
(c) give insight into design of new *in vitro* methods;
(d) reduce the need for testing and hence reduce the number of animals used;
(e) refine the animal testing that is done to avoid unnecessary tests, the outcome of which can be predicted with a reasonable degree of certainty.

REFERENCES

1. Dearden, J. C. (1990) Physico-chemical descriptors. In Karcher, W. and Devillers, J. (eds) *Practical Applications of Quantitative Structure–Activity Relationships (QSAR) in Environmental Chemistry and Toxicology*, pp. 25–59. Kluwer Academic, Dordrecht, The Netherlands.
2. Barratt, M. D., Basketter, D. A. and Roberts, D. W. (1994) Skin sensitization structure activity relationship for phenyl benzoates. *Toxicol. In Vitro* **8**: 823–826.

3. Lake, B. G., Lewis, D. F. V., Gray, T. J. B. and Beamand, J. A. (1993) Structure–activity relationships for induction of peroxisomal enzyme activities in primary rat hepatocyte culture. *Toxicol. In Vitro* **7**: 605–614.
4. Mapleson, W. W. (1963) Quantitative predictions of anaesthetic concentrations. In Papper, E. M. and Ritz, R. J. (eds) *Uptake and Distribution of Anaesthetic Agents*, pp. 104–119. McGraw-Hill, New York.
5. Riggs, D. S. (1963) *The Mathematical Approach to Physiological Problems: A Critical Primer.* MIT Press, Cambridge, MA.
6. Fiserova-Bergova, V. and Holaday, D. A. (1979) Uptake and clearance of inhalation anaesthetics in man. *Drug Metab. Rev.* **9**: 41–58.
7. Dedrick, R. L., Forrester, D. D. and Ho, D. H. O. (1971) *In vitro–in vivo* correlation of drug metabolism – deamination of 1-β-D-arabinofuranosylcytosine. *Biochem. Pharmacol.* **21**: 1–16.
8. Green, T., Provan, W. McL., Dugard, P. H. and Cook, S. K. (1988) ECETOC Technical Report No. 32. *Methylene Chloride (Dichloromethane): Human Risk Assessment using Experimental Animal Data.* European Centre for Ecotoxicology and Toxicology of Chemicals, Brussels.
9. Bruner, L. H., Carr, G. J., Chamberlain, M. and Curren, R. D. (1996) Assessing the validity of alternative methods for toxicity testing. In Marzulli, F. N. and Maibach, H. I. (eds) *Dermatotoxicology*, pp. 579–605. Taylor and Francis, Washington D.C.
10. Barratt, M. D. (1995) The role of structure activity relationships and expert systems in alternative strategies for the determination of skin sensitization, skin corrosivity and eye irritation. *ATLA* **23**: 111–122.
11. Chamberlain, M. and Barratt, M. D. (1995) Practical applications of QSAR to *in vitro* toxicology illustrated by consideration of eye irritation. *Toxicol. In Vitro* **9**: 543–547.
12. Whittle, E. G., Barratt, M. D., Carter, J. A., Basketter, D. A. and Chamberlain, M. (1995) The skin corrosivity potential of fatty acids: *in vitro* rat and human skin testing and QSAR studies. *Toxicol. In Vitro* **10**: 95–100.
13. Barratt, M. D. (1995) Quantitative structure activity relationships for skin corrosivity of organic acids, bases and phenols. *Toxicol. Lett.* **75**: 169–176.
14. Oliver, G. J. A., Pemberton, M. A. and Rhodes, C. (1986) An *in vitro* skin corrosivity test – modifications and validation. *Food Chem. Toxicol.* **24**: 507–512.
15. Barratt, M. D. (1995) Quantitative structure activity relationships for skin permeability. *Toxicol. In Vitro* **9**: 27–37.
16. Oliver, G. J. A. and Pemberton, M. A. (1986) The identification of corrosive agents for human skin *in vitro*. *Food Chem. Toxicol.* **24**: 513–515.
17. Whittle, E. and Basketter, D. A. (1993) The *in vitro* corrosivity test: comparison of *in vitro* human skin with *in vivo* data. *Toxicol. In Vitro* **7**: 269–274.
18. Cronin, M. T. D., Basketter, D. A. and York, M. (1993) A quantitative structure–activity relationship (QSAR) investigation of a Draize eye irritation database. *Toxicol. In Vitro* **8**: 21–28.
19. Ridings, J. E., Manallack, D. T., Saunders, M. R., Baldwin, J. A. and Livingstone, D. J. (1992) Multivariate quantitative structure–toxicity relationships in a series of dopamine mimetics. *Toxicology* **76**: 209–217.
20. Barratt, M. D. (1994) A quantitative structure activity relationship (QSAR) for prediction of α-2μ-globulin nephropathy. *Quantitative Structure Activity Relationships* **13**: 275–280.
21. Barratt, M. D. (1995) A quantitative structure activity relationship for the eye irritation potential of neutral organic chemicals. *Toxicol. Lett.* **80**: 69–74.
22. Bagley, D. M., Bruner, L. H., de Silva, O., O'Brien, K. A. F., Uttley, M. and Walker, A. P. (1992) An evaluation of five potential alternatives *in vitro* to the rabbit eye irritation test *in vivo*. *Toxicol. In Vitro* **6**: 275–284.
23. Jacobs, G. A. and Martens, M. A. (1989) An objective method for the evaluation of eye irritation *in vivo*. *Food Chem. Toxicol.* **27**: 255–258.
24. Johnson, S. M. and Bangham, A. D. (1969) The action of anaesthetics on phospholipid membranes. *Biochim. Biophys. Acta* **193**: 92–104.
25. Cherry, R. J., Dodd, G. H. and Chapman, D. (1970) Small molecule-lipid membrane interaction and the puncturing theory of olfaction. *Biochim. Biophys. Acta* **211**: 409–416.
26. Botham, P. A., Chamberlain, M., Barratt, M. D. *et al.* (1995) A prevalidation study on *in vitro* skin corrosivity testing. The report and recommendations of ECVAM workshop 6. *ATLA* **23**: 219–255.
27. EEC (1993) Annexes I, II, III and IV to Commission Directive 93/21/EEC of 27 April 1993 adapting to technical progress for the 18th time. Council Directive 67/548/EEC on the

approximation of the laws, regulations and administrative provisions relating to the classification, packaging and labelling of dangerous substances. *Official Journal of the European Communities*, L110A.

28. ECETOC (1995) *ECETOC Technical Report No. 66. Skin Irritation and Corrosion.* Reference Chemicals Data Bank, European Centre for Ecotoxicology and Toxicology of Chemicals, Brussels.
29. Balls, M., Blaauboer, B. J., Brusick, D. *et al.* (1990) The report and recommendations of the CAAT/ERGATT workshop on the validation of toxicity test procedures. *ATLA* **18:** 313–337.
30. Balls, M., Blaauboer, B. J., Fentem, J. H. *et al.* (1995) Practical aspects of the validation of toxicity test procedures. The report and recommendations of ECVAM workshop 5. *ATLA* **23:** 129–147.
31. Basketter, D. A., Scholes, E. W., Kimber, I. *et al.* (1991) Interlaboratory evaluation of the local lymph node assay with 25 chemicals and comparison with guinea pig test data. *Toxicol. Methods* **1:** 30–43.
32. Whittle, E., Basketter, D., York, M. *et al.* (1992) Findings of an interlaboratory trial of the enucleated eye method as an alternative eye irritation test. *Toxicol. Methods* **2:** 30–41.
33. EEC (1990) *Collaborative Study on the Evaluation of Alternative Methods to the Eye Irritation Test.* Directorate-General, Employment, Industrial Relations and Social Affairs, Health and Safety Directorate. DGV and DGXI, Brussels.
34. Purchase, I. F. H. (1990) An international reference chemical data bank would accelerate the development, validation and regulatory acceptance of alternative toxicology tests, *ATLA* **18:** 345–348.
35. Bagley, D. M., Botham, P. A., Gardner, J. R. *et al.* (1992) Eye irritation: reference chemicals data bank. *Toxicol. In Vitro* **6:** 487–491.
36. ECETOC (1992) *ECETOC Technical Report No. 48. Eye Irritation.* Reference Compounds Data Bank, European Centre for Ecotoxicology and Toxicology of Chemicals, Brussels.
37. OECD (1987) Test guideline 405: acute eye irritation/corrosion. In *Guidelines for the Testing of Chemicals.* OECD, Paris.
38. Kristen, V., Hoppe, V. and Pape, W. (1993) The pollen tube growth test: a new alternative to the Draize eye irritation test. *Journal of the Society of Cosmetic Chemists* **44:** 153–162.
39. Barratt, M. D. and Brown, K. R. (1985) Photochemical binding of photoallergens to human serum albumin; a simple *in vitro* method for screening potential photoallergens. *Toxicol. Lett.* **24:** 1–6.
40. Burton, A. B. G., York, M. and Lawrence, R. S. (1981) The *in vitro* assessment of severe eye irritants. *Food Chem. Toxicol.* **19:** 471–480.
41. Barratt, M. D., Castell, J. V., Chamberlain, M. *et al.* (1995) The integrated use of alternative approaches for predicting toxic hazard. The report and recommendations of ECVAM workshop 8. *ATLA* **23:** 410–429.
42. Hermens, J. L. M. (1989) Quantitative structure activity relationships of environmental pollutants. In Hutzinger, O. (ed.) *Handbook of Environmental Chemistry*, Vol. 2E, pp. 111–162. Springer, Berlin.
43. McCarty, L. S. (1987) Relationship between toxicity and bioconcentration for some organic chemicals. I. Examination of the relationship. In Kaiser, K. L. E. (ed.) *QSAR and Environmental Toxicology – II*, pp. 207–220. D. Reidel Publishing, Dordrecht, The Netherlands.
44. Basketter, D. A., Roberts, D. W., Cronin, M. and Scholes, E. W. (1992) The value of the local lymph node assay in quantitative structure activity investigations. *Contact Dermatitis* **27:** 137–142.
45. Balls, M., Botham, P. A., Bruner, L. H. and Spielmann, H. (1995) The EC/HO international validation study on alternatives to the Draize eye irritation test. *Toxicol. in Vitro* **9:** 871–929.
46. Gordon, V. (1992) The scientific basis of the EYTEX system. *ATLA* **20:** 537–548.
47. Potts, R. O. and Guy, R. (1992) Predicting skin permeability. *Pharm. Res.* **9:** 663–669.
48. Barratt, M. D., Dixit, M. B. and Jones, P. A. (1996) The use of in vitro cytotoxicity measurements in QSAR methods for the prediction of the skin corrosivity potential of acids. *Toxicol. In Vitro* **10:** 283–290.

3

Continuous Cell Lines as a Model for Drug Toxicity Assessment

FRANK A. BARILE

I. Introduction 34
A. *In vitro* toxicology 34
B. Test systems 34
II. Cell culture systems in toxicity testing 35
A. Finite cell lines 35
B. Continuous cell lines 35
C. Static and perfusion cell systems 35
D. Criteria for identification and monitoring of growth 36
1. Karyotyping 36
2. Aging in culture 36
3. Contact inhibition 37
4. Measurement of growth and viability 37
5. Sources of cell lines 37
6. Summary 37
III. General cytotoxicity assessment of xenobiotics using cell lines 38
A. General toxicity criteria 38
B. Use of continuous cell lines 39
C. Acute versus chronic cell tests 40
D. When are cell lines used in acute toxicity testing? 41
1. Neutral red uptake assay 41
2. MTT assay 43
E. Summary 43
IV. Cell lines for target organ toxicity 44
A. Differential toxicity 44
B. Traditional cell lines used for target organ toxicity testing 44
1. Continuous renal cell lines 44
2. Continuous lung cell lines 45
3. Continuous cell lines of lymphocytic origin 45
4. Continuous cell lines for local toxicity 46
V. Experimental design 48
A. Experimental setup and design 48
B. Incubation medium and test chemical incompatibility 49
1. Micronization 49
2. Use of solvents to improve solubility 49

IN VITRO METHODS IN PHARMACEUTICAL RESEARCH
ISBN 0-12-163390-X

3. Sonication . . . 50
4. Use of paraffin (mineral) oil overlay . . . 50
C. Determination of dosage range . . . 50
D. Determination of inhibitory concentrations . . . 51
VI. Future perspectives . . . 51
References . . . 51

I. INTRODUCTION

A. *In vitro* toxicology

The techniques to grow animal and human cells and tissues on plastic surfaces or in suspension have contributed significantly to the development of biomedical science. Thus the term *in vitro* refers primarily to the handling of cells and tissues outside of the body under conditions which support their growth, differentiation, and stability.

Cell culture technology, as an important constituent of *in vitro* methodologies, is fundamental for understanding the basis of cell and molecular biology, and have been used with increasing frequency in medicinal chemistry, pharmacology, genetics, reproductive biology and oncology. The technology has improved throughout the decades, partly as a result of the interest in the methods, rather than through its applications, and much of the mystery originally surrounding the techniques has waned. Today, tissue culture (often used interchangeably with cell culture) represents a tool where scientific questions in the biomedical sciences can be answered through the use of isolated cells or tissues, without the influence of other organ systems. With this understanding, the use of continuous cell lines, as a model cell culture system, does not purport to represent the whole human organism, but can contribute to our understanding of the workings of its components.

B. Test systems

The use of cell culture techniques in toxicological investigations is referred to as *in vitro cytotoxicology.*[1] The techniques have gained increasing popularity since the growth of the first mammalian cells was described in capillary glass tubes. Since then, the technology has progressed rapidly and has been extensively refined. In addition, *in vitro* cytotoxicological methods have demonstrated that the direct interaction of chemicals with human and animal cells are responsible for the toxic effects. The necessity to determine the effects of industrial chemicals and pharmaceuticals that are developed and marketed at rapid and unprecedented rates has provoked the need for fast, simple, and effective test systems. Although the normal rate of progression of any scientific discipline is dictated by the progress within the scientific community, some areas have experienced more encouragement than others. As a result political and societal pressures have influenced research initiatives toward the development of alternative methods of toxicity testing.

To understand the possibilities for and, more importantly, the limitations of continuous cell line methods in toxicology, it is necessary to be acquainted with the main features of the techniques. Unlike other types of biomedical research, continuous care of the cells in culture is required for extended periods, which necessitates planning.

II. CELL CULTURE SYSTEMS IN TOXICITY TESTING

A. Finite cell lines

When a primary culture (that is, the initial cells arising from an explanted tissue or organ) is transferred to a new culture vessel with fresh medium, it is designated as a *cell line*. The subcultivation (passage) is made by detaching the cells from the glass or plastic using chemical or enzymatic methods; the cells are then dispersed and inoculated in a number of new vessels.[2] Because of selective survival of viable cells, the cell line will be more homogeneous and dedifferentiated with time. A culture which is demonstrating adequate growth is harvested every 3–7 days and subdivided to several new flasks, indicating a doubling rate of 56–84 hours. After 40–50 cell divisions (also referred to as population doubling level and may require months in culture depending on growth rate), most cell lines stop growing and ultimately die, possibly due to the timing of the genetic program. Such a *finite cell line* displays the diploid number of chromosomes and exhibits an orderly orientated growth pattern, including contact inhibition.[3]

B. Continuous cell lines

A small proportion of cell lines will not die out with time, but are *transformed* to *continuous cell lines*, with a growth pattern often referred to as immortal. Transformation occurs either spontaneously or as a result of incubation with viruses or chemicals. The exact mechanism of the transformation is still undefined but a continuous cell line has acquired a set of characteristics, such as varied chromosome number (heteroploidy) and loss of contact inhibition. Moreover, continous cell lines are able to form colonies in soft agar media, and induce tumors if implanted in immunologically nude animals. In spite of this, some highly differentiated functions, which mimic those of specialized cells, will persist in continuous cell lines. These differentiated functional markers are used to characterize the line, are relied upon to monitor the progress of the cells in culture, and, most importantly, are used as the parameters for assessing *in vitro* toxicity.

It is possible to select a single cell in a culture and subcultivate this cell to form a *continuous clonal cell line*. Cloning allows for the selection of one type of cell in a culture (for example, cells with specific functional markers) and the establishment of a subculture in which the desired characteristic has been passed onto the progeny.

C. Static and perfusion cell systems

In general, culture conditions during an experiment or assay differ from those used during routine growth and maintenance of stock cultures. Most stock cultures are grown in *static cell systems* which entertain a change of cell medium before or during subcultivation. Normal incubation conditions result in depletion of nutrients and accumulation of metabolic waste in the medium, thus becoming less physiological with time. Cell types that are anchorage dependent are often cultured as monolayers on the bottom surface of a flask which is covered with medium, plus an overlying gas phase consisting of 5–20% carbon dioxide in air. Cells may also be anchored on millipore filters or to polystyrene particles in an attempt to mimic the subcellular stratum. The filters, in particular, offer some advantages during studies of epithelial apical–basolateral–junctional complex communication, by providing exposure to different interfaces. Rotating flasks or tubes are used to increase the culture area by providing contact of the sides and tops of the vessel with medium, which also permits better oxygenation of cells. Some cell types (mainly continuous cell lines) need not adhere to a substratum and may be cultured in magnetically stirred suspension cultures or roller bottles.

Perfusion cultures are more advanced compared with static cell cultures since they allow for uniform flow of fresh medium by continuous irrigation of the flask. In addition to the usual cell culture manipulations, this system also uses positive pressure pumps and micron filters to provide the cultures with oxygenated, waste-free medium. At present these systems are not routinely used in most laboratories. It should be noted that the majority of cultures and test systems are much less oxygenated than animal tissues, and therefore permit anaerobic cell metabolism predominantly.

D. Criteria for identification and monitoring of growth

Several criteria are used for the identification and classification of cells in culture. These methods are employed when the cell line is established and periodically to monitor the genetic purity of the cells.[1,3–5]

1. *Karyotyping*

For a cell line designated as derived from normal tissue, the chromosome complement should be identical to that of the parent cell or species of origin, thus classifying it as diploid. Continuous cell lines derived from tumors, or transformed cells, are designated as aneuploid or heteroploid, with the possible exception of some lymphoblastic cell lines of neoplastic origin.

2. *Aging in culture*

The life span of cells in culture is measured according to the population doubling level (pdl). This criterium refers to the number of times a cell undergoes mitosis since its original isolation *in vitro*. The general formula for assessing pdl is:

$$\text{pdl}_f = 3.32(\log F - \log I) + \text{pdl}_i$$

where pdl_f is the final pdl at the time of trypsinization or at the end of a given subculture; F is the final cell count; I is the initial cell number used as inoculum at the beginning of the subculture; pdl_i is the doubling level of the inoculum used to initiate the subculture.

Cells with finite life spans generally show signs of aging, such as loss of cell shape and increase in the cytoplasmic lipid content. The number of pdls that a particular finite cell line exhibits depends on the age of the donor relative to the species. Continuous cell lines are capable of an indefinite number of mitotic divisions *in vitro*, provided they are maintained under optimum conditions.

3. *Contact inhibition*

Cells which exhibit contact inhibition will arrest their cell cycle in the G_0 phase when the layer of cells completely occupies the surface available for proliferation, thus forming monolayer cultures. Cells which do not exhibit contact inhibition will grow in multilayers.

4. *Measurement of growth and viability*

There are important considerations when determining the integrity of a cell line. The judgment required is generally based on knowledge and experience that the individual has with cell culture in general. Overall, several criteria are assessed to determine the potential of the cells for future toxicological investigations, including: the viability of the cultures, the appearance of the cells under the phase-contrast microscope, especially as a finite cell line approaches the anticipated maximum number of doublings, and the ability of the cells to retain as many of the morphological and biochemical features as the original parent cell or primary culture.

The techniques used to monitor cell growth and viability on a daily basis include: cell counting, exclusion of the vital dye, trypan blue, the ability to survive normal culture conditions, and the proportion of cells inoculated into the culture vessel with passage that will attach to the culture surface. Most of these features can be determined under the phase-contrast microscope, assuming that the individual responsible for the cultures has familiarity with the cells in question.

5. *Sources of cell lines*

Sources of cell lines include certified cell banks, such as the American Type Culture Collection (ATCC, Rockville, Maryland, USA) and the European Collection of Animal Cell Cultures (ECACC, Porton Down, UK). These facilities operate as non-profit institutions and stock thousands of cell types classified as either certified cell lines (CCLs) or cell repository lines (CRLs). CCLs have more information available as to the donor, karyotypic analysis, expected population doublings, cell structural features and enzyme markers. In addition, the ATCC also houses repositories for viruses, fungi, bacteria, and genetic probes and vectors.

6. *Summary*

Other methods of cell classification are not necessarily routinely performed. These include analysis of tissue-specific differentiated properties, such as secretion of macromolecules, the presence of intracellular enzymes, ultrastructural identification, fluorescent labeling for identifiable structural proteins, or the ability of the cells to form an invasive malignant tumor when injected into immunologically deficient (*nude*) mice.

Because of the risk of cross contamination in a laboratory that is accustomed to handling several cell lines by various individuals, it is necessary to verify the original cell type in use. Some methods used for identification of characteristic cell markers include labeling with fluorescent antibodies, cytogenetic karyotypic studies and isoenzyme profiles. In addition, it is also necessary to check for the possibility of specific mycoplasma infections of the cultures.

This contaminant is described as a bacteria, lacking a cell wall, which tenaciously adheres to cell membranes and cannot be eliminated with routine addition of antibiotics to the media. In fact, the indiscriminate addition of penicillin and streptomycin to the growth and saline-buffered wash media have been blamed for mycoplasma contamination, resulting in the misinterpretation of information generated by the use of the cell lines. Tests for the detection of mycoplasma are commercially available through suppliers of cell culture products.

III. GENERAL CYTOTOXICITY ASSESSMENT OF XENOBIOTICS USING CELL LINES

A. General toxicity criteria

The data obtained from animal experiments yield information pertaining to the dose for lethal or sublethal toxicity, which corresponds to many different general toxic mechanisms and effects.[6] Similarly, cell systems also detect a wide spectrum of unspecified mechanisms and effects.[7] In contrast to animal experiments, however, all cell tests of general toxicity in current use measure the concentration of a substance which damages components, structures, or biochemical pathways within the cells. This range of injury is further specified by the length of exposure to the chemical, thus allowing the test to be predictive for risks associated with toxic effects *in vivo*, for those doses of the tested substance. This assumes that similar concentrations can be measured in the corresponding human tissue for comparable exposure periods.

About 20 methods used for general toxicity testing have filtered through from those traditionally used in mechanism studies and are referenced in several texts available in the *in vitro* toxicology literature.[1,8,9] Their validity has been established usually as a result of frequent use in one laboratory, followed by repetition and confirmation by others. This method of evaluation thus proceeds more as a matter of convenience for the laboratory, particularly if the assay can be easily accommodated to the routine of the testing facilities. The methods are necessarily similar: cells are exposed to different concentrations of the substance for a predetermined period of time, after which the degree of inhibition of viability or functional condition is measured. This indicator as the standard of measurement then becomes the toxic end-point. The most common general toxicity criteria for cell lines are listed in Table 3.1. Several tests are described below.

The first and most readily observed effect following exposure of cells to toxicants is phase-contrast morphological alteration in the cell layer and/or cell shape in monolayer culture. Therefore, it is not surprising that morphologic alterations are used as an index of toxicity. Different types of toxic effects, however, may also require investigative tools at different levels of sensitivity. Gross modifications such as blebbing or vacuolization are observed using light microscopy whereas ultrastructural modifications require analysis by transmission or scanning electron microscopy.

Another indicator of toxicity is altered cell growth. The effect of chemicals on the ability of cells to replicate is used as an index of toxicity; the concentration of the substance at which 50% of the cells do not multiply is called the median inhibitory dose (ID_{50}). A more specific measure of replication is plating efficiency: the ability of cells to form colonies after 10–15 days in culture in the presence of a toxic agent. The information obtained with this parameter, together with cell growth, yields more complete information since both cell

Table 3.1 Some common general toxicity criteria for cell lines in culture. (Adapted from Barile.[1])

Criterion	Method for determining the degree of inhibition or injury
Cell morphology	Histological analysis using light microscopy; ultrastructural analysis using transmission electron microscopy
Cell growth	Cell counts; mitotic frequency using karyotypic analysis; DNA synthesis
Cell division	Clone formation; plating efficiency
Cell metabolism	Anaerobic glycolysis; uptake of isotope-labeled precursors as indicators for newly synthesized macromolecules; assays for specific proteins, hormones, and enzymes (collagen, steroids, neurotransmitters)
Cell staining	Immunohistochemical or cytochemical stains for proteins, enzymes, and carbohydrates
Cell membrane	Leakage of isotope-labeled markers; leakage of enzymes (lactate, dehydrogenase-glucuronidase); formation of blebs; uptake of trypan blue
Mitochondria	Mitochondrial integrity (MTT assay)
Lysosomes	Vital staining methods (neutral red assay)
Ribosomes	Synthesis of macromolecules (glycosaminoglycans); induction or inhibition of enzymes (acid and alkaline phosphatases)

survival and ability to reproduce are monitored. Cell reproduction can be measured with several methods including cell count, DNA content, protein content, or enzyme activity. The assay for DNA content using biochemical methods or by monitoring the incorporation of radiolabeled precursors into DNA represents two different methods supplying similar information.[10–12]

Another crude index of toxicity is cell viability. This end-point can easily be measured by using vital stains such as trypan blue, which enters dead cells only, and neutral red uptake, which is actively absorbed by living cells. The latter is commonly used in biomaterial testing in the agar overlay method. A count of dead and vital cells is compared with the control and provides an index of lethality of the test compound.

B. Use of continuous cell lines

Finite and continuous cell lines have traditionally been used for studies of cell biology, biochemistry and, more recently, toxicology. Table 3.2 lists examples of cell lines that have broached the different disciplines and are currently used in cytotoxicity testing. Most retain significant functional markers originally present in the parent cell. Although continuous cell lines offer the advantage of indefinite *in vitro* growth and ease of manipulation, finite cell lines have a diploid karyotype and display *in vitro* aging. For specific purposes, such as the determination of enzymatic activity, the investigator should assess the level of activity before embarking on a bold series of experiments with a particular cell line.[1,13,14]

Table 3.2 Some commonly used cell lines for assessing target organ toxicity. (Adapted from Barile.[1])

Origin	Name	Notes
Human, cervix uteri	HeLa	Continuous
Human, adult lung, epithelial	A549	Continuous
Human, trachea	HEP-2	Continuous
Human, liver	Chang liver	Continuous
Human, epidermoid tumor	KB	Continuous
Human, embryonal lung, fibroblast	HFL1, WI-38, IMR-90, MRC-5	Finite
Human, skin, fibroblast	Detroit 551	Finite
Human, lymphoblasts, Hodgkin's disease	RPMI 6666	Finite
Human, epidermoid carcinoma, larynx	HEP-2	Continuous
Human, neuroblastoma, 'epithelium-like'	SK-N-MC, SK-N-SH	Continuous
Human, adenocarcinoma, colon	Caco-2	Continuous
Mouse, embryo	Balb/c 3T3	Continuous
Mouse, lymphoma	L5178	Continuous
Mouse, neuroblastoma	C1300	Continuous
Rat, hepatoma,	MH1C1, HTC	Continuous
Rat, lung epithelium	L2	Continuous
Rat, intestine	IEC-17	Finite
Chinese hamster, ovary	CHO	Continuous
Hamster, kidney	BHK 21	Continuous
Canine, kidney	MDCK	Continuous
Rabbit, cornea	SIRC	Continuous

C. Acute versus chronic cell tests

A major criticism of *in vitro* cytotoxicity assays is that the procedures measure only acute toxicity, primarily because the exposure is of short duration and occurs through one cellular passage level. This is because occasionally it is difficult to determine the difference between acute and chronic exposure in culture. Since one culture cycle (one passage level) can extend from 3 to 7 days depending on the cell line, it is conceivable to extend the exposure time, within the time of the cycle, to determine the response to a chemical. In this way, exposure to the chemical through at least one cell cycle may differentiate between acute and subacute, or subacute and chronic. This sequence for exposure would also reveal any tolerance developed against a chemical.

The effects of chemicals *in vivo* at the cellular level may also result from repeated exposure and may follow familiar patterns, including: (a) the slow accumulation of the chemical in target tissues until acute toxic concentrations are reached; (b) the slow accumulation of the chemical in blood which subsequently distributes to target tissues; and, (c) the chemical does not accumulate but causes toxicity through low-dose, repeated insults until threshold injury results. To address these mechanisms, repeated and chronic exposure assays could be designed to mimic the *in vivo* situation. Such experiments include: exposure of cultures to *low but increasing doses* of the chemical for at least two to three passages to determine whether the chemical causes toxicity at concentrations below threshold; exposure of proliferating cells to continuous *low* doses of the chemical for three or more passages to determine the mechanism of accumulation at low concentrations and the corresponding toxic response; and short exposure to the test chemical (1–24 h), followed by substitution with fresh medium, thus allowing sufficient time for uncoupling of non-covalently bound substance. In the last experimental setup, incubations are repeated in each of three successive passages. The objective is to determine toxicity occurring at the cellular level after repeated insult.

D. When are cell lines used in acute toxicity testing?

Cell line methods are currently used in academic and industrial research laboratories in a variety of situations. For example, cytotoxicity tests generally precede *in vitro* genotoxicity tests so that mutations and chromosome damage may be ascertained. Cell methods, including the use of primary cultures and *in vitro* pharmacokinetic studies, are used as screening tests for the development of new therapeutic drugs, to assess acute and chronic toxicity. Setting the protocols according to this sequence reduces the number of animals needed for *in vivo* testing. In addition, highly cytotoxic products are screened using cellular methods, thus eliminating the need to expose animals to these compounds.

Similarly, there has been substantial effort into evaluating the potential predictive ability of general cytotoxicity tests for eye and local irritancy. This endeavor is already proving worthwhile for assessing the safety of cosmetic formulations, which would not be tested in animals before human volunteer studies are undertaken.[15] Although such *in vitro* studies have not gained acceptance by the pharmaceutical industry, they can be used for human risk assessment as screening methods.

Cytotoxicity tests are also employed by chemical companies for screening pesticides, food and beverage additives and preservatives, liquids or gases determined to increase the risk of occupational hazards, and chemicals responsible for water, air, and soil pollution. When these chemicals are introduced into the cellular systems, the concentrations necessary to produce toxicity can be compared with those of compounds of a similar or identical class. Table 3.3 lists some commonly used cell tests for general and local cytotoxicity. Two tests commonly employed for the assessment of general cytotoxicity, the MTT assay and the neutral red uptake–release assay, are described below.

1. *Neutral red uptake assay*

The neutral red uptake cytotoxicity assay uses neutral red dye, which is preferentially absorbed into lysosomes.[17,18] The basis of the test is that a cytotoxic chemical, regardless of site or mechanism of action, can interfere with this process and result in a reduction of the number of viable cells. Only viable cells, therefore, are capable of maintaining the process intact. The degree of inhibition of growth, related to the concentration of the test compound, provides an indication of toxicity. Any chemical having a localized effect upon the lysosomes, however, will result in an artificially low reflection of cell number and viability. This factor does make the system useful for detecting chemicals that selectively affect lysosomes, and thus more readily detects a specific mechanism of action. For example, chloroquine phosphate specifically alters lysosomal pH and thus has a greater effect on neutral red uptake than most chemicals, resulting in an overestimation of the toxic concentration.

Table 3.3 Frequently used rapid screening cell culture tests for assessing general cytotoxicity and local irritation.

Test	Toxic end-point	Indication
Neutral red cytotoxicity	Uptake or release	Lysosomal activity or cell viability
Kenacid blue cytotoxicity	Uptake of dye	Total cell protein
MTT assay	Mitochondrial oxidation	Cell viability
LS-L929 cytotoxicity	Uptake of ethidium bromide and fluorescein acetate	Cell viability
V79 cytotoxicity	Nucleic acid leakage	Cell membrane damage
BALB/c 3T3 cytotoxicity	Neutral red uptake	Cell viability
	Kenacid blue R binding	Cell binding
Lung cell assay	Radiolabeling of proteins	Newly synthesized proteins
Pollen tube growth assay	Pollen tube growth	Cell growth
Bovine isolated cornea	Corneal damage	Ocular toxicity
Agar overlay assay	L929 fibroblast viability	Local irritation
EYTEX	Protein aggregation	Corneal opacification or ocular irritation
HET–CAM	Blood vessel changes in chorioallantoic membrane	Local irritation
Fluorescein leakage test	Integrity of junctional complexes	Eye irritancy

From INVITTOX (1994) *Protocol List 7, The ERGATT/FRAME Data Bank of* In Vitro *Techniques in Toxicology*, and Clemedson *et al.*[16]

For these experiments, cells are seeded in microtiter plates and allowed to settle and adhere for 24 h. The medium is then replaced with fresh medium containing the test chemical at increasing concentrations. Some 3 hours before the end of the exposure period, the medium is aspirated from the cells and replaced with neutral red solution (50 μg ml^{-1} in growth medium). The cultures are incubated for an additional 3 h at 37°C. The medium is then removed, the cells are rinsed with phosphate-buffered saline, fixed and destained with 1% acetic acid/50% ethanol. The plates are shaken for 10 min and the absorbance is read at 540 nm with a microplate reader, against a reference well containing no cells. Absorbance correlates linearly with cell number over a specific optical density range of 0.2–1.0.

One major drawback of the assay is precipitation of the dye into visible, fine, needle-like crystals. When this occurs it is almost impossible to reverse and produces inaccurate readings. The precipitation is induced by some chemicals and thus a visual inspection stage during the procedure is important.

2. MTT assay

In the MTT assay, the tetrazolium salt, 3-(4,5-dimethyl-thiazol-2-yl)-2,5-diphenyltetrazolium bromide (MTT), is actively absorbed into cells and reduced in a mitochondrial-dependent reaction to yield a formazan product.[19] The product accumulates within the cell since it cannot pass through the cell membrane. Upon addition of DMSO, isopropanol, or other suitable solvent, the product is solubilized and liberated, and is readily quantified colorimetrically. The ability of the cells to reduce MTT provides an indication of mitochondrial integrity and activity, which is interpreted as a measure of cell viability. The assay is suitable for a variety of cell lines displaying exponential growth in culture and a relatively high level of mitochondrial activity. It should be noted that some known compounds selectively affect mitochondria, resulting in an overestimation of toxicity.

The assay begins as with the neutral red procedure. During the final 2 h of incubation with the test chemical, a 0.5% MTT solution in growth medium replaces the test medium at 37°C. The medium plus MTT is then replaced with DMSO and agitated for 5 min. The plates are read at 550 nm with a microplate reader, against a reference well containing no cells. Absorbance correlates linearly with cell number over a specific optical density range of 0.2–1.0.

Recently, the chemical 2,3-bis[2-methoxy-4-nitro-5-sulphophenyl]-2H-tetrazolium-5-carboxanilide inner salt (XTT) has been substituted for MTT, since the former is already soluble in aqueous media and, consequently, obviates the need for DMSO.

With the MTT assay, the pH of the medium is quickly assessed by the change in color. Phenol red is used as the indicator in the medium and changes to a yellow-orange color when cells are totally inhibited, indicating a lack of MTT reduction. With uninhibited cultures, a violet color develops. This occurs as a result of reduction of the originally yellow MTT solution, yielding the formation of the insoluble formazan product. With partially inhibited cells, the original red-orange color remains unchanged. Initial pH changes caused by test substances and precipitates of water-insoluble substances are also readily visible through the color changes.

E. Summary

To increase comparability of results and optimize testing procedures, standardization and adherence to the experimental approaches and procedures is desirable. The use of well-characterized cell lines, possibly of human origin, is important. Specific toxicity end-points, as well as the most suitable assay methods, should be uniformly established. Cell cultures should be examined periodically for possible contamination with microorganisms and mycoplasmas, for cross contamination with other mammalian cell types, and for karyotypic integrity. Reports should provide details of exposure conditions including information on the purity and source of the test compound. Moreover, the measurement of the concentration of the compound at the beginning and end of the experiment, particularly for insoluble or volatile substances, would facilitate interlaboratory comparison of results.

IV. CELL LINES FOR TARGET ORGAN TOXICITY

A. Differential toxicity

Continuous cell strains and cell lines have traditionally been used for mechanistic studies in cell biology, biochemistry, and toxicology, with the presumption that the cell line is a suitable representative of the donor organ. For the most part, this supposition has been supported by rigorous screening of the sample cultures for the functions whose effects are being demonstrated. For instance, if enzymatic function is monitored in a continuous cell line as an indicator of xenobiotic metabolism, then the presence of critical enzyme levels must be present during the lifetime of the culture. Cellular functions present in the original isolated parent cells, however, do not guarantee that organ-specific effects of chemicals will be observed in the subsequent generations with passage. Flint[20,21] has argued that basal cytotoxicity tests, especially those involving permanent cell lines, are of limited value, because the cells have metabolically distanced themselves from their tissues of origin. Established cell lines, whether continuous or finite, differentiate and lose their organ-specific functions. According to the author, the systems are designed to measure basal cytotoxicity – that is, with the loss of specific functions, the toxin in question affects metabolic processes important to maintain basal activity.

Cell lines can also be used for mechanism studies for chemicals that are known to affect basal cell functions.[12,22] Such substances include antibiotics, chemotherapeutic agents, digitalis, ethanol, organic solvents, and heavy metals. This is an advantage of such a system because methods incorporating cell lines are simpler, do not require repetitive killing of animals, and use cells that are similar from one experiment to the next.

B. Traditional cell lines used for target organ toxicity testing

The use of established cell lines has traditionally been credited with identifying the mechanisms of cellular toxicity. The inference has been added that the cell line is also a reflection of the organ of derivation. This concept, however, should be approached cautiously since it is generally accepted that, with time and passage, cultures lose a significant number of the original characteristics inherited from the parent cell. Thus, although the use of continuous cell lines for target organ toxicity testing is common, the functional markers they retain in culture may not be an accurate reflection of the organ of origin.

1. Continuous renal cell lines

Over the past 20 years, improved methods for maintaining continuous cultures of cells have allowed for the realization of general mechanistic cytotoxicity studies. Renal cell culture technology has benefited primarily from the improved technology in much the same way as in other fields. The problems associated with other continuous cell lines, however, have also plagued the maintenance of continuous cultures of renal cells, the most important of which include the loss of *in vivo* characteristics following isolation and subsequent passage over several generations *in vitro*. This dedifferentiation may be followed by a decrease in the levels of functional markers necessary for identifying the cell type and for assessing cytotoxicity.[23] Nevertheless, the propagation of continuous cell lines has allowed for important contributions to understanding renal cytotoxicology. It is important to remember that, as with the use of continuous cell lines from any organ, cytotoxic effects from a chemical to renal cells may be a reflection of basal cytotoxicity rather than a specific renal toxic effect.[1]

Among the most frequently used continuous cell lines used in renal studies are the transformed cells, including the MDCK (Madin–Darby canine kidney) and LLC-PK_1 renal epithelial cell lines.[9,24]

MDCK cells maintain morphologic features and functional characteristics consistent with cells of distal tubule or collecting duct origin. In addition, they show biochemical evidence of transporting epithelia, although several strains and clones have been established which differ considerably from the parent cell line and from each other. LLC-PK_1 cells are derived from pig proximal tubule cells, and share morphologic features characteristic of their parent cells, including dome formation, presence of apical membrane microvilli, and several junctional complexes. Physiologically, they express high levels of brush border membrane marker enzymes and retain the ability to transport small molecules.

Recently, Bohets *et al.*[25] showed that culture conditions affect MDCK and LLC-PK_1 cell viability, cytotoxicity, and detoxification. In a study measuring neutral red uptake, MTT-dependent cell viability, and glutathione levels on nephrotoxic potential, the authors concluded that, among the factors influencing renal cell cultures, concentrations of fetal calf serum must be taken into consideration when different cytotoxicity studies are compared.

2. *Continuous lung cell lines*

Human fetal lung fibroblasts, such as HFL1, MRC-5, and WI38, have been extensively studied and characterized in aging studies, collagen biosynthesis, and cytotoxicity testing.[26–29] The fibroblasts are easily maintained in culture and exhibit a finite life span. The cells are derived from a first trimester fetus and have a diploid karyotype.

A549 cells, an adult human lung carcinoma continuous cell line, and L2 cells, a rat lung epithelial cell line, are used extensively in studies of pulmonary cell biology. The cells are heteroploid, but retain special characteristics necessary for lung cell biochemistry, including secretion of macromolecules, presence of phospholipid inclusions, and retention of appreciable levels of lung-specific enzymes.[10,30]

3. *Continuous cell lines of lymphocytic origin*

The American Type Culture Collection (ATCC, Bethesda, MD, USA) has many cell lines of human and animal origin as part of the Tumor Immunology Cell Bank. Many of the cell lines, including continuous cultures of myelomas, hybridomas, and lymphomas, have been characterized according to their immunologic properties. Cell-surface markers are identified, and sensitivity or resistance to phytohemagglutinin (PHA), cortisol, thioguanine, and thymidine is noted, as well as any response to or stimulation by significant immuno-regulatory cytokines.[31]

Human placental mast cells,[32] thymocytes,[33] and polymorphonuclear lymphocytes,[34] are finite cell lines that have been used in mechanistic cytotoxicity studies. Continuous cultures of lymphoblasts (RPMI 7666), derived from normal leukocytes from peripheral human blood, and 'lymphoblastoid-like' lymphoblasts (RPMI 6666), derived from leukocytes of a donor with Hodgkin's disease, are frequently used in immunotoxicologic studies.

4. *Continuous cell lines for local toxicity*

Screening techniques to detect local toxicity have been used to investigate the effects of various irritating substances in the lung and on the skin. Agents that have been thoroughly studied in lung cell cultures include tobacco smoke,[35] diesel exhaust,[36] nitrogen dioxide,[37] aldehydes,[38] phorbol esters,[39] and paraquat.[10,40] The isolation of continuous cultures of alveolar epithelial cells and non-ciliated bronchiolar epithelial (Clara) cells has greatly accelerated the underlying mechanisms of the local pulmonary response to xenobiotics. Establishment of initial culture conditions, however, are often labor intensive, and continuous cultures are difficult to maintain in their differentiated state. Despite this, the need for methods to produce continuous cultures is especially necessary in the case of tracheobronchial and bronchial epithelial cell types, particularly since they are known to be sensitive to a variety of inhaled xenobiotics.

A large number of cell culture methods has been developed for screening dental materials. A few standard techniques incorporating cell lines have been established and are widely used. Continuous cell lines, such as L-929 and 3T3 mouse fibroblasts, and primary cultures have been accepted as useful in determining toxicity to dental materials. Examples of these methods include: (1) the agar overlay test;[41–43] (2) Wennberg's millipore filter method;[44] and (3) Spangberg's chromium leakage method.[45] It should be noted, however, that cell culture toxicity testing of dental materials is accompanied by limitations, including lack of simulation to the *in vivo* environment and the difficulty of extrapolating the information to the clinical situation. Schmalz[46] offers a useful review of the current status of toxicity testing of dental materials, presenting both advantages and limitations.

Earlier attempts to assess skin irritation of chemicals *in vitro* met with considerable setbacks. The deficiencies associated with dermal fibroblasts, as a model for skin toxicity studies, center around the continuing controversy of the dedifferentiation of the cells once they are maintained in serial culture.[47] As a result they lose their phenotypic appearance and characteristic features of the original parent cell *in vivo*. Recent progress in toxicological studies has concentrated on the development of human epidermal keratinocytes, in contrast to previously used dermal fibroblasts.

Rheinwald and Green[48] markedly advanced human epidermal keratinocyte culture using mitotically inhibited 'feeder layers' of 3T3 fibroblasts. Improvements on the feeder layer method involved the addition of epidermal growth factor,[49] cholera toxin,[50] and the use of culture dishes coated with extracellular matrix components.[51] In addition, the recent development of serum-free hormone-supplemented media has enhanced the maintenance of keratinocyte cultures.[52] Normal human keratinocytes serially cultivated in defined medium maintained sustained growth and the ability to develop normally into a morphologically differentiated epidermis.

In general, cytotoxicity studies using cultures of keratinocytes have shown conflicting results when correlations are attempted between *in vitro* data and animal skin irritation tests for a large series of chemicals.[47] For skin irritation studies, the effective concentration of a chemical applied to the skin and reaching cells *in vivo* is a function of the pharmacokinetics of the chemical and the epidermal barrier.

More recent studies have shown better correlations between the use of continuous or finite cell lines and *in vivo* studies. Wallace *et al.*[53] used the neutral red uptake assay to show that human epidermal keratinocytes, cultured in serum-free medium, were useful in predicting *generalized* acute lethal toxicity. Ward *et al.*[54] showed that primary human keratinocytes (NHEK) in serum-free medium correlated better with *in vivo* skin irritation data than canine kidney epithelial cells (MDCK) or human skin epithelial derived cell lines (NCTC 2544). Steer *et al.*[55] compared a physicochemical dermal model and a cell-based phototoxicity assay using a human lymphoblast cell line, against available *in vivo* data. Overall, there was general agreement between the two assays when correlated with *in vivo* data.

Many laboratories are currently developing skin organ culture models to assess dermal toxicology, including the use of skin organ cultures,[56] an *in vitro* cell culture epidermis on a collagen matrix,[57] reconstituted human skin models,[58] and a human tissue model composed of neonatal foreskin-derived keratinocytes cultured on permeable cell culture inserts.[59]

Numerous *in vitro* test systems have been developed as potential replacements for ocular toxicity testing in animals.[60,61] However, only a few have managed to survive the rigorous standards demanded for validation or required for general acceptance. Current toxicity testing protocols incorporate either continuous cell culture methods or ocular models designed to mimic the complex arrangement of ocular tissue. Table 3.4 summarizes several recent ocular toxicity testing studies which used either continuous cell lines or ocular models. Most of the studies report good correlations with available Draize eye test data, especially when monolayer cultures were used along with a variety of cytotoxic indicators.

Several ocular models have been developed to evaluate ocular irritancy. The hen's egg test–chorioallantoic membrane (HET–CAM)[67,68] yields information on changes that occur in blood vessels as a response to local injury, rather than monitoring direct cytotoxicity. Combrier and Castelli[42] modified the original protocol for the *in vitro* agarose overlay method[43] to include several classes of agarose classification, such as non-irritant, minimally irritant, mildly irritant, and irritant. The EYTEX system simulates corneal opacification by using a biochemical procedure to measure alterations in the hydration and conformation of an ordered macromolecular matrix to predict *in vivo* ocular irritancy. The EYTEX test is designed to evaluate the decrease in protein hydration associated with changes in protein conformation and aggregation.[70]

Continuous cell lines have enjoyed success because of the ease of manipulation of the cultures, and as a result of the similarity of the test methods.[17,71] In particular, continuous cell lines incorporate several features that are consistent with *in vivo* methods: incubation times *in vitro* are comparable to those used *in vivo*; test substances come in direct contact with the eye epithelium as it does with the isolated cells; the lack of blood vessels in the cornea allows for the attainment of steady-state drug concentrations in contact with the tissue, such that absorption and local pharmacokinetic phenomena do not interfere with results obtained with the test protocols.

Recently, Roguet *et al.*[58] studied 30 surfactants using a cell line derived from rabbit cornea (SIRC) with the neutral red uptake bioassay as the indicator system. Boue-Grabot *et al.*[72] used human fibroblasts cultured on microporous membranes to determine the cytotoxicity of non-hydrosoluble substances. The monolayer rests on the surface of the membrane; the latter acts as an interface between the monolayer above and the test substance dissolved in a non-aqueous non-cytotoxic medium below. Donnelly *et al.*[73] described a three-dimensional human tissue model using co-cultures of dermal fibroblasts and keratinocytes. They reported a high correlation with existing animal eye data when testing surfactants, powders, and creams, using MTT and prostaglandin E_2 as the indicator.

Rougier *et al.*[74] reviewed available toxicity testing protocols and compared the results of several *in vitro* techniques with existing *in vivo* data, including the EYTEX system, the cell membrane integrity test using neutral red uptake assay and the agarose diffusion method, cell growth assessment using total protein content assay, cell metabolism assessment with the Microtox and silicon microphysiometer systems, the bovine corneal opacity and permeability test, and the HET–CAM assay. They suggested that a battery of complementary *in vitro* assays show significant potential for assessing ocular risk from cosmetics and ingredients categories.

Table 3.4 Summary of recent ocular toxicity testing studies. (Adapted from Barile.[1])

Test cells	Assay	Test chemicals	Correlation with *in vivo* data*
Hep G2, BALB/c 3T3, V79, murine macrophages, rabbit corneal epithelial cells	7-day colony formation after 24 h of incubation	34 chemicals	Good agreement among five cell lines[17]
Rabbit corneal cells	7-day colony formation after 24 h of incubation	Surfactants, shampoos	Correlation coefficient 0.9[62]
Baby hamster kidney fibroblasts	4-h cell detachment, 48-h growth inhibition, 7-day cloning efficiency	57 various organic and inorganic chemicals	80% predictive of in vitro classification[63]
BALB/c 3T3	24-h neutral red (NR) uptake	Anionic surfactants, 35 different chemicals	NR uptake in agreement[18]
BALB/c 3T3	24-h protein, 4-h uridine uptake	50 chemicals	Rank correlation in agreement[64]
Enucleated rabbit eyes	Corneal thickness 5-min exposure	11 chemicals	Broad correlation[65]
Primary rabbit corneal epithelial cells	[^{3}H]thymidine incorporation	Antineoplastic agents	Correlation with *in vivo* ocular irritation[66]
Embryonated chicken eggs	HET–CAM assay	60 chemicals and 41 cosmetic formulations	High rank correlation with eye irritants *in vivo*[67]
Isolated rabbit cornea	Changes in electrical impedance	Anionic surfactants	Correlation with *in vivo* ocular irritation[69]

* Correlation with available Draize eye test data.

V. EXPERIMENTAL DESIGN

A. Experimental setup and design

During manipulation of cells in culture, certain details should be established and followed judiciously and uniformly. The rate of inoculating cells depends on the size of the flask or wells. For instance, 6-, 12-, 24-, 48-, and 96-well plates, corresponding to decreasing surface area per well, are routinely employed in screening assays. In general, cells are usually seeded at 10^4 cells per cm^2. Contact-inhibited cultures are grown to confluency, unless cell growth experiments are performed, and subcultured in appropriate complete medium. Depending on the doubling rate of the cell line, the time required for monolayers to reach confluency can be predicted with accuracy. For example, when seeded at one-third the confluent density, most continuous cell lines with appreciable doubling rates reach the stationary phase within 4–8 days.

Monolayers of cells are then incubated with increasing concentrations of each chemical in at least four doses for a predetermined period of time at 37°C in a gaseous atmosphere which is defined by the requirements of the medium. This atmosphere may consist of 5–20% carbon dioxide in air, unless otherwise stated. A stock solution of the test chemical is prepared in the incubating medium and serial dilutions are made from the stock solution. This method of formulating a stock solution decreases the chances of introducing an error when adding chemical to each experimental group. In addition, for experiments requiring longer incubation times, the medium should be sterilized initially, so that aseptic conditions are more easily maintained. A soluble solution of the chemical is sterilized with submicron filters, while insoluble solids are first exposed to ultraviolet light for several minutes in an open test tube before addition of buffer. Before the experiment is terminated, indicators, dyes, fixatives, and reactive substances are added as needed and allowed to incubate. The cells are then counted or processed, and the reaction product is quantified according to the protocol.

B. Incubation medium and test chemical incompatibility

Most of the technical problems associated with the setup and execution of toxicity testing experiments, involve the solubilization or miscibility of the chemicals with the incubation medium. Water-insoluble substances, such as paracetamol (acetaminophen) and acetylsalicylic acid (aspirin), present with dissolution problems, especially at higher dosage levels. The solubility of these chemicals may be improved by the following techniques.

1. Micronization

This procedure increases the surface area of a solid and can improve the solubility of a powder at low doses. A solution of the chemical is prepared in ethanol or dimethylsulfoxide (DMSO) for each group and the solution is evaporated to dryness under a stream of nitrogen gas. The remaining lyophilized powder is then dissolved more readily in medium using constant stirring at 37°C for at least 1 h before incubation.

2. Use of solvents to improve solubility

At times it may be necessary to dissolve the test chemical in a *solvent* which is miscible with the incubation medium, such as ethanol or DMSO. A stock solution of the substance is prepared in the solvent and appropriate aliquots are distributed to the corresponding experimental groups. It is important, however, that individual laboratories determine the toxicity of the solvent, even at its lowest concentration, as part of the incubation medium. Also, all experimental groups should be equilibrated with the same amount of solvent, including controls. This will negate any minor effects of the solvent alone on the cells.

When *high* concentrations of chemicals are dissolved in a solvent and distributed to the corresponding experimental groups, the solution may precipitate in the incubating medium as a result of a 'salting out' effect. This situation nullifies the initial use of the solvent and requires some adjustment of the procedure or concentration.

3. *Sonication*

Other organic liquids used as test chemicals, such as xylene or carbon tetrachloride, are immiscible with water and culture media. Miscibility is improved by *sonicating* a stock solution of the chemical in medium. This usually requires a mechanical homogenizer or an ultrasonic processor equipped with a long probe which is inserted in the immiscible liquids for as little as 10 sec at 10–50 watts of power. This manipulation completely homogenizes the mixture and allows enough time for adequately dispersing an aliquot of the mixture into the incubation medium. On occasion, the liquids still separate out during the incubation time, in which case the medium can be removed, and a fresh resuspended aliquot of test chemical is added again to the cultures.

4. *Use of paraffin (mineral) oil overlay*

More volatile chemicals, such as the alcohols or chloroform, are especially annoying since they permeate the incubator atmosphere and interfere with control wells. The evaporation, and thus the concentration of the chemical in the medium, can be controlled by overlaying the cells with a thin layer of paraffin oil (light mineral oil) after the addition of the volatile chemical. The oil suppresses the evaporation of molecules at the surface by increasing the surface tension. Alternatively, cells can be cultured in 25 cm^2 (T-25) flasks, which are then individually permeated with a stream of gas corresponding to the gaseous atmosphere of the incubator, and sealed with screw caps. This requires some forethought since it is necessary to anticipate which chemical will be tested and which vessels will be used to grow the cells. A separate gas tank, formulated for the incubation medium, is also needed for these studies.

The presence of an oil overlay may produce enough surface tension to prevent evaporation of volatile chemicals partially dissolved in the medium. The partial pressure of the chemical in a liquid, however, may dictate to what extent the test substance partitions between the air and gas phases. Ultimately this partitioning will determine the amount of substance dissolved in the incubating medium and in contact with the cell layer. Essentially, it may be necessary to estimate the actual concentration of the chemical in the liquid and the air space above it in a series of control flasks.

C. Determination of dosage range

Initial concentrations of a chemical used for *in vitro* experiments can be estimated from the known human toxicity data or derived from rodent LD_{50} values[22,75–77] according to the following formula:

$$\text{HETC} = (\text{LD}_{50})/V_d \times 10^{-3}$$

where HETC is the estimated human equivalent toxic concentration in plasma ($mg\,ml^{-1}$), LD_{50} is 50% lethal dose in rodents ($mg\,kg^{-1}$, intraperitoneal or oral), V_d is the volume of distribution ($l\,kg^{-1}$), and 10^{-3} is the constant for conversion into ml ($l\,ml^{-1}$).

This value is an estimate of the toxic human blood concentration equivalent to the LD_{50} dose given to a rodent, based on body weight. The HETC value is then used as a guideline for establishing the dosage range for each group of an experiment. HETC values can also be used as a method of converting animal LD_{50} data into *equivalent* human toxicity information. The calculation facilitates the direct comparison of *in vitro* IC_{50} values and animal LD_{50} data against human lethal concentrations derived from clinical case studies and poison control centers. Essentially, the formula offers a mechanism for converting rodent *in vivo* data to equivalent human toxicity guidelines, in order to compare with *in vitro* data in their ability to predict human toxicity.

D. Determination of inhibitory concentrations

The concentration necessary to inhibit 50% (IC_{50}) of the measured response is calculated based on the slope and linearity of typical concentration–effect curves. The symmetry of the curve is mathematically estimated from *regression analysis* of the plot, 'percentage of control' versus 'log of concentration'. The values for 'percentage of control' are derived by converting the absolute values of the measured response to a fraction of the control value, i.e. the measured value of the group with no chemical. Using the control value as the 100% level, all subsequent groups are transformed into relative percentage values. This has the added advantage that different experiments can be compared, even when the absolute values of the control groups are not identical.[1]

VI. FUTURE PERSPECTIVES

It is conceivable that toxicity testing in the foreseeable future will be regularly performed with continuous and finite cell lines, and some primary cultures. Such testing will be more predictive of human toxicity than current animal tests. If this forecast is realized, many new types of *in vitro* toxicity and toxicokinetic tests will be developed, while many of the present methods will have been validated in refined programs.[78] In addition, the gradual acceptance of new *in vitro* methods should not only depend on formal validation programs, but may be a consequence of the parallel experience of various industrial laboratories using both *in vitro* and *in vivo* methods. Finally, these achievements should not only be based on political or societal attempts to prevent the use of animals in research, but should complement a very efficient and reliable system for protecting the public interest.

REFERENCES

1. Barile, F. A. (1994) *Introduction to* In Vitro *Cytotoxicology: Mechanisms and Methods*. CRC Press, Boca Raton, FL.
2. Bashor, M. M. (1979) Dispersion and disruption of tissues. In Jakoby, W. B. and Pastan, I. H. (eds) *Methods in Enzymology, Cell Culture*, Vol. 53, pp. 119–131. Academic Press, New York.
3. Freshney, R. I. (1994) *Culture of Animal Cells*, 3rd edn. John Wiley, New York.
4. Houser, S., Borges, L., Guzowski, D. E. and Barile, F. A. (1990) Isolation and maintenance of continuous cultures of epithelial cells from chemically-injured adult rabbit lung. *ATLA* **17:** 301–315.

5. Patterson, M. K. (1979) Measurement of growth and viability of cells in culture. In Jakoby, W. B. and Pastan, I. M. (eds) *Methods in Enzymology, Cell Culture*, Vol. 53, pp. 141–152. Academic Press, New York.
6. Ecobichon, D. J. (1992) *The Basis of Toxicity Testing*. CRC Press, Boca Raton, FL.
7. Schou, J. S. (1990) Mechanistic studies in man, laboratory animals and *in vitro* systems. *Food Chem. Toxic.* **28**: 767–770.
8. Gad, S. C. (1994) In Vitro *Toxicology*. Raven Press, New York.
9. Watson, R. R. (1992) In Vitro *Methods of Toxicology*. CRC Press, Boca Raton, FL.
10. Barile, F. A., Arjun, S. and Senechal, J.-J. (1992) Paraquat alters growth, DNA and protein synthesis in lung epithelial cell and fibroblast cultures. *ATLA* **20**: 251–257.
11. Barile, F. A., Ripley-Rouzier, C., Siddiqi, Z-e-A. and Bienkowski, R. S. (1988) Effects of prostaglandin E_1 on collagen production and degradation in human fetal lung fibroblasts. *Arch. Biochem. Biophys.* **265**: 441–446.
12. Barnes, Y., Houser, S. and Barile, F. A. (1990) Temporal effects of ethanol on growth, thymidine uptake, protein and collagen production in human fetal lung fibroblasts. *Toxicol. In Vitro* **4**: 1–7.
13. Barile, F. A., Arjun, S. and Hopkinson, D. (1993) *In vitro* cytotoxicity testing: biological and statistical significance. *Toxicol. in Vitro* **7**: 111–116.
14. Hopkinson, D., Bourne, R. and Barile, F. A. (1993) *In vitro* cytotoxicity testing: 24- and 72-hour studies with cultured lung cells. *ATLA* **21**: 167–172.
15. Balls, M., Reader, S., Atkinson, K., Tarrant, J. and Clothier, R. (1991) Non-animal alternative toxicity tests for detergents: genuine replacements or mere prescreens? *J. Chem. Technol. Biotechnol.* **50**: 423–433.
16. Clemedson, C., McFarlane-Abdulla, E., Andersson, M. *et al.* (1996) MEIC evaluation of acute systemic toxicity for the first 30 reference chemicals: Part I. Methodology of the 68 *in vitro* toxicity assays. *ATLA* **24**: 251–272.
17. Borenfreund, E. and Borerro, O. (1984) *In vitro* cytotoxicity assays: potential alternatives to the Draize ocular irritancy test. *Cell Biol. Toxicol.* **1**: 33–39.
18. Borenfreund, E. and Puerner, J. A. (1985) Toxicity determined *in vitro* by morphological alterations and neutral red absorption. *Toxicol. Lett.* **24**: 119–124.
19. Mossmann, T. (1983) Rapid colorimetric assay for cellular growth and survival: application to proliferation and cytotoxic assays. *J. Immunol. Methods* **65**: 55–63.
20. Flint, O. P. (1990) *In vitro* toxicity testing: purpose, validation, and strategy. *ATLA* **18**: 11–18.
21. Flint, O. P. (1992) *In vitro* test validation: a house built on sand. *ATLA* **20**: 196–198.
22. Barile, F.A., Dierickx, P.J. and Kristen, U. (1994) *In vitro* cytotoxicity testing for prediction of acute human toxicity. *Cell Biol. Toxicol.* **10**: 155–162.
23. Handler, J. S. (1986) Studies of kidney cells in culture. *Kidney Int.* **30**: 208.
24. Williams, P. D., Laska, D. A., Tay, L. K. and Hottendorf, G. H. (1988) Comparative toxicities of cephalosporin antibiotics in a rabbit kidney cell line (LLC-PK_1). *Antimicrob. Agents Chemother.* **32**: 314.
25. Bohets, H. H., Nouwen, E. J., DeBroe, M. E. and Dierickx, P. J. (1994) Effects of foetal calf serum on cell viability, cytotoxicity and detoxification in the two kidney-derived cell lines LLC-PK1 and MDCK. *Toxicol. In Vitro* **8**: 559–561.
26. Barile, F. A., Guzowski, D. E., Ripley, C. R., Siddiqi, Z. and Bienkowski, R. S. (1990) Ammonium chloride inhibits basal degradation of newly synthesized collagen in human fetal lung fibroblasts. *Archives Biochem. Biophys.* **276**: 125–131.
27. Hayflick, L. (1965) The limited *in vitro* lifetime of human diploid cell strains. *Exp. Cell Res.* **37**: 614.
28. Barile, F. A., Siddiqi, Z., Rouzier, C. R. and Bienkowski, R. S. (1989) Effects of puromycin and hydroxynorvaline on production and intracellular degradation of collagen in human fetal lung fibroblasts. *Archives Biochem. Biophys.* **270**: 294–301.
29. Jacobs, J. P., Jones, C. M. and Baillie, J. P. (1976) Characteristics of a human diploid cell designated MRC-5. *Nature* **227**: 168.
30. Raffin, T. A., Simon, L. M., Douglas, W. H. J., Theodore, J. and Robin, E. D. (1980) The effects of variable oxygen tension and of superoxide dismutase on type II pneumocytes exposed to paraquat. *Lab. Invest.* **42**: 205–208.
31. Dean, J. H., Cornacoff, J. B., Rosenthal, G. J. and Luster, M. I. (1989) Immune System: Evaluation of Injury. In Hayes, A. W. (ed.) Principles and Methods of Toxicology, 2nd edn. Raven Press, New York.

32. Purcell, W. M. and Atterwill, C. K. (1994) Human placental mast cells as an *in vitro* model system in aspects of neuro-immunotoxicity testing. *Hum. Exp. Toxicol.* **13:** 429–433.
33. Raffray, M., McCarthy, D., Snowden, R. T. and Cohen, G. M. (1993) Apoptosis as a mechanism of tributyltin cytotoxicity to thymocytes: relationship of apoptotic markers to biochemical and cellular effects. *Toxicol. Appl. Pharmacol.* **119:** 122–130.
34. Governa, M., Valentino, M. and Visona, I. (1994) Chemotactic activity of polymorphonuclear leukocytes and industrial xenobiotics: a brief review. *Toxicology* **91:** 165–177.
35. Ryrfeldt, A., Kroll, F., Berggren, M. and Moldeus, P. (1988) Hydroperoxide and cigarette smoke induced effects on lung mechanics and glutathione status in rat isolated perfused and ventilated lungs. *Life Sci.* **42:** 1439–1445.
36. Zamora, P. O., Gregory, R. E., Li, A. P. and Brooks, A. L. (1986) An *in vitro* model for the exposure of lung alveolar epithelial cells to toxic gases. *J. Environ. Pathol. Toxicol. Oncol.* **7:** 159–168.
37. Patel, J. M. and Block, E. R. (1986) Nitrogen dioxide-induced changes in cell membrane fluidity and function. *Am. Rev. Respir. Dis.* **134:** 1196–1202.
38. Saladino, A. J., Willey, J. C., Lechner, J. F., Grafstrom, R. C., LaVeck, M. and Harris, C. C. (1985) Effects of formaldehyde, acetaldehyde, benzoyl peroxide and hydrogen peroxide on cultured human bronchial epithelial cells. *Cancer Res.* **45:** 2522–2526.
39. Carpenter, L. J., Johnson, K. J., Kunkel, R. G. and Roth, R. A. (1987) Phorbol myristate acetate produces injury to isolated rat lungs in the presence and absence of perfused neutrophils. *Toxicol. Appl. Pharmacol.* **91:** 22–32.
40. Wyatt, I., Soames, A. R., Clay, M. F. and Smith, L. L. (1988) The accumulation and localisation of putrescine, spermidine, spermine and paraquat in the rat lung: *in vitro* and *in vivo* studies. *Biochem. Pharmacol.* **37:** 1909–1918.
41. Autian, J. (1973) The new field of plastics toxicology: methods and results. In Goldberg, L. (ed.) *CRC Critical Reviews in Toxicology*, Vol. 2, pp. 1–40. CRC Press, Cleveland, Ohio.
42. Combrier, E. and Castelli, D. (1992) The agarose overlay method as a screening approach for ocular irritancy: application to cosmetic products. *ATLA* **20:** 438–444.
43. Rosenbluth, S. A., Weddington, G. R., Guess, L. W. and Autian, J. (1965) Tissue culture method for screening toxicity of plastics to be used in medical practice. *J. Pharm. Soc.* **54:** 156–159.
44. Wennberg, A., Hasselgren, G. and Tronstad, L. (1979) A method for toxicity screening of biomaterials using cells cultured on millipore filters. *J. Biomed. Mater. Res.* **13:** 109–120.
45. Pascon, E. A. and Spangberg, L. S. W. (1990) *In vitro* cytotoxicity of root canal filling materials: 1. Gutta-percha. *J. Endodontics* **16:** 429–433.
46. Schmalz, G. (1994) Use of cell cultures for toxicity testing of dental materials – advantages and limitations. *J. Dent.* **2 (supplement):** S6–S11.
47. Ekwall, B. and Ekwall, K. (1988) Comments on the use of diverse cell systems in toxicity testing. *ATLA* **15:** 193–200.
48. Rheinwald, J. G. and Green, H. (1975) Serial cultivation of strains of human epidermal keratinocytes: the formation of keratinizing colonies from single cells. *Cell* **6:** 331–343.
49. Gilchrest, B. A., Marshall, W. L., Karassik, R. L., Weinstein, R. and Maciag, T. (1984) Characterization and partial purification of keratinocyte growth factor from the hypothalamus. *J. Cell. Physiol.* **120:** 337.
50. Green, H. (1978) Cyclic AMP in relation to the proliferation of the epidermal cell. A new view. *Cell* **15:** 1801.
51. Gilchrest, B. A., Nemore, R. E. and Maciag, T. (1980) Growth of human keratinocytes on fibronectin-coated plates. *Cell Biol. Int. Rep.* **4:** 1009.
52. Johnson, E. W., Meunier, S. F., Roy, C. J. and Parenteau, N. L. (1992) Serial cultivation of normal human keratinocytes: a defined system for studying the regulation of growth and differentiation. *In Vitro Cell. Dev. Biol.* **28A:** 429.
53. Wallace, K. A., Harbell, J. H., Accomando, N., Triana, A., Valone, S. and Curren, R. D. (1992) Evaluation of the human epidermal keratinocyte neutral red release and neutral red uptake assay using the first 10 MEIC test materials. *Toxicol. In Vitro* **6:** 367–371.
54. Ward, R. K., Agrawalla, S. and Clothier, R. H. (1994) Investigation of an *in vitro* cytotoxicity assay for prediction of skin irritation. *Toxicol. In Vitro* **8:** 659–660.
55. Steer, S., Balls, M., Clothier, R. H. and Gordon, V. (1994) The development and evaluation of *in vitro* tests for photoirritancy. *Toxicol. In Vitro* **8:** 719–721.
56. Rutten, A. A. J. J. L. and van de Sandt, J. J. M. (1994) *In vitro* dermal toxicology using skin organ cultures. *Toxicol. In Vitro* **8:** 703–705.

57. Cohen, C., Dossou, K. G., Rougier, A. and Roguet, R. (1994) Episkin: an *in vitro* model for the evaluation of phototoxicity and sunscreen photoprotective properties. *Toxicol. In Vitro* **8:** 669–671.
58. Roguet, R., Regnier, M., Cohen, C., Dossou, K. G. and Rougier, A. (1994) The use of *in vitro* reconstituted human skin in dermotoxicity testing. *Toxicol. In Vitro* **8:** 635–639.
59. Cannon, C. L., Neal, P. J., Southee, J. A., Kubilus, J. and Klausner, M. (1994) New epidermal model for dermal irritancy testing. *Toxicol. In Vitro* **8:** 889–891.
60. Balls, M. (1991) The replacement of animal testing: ethical issues and practical realities. *Int. J. Cosm. Sci.* **13:** 23–28.
61. Shaw, A. J., Clothier, R. H. and Balls, M. (1990) Loss of transepithelial impermeability of confluent monolayer or Madin-Darby Canine Kidney (MDCK) cells as a determinant of ocular irritancy potential. *ATLA* **18:** 145–151.
62. North-Root, H., Yackovich, F., Demetrulias, J., Gacula, M. and Heinze, J. E. (1982) Evaluation of an *in vitro* cell toxicity test using rabbit corneal cells to predict the eye irritation potential of surfactants. *Toxicol. Lett.* **14:** 207–212.
63. Reinhardt, C. A., Pelli, D. A. and Zbinden, G. (1985) Interpretation of cell toxicity data for the estimation of potential irritation. *Fd. Chem. Toxicol.* **23:** 247.
64. Shopsis, C., Borenfreund, E., Walberg, J. and Stark, D. M. (1985) A battery of potential alternatives to the Draize test: uridine uptake inhibition, morphological cytotoxicity, macrophage chemotaxis and exfoliate cytology. *Fd. Chem. Toxicol.* **23:** 259–266.
65. Burton, A. B. G., York, M. and Lawrence, R. S. (1981) The *in vitro* assessment of severe eye irritants. *Food. Cosmet. Toxicol.* **19:** 471–480.
66. Lazarus, H. M., Imperia, P. S., Botti, R., Mack, R. J. and Lass, J. S. (1989) An *in vitro* method which assesses corneal epithelial toxicity due to antineoplastic, preservative and antimicrobial agents. *Lens Eye Toxic. Res.* **6:** 59–85.
67. de Silva, O., Rougier, A. and Dossou, K. G. (1992) The HET–CAM test: a study of the irritation potential of chemicals and formulations. *ATLA* **20:** 432–437.
68. Leupke, N. P. and Kemper, F. H. (1986) The HET/CAM test: an alternative to the Draize eye test. *Fd. Chem. Toxicol.* **24:** 495–496.
69. Scaife, M. C. (1983) *In vitro* studies on ocular irritancy. In Balls, M., Ridell, R. G. and Worden, A. (eds) *Animals and Alternatives in Toxicity Testing*, pp. 367–371. Academic Press, London.
70. Kruszewski, F. H., Hearn, L. H., Smith, K. T., Teal, J. T., Gordon, V. C. and Dickens, M. S. (1992) Application of the EYTEX system to the evaluation of cosmetic products and their ingredients. *ATLA* **20:** 146–163.
71. Gettings, S. D. (1993) Towards validation: an update on *in vitro* eye irritation testing. *Newsletter of the Johns Hopkins Center for Alternatives to Animal Testing* **11:** 4.
72. Boue-Grabot, M., Halaviat, B. and Pinon, J.-F. (1992) Cytotoxicity of non-hydrosoluble substances towards human skin fibroblasts cultured on microporous membrane: a model for the study of ocular irritancy potential, *ATLA* **20:** 445–450.
73. Donnelly, T., Decker, D., Stemp, M., Rheins, L. and Logemann, P. (1994) A three-dimensional *in vitro* model for the study of ocular cytotoxicity and irritancy. *Toxicol. In Vitro* **8:** 631–633.
74. Rougier, A., Cottin, M., de Silva, O., Catroux, P., Roguet, R. and Dossou, K. G. (1994) The use of *in vitro* methods in the ocular irritation assessment of cosmetic products. *Toxicol. In Vitro* **8:** 893–905.
75. Baselt, R.C. and Cravey, R.H. (1989) *Disposition of Toxic Drugs and Chemicals in Man*, 3rd edn. Year Book Medical, Chicago.
76. Budvari, S., O'Neil, M. J., Smith, A. and Heckelman, P. E. (eds) (1989) *Merck Index*, 11th edn., pp. 1606. Merck and Co. Ltd, Rahway.
77. Lewis R. J. (1993) *Hazardous Chemicals Desk Reference*, 3rd edn. Van Nostrand Reinhold, New York.
78. Ekwall, B. and Barile, F.A. (1994) Standardization and validation. In Barile, F. A. *Introduction to* In Vitro *Cytotoxicology: Mechanisms and Methods*, pp. 189–208. CRC Press, Boca Raton, FL.

4

In Vitro Models for Nephrotoxicity Screening and Risk Assessment

PETER H. BACH, DAVID K. OBATOMI AND STEPHEN BRANT

- I. Introduction . . . 56
  - A. The kidney . . . 56
  - B. Nephrotoxicity . . . 56
  - C. Renal injury . . . 58
- II. The choice of *in vitro* system . . . 59
  - A. Which *in vitro* system is appropriate? . . . 61
  - B. Conditions that affect phenotypic expression of cellular systems . . . 62
    - 1. Cell culture media . . . 62
    - 2. Substratum and cell support . . . 63
    - 3. Other *in vitro* renal systems . . . 63
    - 4. Consequences of changing the phenotypic expression of cells . . . 63
  - C. What concentration of nephrotoxin? . . . 63
  - D. End-points . . . 64
    - 1. Marker enzymes . . . 65
  - E. Micromethods for studying cells . . . 66
    - 1. Fluorescent probes . . . 66
  - F. Non-invasive methods for the repeated screening of cells . . . 68
    - 1. Epithelial barrier function . . . 68
    - 2. Alamar blue . . . 69
- III. Intact renal cellular systems *in vitro* . . . 69
  - A. Isolated perfused kidney . . . 69
  - B. Microperfusion . . . 70
  - C. Renal cortical slices . . . 70
    - 1. Conventional renal slices . . . 70
    - 2. Precision-cut renal slices . . . 71
  - D. Isolated nephron segments . . . 71
    - 1. Isolation by enzymic dispersion . . . 72
    - 2. Isolation by mechanical shearing . . . 72
  - E. Proximal tubular fragments . . . 72
  - F. Glomeruli . . . 73

IN VITRO METHODS IN PHARMACEUTICAL RESEARCH
ISBN 0-12-163390-X

IV. Cells and cell-free systems 73
A. Freshly isolated renal cells 74
B. Primary renal proximal tubule cultures 74
C. Primary distal tubule cultures 75
D. Primary renal glomerular cell cultures 75
E. Renal medullary interstitial cell cultures 75
F. Renal cell lines 75
1. The forgotten cell lines 76
2. New cell lines 76
G. Cell-free systems: the use of subcellular fractions 78
1. Renal cell organelles 78
2. Metabolism in cytosolic systems 78
V. Mechanistic studies and toxicity screening 79
A. Mechanisms of injury 79
B. How does cytotoxicity relate to nephrotoxicity? 79
C. The use of human tissue 80
VI. Integrated mechanisms of renal injury *in vitro* 81
A. Chloroform nephrotoxicity 81
B. Haloalkene nephrotoxicity 81
C. Antibiotic-induced injury 82
D. Glomerular injury 82
E. Heavy metal toxicity 83
F. Reactive oxygen species and lipid peroxidation 84
G. Hydroperoxidase-mediated nephrotoxicity 84
H. Bile acid-related renal injury 85
VII. Conclusions 85
Acknowledgements 87
References 87

I. INTRODUCTION

A. The kidney

The kidney is a complex organ composed of over 20 different cell types, each with diverse morphological, biochemical and functional heterogeneity, but they work in concert to maintain normal renal function.[1,2] It is this heterogeneity that provides a basis for renal injury and also ensures that *in vitro* methods offer the key to understanding these processes.

B. Nephrotoxicity

Exposure to chemicals and medicines contributes directly to over 20% of end-stage renal disease[2–5] due to the kidney's small mass and the large cardiac output it handles. Many nephrotoxins (Table 4.1) produce distinct patterns of injury localized to discrete cell types. This 'target selective toxicity' can be ascribed to one or more of the biophysiological characteristics expressed by the injured cells (Table 4.2). Thus, for example, the presence of an appropriate membrane transport pathway and a bioactivation system could predispose a single cell type to selective injury. Morphologically different, but adjacent, cells (which lack these biophysiological characteristics) are unaffected in the first instance, although they may subsequently undergo degenerative changes as a result of loss of the target cells and the key functions they undertake.

Table 4.1 Groups of nephrotoxic compounds to which humans are exposed.

Therapeutic agents	**Chemicals**
Analgesics	Ethylene glycol
Non-steroidal anti-inflammatory drugs	Organic chemicals and solvents
Paracetamol (acetaminophen)	Volatile hydrocarbons
Antibiotics	Chloroform
Aminoglycosides	Halogenated alkenes
Cephalosporins	Light hydrocarbon
Amphotercin B	Bipyridyl herbicides
Tetracyclines	**Mycotoxins**
Penicillamine	Aflatoxins
Lithium	Ochratoxin A
Urographic contrast media	Citrinin
Anticancer drugs	**Silicon**
Cisplatin	**Metals**
Adriamycin	Lead
Immunosuppressive agents	Cadmium
Cyclosporin A	Mercury
Heroin	Gold
Puromycin aminonucleoside	Bismuth
Plant toxins	Uranium
Atractyloside	Chromium
Recombinant peptides	Arsenic
Interferon	Germanium

Table 4.2 Functional characteristics of the kidney that predispose to target selective nephrotoxicity.

Accumulation
Active transport
Specific membrane binding sites
Intracellular binding sites
pH or ionic concentration differential
} may result in accumulation

Generation of reactive species or intermediates
Many renal cells can generate reactive intermediates and/or reactive oxygen species.
Toxicological consequences depend on:
- Compartmentalization of the chemical (its metabolites) within target cells
- Type of reactive species formed
- Presence of systems that inactivate the reactive species
- 'Silent' receptors (macromolecule) to which reactive species can bind cellular antioxidants, nucleophiles, free radical scavengers, etc.
- Compartmentalization within the cell

Modulation of other cellular processes
Specific examples of effects on metabolic pathways or organelle disruption are documented but little is known about such interactions in the broad context of nephrotoxicity.

Membrane, junction and cytoskeletal changes
Renal cell membranes have a vital role in selective transport and exclusion of substances.
Little is known about normal membrane functions, fluidity and turnover, and cytoskeletal functions in toxicology.
Changes in tight junctions are known to cause profound changes in cell function.

C. Renal injury

Injury is a dynamic process. If the affected cells can and do repair, then the effect may be transient and have no long-term clinical consequences. Even when the kidney is irreversibly damaged, both renal or extrarenal compensation does occur, so that functional changes may go unnoticed, and a severely damaged kidney may maintain homoeostasis for long periods. Not all renal cells have the same capacity to repair. Proximal tubules will normally undergo rapid repair,[6] but more highly differentiated glomerular epithelial and mesangial cells and the medullary interstitial cells do not.[7] One of the best examples of a degenerative cascade that follows the loss of renal medullary interstitial cells is associated with analgesic abuse.[8] The underlying mechanism associated with such change is not clear, but probably relates to perturbation of a number of processes including endocrine, paracrine and autocrine

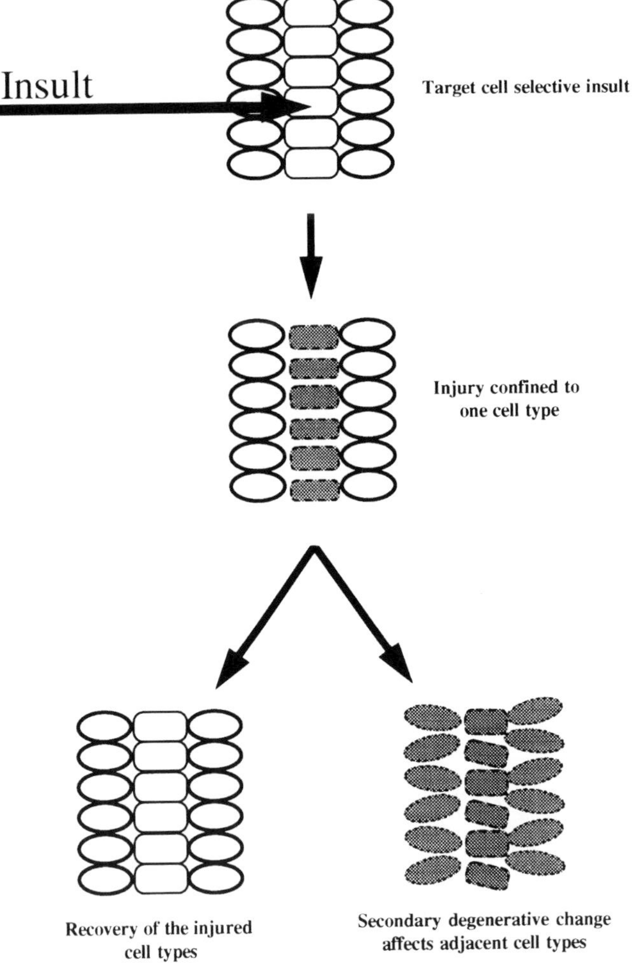

Fig. 4.1 Schematic representation of the different types of renal response to injury, showing target selective injury leading to either recovery or secondary degenerative changes in renal cells not affected by the primary injury. These secondary degenerative changes are thought to be mediated by loss of autocrine and paracrine function, and are a key part of the degenerative cascade.

functions (Fig. 4.1). Changes in receptors and cell signalling as a result of ion modulation[9–12] are also probably important.

Several inter-related processes take place during renal injury. The chemical injures the 'target cells' and causes damage, resulting in the release of cytoplasmic and organelle enzymes, structural and functional immunoreactive markers. Then a *repair phase* is associated with functional adjustment in damaged cells and adjacent unaffected regions compensate for loss of parenchyma. The proximal tubule has a very significant repair capacity, associated with anabolic metabolism for cell growth and division, but little is known about the repair capacity of glomerular cells. In the *post-repair phase* many functions return to normal, but in still inadequately defined circumstances (perhaps repeated insult or physiological stress) the kidney may lose functional reserve or undergo a slow degenerative cascade which leads to end-stage renal disease. The rate, type and progression of the degenerative changes explain (in part) the development of renal failure or maintenance of 'normal' renal function, even when there is considerable loss of functional reserve. The renal medulla and glomeruli consist of small numbers of highly differentiated and slow growing cells,[13,14] and the proximal tubular cells de-differentiate rapidly and facilitate growth and repair.[15] The long-term consequences may be where anatomical regions such as the medulla and glomeruli show irreversible degenerative changes, the proximal tubule repairs significantly. Once medullary interstitial cells have necrosed (in the case of renal papillary necrosis), they do not repair, despite the presence of viable cells of this type in adjacent tissue.[7] Thus medullary necrosis almost invariably leads to gross functional changes that produces a cascade of secondary effects, some of which may contribute to the development of chronic renal failure or extrarenal pathology. These changes cannot be reproduced in short-term *in vitro* studies.

Loss of renal parenchyma increases the toxicity of exogenous agents by removing tissue that could otherwise provide functional reserve capacity and by increasing the renal workload and the ratio of toxic agent to cell. Other factors that may predispose to a primary injury or speed progressive degenerative changes in the kidney include dehydration, high protein intake, reduced extrarenal detoxification (in the liver and lung), pre-existing nephropathy and chemical interactions arising from multiple exposures.

II. THE CHOICE OF *IN VITRO* SYSTEM

In vitro methods (Table 4.3) offer a rapid and economical method of screening specific cell types for specific effects.[16,17] They offer systems in which the direct effects of chemicals can be evaluated and manipulated under precisely controlled conditions, in order to distinguish direct and indirect effects at a cellular and subcellular level. *In vitro* methods have been invaluable in helping to understand the mechanisms of well-established nephrotoxins. This insight has also been used to help screen new chemicals for their potential nephrotoxicity.[5, 17–30] The complexity of the kidney does, however, demand a careful match between the *in vitro* system and the *in vivo* situation. This is not as straightforward as it may at first appear, as there are a number of considerations (Table 4.4) that need to be addressed before designing and interpreting an *in vitro* experiment for studying nephrotoxicity of chemicals, including:

1. Which of the different systems (Table 4.3) provides the most reliable data?
2. Which system really represents the renal tissue of interest?

3. What concentration of chemical should be used and how this can be related to the *in vivo* situation in animals and humans?
4. What end-point is most appropriate?
5. How does this relate to the situation *in vivo* and how relevant it is to pathological injury?
6. What are the advantages of using human renal tissue as the source of material for investigations?

Table 4.3 Different approaches to investigating nephrotoxicity *in vitro*.

Technique for assessing nephrotoxicity	Advantages and limitations
Anatomical relationship between cells maintained	
Perfusion, micropuncture	Technically difficult, requires sophisticated equipment, subject to artefact in inexperienced hands and difficult to interpret
Slices	Technically easier, no sophisticated equipment, less artefact and easier to interpret
Glomeruli and tubular fragments	Technically easy, some sophisticated equipment subject to artefact and easy to interpret
Anatomical relationship between cells lost	
Cell culture	
Freshly isolated cells	Dispersal may damage cells and make it difficult to establish their anatomical identity unless there are clearly defined histochemical and immunocytochemical markers. Isolated cells are generally mixtures but may be enriched. Must be used within a few hours
Primary cell cultures	De-differentiate rapidly or change characteristics which may obfuscate their anatomical origins. Loss of a key biochemical characteristic may invalidate *in vitro* studies or alter sensitivity and selectivity
Established renal cell lines	Properties reminiscent of specific parts of the nephron. Often heterogeneous. Need to be characterized more systematically
Cell-free systems	
Vesicles, nuclei, lysosomes and microsomes	Study subcellular distribution, interactions between cellular compartments and a chemical, and the kinetics of binding or release of substances. Enzyme inhibition, metabolic activation, covalent binding and modulation of lipid peroxidation using purified or commercially available chemicals with appropriate cofactors

Table 4.4 Some of the key considerations that have to be addressed when undertaking *in vitro* investigations on nephrotoxicity.

Identification of compounds with well-documented *in vivo* nephrotoxicity, sequence of pathological functional changes, metabolites formed, quantities excreted and cellular pharmacodynamic effects
Chemicals that target specifically for one anatomically discrete cell type *in vivo*
Use analogues for structure–activity relationship
Systematic study of compounds by several different *in vitro* methods
Use of several criteria for assessing *in vitro* nephrotoxicity for each system

There is no simple answer to any of these questions, but the applications of *in vitro* methods below attempt to illustrate why each must be considered (Fig. 4.2) to answer the important questions of risk assessment.

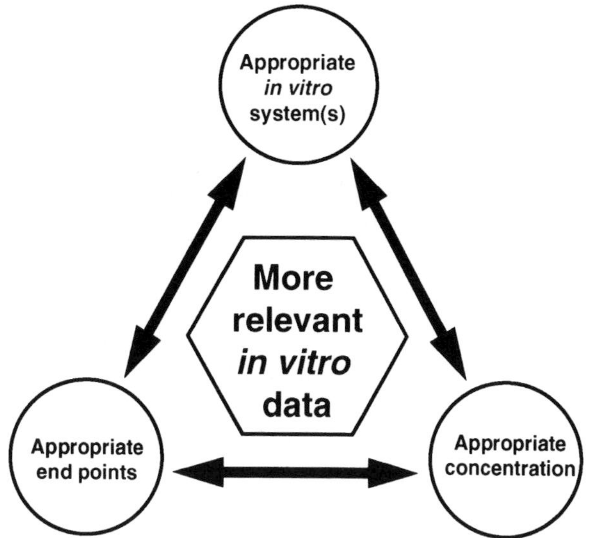

Fig. 4.2 The key factors that have to be considered when designing an *in vitro* experiment for assessing nephrotoxicity.

A. Which *in vitro* system is appropriate?

A variety of *in vitro* techniques are available (Table 4.3), and include those where anatomical integrity is well maintained (perfusion, micropuncture and slices) and simple models such as isolated fragments (glomeruli and tubular fragments), cultures primary and continuous lines, and cell-free systems (Fig. 4.3). These *in vitro* systems have helped

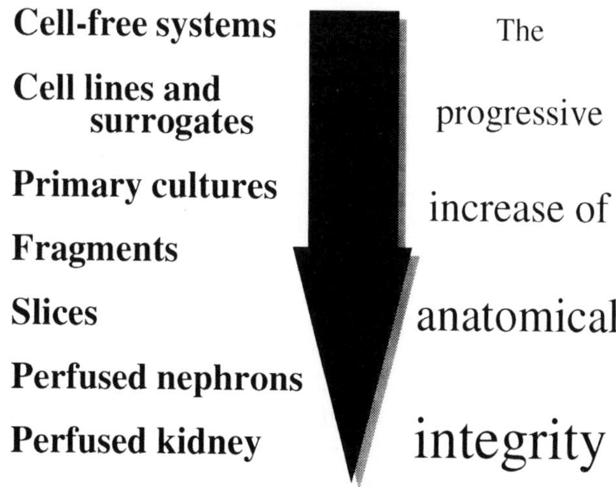

Fig. 4.3 Spectrum of *in vitro* systems used for assessing nephrotoxicity progressing from an intact anatomy to subcellular components.

understand the physiological processes in renal cells; each has strengths and weaknesses[5,17,19,20,24] and some are technically difficult. Thus, data must be interpreted in relation to each method used. In general, it is most desirable to use complementary techniques to provide a rational basis upon which to predict nephrotoxicity *in vivo*.

B. Conditions that affect phenotypic expression of cellular systems

The kidney is a complex organ, the integrity of which is the quintessence of function. Altering this integrity may dramatically change the function. It is generally agreed that, if *in vitro* toxicological data are to be relevant, then phenotypic expression of cells should closely parallel the situation *in vivo*. Cell culture protocols often ignore well-documented biophysiological characteristics of cells. This is best appreciated by the rapid dedifferentiation of primary cultured renal cells,[31] which lose those biochemical characteristics that form part of the molecular basis for target cell toxicity. The modulation of culture medium has long been known to alter cell biochemistry and morphology.[32] The expression of cells in culture can be affected by choice of medium, substratum and other factors.[33,34]

1. *Cell culture media*

Tradition is used to determine what should be used for culturing cells, but the obvious is often ignored. Phenol red is widely used in cell culture media as a pH indicator, but it was the first visual indicator of active proximal tubule transport used by Marshall in the 1940s. Phenol red interacts with a number of biological systems (Table 4.5), which raises concern about the validity of *in vitro* data where phenol red has been used. Thus, phenol red should be omitted from all culture media used to study renal tubular cells.

Table 4.5 Effects of phenol red on renal proximal tubular cells.

Competes with the uptake of other organic anions, including drugs
Induces glutathione peroxidases, glutathione-*S*-transferases and glutathione reductase
Inhibits mitochondrial succinate dehydrogenase, glycolysis markers such as hexokinase and lactate dehydrogenase, and lysosomal markers such as *N*-acetyl-β-D-glucosaminidase and cathepsin B
Has no effect on Na^+–K^+-ATPase

'Standard' culture medium has a high glucose level, which prevents expression of the gluconeogenic function present in the proximal tubule *in vivo*. LLC-PK_1 and OK cell lines grown in low or glucose-free media re-express gluconeogenic activity. OK and LLC-RK_1 cells have been used most widely to represent the proximal tubule, but their apical membrane microvilli are poorly developed, and receptors, marker enzymes and transport activities are missing or differ from those reported *in vivo*. By contrast, LLC-PK_1 cells, optimized primary cultures of rat and rabbit and, to a lesser extent, human proximal tubule cells marker enzyme levels (e.g. alkaline phosphatase and γ-glutamyl transpeptidase) and active glucose transport are very similar to those reported *in vivo*. Similarly, phase II biotransformation is low in LLC-PK_1, NRK and OK cells, intermediate in LLC-RK_1 cells, but similar to the *in vivo* levels in primary rabbit, rat and human proximal tubule cells grown in hormonally defined culture media.[34] MDCK in high osmolality media change their phenotype[35,36] to represent the collecting duct more closely.

2. *Substratum and cell support*

Epithelial architecture is much more similar to the *in vivo* situation when epithelial cells are grown on collagen-coated[37] microporous[38] supports that provide nutrients to both apical and basolateral sides and allow polarity to be expressed[27,39] than cells grown on plastic surfaces.

3. *Other* in vitro *renal systems*

The addition of amino acids to perfusion medium dramatically improves kidney viability and function,[40] and there is indication that the methods used for isolating cells,[41–43] and renal slices (D. K. Obatomi and P. H. Bach, unpublished results) can significantly affect the behaviour of such cells *in vitro*, especially long-term studies. The addition of antioxidants to freshly prepared slices can improve viability (D. K. Obatomi and P. H. Bach, unpublished results), but could also interfere with mechanistic studies involving the use of nephrotoxins that act by causing oxidative damage.

4. *Consequences of changing the phenotypic expression of cells*

The correct phenotypic expression has been shown to affect quantitative and qualitative toxicity data from gentamicin and *cis*-platinum. The intracellular uptake of gentamicin by adsorptive pinocytosis is related to apical brush-border membrane structure and function. Thus gentamicin is taken up more effectively and is therefore more cytotoxic in cells with well-developed apical membrane microvilli, LLC-PK_1 and rabbit PTC grown in glucose-free culture medium, and closely represents the *in vivo* situation, compared with OK cells or in rabbit PTC grown in the presence of insulin and glucose.[44,45]

C. What concentration of nephrotoxin?

It is still not certain what concentration of the 'ultimate' toxin reaches the target cells during renal injury. Some chemicals are concentrated (to several times the plasma level) selectively in discrete areas of the kidney, and others are excluded from selected cells.[46–48] In addition, the enzymes responsible for xenobiotic metabolism are localized in discrete compartments. Each cell type (Table 4.6) has a different profile of transport systems, antioxidants and metabolic systems, such that the xenobiotic dynamics between these different 'cellular compartments' contribute to the uncertainty of the structure of the proximate and ultimate nephrotoxins *in vitro*. It is likely that higher systems (such as slices) have physiological processes working more similarly to the intact kidney, which will contribute to localized accumulation or exclusion from cells, whereas cultured cells may not, especially if grown on solid supports.

Standard analytical techniques cannot establish data on such distribution, and light microscopic autoradiography shows only the localization of labelled material and provides no indication of what it represents. Thus, the Paracelsus' axiom 'all things are toxic in high enough concentrations' also becomes a 'Gordian knot'. There are always problems establishing what concentration, of which metabolite, for what period of time, on which cell(s) is relevant to screening for a specific effect on the kidney. The use of concentrations that are too high will produce spurious results that represent non-specific cytotoxicity; and the use of low concentrations will miss potentially nephrotoxic compounds.

Table 4.6 Factors that affect the experimental design of *in vitro* nephrotoxicity investigations.

Choice of chemical concentrations for *in vitro* studies
Impossible to establish the concentration of a xenobiotic (or its metabolites) in any one cell because:
Intact functioning kidney, highly compartmentalized
Different transport systems
Transcellular pH gradients
Selective accumulation in, and exclusion from, a discrete area of the kidney
Drug-metabolizing systems distributed heterogeneously
Xenobiotic products may concentrate selectively in specific cell types
Autoradiography shows only the distribution of labelled molecules and not their chemical nature
Identifying proximate and ultimate nephrotoxins *in vitro*
Important to choose:
Anatomical integrity of the kidney
Consider how chemical is delivered to the cells (i.e. free or bound)
Physicochemical characteristics of the solution in which the chemical is delivered (its pH, ionic concentration, endogenous and exogenous micromolecules or macromolecules)
Kinetics of delivery

These uncertainties can be addressed by:

(i) building up expertise on chemicals that cause a primary effect specifically in one anatomically discrete cell type *in vivo*;
(ii) studying the sequence of pathological and functional changes caused by these model toxins both *in vivo* and *in vitro*;
(iii) documenting the metabolites formed, quantities excreted and cellular pharmacodynamic effects of these chemicals;
(iv) using both more and less nephrotoxic analogues of these model chemicals to help define structure–activity relationships and computer-based simulations;
(v) using several cytotoxicity criteria for assessing nephrotoxicity *in vitro*; and
(vi) the systematic investigation of 'model' compounds in several *in vitro* systems.

When novel chemicals are assessed it may be necessary to choose chemical concentrations over a larger range than might otherwise be used.

D. End-points

There are a number of end-points depending on the uptake (such as anion, cation, glucose or chemical) and release (e.g. enzyme, anion, cation, chemical), presented schematically in Fig. 4.4.[18,22,49–51] In addition, the distribution of molecules, energy metabolism, and the synthesis, expression and turnover of specific markers, as well as light and ultrastructural morphology,[52] have been applied to each of the *in vitro* techniques (Table 4.7).

Table 4.7 Criteria commonly used to measure normal cellular function and to assess cytotoxicity in renal cell types. These effects are then related to nephrotoxicity *in vivo*.

Electrolyte and enzyme exclusion
Electrophysiology
Leakage and intracellular concentration
Incorporation of labelled precursors into macromolecules
Degradation of marker molecules
Oxidation of carbohydrates and lipids to labelled carbon dioxide
Intermediary and xenobiotic metabolism
Ultrastructural morphological
Histochemical changes

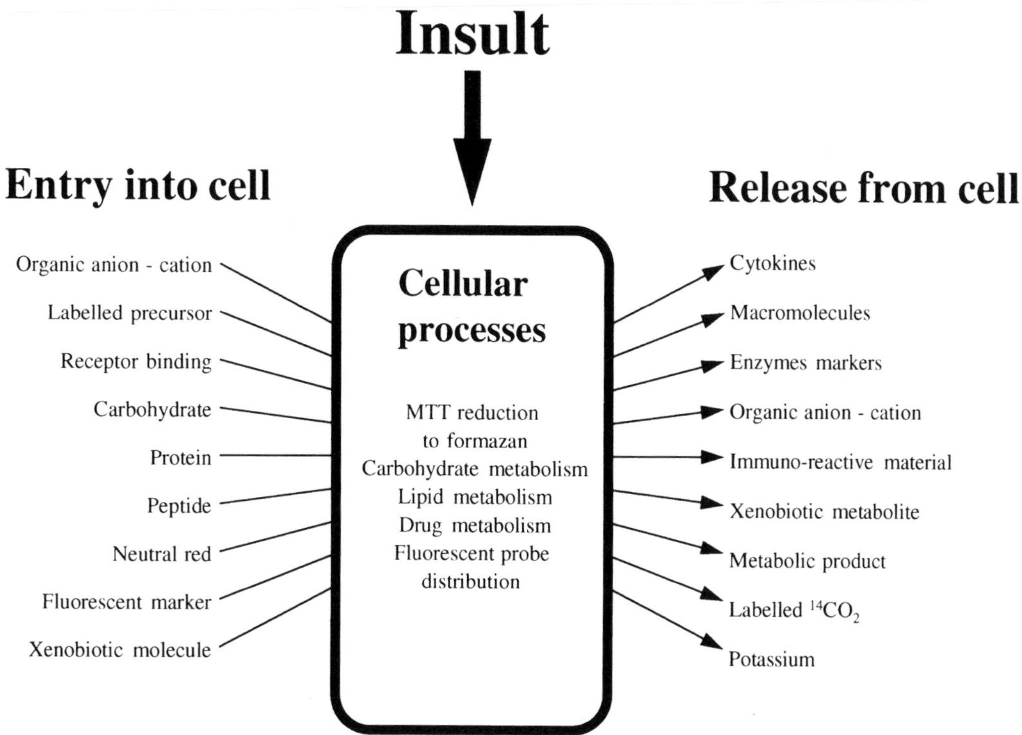

Fig. 4.4 Schematic representation of the end-points that can be used to assess cellular injury *in vitro*.

1. *Marker enzymes*

Enzyme distribution along the nephron has been well documented by microdissection[53,54] and enzyme histochemistry.[55,56] Despite the wide range of enzymes that has been reported, only relatively few have been used for *in vitro* investigations.[57] This is based on the fact that most of the short-term methods of assessing renal tissues induce some cellular injury, which may reflect as increased membrane fragility, leakage of markers and altered genetic control of enzyme systems. Some of the failure to realize the fuller potentials of this approach revolves around technical difficulties. Enzyme leakage is assessed in terms of the total activity that is available from the tissue at time zero, but this normally requires the use of sonication, detergents, etc., and there does not appear to be a clear idea of how to deal with the anomalies that are encountered, but rarely reported. This includes greater enzyme leakage than that which appears to be totally available, denaturation of proenzymes, etc. In addition, there is the same problem that pervades the use of urinary enzymes as markers of injury *in vivo*, i.e. the presence of proteolytic enzymes and temperature-related instability, which may, under *in vitro* incubation conditions, promote the loss of enzymic activity. Some of the compounds studied in nephrotoxicity assessment, especially the heavy metals and reactive intermediates, may also inactivate enzymes, and many chemicals interfere with spectrophotometric assays. This could explain the high background and variance of data that are so often encountered, and why most researchers appear to have opted for technically simple methods (such as lactate dehydrogenase and *N*-acetyl-*β*-D-glucosaminidase) that can process large numbers of specimens.

Enzyme leakage from specific cells in mixed cell populations Simple measures of cell injury suffice for monocultures (a single cell type in culture), but may not be adequate in mixed cell cultures, slices and perfused organs. Despite the extensive data on renal enzyme distribution, there are still some areas of ignorance on the distribution of enzymes in individual cell types. For example, Takahashi *et al.*[58] have shown very high levels of adenosine deaminase and purine nucleoside phosphorylase in glomeruli, but it would be necessary to define which of the five morphologically and biochemically distinct glomerular cell types express this enzyme if it were to be a useful marker.[59] The commercial availability of the major isoforms of glutathione-*S*-transferase (GST) α and π are selectively present in the proximal and distal tubule respectively (Plate 1), allowing target cell injury to be identified *in vivo*[60] and offering the significant potential for a number of different *in vitro* techniques, especially renal tissue slices (Vickers A.E.M., unpublished results) and the perfused kidney.

E. Micromethods for studying cells

Microdissection (using nanogram quantities of tissue) has been an essential tool for identifying the distribution of enzymes along the nephron to demonstrate specific enzymes by 'cycling' radiolabelled or fluorescent assays.[61] Such techniques have not been used for *in vitro* studies, but cytochemistry typically uses 10–1000 cells[62] and increasingly the application of quantitative fluorescent analysis allows nanogram quantities of materials and cellular changes to be assessed in single cells.

Microscopy circumvents many of the problems that limit the use of isolated cells to study subcellular mechanisms of 'cytotoxicity'. Normarski (differential interference contrast) optics offer excellent image contrast and details, at a resolution greater than 0.2 μm in a single plane of unstained live cells. Interference from other cellular material is minimal, and nuclei and their contents, intracellular organelles, aspects of the cytoskeleton and cell surface features in living cells that could otherwise be studied only from the differential staining of fixed (dead) cells, or ultrastructure. This offers a most important time-saving technique of establishing where chemically induced cell changes warrant further ultrastructural evaluation.

1. Fluorescent probes

Fluorescent probes are much more versatile and can be used to study a diverse array of biochemical processes.[63] Selective fluorescent probes can be used to assess biomorphological changes within cells and quantified at concentrations as low as 0.01 μM. The use of time-lapse video can be used to study the sequence of subcellular changes and hence time-course changes in live cells. This technique provides *dynamic data* on live cells exposed to chemicals.

Also, these fluorophores offer several orders of magnitude more sensitivity with which to link morphological change closely to biochemical events (Table 4.8). Discrete biochemical perturbations in specific organelles, membranes or the cytoplasm can be linked to subcellular morphological changes. The origin of any one cell type in a mixed population can be established by using antibody-tagged probes or other selective biochemical criteria such as specific enzymes, large numbers of mitochondria, etc. Changes in adjacent but different cell types can be compared and contrasted; this is especially important where one cell type forms

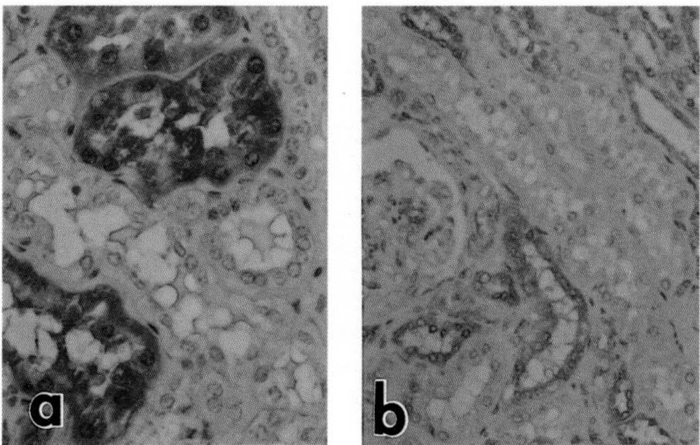

Plate 1 The cell selective distribution of the isoforms of glutathione-*S*-transferase (GST) in the kidney. Immunohistochemical staining of wax embedded, fixed renal tissue show the selective localization of (a) α-GST in the proximal and (b) π-GST in the distal tubule. (Alkaline phosphatase, magnification $\times 10$, objective.)

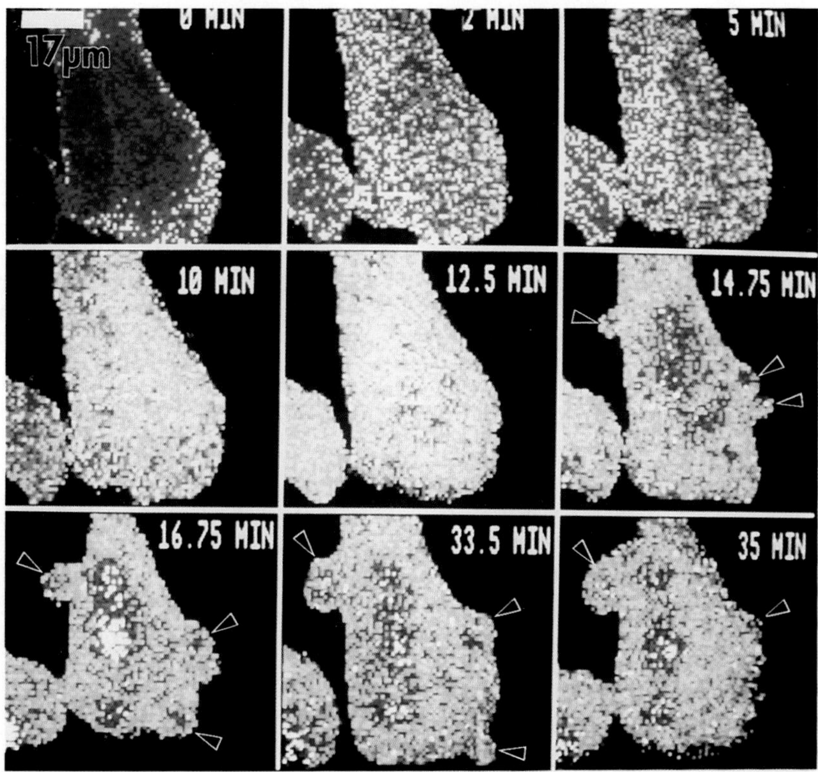

Plate 2 Changes in cytosolic calcium ($[Ca^{2+}]_i$) in Fura-2-loaded cultured rabbit renal proximal tubule epithelial cells at zero time and following treatment with $HgCl_2$. Analysis was determined by digital imaging fluorescence microscopy and images were generated by 'ratioing' images collected at 340–380 nm excitation. Images are displayed in pseudocolour to indicate $[Ca^{2+}]_i$ ranging from approximately 50 nM (dark blue) to more than 1200 nM (red/white). The $[Ca^{2+}]_i$ had increased significantly by 10 min after the addition of 50 μM $HgCl_2$ and cytoplasmic bleb formed by 14 min (as shown by arrowheads). This is thought to be a vehicle for removing free calcium. (Reprinted from Trump *et al.*,[12] with permission.)

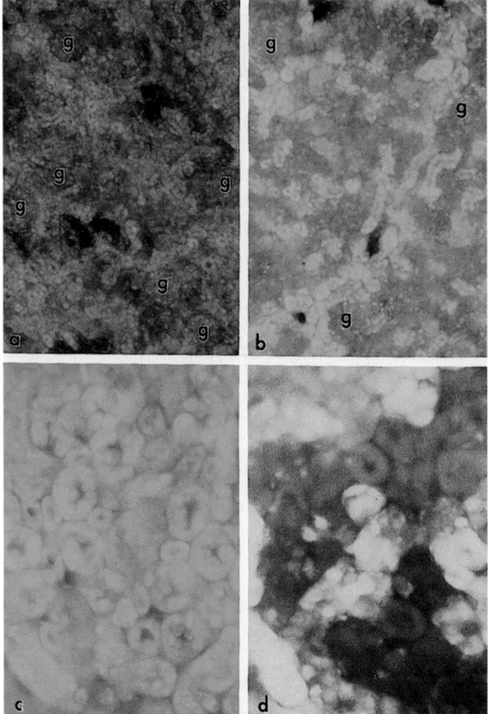

Plate 3 Changes in mitochondrial staining in precision-cut kidney slices following exposure to bile acids. The fluorescent probe 4(4-dimethylaminostyryl)-*N*-methylpyridinium iodide shows mitochondrial staining in the proximal tubules (pars recta) and glomeruli (a) in control slices whereas (b) exposure to 50 μM lithocholic acid for 2.5 h reduced glomerular staining intensity and that of the proximal tubules (pars recta), and also maintained staining intensity in distal tubules and convoluted proximal tubules. g, Glomeruli. (Objective, magnification ×4.) The fluorescent probe 2(4-dimethylaminostyryl)-*N*-methylpyridinium iodide showed similar mitochondrial staining in proximal and distal tubular cells of (c) control precision-cut slice and (d) reduced glomerular and pars recta of proximal tubule, whereas convoluted proximal and distal tubule stained strongly staining following treatment with 50 μM lithocholic acid. (Objective, magnification ×10.)

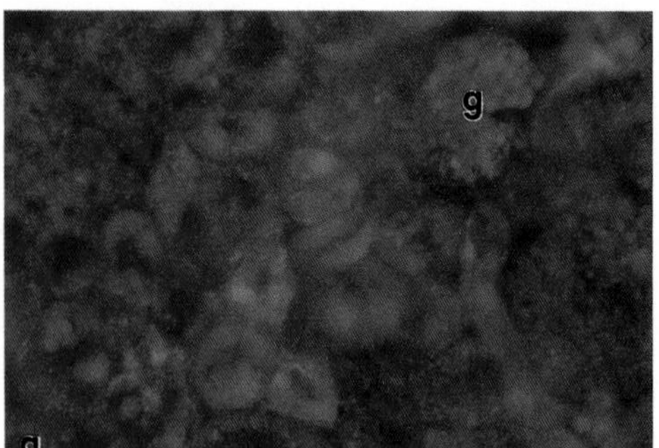

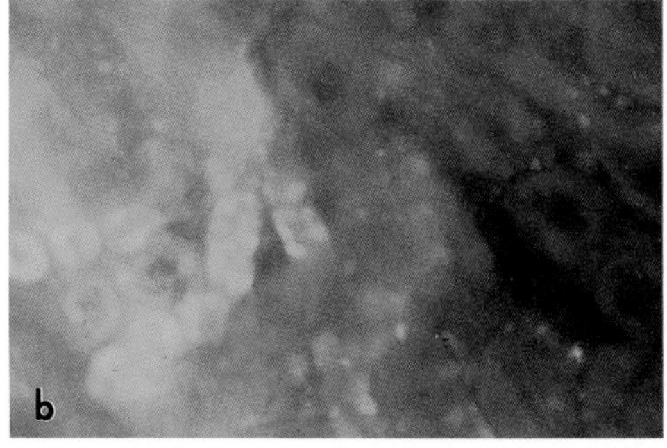

Plate 4 Changes in intracellular peroxide levels stained with 2′,7′-dihydrodichlorofluorescein in precision-cut kidney slices following exposure to bile acids. In control tissue (a) the glomeruli and all tubular cells (especially proximal tubules, pars recta) showed similar levels of peroxide, whereas (b) exposure to 50 μM lithocholic acid (2.5 h) diminished peroxide levels in the proximal tubules, had no effect on glomeruli, but enhanced staining in distal tubules (pars recta and pars convoluta). g, Glomeruli. (Objective, magnification ×10.)

Table 4.8 Fluorescent probes linking subcellular biochemistry and morphology.

Parameter	Probes used to assess or measure
Enzymes	4-Methylumbelliferyl acetate, 4-ethylumbelliferyl-*N*-acetyl-*β*-D-glucosaminide, 4-methylumbelliferyl palmitate
Mixed function oxidase	Fluorescein monoethylether ethyl ester, 5(and 6)ethoxycarbonylfluorescein ethyl ether ethyl ester, 7-pentoxy resorufin
Peroxidase substrate	2′-7′-Dichlorodihydrofluorescein diacetate, 5(and 6)carboxy-2′,7′-dichlorofluorescin diacetate
Protein kinase C	Rhodamine bisindolylmaleimide 1
Hydrolytic substrate	8-Hydroxypyrene-1,3,6-trisulfonic acid, 8-butyroxypyrene-1,3,6-trisulphonic acid, 8-oleoyloxypyrene-1,3,6-trisulfonic acid, 8-acetoxypyrene-1,3,6-trisulfonic acid
Cathepsin D	3-(2,4-Dinitroanilino)-3′-amino-*N*-methyldipropylamine
Oxygen detectors	Napthalene-1,4-dipropionic acid, anthracene-9,10-dipropionic acid, acridine orange
Superoxide anion (O_2^-)	Hydroethidine
Peroxide	2′,7′-Dichlorodihydrofluorescein
Calcium ion	Photoproteins: Aequorin, Indo-1, Quin-2, Fura-2 or Fluo-3
pH	2′,7′-*bis*-(2-Carboxyethyl)-5(6)-carboxyfluorescein (BCECF), seminaphtho-rhodafluor-1-acetoxymethylester (SNARF-1-AM)
Other ions	Selective probes for potassium, sodium and magnesium ions
Drugs	Tetracycline, chloroquine, anthrcyclines such as Adriamycin
Receptor	Tetramethylrhodamine *α*-bungarotoxin, tetramethylrhodamine epidemal growth factor, histamine fluorescein
Ionophore	4,4′-Diisothiocyanatostilbene-2,2-disulfonic acid, 4-acetamido-4′-isothiocyanato-stilbene-2,2-disulfonic acid
Lipid	Nile red, 4,4-difluoro-5-methyl-4-bora-3a,4a-diaza-*s*-indacene-3-dodecanoic acid
Lipophylic	1,1′-Dioctadecyl-3,3,3′,3′-tetramethyl-indocarbocyanine perchlorate, FluoroBora P
Membrane	8-Dodecanoyloxy-1,3,6-trisulfonic acid
Membrane surfaces	FluoroBora T
Transmembrane potentials	Oxonol dyes such as DiBAC4(3), carbocyanine dyes such as DiOC5(3), rhodamine 123, *N*-(3-triethylammonium)propyl-4-(4-(*p*-dibutylaminophenyl)butadienyl)-pyridinium
Cell surface carbohydrates	Lectins differentiate cell surface carbohydrate
Transport processes	Cationic rhodamine ester, cyanine and styrylpyridinium dyes
Nucleoside transporter	5′-S-(2-Aminoethyl)-*N*-6-(4-nitrobenzyl)-5′-thioadenosine-x-2-fluorescein
Anion transporter	*N*-(7-Nitrobenz-2-oxa-1,3-diazol-4-yl)-aminoethanesulfonic acid
Cl transporter	4,4′-Diisothiocyanatostilbene-2,2′-disulfonic acid
F-actin	Rhodamine phalloidin
Gap junction	Lucifer yellow
Lysosomes	FluoroBora I
Acidic organelles	*N*-(3-((2,4-dinitrophenyl)amino)propyl)-*N*-(3-aminopropyl)methylamine
Mitochondria	2-(4-Dimethylaminostyryl)-*N*-ethyl-pyridinium, 2-(4-dimethylaminostyryl)-*N*-methyl-pyridinium, 4-(4-dimethylaminostyryl)-*N*-methyl-pyridinium, rhodamine 6G, tetramethylrhodamine
Mitochondria (requires oxidation)	Dihydrorhodamine 6G, dihydrorhodamine 123
Mitochondria	3,3′-Dihexyloxacarbocyanine iodide (DiOC6(3))
Endoplasmic reticulum	Dihydrorhodamine 6G, rhodamine 6G, (at high concentrations) 3,3′-dihexyloxacarbocyanine iodide (DiOC6(3))
Golgi apparatus	*N*-(4,4-difluoro-5,7-dimethyl-4-bora-3a,4a-diaza-s-indacene-3-pentonoyl)sphingosylphosphocholine, FluoroBora II, *N*-(4,4-difluoro-5,7-dimethyl-4-bora-3a,4a-diaza-s-indacene-3-pentanoyl) sphingosine,
DNA	Hydroethidine, Hoechst 33258, DAPI
Nucleic acids	Fluorescence-labelled oligonucleotide or nucleic acid identify complementary sequences of DNA and mRNA and distinguish intron and exon sequences. Fluorescence *in situ* hybridization (FISH)

the target for chemical injury *in vitro* and the other(s) do not. Some of the subcellular characteristics that can be vizualized are shown schematically in Fig. 4.5.

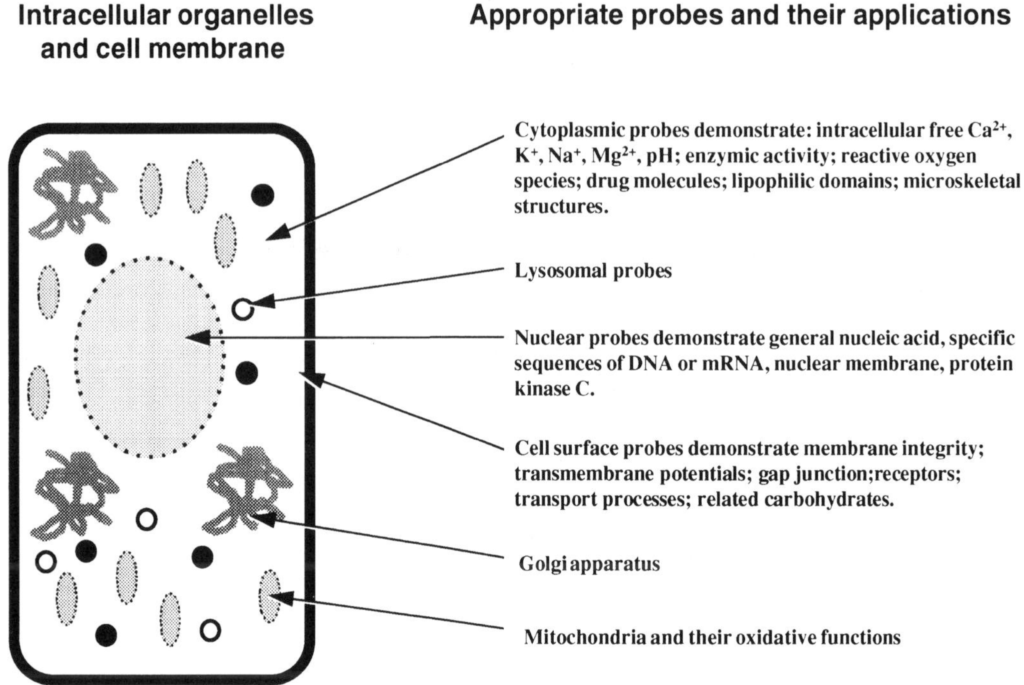

Fig. 4.5 Schematic representation of the subcellular components identified by different fluorescent probes in Table 4.8.

F. Non-invasive methods for the repeated screening of cells

There is a great advantage in using methods that allow cells to be reassessed over an interval of time to help study long-term changes *in vitro*.

1. *Epithelial barrier function*

Measurement of barrier function offers a novel criterion by which to assess cell injury in epithelial monolayers that separate two fluid compartments. Solute transport provides a transepithelial potential difference, where the electrical resistance depends on the tightness of the junctional complexes between cells. The greater the unidirectional transport of charged particles across an epithelial barrier, the higher the potential difference. Pfaller (see reference 5) has described a most efficient and rapid approach using a specific voltage-clamping unit, which allows repeated measurement on the same culture and allowed the ranking of β-lactam antibiotic toxicity as cephloridin > ceftazidime > cefotaxime. In addition, barrier function changes were more sensitive than enzyme release or ultrastructural alterations in confluent LLC-PK_1 monolayer cultures exposed to interferon α.

2. *Alamar blue*

Alamar blue is a proprietary tetrazolium salt that is converted to a fluorescent product. Unlike many of the other tetrazolium salts, including MTT (3-[4,5-dimethylthiazol-2-yl]-2,5-diphenyltetrazolium bromide) which deposits as an insoluble formazan, the reduced product of Alamar blue is freely soluble, is in equilibrium with the medium and is reported to be a vital stain that has no adverse effects on cells.[64,65] This means that it is possible repeatedly to assess the mitochondrial and cytoplasmic reduction over a period of time.

III. INTACT RENAL CELLULAR SYSTEMS *IN VITRO*

Isolated renal perfusion, micropuncture and perfused nephron segments are highly specialized, and are both labour and cost intensive. They have an essential place in studying intact cellular architecture within the organ, but are currently not widely used due to the high degree of expertise required to reproduce the *in vivo* system most closely.

A. Isolated perfused kidney

The isolated perfused kidney is the only *in vitro* system that maintains the full anatomical integrity of the kidney and has therefore been used frequently to evaluate the physiological basis of renal function and the factors that affect it. The detailed methodology for the preparation of isolated, perfused kidney has been described.[40,66–71] The minimum condition which should be met for this preparation includes keeping the perfusion pressure between 80 and 110 mmHg, keeping the perfusate flow at 20–35 ml min^{-1} and ensuring that the glomerular filtration rate is greater than 0.5 ml per g kidney. Routinely measured parameters include glomerular filtration, perfusate flow and pressure, electrolyte excretion and reabsorption, and water reabsorption.[68,69] Apart from studying the direct toxicity of chemicals such as cadmium[72] or mercury,[73] the main application of the isolated perfused kidney in nephrotoxicity studies lies in the ability to investigate the renal handling and biotransformation of xenobiotics[74,75] at concentrations of drugs or metabolic inhibitors that would not be possible *in vivo*. In addition there are no extrarenal (such as nervous, hormonal and blood-borne factors) effects and known concentrations of specific chemicals, including metabolites, can be presented to the cells. For example, the model of the non-filtering kidney has provided evidence for the luminal uptake of aminoglycosides[76] and has shown that filtration of cisplatin is not a prerequisite for the induction of toxicity.[77] Renal metabolism of several chemicals including paracetamol (acetaminophen) and the subsequent formation of reactive metabolites has also been evaluated in this system[78,79] and alcohol and methyltetrahydrofolate.[80] The characterization of *N*-acetyl-β-glucosaminidase from the isolated perfused kidney at a similar rate as *in situ* has helped to confirm its renal origin.[81]

The main limitations preventing a more widespread application of this system are that it requires experience, considerable technical skill and an elaborate technical set-up (such as carrying out experiments using sterile materials and solutions), and its function is crucially dependent on the composition of the perfusion medium,[68,82] which could be a determining factor in the viability of the preparation. Not all of the systems that have been reported provide physiologically or morphologically sound kidneys, and the application is limited to rodents. Although glomerular and tubular functions may be well preserved, there are defects in the distal tubule leading to an impaired electrolyte reabsorption and urinary concentration capacity.[68] Anoxic damage to the thick ascending limb of Henle during cell-free perfusion has been described.[83,84] Such unavoidable artefacts could cause brush border loss and membrane fragility. The isolated perfused kidney could therefore be a valuable tool for the study of nephrotoxicity, provided the technical limitations are taken into account.

B. Microperfusion

It is possible to isolate single nephron segments (normally from young rabbits) and connect these to two microsyringes (one at either end) and perfuse the tubule. Microperfusion is technically most difficult and requires sophisticated equipment; data are painstakingly produced and difficult to interpret in inexperienced hands. These methods have been applied to toxicological questions relating to membrane permeability changes, transport processes and the significance of luminal versus peritubular uptake of toxins.[85–90]

C. Renal cortical slices

The earliest renal biochemical investigations in the 1940s used hand-cut slices for the investigation of tubular transport processes. This relatively simple technique offers the opportunity to study both renal function and toxicity in different regions of the kidney (i.e. cortex, medulla or papilla) in an *in vitro* system that exhibits many of the characteristics seen *in vivo*. Tissue slices provide a system where renal-specific parameters are maintained and several functional parameters can be assessed. The use of slices is accomplished by few limitations such as limited life span, lack of reproducibility of nephron segments and the surface of the slices represents damaged area. The cellular heterogeneity of renal slices makes it difficult to discriminate between toxicity to the proximal tubules and other nephron segments such as the glomerulus or distal tubule.[70,75]

1. *Conventional renal slices*

Renal slices have been frequently used for the study of nephrotoxicity. They are relatively straightforward and easy to prepare and do not require major technical apparatus;[91] the technique can be applied to a number of different species including humans.[92] The preparation does not require enzyme digestion. The normal anatomical integrity of adjacent nephron segments is, at least partially, maintained and it is possible to prepare slices with a particular orientation (three-dimensional structure) from major regions of the kidney.[93] Cell–cell contacts are maintained and site-specific effects can be studied. The main use of slices in toxicological studies is related to the transport of organic ions such as *p*-aminohippurate (PAH) and tetraethylammonium (TEA) in the proximal tubule. Effects of toxins such as mercuric chloride,[94] potassium dichromate or cephaloridine[95] on PAH and TEA transport are among the most sensitive indicators of tubular damage. Other measurements include oxygen consumption, morphological assessment following exposure to toxins such as heavy metals,[96,97] or cisplatin and potential cellular protectants,[98–103] halogenated chemicals,[104–108] branch-chain hydrocarbon metabolites,[109] and age- and sex-related differences in rat tissue.[110] Specific changes have also been reported for paracetamol metabolism[111] and intermediary metabolism such as decreased gluconeogenesis when slices are exposed to gentamicin,[112] cephalosporins[113,114] and ochratoxin A.[115] There is also decreased ammoniagenesis with gentamicin,[112] and increased pentose phosphate metabolism, with decreased fatty acid synthesis, in the presence of paraquat.

In addition, the importance of contraluminal transport may be overemphasized in the light of limited access of chemicals to the luminal membrane, due to collapsed tubules.[116]

2. *Precision-cut renal slices*

The major sources of error in tissue slice work, namely the use of uneven thickness with irregular, non-reproducible damage at the cut surface, are being overcome with the recent introduction of a mechanical device able to provide reproducible sections of cores of renal tissue. The Krumdieck precision tissue slicer[117] has revitalized the use of tissue slices. This approach uses cores of fresh tissue 5–10 mm in diameter to prepare slices in an aqueous environment more rapidly and reproducibly, and with less cell trauma, than hand slicing.[118,119] The precision-cut slices are viable for up to 96 h and retain normal histological architecture, cell–cell and cell–matrix interactions, and expression of receptors. It is possible to select regions (such as the inner and outer medullary stripe) of large porcine and human kidneys and to include all of the cortex in rat renal slices. The 'functional' integrity of rat renal slices is shown by the maintenance of target selectivity of a whole range of chemicals that affect the same region *in vivo*.[75,93,120] Tissue can be harvested from most species, and also at different stages in the progression of a model lesion. The method therefore offers the first possibility of extrapolation between species and from *in vitro* to *in vivo*. The application to human kidney slices has shown the importance of interspecies comparisons using this approach. Both cisplatin and mercury chloride have been shown to be toxic in human tissue.[121]

Renal slices have been successfully cryopreserved,[122,123] which enables more efficient use of human tissue and also permits the transfer of material between research groups. The preparations of slices between investigators are also minimized by using commercially available tissue slices.

D. Isolated nephron segments

The most frequently used methods are enzymatic dispersion,[124] differential sieving[125] and gradient centrifugation.[126] These renal fragments retain the architecture of the proximal tubule and whole decapsulated glomeruli and offer a simple, rapid, inexpensive and flexible method for toxicological studies. Proximal tubular fragments (which are easier to isolate than distal tubule fragments or glomeruli) and glomeruli have been used from rat, rabbit, pig, dog and human kidneys. It is also possible to isolate 'superficial' and 'juxtamedullary' glomeruli and show the subtle difference in the sensitivity of each to a toxin. Fragments can be used to assess biochemical functions at various times after injury and provide useful information about mechanisms of toxicity.[127] The major limitation of isolated nephron fragments is their limited viability *in vitro*, which makes it difficult to study effects for longer than 4–6 h.[19]

A number of freshly isolated glomeruli and tubular systems exhibit high initial viability[15,128–130] and have been used to study the metabolism of xenobiotics[129] and intermediary metabolism in different species including humans,[131–139] and have found applications for assessing toxicology.[140] It is also possible to prepare fragments from a selected region of the nephron such as the thick ascending limb[133,141,142] and collecting tubules.[141] Fresh tubule or cell suspensions thus offer an important way of studying the mechanisms of nephrotoxicity and screening novel compounds, but have a limited *in vitro* lifespan and cells lack polarity, as a result of which some key transport processes may be lost.[143] A spectrum of proximal tubule toxins (ochratoxin A, citrinin, furosemide, cephalosporins, cisplatin, mercuric chloride and potassium chromate) release enzyme markers[144] and affect intermediary metabolism[145,146] in a time- and dose-dependent manner.

1. *Isolation by enzymic dispersion*

Enzymically isolated renal tubular fragments[124,147] are mixtures of different cell types, but they are active in intermediary metabolism[131,132] and in phase I and II drug metabolism.[124] These tubular preparations have been used to study the metabolism and conjugation of paracetamol,[138] together with glutathione synthesis and turnover.[148] Methods have been developed for separating mixed tubule populations by gradient centrifugation,[149] but this leads only to an enrichment and not to a purified population of proximal tubule cells. Other cell isolation and purification processes include centrifugal elutriation and immunomagnetic separation.[150,151]

2. *Isolation by mechanical shearing*

One advantage of dispersing cells by mechanical shearing is the ability to isolate medullary cells, glomeruli and proximal tubular fragments (PTFs), respectively, from the same kidney.[20] Apart from the economy of tissue and effort, this also allows the effects of one chemical to be studied on different renal cell types, which is particularly important when establishing whether target cell toxicity is maintained *in vitro*. The medulla is dissected free for culturing renal medullary interstitial cells,[152] and glomeruli and PTFs are both isolated and separated[20] to give fresh fragments that maintain a wide variety of normal functions and are not subject to de-differentiation, as is the case for cultured renal cells.[15] The organic ion transport system is very insensitive to nephrotoxins,[153] and many non-nephrotoxic agents (e.g. probenecid) interfere with organic ion transport. A pronounced degree of cell-selective toxicity has been documented for several established *in vivo* nephrotoxins using *de novo* protein synthesis from labelled amino acids to measure cytotoxicity. The use of these labelled precursors measures a variety of different processes, such as the uptake and incorporation into macromolecules. Proline, for example, is preferentially incorporated into glomerular and proximal tubular basement membranes.

E. Proximal tubular fragments

The purity of proximal tubular fragments is high, greater than 90%, and if carefully prepared they are largely free of both glomeruli and distal tubules. Methods for further division of PTFs into proximal straight and convoluted segments have been described.[154] The viability can be assessed rapidly by ethidium bromide–fluorescein diacetate exclusion.[155] A range of end-points can be used to quantify viability and the effect of chemicals. This includes organic anion (e.g. *p*-aminohippurate) uptake, enzyme (e.g. γ-glutamyl transpeptidase) leakage and *de novo* protein synthesis,[20,156,157] or metabolic processes such as cellular ATP content which show that mercuric chloride predominantly affects the S2 segment[146] and ochratoxin A both S2 and S3.[145]

The measurement of marker enzymes has been used mainly for characterization of the tubular preparation. For example, the ratio between alkaline phosphatase, a proximal brush border enzyme, and hexokinase, which is located predominantly in distal tubular segments, is a good indicator of the purity of a tubular suspension.[41,154] The pattern of urinary enzyme release after $HgCl_2$ correlates with the intracellular enzyme activities in the tubule fragments. By contrast, the pattern of urinary enzyme release following gentamicin treatment resembles more the profile found in the S1 segment, although no significant changes in intracellular enzyme activity were found in the microdissected segments following gentamicin treatment. It seems, therefore, that urinary enzyme levels are a more sensitive indicator of tubular damage than the determination of the (remaining) tissue enzyme activity.[158,159] Release of alanine aminopeptidase, leucine aminopeptidase and alkaline phosphatase in tubule suspensions after *in vitro* exposure to the fungal toxin ochratoxin A is similar to effects seen in microdissected proximal straight tubules, but the measured enzyme activities are decreased by 30–50% in the tubular suspension, indicating a loss of enzyme activity following the isolation procedure.[158] The significance of these findings for studies with other nephrotoxins, as well as the question whether the use of different isolation procedures has an influence on the enzyme loss, remains to be assessed systematically.

F. Glomeruli

Glomeruli can be isolated by the same procedure as proximal tubular fragments, using the sieving method,[160] and shown to metabolize various fatty acids.[161] They have been widely used in physiological studies on basement membrane synthesis,[162] prostaglandin metabolism[135,163] or action of hormones such as angiotensin II[164] and atrial natriuretic peptide.[165] Glomeruli have also been isolated from normal and diseased human kidneys,[166] and their capacity for prostaglandin synthesis[135] studied and compared with that of rodent glomeruli.[137] Only recently, isolated glomeruli have been evaluated as a tool to study mechanisms of nephrotoxicity and to be sensitive to puromycin aminonucleoside.[14]

IV. CELLS AND CELL-FREE SYSTEMS

There are a number of advantages to studying renal cells in culture, cell-free systems and renal organelles. Primary cells (with a limited life span) and continuous lines (unlimited life span) express varying degrees of characteristics seen in their *in vivo* counterparts. Primary cells de-differentiate rapidly and lines often lack specific functions (such as xenobiotic metabolism or organic anion transport across the basolateral membrane into the cell) which are prerequisites for the toxic effects of many established nephrotoxins. The need to develop renal cell lines that more closely resemble specific cells from the nephron is being met in a number of ways. Provided they retain key characteristics of renal cells, and 'appropriate' methods are used to study them, they offer a useful tool for understanding primary mechanisms and screening novel compounds. They can be used to study mechanisms of toxicity at cellular level and to design strategies for reducing or protecting against cell toxicity. Relevant *in vitro* to *in vivo* extrapolations can be made between species. In common with isolated fragments, the use of isolated cells is limited by their relatively short-lived viability in suspension.[19] One of the major problems in studying 'target cells' is how to obtain the correct cell type which then maintains the key properties that predispose to nephrogenic injury.

A. Freshly isolated renal cells

The isolation procedure for glomeruli and tubular fragments can be extended, for example by collagenase digestion[167] or Percoll density gradient centrifigation,[168] to yield single cells in suspension. Attempts to isolate appropriate cells have used a wide variety of approaches such as immunodissection,[169] free-flow electrophoresis[170] and centrifugation.[128,149] Irrespective of the combination of these methods, the cells then require extensive characterization.[171–174] Primary renal cell cultures that have been derived from glomeruli,[14,160,166,175–181] proximal tubules[15,31,182–185] and distal tubular cells[88,142,186–190] are sensitive to compounds that target for these regions *in vivo*. The combined use of different renal cell types has facilitated the investigation of cyclosporin A on glomeruli[191] and proximal tubule cells.[192]

These have been used, for example, in studies to characterize the transport of nephrotoxic halogenated hydrocarbons into tubular epithelial cells.[193,194] Isolated tubular epithelial cells can be characterized using marker enzymes such as γ-glutamyl transpeptidase,[195] receptor responsiveness and transport characteristics[139] or specific molecules such as glutathione or cytochrome P450.[167] Recently, a method has been described to separate cells from the convoluted and straight segments of the proximal tubule by free-flow electrophoresis,[196] where a knowledge of the enzyme distribution in renal cells was used as the basis for choosing fractions that represented specific regions of the nephron.

B. Primary renal proximal tubule cultures

Proximal tubular cells account for 65% of the renal volume and are major targets for xenobiotic injury because of high metabolic activity, active transport systems, well-developed apical microvilli (which provide a huge area for xenobiotic contact and uptake) and enzymes that metabolically activate chemicals.[34,197,198] It is for these reasons that significant effort has focused on *in vitro* evaluation of proximal tubule models for xenobiotic safety (see below).

Primary culture of epithelial cells is possible for several weeks and cells can be passaged a number of times, thus yielding much more cellular material. However, the continued growth is paralleled by de-differentiation of specific cellular functions, which makes it more difficult to extrapolate data to the *in vivo* situation.[199] The medium and time-related de-differentiation of cells has also been shown by the changes in several marker enzymes in primary rat proximal tubule cultures;[15] data that show how labile the total concentration of enzyme markers can be in cells. Morin *et al.*[200] recently described the change in expression of characteristic marker enzymes in rabbit tubular epithelial cells with increasing time in culture. They showed that the activity of brush border enzymes decreased slightly over the first 6 days in culture, but glycolytic enzymes increased 17- to 50-fold compared with freshly isolated proximal tubules, indicating a shift in energy metabolism towards glucose utilization. Similar changes have also been reported in cell lines grown in media containing different carbohydrates.[201]

Primary cell cultures allow long exposure to xenobiotics and the choice of appropriate metabolites, as well as ease of manipulating and monitoring functional or morphological responses in a dose- and time-related manner.[15,92,124,183,192,202–205]

C. Primary distal tubule cultures

Distal tubular cells[88,142,186–190] have been cultured but not yet widely used for pharmacotoxicology studies.

D. Primary renal glomerular cell cultures

Homogeneous glomerular mesangial and epithelial cells may be co-cultured or each derived separately,[14,39,137,149,160,166,175–181,191,206,207] and maintain their sensitivity to glomerular toxins (see below).

E. Renal medullary interstitial cell cultures

The renal medullary interstitial cells are the target of most papillotoxic chemicals in animals and probably in humans.[208–210] The unique characteristics of these cells include the high osmolality in which they exist *in vivo*, and the fact that they have an exceptionally high prostaglandin synthetase capacity and a large number of polyunsaturated lipid droplets.[211] The mechanism of renal medullary necrosis is thought to be linked to the peroxidative activation of agents to form reactive intermediates (see below), and cultured rat interstitial cells are sensitive to compounds that cause papillary necrosis.[152]

F. Renal cell lines

Established renal lines have properties reminiscent of specific parts of the nephron such as LLC-PK_1 and OK (of proximal tubule type) and MDCK (of distal tubule type[212,213]), but the exact site of origin is not known and the cells do not totally represent the normal physiological state. The use of cell lines in nephrotoxicity studies has been reviewed.[21] LLC-PK_1 cells are sensitive to a variety of haloalkene conjugates[214–216] due to the presence of the brush border enzyme γ-glutamyl transpeptidase, which catalyses the breakdown of the conjugate to the proximate toxin, and an organic anion transport system,[217] which facilitates the entry of the chemicals into cells.

The use of continuous cell lines has become increasingly popular because of the virtually unlimited material available. The most commonly used renal cell lines are the LLC-PK_1 and the MDCK cells, epithelial cells derived from the pig and dog kidney, respectively. The problem of de-differentiation of normal cellular functions is much more evident with cell lines, and much work has been done to characterize these cells and define their likely origin within the nephron.[218] The enzymatic profiles of these two cell lines suggest a proximal tubular origin for LLC-PK_1 and a distal tubular origin for MDCK cells, although the expression of some marker enzymes notably differ from *in vivo* data.[130] Examples of recent toxicological studies using LLC-PK$_1$ cells include studies on lipid alterations after exposure to mercuric chloride,[219] cellular viability on aminoglycoside exposure,[220] uptake studies with radiolabelled cisplatin,[221] effects of hexachlorobutadiene conjugates on organic ion transport and measurement of unscheduled DNA synthesis after exposure to halogenated hydrocarbons.[222] Despite detailed information on the enzymatic profile of LLC-PK$_1$ cells, this knowledge has so far not been employed for toxicity studies.

In addition, there has been the widespread use of continuous renal cell lines. Several established renal cell lines have properties reminiscent of specific parts of the nephron. These lines are, however, often heterogeneous and they are still not characterized systematically to establish their usefulness in screening chemicals for toxicity and in understanding the mechanisms of target cell toxicity. In recent years LLC-PK$_1$, OK, LLC-RK$_1$ (of proximal tubular origin) and MDCK (of distal tubule and collecting duct origin) cells have been characterized under controlled conditions and following exposure to nephrotoxins.[35,36,212]

Cell lines derived from the kidneys of various species are commercially available. The cell lines most used in toxicological studies are those which exhibit *in vitro* some of the properties of the proximal tubular epithelium *in vivo* such as LLC-PK$_1$, LLC-RK$_1$ and OK cells. In culture, these cells grow to form a confluent monolayer, and they exhibit some degree of differentiation. They have been shown to exhibit apical–basolateral polarization, with brush border microvilli and basolateral infoldings being present.[218]

The use of isolated and cultured primary cells or lines is based on the presence and absence of a range of functional and biochemical characteristics, such as transport systems, and an array of structural and functional molecules and those biochemical characteristics that predispose these target cells to the effects of the toxin.

1. *The forgotten cell lines*

It is worth considering that there are over 20 renal cell lines (some of which are listed in Table 4.9) described in the literature, but only OK, MDCK and LLC-PK$_1$ have been widely characterized physiologically and therefore continue to be used as the 'easy option' for toxicology studies. It is the major logistical problem of characterizing these cells that could prevent better cell lines being identified. It is, however, worth noting that MDBK cells express more of the phenotypic characteristics commonly ascribed to the distal tubule than is the case for MDCK. These similarities between MDBK cells and the distal nephron have been derived from routine culture protocols, where there has been no attempt to optimize the culture conditions to maximally express any other characteristics.

2. *New cell lines*

Cell hybrids formed by electrofusion have already been used to produce monoclonal antibodies.[223] No single cell type contains all of the factors that may predispose them to 'target-selective' injury. Thus the possibility of using the cell biological approach of fusing two different cells to combine desirable functions (such as a transport process and a metabolic activation system) is already being investigated. Combining human renal primary cells with stable lines could provide hybrids that reflect the characteristic of each cell type for nephrotoxicity testing. Hybrid cell lines expressing functions lost in primary cells are being developed by fusing permanent, non-tumorigenic cell lines with primary human or rat proximal tubule cells. Several clones have been produced, and now need a substantial

Table 4.9 Comparison of the origins and anatomical representation of the cell lines that are reported to be derived from renal tissues.

Cell line	Species	Full name	Derived from	Origins
Widely used renal cell lines				
MDCK (NBL-2)	Dog	Madin-Darby Canine Kidney	Cocker Spaniel	Distal tubular
OK	Opossum	Opossum Kidney	Opossum	Proximal tubular
LLC-PK_1	Pig	Pig Kidney	Large White Pig	Proximal tubular
Poorly characterized renal cell lines				
BGM	Monkey	Buffalo green monkey kidney	Buffalo green monkey	Not defined
CRFK	Cat	Crandall feline kidney fibroblasts	Cat	Not defined
CV-1	Monkey	Not defined	Not defined	Not defined
FRhK-4	Monkey	Fetal rhesus monkey kidney cells	Rhesus monkey	Not defined
KASZA	Pig	Not defined	Not defined	Not defined
LLC-MK_1	Monkey	Not defined	Not defined	Not defined
LLC-MK_2	Monkey	Not defined	Not defined	Not defined
LLC-RK_1	Rabbit	Not defined	Not defined	Not defined
MA104	Monkey	African green monkey kidney	African green monkey	Not defined
MDBK (NBL-1)	Bovine	Madin-Darby Bovine Kidney	Cattle	Appears to be distal
NRK-52E	Rat	Normal rat kidney	Rat fibroblast with epithelial characteristics	Endothelial
NBL-1	Bovine	Normal Bovine Line	Not defined	Proximal tubule
NRL-3 (Pt K1)	Potoroo	Not defined	Female Potoroo tridactylis	Not defined
NRL-5 (Pt K2)	Potoroo	Not defined	Male Potoroo tridactylis	Not defined
PAP-HT25	Rabbit	Rabbit renal papillary epithelial	Not defined	Collecting duct
PK(15)	Pig	Pig kidney epithelial	Not defined	Subclone of PK-2a
RhMK	Monkey	Secondary rhesus monkey kidney	Rhesus monkey	Not defined
RK13	Rabbit	Rabbit kidney epithelial	Derived from 5-week-old rabbit	Not defined
RMK	Monkey	Rhesus monkey kidney	Rhesus monkey	Not defined
SV40 viral transformed cell lines				
COS-1	Monkey	CV-1 transformed with SV40		
COS-7	Monkey	CV-1 transformed with SV40		
PyY	Hamster	BHK/C13 transformed with SV40		

Renal fibroblast lines such as Vero, Normal rat kidney (NRK-49F) and Crandall feline kidney fibroblasts (CRFK) have been omitted.

investment to characterize them, to establish whether they are stable and immortal, and to clarify whether they are more useful for *in vitro* testing than cells that are currently available. Similarly, cells transfected with genes coding for specific characteristics (xenobiotic metabolism, organic anion transport, etc.) that are absent from the original cell line will be an area of important future advancement.

The ability to establish an array of tailored cells that represent each of the different regions of the kidney, by fusion, transfection or nuclear injection with selected properties will provide the potential to learn a great deal more about the mechanisms of injury in model chimeric systems. The newly tailored cell lines need to be rapidly characterized by molecular and cellular biology techniques such as immunocytochemistry and fluorescent probes to document biochemical, metabolic and transport properties, to establish their hormone responsiveness, handling of macromolecules, as well as to document their ultrastructural features.

G. Cell-free systems: the use of subcellular fractions

The main potential for the use of subcellular fragments lies in the study of known *in vivo* effects under well-defined experimental conditions; this has helped to characterize some of the effects of proximal tubular toxins. The appropriate choice of enzymes can be used to screen for chemicals that are likely to undergo parallel metabolic activations *in vitro*.

1. Renal cell organelles

Fractionated organelles, membranes or cytoplasm from defined cells or from kidney in general can be used for specific cell-free investigations, to study chemical distribution, interaction between a cellular compartment and a chemical and/or the kinetics of binding or release of substances. This includes specific enzyme inhibition, metabolic activation, covalent binding, or the modulation of lipid peroxidation, etc., using purified or commercially available biochemicals. These *in vitro* systems are usually prepared by differential centrifugation,[224,225] nuclei and membrane vesicles.[226,227] The purity of the preparations is usually confirmed by marker enzyme assays, by transmission and scanning electron microscopy and, more recently, by the application of fluorescent probes that specifically identify organelles. Isolated brush border membrane vesicles have been used to study aminoglycoside binding and the effects of a range of molecules on the transport systems that remain intact in the vesicles.

The knowledge of compartmentalization of specific functions to discrete cell types and within specific organelles in renal cells has led to the development of sensitive tests for the assessment of nephrotoxicity in particular fragments of renal cells isolated by differential centrifugation. Enzyme measurement is an important parameter frequently used in studies with subcellular fragments. For example, isolated renal microsomes have been used for the study of CYP450.[228,229] Aminoglycoside antibiotics have a membrane stabilizing effect on isolated lysosomes at low concentrations as assessed by the release of *N*-acetyl-β-glucosaminidase, while higher concentrations lead to a dose-dependent release of this enzyme paralleling the clinically observed potential for producing nephrotoxicity.[230] Comparable results were obtained measuring the inhibitory effect of aminoglycosides on the lysosomal phospholipase activity *in vitro*.[231] Marker enzymes have been used to characterize brush border membrane vesicles, which have been used to study the effect of aminoglycosides on calcium binding and transport.[226] The comparison of effects on brush border membrane and basolateral vesicles has been useful in the characterization of tubular transport of aminoglycosides.[232] The potential of cyclosporine A to cause lipid peroxidation has been evaluated in studies with renal microsomes.[233]

2. Metabolism in cytosolic systems

Metabolic activation of chemicals is important for nephrotoxicity, as enzymes responsible are localized to regions that are affected.[234] Thus the use of an appropriate commercially available enzyme can give information *in vitro* on the metabolic activation of a chemical, and it is likely that the sophistication of such systems, and the parallel use of the appropriate cell type in culture, could help screen for chemicals with the potential to cause toxicity.

V. MECHANISTIC STUDIES AND TOXICITY SCREENING

The major limitations in interpretation of data obtained using the above-mentioned methods include: species and strain differences in the renal response to chemicals, disruption of the anatomical integrity during the isolation procedure, absence of normal renal and extrarenal xenobiotic metabolism (which may form a proximate toxin), de-differentiation of cellular functions *in vitro*, an inappropriately high or low concentration of toxins in the incubation media, and an abnormal route of administration of chemicals and arbitrary choice of exposure time and vehicle.[24,235] These limitations are valid for all parameters measured *in vitro* and, to a varying degree, for the various systems in use. Their implications are better considered in terms of a number of other factors.

A. Mechanisms of injury

An understanding of the mechanisms of renal injury is fundamental to an appreciation of how to screen for nephrotoxicity *in vivo* and *in vitro*, and to making rational extrapolations between species and to assessing risk. Many of the changes caused by nephrotoxic agents are closely parallelled in both laboratory animals and humans, despite the marked species differences in the structure and function of the kidney.[63] The mechanistic basis for nephrotoxicity in target cells generally depends on direct interaction of a chemical with a discrete cell type. These target cells have a series of biochemical characteristics that predispose to perturbation of those molecular processes that lead to cell injury and/or death. The site of renal injury relates to the sum of a series of interactions, depending on the physicochemical properties and metabolism of the chemical and its metabolites, their cellular and subcellular distribution, and the biochemical properties of the target cell. Most nephrotoxic lesions are thought to occur as a result of a limited number of processes.

The exact mechanism of cell death is not clear; even two closely related compounds could damage the same region of the kidney by different mechanisms and it is not uncommon for structural analogues to target for different cell types. Such uncertainties compromise the simplistic concept of finding a ‘good or valid’ test and using it to screen blindly for the toxicity of a series of analogues or for compounds that damage a discrete cell type. It is thus apparent that cytotoxicity should not be assessed by only one method and both general (enzyme leakage and protein synthesis) and specific (metabolism of specific molecules, organelle function or changes in a cell specific marker) assays should be used. *In vitro* methods offer a very powerful system in which the mechanistic basis of target selective renal cell injury can be assessed. It is possible to use both target and non-target cells to compare interaction between a cell with well-defined characteristics and a toxin.

B. How does cytotoxicity relate to nephrotoxicity?

Cytotoxicity in renal cells or tissue does not necessarily equal nephrotoxicity. Many of the end-points chosen for routine screening procedures are, however, developed to facilitate handling a large number of samples, rather than being the most relevant marker of cell specific injury. There is a need to choose between sensitive and selective methods in relation to the lesion that occurs *in vivo*. Ideally there should be an appropriate mechanistic link between cell type, the toxic chemical and its mechanism of action – a priori this is rarely possible. The rational choice of methods for the study of target selective nephrotoxicity has therefore to be based on the individual strengths and weaknesses of the various systems available.

De novo protein synthesis is widely used as it is generally sensitive. However, ranking toxicity according to the inhibition of protein synthesis may show no or an inverse relationship with clinical effects, as seen for aminoglycosides,[157] where fatty acid oxidation is more specific, but less sensitive, than protein synthesis for identifying toxicity *in vivo*. Similar results were obtained with heavy metals[236] and atractyloside, which has almost no effects on protein synthesis at concentrations that are profoundly cytotoxic.[237,238] These data underline the importance of the choice of suitable parameters for all *in vitro* toxicity studies. The method of assessment may often depend on whether monocultures, co-cultures and renal tissue are in use. If *in vitro* systems are heterogeneous, there is an increasing awareness of the need to use methods that identify the integrity of one cell type selectively.

Bearing these potential problems in mind, the use of *in vitro* techniques offers unique advantages in the study of the mechanistic basis of nephrotoxicity. Thus, direct effects of chemicals and their interactions with renal tissue can be evaluated, the experimental conditions can be precisely controlled and manipulated, samples may be obtained from individual animals, and effects can be tested in well-defined areas of the kidney.[24,75]

C. The use of human tissue

There are several reasons for the preferred use of human renal tissue as the source of cells for *in vitro* toxicity studies. The rat kidney differs significantly from that of humans, as shown in Table 4.10. More importantly, it is assumed that most experimental animals are free of pre-existing renal disease, but this is not the case in humans, where decreased functional reserve may be one of the least adequately studied aspects of comparative nephrotoxicity. Thus the use of human renal cells could offer the potential to circumvent the need to extrapolate animal *in vitro* studies to humans. There have already been a number of published studies on human kidneys. These have been characterized in terms of normal and diseased tissue[92,203] and glomeruli.[137,160,166,206,207] Recently, there has been a trend towards studying cultured human renal proximal tubular cells exposed to nephrotoxins.[183–185]

Warning: The potential to use human tissues as a source of cells for *in vitro* investigations has been widely reported (see meeting report by Jeremy[239]). Human renal tissue used as the source of cells is rarely adequately assessed in terms of pre-existing pathology, using routine assessment or the powerful techniques of immuno-histochemistry or conventional histochemistry. The cells are therefore isolated from inadequately defined origins. All too often these cells are cultured under inappropriate conditions; they are rarely adequately characterized. Thus it is still not certain whether these human renal cells provide more relevant data than any other *in vitro* system.

The recent introduction of precision-cut human tissue slices[121] may prove to be a powerful tool, as the need to disrupt cells is avoided. It is important to be aware of the fact that all the constraints defined for each of the *in vitro* systems may apply to slices, and additional characterization is needed before their full potential can be realized.

Table 4.10 Comparison between renal structure and function in man and commonly used laboratory species.

	Man	Rat	Dog
Cortical structure			
Nephrons (per g body-weight)	16	128	45
Glomerular radius (μm)	100	61	90
Proximal tubular length (mm)	16	12	20
Tubular radius (μm)	36	29	33
Cortical function			
Insulin clearance (ml min^{-1} kg body-$weight^{-1}$)	2.0	6.0	4.3
p-Aminohippurate transport maxima (mg min^{-1} kg body-$weight^{-1}$)	1.3	3.0	1.0
Drug metabolizing enzymes*			
Mixed functional oxidase	4	5	—
NADPH–cytochrome *c* reductase	15	48	—
Medullary structure			
Percent long loops	14	28	100
Relative medullary thickness	3.0	5.8	4.3
Medullary function			
Maximum urine osmolality (mOsmol kg^{-1})	1400	2610	2610

* Renal enzyme activity expressed as a percentage of liver activity.

VI. INTEGRATED MECHANISMS OF RENAL INJURY *IN VITRO*

These systems have been studied *in vitro* using a full range of renal slices or cells/fragments, organelles and progressively appropriate cytosolic, mitochondrial or microsomal enzymes. The intensive study of each compound has helped establish how to screen better for nephrotoxins and also to understand mechanisms.

A. Chloroform nephrotoxicity

Isolated renal microsomes (a source of mixed functional oxidase) cause metabolic activation and protein binding of radiolabelled chemicals. The inhibition of such binding may be manipulated by substances known to block these enzymes. There is a sex-related sensitivity of male mice to chloroform nephrotoxicity,[240] which is based on the mixed functional oxidase (cytochrome P450)-mediated metabolic activation of this compound. Both cortical slices and microsomes from male mice[241] generate the reactive intermediate phosgene (which binds to macromolecules) in the presence of NADPH and oxygen, a process that can be inhibited by carbon monoxide,[228,242] which is an effect that can be shown to be induced by phenobarbital in rabbit microsomes.[229]

B. Haloalkene nephrotoxicity

Proximal tubular cells are also sensitive to the haloalkene glutathione conjugate formed in the liver. During its renal excretion, it is degraded to a cysteine conjugate, which accumulates in renal cells by an anion transport mechanism and is activated by the renal enzyme cysteine conjugate β-lyase (glutamine transaminase K) which cleaves the C–S bond, generating 1 mole of pyruvate and 1 mole of ammonia plus a reactive mercaptan moiety that binds to biological macromolecules producing a discrete necrosis of the straight portion (*pars recta*) of the proximal tubule which resolves within 21–28 days.[215,216,243–258] These processes have all been studied *in vitro*,[247,248,259–266] where the use of inhibitors such as amino-oxyacetic acid (pyridoxal phosphate-dependent inhibitor of β-lyase), phenylalanylglycine (competitively blocks cysteinglycine dipeptidase) and AT-125 (irreversible inhibitor of γ-glutamyltransferase) have all served to help elucidate the mechanism of haloalkene toxicity and *in vitro* test systems.

C. Antibiotic-induced injury

Use of a combination of *in vivo* and *in vitro* techniques has made it possible to show that aminoglycosides bind to the anionic membrane receptor phospholipid (such as phosphatidylinositol[267]). The antibiotic–membrane complex is taken up by adsorptive endocytosis and sequestrated in lysosomes[268,269] where it accumulates to high concentrations[270] and inhibits the enzymes that normally degrade membrane phospholipid[271,272] and causes an increase in the level of renal cortical phosphatidylinositol,[270,273] seen ultrastructurally by the accumulation of lysosomal myeloid bodies.[269] Polyaspartic acid protects animals from aminoglycoside nephrotoxicity without inhibiting the proximal tubular cell uptake of the antibiotic.[220,274,275] *In vitro* studies show the binding interaction between the polyanionic peptide and aminoglycoside, and suggest this prevents electrostatical interactions between the antibiotic and cellular targets (such as anionic phospholipids) that are central to the development of nephrotoxicity.[276]

The exact cause of cell necrosis is still not clear, but lysosomal phospholipidosis is a critical first step,[277] dependent on a threshold concentration of aminoglycoside, which if it is not reached does not cause biochemical or morphological evidence of cellular necrosis.[278] In addition, aminoglycosides may also inhibit agonist activation of the phosphatidylinositol cascade,[279] depress Na^+–K^+-ATPase, adenylate cyclase, alkaline phosphatase and calcium binding,[268,280,281] impair mitochondrial respiration[282] and decrease incorporation of leucine into microsomal protein, all of which could contribute to cell injury.

The inhibition of protein synthesis by aminoglycosides *in vitro* does not reflect their potential to cause nephrotoxicity *in vivo*,[157] which argues against a major role of this metabolic pathway in the molecular mechanism of the lesion. Similarly, examination of the oxidation of fatty acids also failed to show a good correlation between *in vitro* effects and *in vivo* toxicity.[157] Because renal cortical accumulation of aminoglycosides is believed to be of major importance in the development of renal failure, the absence of close clinical toxicity and lack of predictiveness of a single general method for assessing cytotoxicity without relating it to an *in vivo* situation and in the intact kidney is not surprising.

In vitro methods have also been essential for the understanding of the mechanisms by which cephalosporines accumulate, injure cells and as a way to screen for the least toxic in a series of novel compounds.[283–286]

D. Glomerular injury

Adriamycin selectively injures glomerular epithelial cells in rodents and causes nephrotic syndrome within days of a single dose.[287] This model nephrotic syndrome is characterized by proteinuria, hypoalbuminaemia and peripheral oedema,[287–292] which occur a few weeks after treatment[293,294] in susceptible species such as rats and rabbits. Fibrosis or sclerosis of glomeruli develops after extended periods.[295] The ultrastructural pathology of the Adriamycin-exposed kidney shows early glomerular epithelial cell changes leading to increased protein permeability and high molecular weight proteinuria.[287,288,290] The use of glomerular fragments has helped understand the mechanistic basis of this lesion.[296]

Micropuncture studies in animals have shown that the proteinuria originates predominantly from juxtamedullary glomeruli, indicating that cortical glomeruli are less sensitive to the effect of the compound.[297] Cortical and juxtamedullary glomeruli from Adriamycin-treated animals were separated and incubated with radiolabelled precursors to study protein synthesis and glucose oxidation. Glucose oxidation was stimulated in juxtamedullary, but not superficial, glomeruli,[296] which may be a metabolic expression of the increased protein excretion from juxtamedullary nephrons *in vivo*.[297] Thus glomerular damage by Adriamycin was associated with a stimulating effect on glomerular metabolism, which was significantly more pronounced in juxtamedullary than in cortical glomeruli. Isolated glomeruli are able to contract, an observation that is thought to be related to the contraction of the mesangial cells[298] and which may affect the glomerular microcirculation *in vivo*.[299] Cyclosporin A has profound effects on the renal vascular resistance,[300] resulting in a reduction of the glomerular surface area of superficial glomeruli within 5 min of the beginning of incubation, whereas isolated juxtamedullary glomeruli were not affected.[191] The underlying differences in structure and/or function between juxtamedullary and superficial glomeruli which may cause the differences in response to toxins remain to be elucidated.

The mechanistic basis of this heterogeneity of glomerular injury is not fully understood but may be related to differences in oxygen pressure in the outer and inner cortex. The inner cortical partial pressure of oxygen is considerably higher than that of the subcapsular region,[84] which would enhance oxidative stress on membrane components mediated by Adriamycin semiquinone radicals in juxtamedullary glomerular epithelial cells due to the more abundant oxygen supply. Lipid oxidation is one step in the cascade of Adriamycin nephrotoxicity, leading to metabolic alterations in the epithelial cells, which in turn could lead to structural alterations in the glomerular filtration barrier.

Fluorescent illumination of cultured glomeruli (with outgrowths of both mesangial and epithelial cells) suggests the preferential uptake of Adriamycin into epithelial, but not mesangial, cell nuclei (P. H. Bach, unpublished results). The effect of Adriamycin could also relate to its preferential accumulation in the juxtamedullary nephrons, data that can be obtained only from *in vivo* investigations.

E. Heavy metal toxicity

Many heavy metals are potently nephrotoxic and generally target the proximal tubule.[301] Glomeruli are markedly sensitive to mercury *in vitro*.[236] Protein synthesis and fatty acid oxidation in isolated glomeruli are inhibited by heavy metals with the greatest potential to cause acute renal failure, such as mercuric chloride and potassium dichromate,[236] suggesting a role of direct glomerular toxicity in acute renal failure. This was originally thought to be artefact as mercury is generally thought to target the proximal tubule. The combination of *in vivo* and *in vitro* techniques (M. F. Wilks, unpublished results) has shown a distinct, but subtle, primary effect of mercury on glomeruli, followed by a secondary and more dramatic effect on the proximal tubule. This shows how long-established mechanisms of nephrotoxicity (i.e. of mercury on the proximal tubule) are in fact more complex. Indeed, parallel *in vivo* experiments have shown that the distribution of mercury in the early phases of insult is in fact also predominant in the juxtamedullary glomerular population.[302]

There is also evidence that the incubation of isolated glomeruli with several heavy metals leads to an impairment of ^{35}S incorporation into proteoglycans in a manner similar to the inhibition of total protein synthesis.[303] 'Softer' metal ions such as Cd^{2+} and Hg^{2+} caused a preferential decrease in the production of the more highly charged dermatan sulphate, indicating a possible effect on mesangial cells.

F. Reactive oxygen species and lipid peroxidation

In vitro systems are also being used to understand other processes that injure proximal tubular cells by reactive chemical intermediates or oxygen species.[304–306] Puromycin aminonucleoside causes a morphologically similar lesion. Kawaguchi *et al.*[307] have shown the formation of reactive oxygen species in glomerular epithelial cells and Adriamycin produces similar effects in isolated glomeruli and glomerular cells,[308] although it seems likely that there are also other effects.[309] There is increasing evidence from isolated cells and mitochondria that mercury produces hydrogen peroxide and lipid peroxidation.[310,311] It is likely that these mediators play a role in the increased release of free calcium in proximal tubule cells, which can be seen with the fluorescent indicator Fura-2,[11,12] as major degenerative changes have occurred within minutes of exposure (Plate 2); it is thought that the cell attempts to remove some of the free calcium by enclosing it in 'blebs' that are exocytosed from the cell surface.

G. Hydroperoxidase-mediated nephrotoxicity

Prostaglandin synthase consists of two enzymic activities: cyclo-oxygenase and hydroperoxidase. The hydroperoxidase (and other peroxidases) convert a number of chemicals to reactive intermediates, explaining those toxicological processes that cannot be mediated by CYP450.[312] The prostaglandin synthase (and therefore peroxidase) localization to the inner medulla has been strongly implicated in analgesic nephropathy.[313] The metabolic activation of acetaminophen is dependent on arachidonic acid in the papilla and forms reactive intermediates which bind covalently to medullary microsomes. Metabolic activation is reduced by inhibitors of prostaglandin synthase and by antioxidants, and is thought to be mediated by a reactive intermediate of the quinone–imine type[314] which can also bind nucleic acid covalently. Prostaglandin-mediated peroxidation is closely paralleled by horseradish peroxidase[315] which, because of its commercial availability, has become the simple model system for studying such processes.

In vitro methods have been used to show that cultured rodent renal medullary interstitial cells (RMICs) are sensitive to established papillotoxins *in vitro*.[152] The responses of cultured RMICs were scored for cytotoxic change from 0 to +++ in the presence of 2-bromoethanamine, and paracetamol and its major metabolites; and maintained the same spectrum of *in vivo* toxicity. However, cell death gives no indication of the mechanism. Time-lapse studies on RMICs suggest that cells with most lipid droplets are the most sensitive to 2-bromoethanamine.[20] In an attempt to confirm an association between peroxidase activity and lipid material, we have also studied the sensitivity of cell lines to papillotoxins. Both RMICs and 3T3 fibroblasts are sensitive to 2-bromoethanamine,[20] but there are no cytotoxic changes in MDCK or HaK cells exposed to a tenfold increased concentration of 2-bromoethanamine for four times as long. RMICs are thought to be fibroblastic in origin,[13] hence the comparison with 3T3 cells, whereas HaK[316] and MDCK[317] represent proximal and distal renal epithelial cells, respectively. The absence of lipid droplets and peroxidase activity from HaK and MDCK cells may explain the lack of 2-bromoethanamine cytotoxicity. Fluorescent probes have revealed high levels of peroxidase activity and/or peroxides in RMICs,[318] and Nile red[319] confirms the presence of lipid droplets[13,211] in medullary and 3T3 cells.

H. Bile acid-related renal injury

Death from postoperative renal failure is more common in patients with jaundice than in any other group. Chronically bile duct-ligated rodents also show changes in urinary enzymes that suggest selective proximal tubular injury.[320] Glomeruli and proximal tubule fragments are both more sensitive to the hydrophobic bile acids (such as lithocholic acid) than has been reported for hepatocytes or erythrocytes.[321] Cell injury also occurs at lower concentrations of chenodeoxycholic acid for precision-cut renal slices than for liver slices (B. Kaler *et al.*, unpublished results), suggesting that part of the sensitivity of jaundiced patients to surgery relates to pre-existing renal cell compromise caused by bile acids.

Krumdieck precision-cut kidney slices from male Wistar rats (200 μm thick), exposed to lithocholic acid at IC_{50} 50 μM for 2.5 h have been assessed by fluorescent probes staining for mitochondrial function (the carbocyanine dye 3,3′-dihexyloxacarbocyanine iodide, and the styryl dyes 2-(4-dimethylaminostyryl)-*N*-methylpyridinium and 4-(4-dimethylaminstyryl)-*N*-methylpyridinium iodide). These probes showed an enhanced mitochondrial staining in the proximal and distal tubule (Plate 3), suggesting regioselective membrane changes in these regions and/or an increased mitochondrial function. In addition, the resting levels of peroxide formation (shown by 2′,7′-dichlorofluorescein) demonstrated an increase peroxide staining (Plate 4) in the distal tubule (I. Seefeldt *et al.*, unpublished results).

Taken together, the data suggest that the primary sites of injury following lithocholic acid exposure are the proximal and especially distal tubular cells. There is also an enhanced level of peroxide present in these regions, which suggests that oxidative injury may be involved in the early genesis of bile acid-related nephrotoxicity.

Thus the combination of precision-cut renal slices and fluorescent probes provides an immediate insight into the biochemical mechanism of bile acid effects on the intact kidney that could not otherwise be easily identified.

VII. CONCLUSIONS

Inevitably, *in vitro* investigations must produce artefacts, because the complex renal system has been disrupted and extrarenal processes (such as hepatic metabolism of haloalkanes to their cystine derivatives), haemodynamic factors, compartmentalization of the multicellular organ have been lost or changed. Thus disruption of anatomical integrity and cell–cell interactions leads to the disordering of a highly compartmentalized system. It is therefore likely that some *in vitro* data will be anomalous, but thus far many changes in renal cell systems do reflect *in vivo* processes and are highly relevant to nephrotoxicity. This augers well for the future of *in vitro* nephrotoxicity studies, but several factors still make it difficult to distinguish between non-specific cytotoxicity that is irrelevant to *in vivo* damage and target selective injury affecting discrete anatomical regions in the kidney. Any attempt to define the mechanism(s) of target selective toxicity *in vitro* depends on the ability to show, a priori, that the same cellular injury occurs specifically in isolated cells. The selective targeting of chemicals for discrete cells within the kidney can be a useful means of developing two strategies for *in vitro* renal research:

1. To establish what biochemical functions are changed at an early stage after exposure to chemicals that target for them, or a biochemical change that is a selective indicator of the type of injury (e.g. lipid changes in cyclosporin and cytosegrosomes in aminoglycoside-exposed cells). Once these criteria are defined, they will offer the most useful biochemical basis by which to undertake routine toxicological screening on these cells.
2. To define what biochemical functions are perturbated. This will give a rational basis to study the primary mechanism of target cell toxicity.

It would be unwise (and undesirable) to focus on either of these approaches to the exclusion of the other. The characterization of biochemical criteria that are indicative of injury in the presence of chemicals with well-defined positive or negative *in vivo* toxicity, together with concentration data and other variables that relate to *in vivo* toxicity, should be used to identify possible areas of mechanisms. The more we understand about mechanisms, the better will be the rational basis for developing valid screening criteria, which are reliable and can be used to investigate interspecies differences. This will serve to help validate where extrapolation can be undertaken, in order to assess human health hazards. Furthermore, the development of cell-free methods for screening for toxicity could be greatly expedited by better understanding of which primary mechanisms are involved in target cell selective toxicity.

While it is possible to separate target from non-target cells and culture these individually, it may be inappropriate to study them in isolation because of cell–cell interactions in the intact organ. Furthermore, the separation of mixed cells is very complex, and while there are good methods to separate blood cells, this is much more difficult to achieve from solid organs. The tissue has to be dispersed into free cells, the identity of which then becomes uncertain.[322] Inevitably many cells are damaged by the mechanical or enzymic methods of dispersion, and the anoxia that develops during some of the separation procedures may compromise cell viability. The different approaches used to separate heterogeneous cells are also time-consuming, costly, generally of low efficiency and may yield high proportions of non-viable cells.[323] In addition, there may still be marked heterogeneity in these 'purified' populations[324] and even in cell lines.[212,213,325] This impure cell population may arise because the criteria used to separate different cells generally make use of only one of a number of determinants. These include size and/or density,[149] cell surface charge, the presence or absence of surface lectin or antibody binding sites, attachment and osmotic stability;[19] all of these are characteristics that may be shared by morphologically different cell types. Mixed populations of cells can be isolated and grown, but conventional biochemical methods cannot be used to study the target cell type in the presence of a non-target population.

The potential future uses of the single cell approach to understanding the mechanisms of selective injury and general cytotoxicity (and hence to develop rational *in vitro* tests for evaluating chemical safety and improving drug design) are exciting. Most of the future techniques that can answer the important questions are well-established parts of the cell biologist's armamentarium. Recent advances in cell biology have included computer-based image analysis of the movement and changes in shapes of cells, which will allow us to understand better the role the cytoskeleton plays in normal cell function, real-time multioptical system imaging and image manipulation to combine the most relevant and productive features of different illumination systems used for viewing.

On the premise that no single *in vivo* or *in vitro* method can elucidate the mechanistic basis of toxicity, there will be inherent uncertainty as to what should be studied in *in vitro* renal systems. It is therefore advisable not to separate whole animal studies from *in vitro* alternatives, or mechanistic investigations from screening procedures. The complexity of the kidney needs to be answered using a holistic integrated approach. *In vitro* methods provide information on the mechanism of primary insult and the effect on cell viability for screening methods. This approach can also be used to develop an understanding of the basis of secondary renal changes that contribute to the cascade of chronic renal degeneration if tissue is harvested over a period of time.

The last comment: *In vitro* technologies are advancing rapidly, improving the scientific validity of this approach, and extending their use.[5,17] The future is therefore one in which more *in vitro* techniques will be used, better to answer questions regarding how to understand disease and improve health for animals and humans.

ACKNOWLEDGEMENTS

The authors acknowledge financial support from the European Union, UFC, Dr Hadwen Trust for Humane Research, Humane Research Trust, FRAME, British Council and, in part, the Wellcome Trust. They are grateful to M. E. van Ek for typing, Professor Benjamin Trump for providing the figures illustrating calcium demodulation in cultured renal cells and Drs Cormick McKilty and Sean Doyle for the figures on the cell-specific localization of the glutathione-*S*-transferase isoforms. Thanks to Mr Seefeldt for providing Plates 3 and 4.

REFERENCES

1. Walker, L. A. and Valtin, H. (1982) Biological importance of nephron heterogeneity. *Annu. Rev. Physiol.* **44:** 203–219.
2. CEC-IPCS (1989) International Workshop on the Health Significance of Nephrotoxicity. *Toxicol. Lett.* **46:** 1–301.
3. WHO (1991) *Environmental Health Criteria Series Number 119, Principles and Methods for the Assessment of Nephrotoxicity Associated with Exposure to Chemicals.* WHO, Geneva.
4. US Academy of Science (1995) *Task Force on Nephrotoxicity: Implications for US Health Care.* US Academy of Science, Washington, DC.
5. Bach, P. H., Morin, J. -P. and Pfaller, W. (1996) Nephrotoxicity – What we have learned and what we still need to know? *Toxicol. Ecotoxicol. News* **3:** 4–13.
6. Venkatachalam, M. J., Bernard, D. B., Donohoe, J. F. and Levinsky, N. G. (1978) Ischemic damage and repair in the rat proximal tubule: differences among the S_1, S_2, and S_3 segments. *Kidney Int.* **14:** 31–49.
7. Bach, P. H. and Bridges, J. W. (1985) Chemically induced renal papillary necrosis and upper urothelial carcinoma. *Crit. Rev. Toxicol.* **15:** 217–439.
8. Bach, P. H., and Gregg, N. J. (1988) Experimentally induced renal papillary necrosis and upper urothelial carcinoma. *Int. Rev. Exp. Pathol.* **30:** 1–54.
9. Orrenius, S. (1985) Biochemical mechanisms of cytotoxicity, *TIPS FEST Suppl.* **November** 15–20.

10. Orrenius, S., McConkey, D. J., Bellomo, G. and Nicotera, P. (1989) Role of Ca^{2+} in toxic cell killing. *TIPS* **10:** 281–285.
11. Trump, B. F., Berezesky, I. K., Elliget, K. A., Smith, M. A. and Phelps, P. C. (1990) Nephrotoxicity *in vitro*: role of ion deregulation in signal transduction following injury – studies utilizing digital imaging fluorescence microscopy. *Toxicol. In Vitro* **4:** 409–414.
12. Trump, B. F., Berezesky, I. K. and Smith, M. W. (1993) Cellular calcium and mitochondrial dysfunction. In Lash, L. H. and Jones, D. P. (eds) *Methods in Toxicology, Vol. 2: Mitochondrial Dysfunction*, Section V, pp. 337–386. Academic Press, New York.
13. Bohman, S.-O. (1980) The ultrastructure of the renal medulla and the interstitial cells. In Mandal, A. K. and Bohman, S.-O., (eds) *The Renal Papilla and Hypertension*, pp. 7–34. Plenum, New York.
14. Kreisberg, J. I. and Karnovsky, M. J. (1983) Glomerular cells in culture. *Kidney Int.* **23:** 439–447.
15. Belleman, P. (1980) Primary monolayer cultures of liver parenchymal cells and kidney tubules as a useful new model for biochemical pharmacology and experimental toxicology. Studies *in vitro* on hepatic membrane transport, induction of liver enzymes and adaptive changes in renal cortical enzymes. *Arch. Toxicol.* **44:** 63–84.
16. Purchase, I. F. H. and Conning, D. (eds) (1986) International Conference on Practical *In Vitro* Toxicology. *Food Chem. Toxicol.* **24:** 447–818.
17. Hawkesworth, G. M., Bach, P. H., Nagelkerke, J. F. *et al.* (1995) Nephrotoxicity testing *in vitro*. The report and recommendation of ECVAM workshop 10. *ATLA* **23:** 713–727.
18. Acosta, D., Sorensen, E. M. B., Anuforo, D. C. *et al.* (1985) An *in vitro* approach to the study of target organ toxicity of drugs and chemicals. *In Vitro Cell. Dev. Biol.* **21:** 495–504.
19. Bach, P. H., Ketley, C. P., Benns, S. E., Ahmed, I. and Dixit, M. (1985) The use of isolated and cultured renal cells in nephrotoxicity – practice, potential and problems. In Bach, P. H. and Lock, E. A. (eds) *Renal Heterogeneity and Target Cell Toxicity*, pp. 505–518. Wiley, Chichester.
20. Bach, P. H., Ketley, C. P., Dixit. M. and Ahmed, I. (1986) The mechanisms of target cell injury in nephrotoxicity. *Food Chem. Toxicol.* **24:** 775–779.
21. Wilson, P. D. (1986) Use of cultured renal tubular cells in the study of cell injury. *Mineral Electrol. Metab.* **12:** 71–84.
22. Smith, M. A., Acosta, D. and Bruckner, J. V. (1986) Development of a primary culture system of rat kidney cortical cells to evaluate the nephrotoxicity of xenobiotics. *Food Chem. Toxicol.* **24:** 551–556.
23. Kreisberg, J. I. and Wilson, P. D. (1988) Renal cell culture. *J. Electron Micros. Techn.* **9:** 235–263.
24. Bach, P. H. and Kwizera, E. N. (1988) Nephrotoxicity: a rational approach to *in vitro* target cell injury in the kidney. *Xenobiotica* **16:** 685–698.
25. Williams, P. D. (1989) The application of renal cells in culture in studying drug-induced nephrotoxicity. *In Vitro Cell. Dev. Biol.* **25:** 800–805.
26. Gandolfi, A. J. and Brendel, K. (1990) *In vitro* systems for nephrotoxicity studies. *Toxicol. In Vitro* **4:** 337–345.
27. Gstraunthaler, G., Steinmassl, D. and Pfaller, W. (1990) Renal cell cultures: a tool for studying tubular function and nephrotoxicity. *Toxicol. Lett.* **53:** 1–7.
28. L'Eplattenier, H. F., Zhao, J., Pfannkuch, F., Scholtysik, G. and Wüthrich, A. (1990) Cell culture in nephrotoxicity testing. *Toxicol. Lett.* **53:** 227–229.
29. Simmons, N. L. (1990) Tissue culture of established renal cell lines. *Methods Enzymol.* **191:** 426–436.
30. Pfaller, W., Gstraunthaler, G. and Willinger, C. C. (1990) Morphology of renal tubular damage from nephrotoxins. *Toxicol. Lett.* **53:** 39–43.
31. Curthoys, N. P. and Bellemann, P. (1979) Renal cortical cells in primary monolayer culture. Enzymatic changes and morphological observations. *Exp. Cell Res.* **121:** 31–45.
32. Sato, G. (1980) Methods for growth of cultured cells in serum-free medium. *Anal. Biochem.*, **102:** 255–270.
33. Lelongt, B., Vandewalle, A., Brenchley, P. E. C. *et al.* (1993) Major influence of cell differentiation status on characteristics of proteoglycans synthesized by cultured rabbit renal proximal tubule cell: role of insulin and dexamethasone. *J. Cell. Physiol.* **154:** 175–191.
34. Morin, J. P., Leclere C., Marouillat, S. and Monteil C. (1996) Some milestones in *in vitro* organ toxicity assessment: the kidney as a case study. *Toxicol. In Vitro* **9:** 795–814.

35. Gstraunthaler, G. and Pfaller, W. (1992) Continuous renal cell lines as *in vitro* tools to study nephrotoxicity. In Watson, R. R. (ed.) In Vitro *Methods in Toxicology*, pp. 93–114. CRC Press, Florida.
36. Gstraunthaler, G. and Pfaller, W. (1992) The use of cultured renal epithelial cells in *in vitro* assessment of xenobiotic-induced nephrotoxicity. In Anders, M. W., Dekant, W., Henschler, D., Oberleithner, H. and Silbernagl, S. (eds) *Renal Disposition and Nephrotoxicity of Xenobiotics*, pp. 27–62. Academic Press, New York.
37. Chang, S.-G., Toth, K., Black, J. D. *et al.* (1992) Growth of human renal cortical tissue on collagen Gel. *In Vitro Cell. Dev. Biol.* **28A:** 128–135.
38. Palmoski, M. J., Masters, B. A., Flint, O. P., Ford, S. M. and Oleson, F. B. (1992) Characterization of rabbit primary proximal tubule kidney cell cultures grown on Millicell-HA membrane filters. *Toxicol. In Vitro* **6:** 557–567.
39. Jakoby, W. B. and Pastan, I. H. (ed.) (1979) *Cell Culture, Methods in Enzymology*, Vol. 58. Academic Press, New York.
40. Epstein, F. H., Brosnan, J. T., Tange, J. D. and Ross, B. D. (1982) Improved function with amino acids in the isolated perfused kidney. *Am. J. Physiol.* **243:** F284–F292.
41. Green, C. E., Dabbs, J. E., Allen, K. L., Tyson, C. A. and Rauckman, E. J. (1989) Characterization of isolated renal proximal tubules for nephrotoxicity studies. In Bach, P. H. and Lock, E. A. (eds) *Nephrotoxicity:* In Vitro *to* In Vivo, *Animals to Man*, pp. 719–723. Plenum Press, New York.
42. Green, C. E., Dabbs, J. E., Tyson, C. A. and Rauckman, E. J. (1990) Stress initiated during isolation of rat renal proximal tubules limits *in vitro* survival. *Ren. Fail.* **12:** 147–156.
43. Gower, J. D., Lane, N. J., Goddard, J. G., Manek, S., Ambrose, I. J. and Green, C. J. (1992) Antioxidant capacity in renal preservation. *Biochem. Pharmacol.* **43:** 2341–2348.
44. Toutain, H. and Morin, J. P. (1992) Renal proximal tubule cell-cultures for studying drug-induced nephrotoxicity and modulation of phenotype expression medium components. *Renal Fail.* **14:** 371–383.
45. Toutain, H. and Courjault, F. (1993) The use of the epithelial kidney OK cell-line for studying the nephrotoxicity of anticancer platinum coordination complexes. *ATLA* **21:** 30–37.
46. Mudge, G. H. (1985) Pathogenesis of nephrotoxicity: pharmacological principles. In Bach, P. H. and Lock, E. A. (eds) *Renal Heterogeneity and Target Cell Toxicity*, pp. 1–12. Wiley, Chichester.
47. Moffat, D. B. (1981) New ideas on the anatomy of the kidney. *J. Clin. Pathol.* **34:** 1197–1206.
48. Ullrich, K. J., Rumrich, G., Gemborys, M. W. and Dekant, W. (1991) Renal transport and nephrotoxicity. In Bach, P. H., Gregg, N. J., Wilks, M. F. and Delacruz, L. (eds) *Nephrotoxicity. Mechanisms, Early Diagnosis, and Therapeutic Management*, pp. 1–8. Marcel Dekker, New York.
49. Viano, I., Eandi, M. and Santiano, M. (1983) Toxic effects of some antibiotics on rabbit kidney cells. *Int. J. Tissue React.* **5:** 181–186.
50. Smith, M. A. and Acosta, D. (1987) Cephaloridine toxicity in primary cultures of rat renal cortical epithelial cells. *Toxicol. In Vitro* **1:** 23–29.
51. Tay, L. K., Bregman, C. L., Masters, B. A. and Williams, P. D. (1988) Effects of *cis*-diamminedichloroplatinum (II) on rabbit kidney *in vivo* and on rabbit renal proximal tubule cells in culture. *Cancer Res.* **48:** 2538–2543.
52. Rees, J. A., Evans, J. G., Blackmore, M., Spencer, A. J. and Gray, T. J. B. (1994) Use of scanning electron microscopy in the study of nephrotoxin-induced renal proximal tubular damage *in vitro*. *Toxicol. In Vitro* **8:** 601–603.
53. Ross, B. D. and Guder, W. G. (1982) Heterogeneity and compartmentation in the kidney. In Sies, H. (ed.) *Metabolic Compartmentation*, pp. 363–409. Academic Press, New York.
54. Guder, W. G. and Ross, B. D. (1984) Enzyme distribution along the nephron. *Kidney Int.* **26:** 101–111.
55. Wachsmuth, E. D. (1985) Renal heterogeneity at a light microscopic level. In Bach, P. H. and Lock, E. A. (eds) *Renal Heterogeneity and Target Cell Toxicity*, pp. 13–30. Wiley, Chichester.
56. Bach, P. H., Gregg, N. J. and Wachsmuth, E. D. (1987) The application of histochemistry at the light microscopic level to the study of nephrotoxicity. In Bach, P. H. and Lock, E. A. (eds) *Nephrotoxicity in the Experimental and the Clinical Situation*, pp. 19–84. Nijhoff, Dordrecht.
57. Wilks, M. L. and Bach, P. H. (1992) Renal enzymes as the basis for alternative methods of safety screening *in vitro* and understanding the mechanism of nephrotoxicity. In Jung, K., Burchardt, U. and Mattenheimer, H. (eds) *Urinary Enzymes in Clinical and Experimental Medicine*, pp. 299–317. Springer, Heidelberg.

58. Takahashi, T., Kakuno, K., Yamada, H. and Endou, H. (1989) Intranephron distribution of purine-metabolizing enzymes in rats. *Renal Physiol. Biochem.* **12:** 287–294.
59. Striker, G. E., Lange, M. A., MacKay, K., Bernstein, K. and Striker, L. J. (1987) Glomerular cells *in vitro*. *Adv. Nephrol.* **16:** 169–186.
60. Beckett, G. J. and Hayes, J. D. (1993) Glutathione *S*-transferase: biomedical applications. *Adv. Clin. Chem.* **30:** 281–380.
61. Neuhoff, V. (ed.) (1973) *Micromethods in Molecular Biology*. Chapman and Hall, London.
62. Chayen, J. (1985) Quantitative cytochemistry: a precise form of cellular biochemistry. *Biochem. Soc. Trans.* **12:** 887–898.
63. Bach, P. H. (1990) Fluorescent probes for understanding the mechanisms of chemically induced cellular injuries. *Marine Environ. Res.* **28:** 351–356.
64. Fields, R. D. and Lancaster, M. V. (1993) Dual attribute continuous monitoring of cell proliferation/cytotoxicity. *Am. Biotech. Lab.* **11:** 48–50.
65. DeFries, R. and Mitsuhashi, M. (1995) Quantification of mitogen induced human lymphocyte proliferation: comparison of Alamar Blue assay to ^{3}H-thymidine incorporation assay. *J. Clin. Lab. Anal.* **9:** 89–95.
66. Ross, B. D. (1978) The isolated perfused rat kidney. *Clin. Sci. Mol. Med.* **55:** 513–521.
67. Schurek, H. J. (1980) Application of the isolated perfused rat kidney in nephrology. *Contrib. Nephrol.* **19:** 176–190.
68. Maack, T. (1980) Physiological evaluation of the isolated perfused rat kidney. *Am. J. Physiol.* **238:** F71–F78.
69. Newton, J. F. and Hook, J. B. (1981) Isolated perfused rat kidney. *Methods Enzymol.* **77:** 94–105.
70. Bach, P. H. and Lock, E. A. (1982) The use of renal tissue slices, perfusion and infusion techniques to assess renal function and malfunction. In Bach, P. H., Bonner, F. W., Bridges, J. W. and Lock, E. A. (eds) *Nephrotoxicity: Assessment and Pathogenesis*, pp. 128–143. Wiley, Chichester.
71. Schramek, H., Willinger, C. C., Gstraunthaler, G. and Pfaller, W. (1992) Endothelium-3 modulates glomerular filtration rate in the isolated perfused rat kidney. *Renal Physiol. Biochem.* **15:** 325–333.
72. Abel, J., Hohr, D. and Schurek, H. J. (1987) Renal handling of cadmium and cadmium–metallothionein: studies on the isolated perfused rat kidney. *Arch. Toxicol.* **60:** 370–375.
73. Endre, Z. H., Nicholls, L. G., Ratcliffe, P. J. and Ledingham, J. G. G. (1989) Prevention and reversal of mercuric chloride-induced increases in renal vascular resistance by captopril. In Bach, P. H. and Lock, E. A. (eds) *Nephrotoxicity:* In Vitro *to* In Vivo, *Animals to Man*, pp. 103–106. Plenum Press, New York.
74. Bekersky, I. (1983) Use of the isolated perfused kidney as a tool in drug disposition studies. *Drug Metab. Rev.* **14:** 931–960.
75. Smith, M. A., Hewitt, W. R. and Hook, J. B. (1988) *In vitro* methods in renal toxicology. In Atterwill, C. K. and Steele, C. E. (eds) In vitro *Methods in Toxicology*, pp. 13–35. Cambridge University Press, Cambridge.
76. Collier, V. U., Lietman, P. S. and Mitch, W. E. (1979) Evidence for luminal uptake of gentamicin in the perfused rat kidney. *J. Pharmacol. Exp. Ther.* **210:** 247–251.
77. Miura, K., Goldstein, R. S., Pasino, D. A. and Hook, J. B. (1987) Cisplatin nephrotoxicity: role of filtration and tubular transport of cisplatin in isolated perfused kidneys. *Toxicology* **44:** 147–158.
78. Emslie, K. R., Smail, M. C., Calder, I. C., Hart, S. J. and Tange, J. D. (1981) Paracetamol and the isolated perfused kidney: metabolism and functional effects. *Xenobiotica* **11:** 43–50.
79. Emslie, K. R., Calder, I. C., Hart, S. J. and Tange, J. D. (1981) Induction of paracetamol metabolism in the isolated perfused kidney. *Xenobiotica* **11:** 579–587.
80. Muldoon, R. T. and McMartin, K. E. (1994) Ethanol acutely impairs the renal conservation of 5-methyltetrahydrofolate in the isolated perfused rat kidney. *Alcohol Clin. Exp. Res.* **18:** 333–339.
81. Lockwood, T. D. and Bosmann, H. B. (1979) The use of urinary *N*-acetyl-beta-glucosaminidase in human renal toxicology. I. Partial biochemical characterization and excretion in humans and release from the isolated perfused rat kidney. *Toxicol. Appl. Pharmacol.* **49:** 323–336.
82. Schurek, H. J. and Alt, J. M. (1981) Effect of albumin on the function of perfused rat kidney. *Am. J. Physiol.* **240:** F569–F576.
83. Alcorn, D., Emslie, K. R., Ross, B. D., Ryan, G. B. and Tange J. D. (1981) Selective distal nephron damage during isolated kidney perfusion. *Kidney Int.* **19:** 638–647.

84. Schurek, H. J. (1988) Die Nierenmarkhypoxie: ein Schlüssel zum Verständnis des akuten Nierenversagens? *Klin. Wochenschr.* **66:** 828–835.
85. Gottschalk, C. W. and Lassiter, W. E. (1973) Micropuncture methodology. Chapter 6. In Orloff, J. and Berliner, W. R. (eds) *Handbook of Physiology*, pp. 129–143. American Physiological Society, Washington, D.C.
86. Lewy, J. E. and Pesce, A. (1973) Micropuncture study of albumin transfer in aminonucleoside nephrosis in the rat. *Pediat. Res.* **7:** 553–559.
87. Landwehr, D. M., Carvalho, J. S. and Oken, D. E. (1977) Micropuncture studies of the filtration and absorption of albumin by nephrotic rats. *Kidney Int.* **11:** 9–17.
88. Burg, M., Green, N., Sohraby, S., Steele, R. and Handler, J. (1982) Differentiated function in cultured epithelia derived from thick ascending limbs. *Am. J. Physiol.* **242:** C229–C233.
89. Diezi, J. and Roch-Ramel, F. (1987) The use of single nephron techniques in renal toxicity studies. In Bach, P. H. and Lock, E. A. (eds) *Nephrotoxicity in the Experimental and the Clinical Situation*, pp. 317–358. Nijhoff, Dordrecht.
90. Ullrich, K. J. and Greger, R. (1985) Approaches to the study of tubular transport function. In Seldin, D. G. and Giebisch, G. (eds) *The Kidney, Physiology and Pathology*, pp. 427–455. Raven Press, New York.
91. Berndt, W. O. (1976) Use of renal slice technique for evaluation of renal tubular transport processes. *Environ. Health Perspect.* **15:** 73–88.
92. Roth, K. S., Holtzapple, P., Genel, M. and Segal, S. (1979) Uptake of glycine by human kidney cortex. *Metabolism* **18:** 677–681.
93. Ruegg, C. E., Gandolfi, A. J., Nagle, R. B., Krumdieck, C. L. and Brendel, K. (1987) Preparation of positional renal slices for study of cell-specific toxicity. *J. Pharmacol. Methods* **17:** 111–123.
94. Kyle, G. M., Luthra, R., Bruckner, J. V., Mackenzie, W. F. and Acosta, D. (1983) Assessment of functional, morphological and enzymatic tests for acute nephrotoxicity induced by mercuric chloride. *J. Toxicol. Environ. Health* **12:** 99–117.
95. Miyajima, H., Hewitt, W. R., Cote, M. G. and Plaa, G. L. (1983) Relationships between histological and functional indices of acute chemically induced nephro toxicity. *Fund. Appl. Toxicol.* **3:** 543–551.
96. Kacew, S. and Hirsch, G. H. (1981) Evaluation of nephrotoxicity of various compounds by means of *in vitro* techniques and comparison to *in vivo* methods. In Hook, J. B. (ed.) *Toxicology of the Kidney*, pp. 77–98. Raven Press, New York.
97. Ruegg, C. E., Gandolfi, A. J., Nagle, R. B. and Brendel, K. (1987) Differential patterns of injury to the proximal tubule of renal cortical slices following *in vitro* exposure to mercuric chloride, potassium dichromate or hypoxic conditions. *Toxicol. Appl. Pharmacol.* **90:** 261–273.
98. Hannemann, J. and Baumann, K. (1988) Cisplatin-induced lipid peroxidation and decrease of gluconeogenesis in rat kidney cortex: different effects of antioxidants and radical scavengers. *Toxicology* **51:** 119–132.
99. Zhang, J.-G., Zhong, L. F., Zhang, M. and Xia, Y. X. (1992) Protection effects of procaine on oxidative stress and toxicities of renal cortical slices from rats caused by cisplatin *in vitro*. *Arch. Toxicol.* **66:** 354–358.
100. Zhang, J.-G., Zhong, L. F., Zhang, M., Ma, X. L., Xia, Y. X. and Lindup, W. E. (1994) Amelioration of cisplatin toxicity in rat renal cortical slices by dithiothreitol *in vitro*. *Hum. Exp. Toxicol.* **13:** 89–93.
101. Zhang, J.-G. and Lindup, W. E. (1993) Role of mitochondria in cisplatin-induced oxidative damage exhibited by rat renal cortical slices. *Biochem. Pharmacol.* **45:** 2215–2222.
102. Zhang, J.-G. and Lindup, W. E. (1994) Effects of procaine and two of its metabolites on cisplatin-induced kidney injury *in vitro*: mitochondrial aspects. *Toxicol. In Vitro* **8:** 477–481.
103. Zhang, J.-G. and Lindup, W. E. (1994) Cisplatin nephrotoxicity: decreases in mitochondrial protein sulphydryl concentration and calcium uptake by mitochondria from rat renal cortical slices. *Biochem. Pharmacol.* **47:** 1127–1135.
104. Rankin, G. O., Shih, H-C., Teets, V. J., Yang, D. J., Nicoll, D. W. and Brown, P. I. (1991) *N*-3,5-dichlorophenyl)succinimide nephrotoxicity: evidence against the formation of nephrotoxic glutanione or cysteine conjugates. *Toxicology* **68:** 307–325.
105. Rankin, G. O., Valentovic, M. A., Beers, K. W. *et al.* (1993) Renal and hepatic toxicity of monochloroacetanilides in the Fischer 344 rat. *Toxicology* **79:** 181–193.
106. Rankin, G. O., Valentovic, M. A., Nicoll, D. W., Ball, J. G. *et al.* (1994) *In vivo* and *in vitro* 4-amino-2,6-dichlorophenol nephrotoxicity and hepatotoxicity in the Fischer 344 rat. *Toxicology* **90:** 115–128.

107. Stijntjes, G. J., Commandeur, J. N. M., Te-Koppele, J. M., McGuinness, S., Gandolfi, A. J. and Vermeulen, N. P. E. (1993) Examination of the structure–toxicity relationships of L-cysteine-*S*-conjugates of halogenated alkenes and their corresponding mercapturic acids in rat renal tissue slices. *Toxicology* **79:** 67–79.
108. Trevisan, A., Meneghetti, P., Maso, S. and Troso, O. (1993) *In vitro* mechanisms of 1,2-dichloropropane nephrotoxicity using the renal cortical slice model. *Hum. Exp. Toxicol.* **12:** 117–121.
109. Lock, E. A., Strasser, J. Jr., Bus, J. S. and Charbonneau, M. (1993) Studies on the renal transport of trimethylpentanoic acid metabolites of 2,2,4-trimethylpentane in rat renal cortical slices. *J. Appl. Toxicol.* **13:** 291–296.
110. Trevisan, A., Meneghetti, P., Maso, S., Secondin, L. and Nicoletto, G. (1992) Sex- and age-related nephrotoxicity due to 1,2-dichloropropane *in vitro*. *Arch. Toxicol.* **66:** 641–645.
111. Carpenter, H. M. and Mudge, G. H. (1981) Acetaminophen nephrotoxicity: studies on renal acetylation and deacetylation. *J. Pharmacol. Exp. Ther.* **218:** 161–167.
112. Kluwe, W. M. and Hook, J. B. (1978) Functional nephrotoxicity of gentamicin in the rat. *Toxicol. Appl. Pharmacol.* **45:** 163–175.
113. Wold, J. S., Turnipseed, S. A. and Miller, B. L. (1979) The effect of renal cation transport inhibition on cephaloridine nephrotoxicity. *Toxicol. Appl. Pharmacol.* **47:** 115–122.
114. Cojocel, C., Gottsche, U., Tollt, K. and Baumann, K. (1988) Nephrotoxic potential of first-, second- and third-generation cephalosporins. *Arch. Toxicol.* **62:** 458–464
115. Meisner, H. and Selanik, P. (1979) Inhibition of renal gluconeogenesis in rats by ochratoxin. *Biochem. J.* **180:** 681–684.
116. Arthus, M. F., Bergeron, M. and Scriver, C. R. (1982) Topology of membrane exposure in the renal cortex slice. Studies of glutathione and maltose cleavage. *Biochim. Biophys. Acta* **692:** 371–376.
117. Krumdieck, C. L., dos Santos, J. E. and Ho, K. (1980) A new instrument for the rapid preparation of tissue slices. *Anal. Biochem.* **104:** 118–123.
118. McGuinness, S., Gandolfi, A. J. and Brendel, K. (1993) Use of renal slices and renal tubule suspensions for *in vitro* toxicity studies. *In Vitro Toxicol. J. Mol. Cell. Toxicol.* **6:** 1–24.
119. Ruegg, C. E. (1994) Preparation of precision-cut renal slices and renal proximal tubular fragments for evaluating segment-specific nephrotoxicity. *J. Pharmacol. Toxicol. Methods* **31:** 125–133.
120. Phelps, J. S., Gandolfi, A. J., Brendel, K. and Dorr, R. T. (1987) Cisplatin nephrotoxicity: *in vitro* studies with precision-cut rabbit renal cortical slices. *Toxicol. Appl. Pharmacol.* **90:** 501–512.
121. Fisher, R. L., Sannik, J. T., Gandolfi, A. J. and Brendel, K. (1994) Toxicity of cisplatin and mercuric chloride in human kidney cortical slices. *Hum. Exp. Toxicol.* **13:** 517–523.
122. Fisher, R. L., Halal, S. J., Sanuik, J. T., Scott, K. S., Gandolfi, A. J. and Brendel, K. (1993) Cold and cryopreservation of human liver and kidney slices. *Cryobiology* **30:** 250–261.
123. de Kanter, R. and Koster, H. J. (1995) Cryopreservation of rat and monkey liver slices. *ATLA* **23:** 653–665.
124. Fry, J. R. and Perry, N. K. (1981) The effect of Aroclor 1254 pretreatment on the phase I and phase II metabolism of 7-ethoxycoumarin in isolated viable rat kidney cells. *Biochem. Pharmacol.* **30:** 1197–1201.
125. Brendel, K. and Meezan, E. (1975) Isolation and properties of proximal kidney tubules obtained without collagenase treatment. *Fed. Proc.* **34:** 308.
126. Norgaard, J. O. R. (1976) A new method for the isolation of ultrastructurally preserved glomeruli. *Kidney Int.* **9:** 278–285.
127. McGuiness, S. J. and Ryan, M. P. (1994) Mechanism of cis-platin nephrotoxicity in rat proximal tubule suspension. *Toxicol. In Vitro* **8:** 1203–1212.
128. Vinay, P., Gougoux, A. and Lemieux, G. (1981) Isolation of a pure suspension of rat proximal tubules. *Am. J. Physiol.* **241:** F403–F411.
129. Jones, D. P., Sundby, B., Ormstad, K. and Orrenius, S. (1979) Use of isolated kidney cells for study of drug metabolism. *Biochem. Pharmacol.* **28:** 929–935.
130. Gstraunthaler, G. J. A., Pfaller, W. and Kotanko, P. (1985) Biochemical characterization of renal epithelial cell cultures (LLC-PK_1 and MDCK). *Am. J. Physiol.* **248:** F536–F544.
131. Stumpf, B. and Kraus, H. (1978) Inhibition of gluconeogenesis in isolated rat kidney tubules by branched chain alpha-ketoacids. *Pediatr. Res.* **12:** 1039–1044.
132. Baverel, G., Bonnard, M., D'Armagnac de Castanet, E. and Pellet, M. (1978) Lactate and pyruvate metabolism in isolated renal tubules of normal dogs. *Kidney Int.* **14:** 567–575.

133. Baverel, G., Forissier, M. and Pellet, M. (1980) Lactate and pyruvate metabolism in dog renal outer medulla. Effects of oleate and ketone bodies. *Int. J. Biochem.* **12:** 163–168.
134. Baverel, G., Genoux, C., Forissier, M. and Pellet, M. (1980) Fate of glutamate carbon and nitrogen in isolated guinea-pig kidney-cortex tubules. Evidence for involvement of glutamate dehydrogenase in glutamine synthesis from glutamate. *Biochem. J.* **188:** 873–880.
135. Schlondorff, D., Roczniak, S., Satriano, J. A. and Folkert, V. W. (1980) Prostaglandin synthesis by isolated rat glomeruli: effect of angiotensin II. *Am. J. Physiol.* **239:** F486–F495.
136. Stollenwerk Petrulis, A., Aikawa, M. and Dunn, M. J. (1981) Prostaglandin and thromboxane synthesis by rat glomerular epithelial cells. *Kidney Int.* **20:** 469–474.
137. Sraer, J., Rigaud, M., Bens, M., Rabinovitch, H. and Ardaillou, R. (1983) Metabolism of arachidonic acid via the lipoxygenase pathway in human and murine glomeruli. *J. Biol. Chem.* **258:** 4325–4330.
138. Ormstad, K. (1987) Metabolism of glutathione in the kidney. In Bach, P. H. and Lock, E. A. (ed.) *Nephrotoxicity in the Experimental and the Clinical Situation*, pp. 405–428. Nijhoff, Dordrecht.
139. McLaren, J., Whiting, P. H., Simpson, J. G. and Hawksworth, G. M. (1995) Isolation and characterization of human proximal tubular cells derived from cortical segments. *Hum. Exp. Toxicol.* **14:** 916–922.
140. Savin, V., Karniski, L., Cuppage, F., Hodges, G. and Chanko, A. (1985) Effect of gentamicin on isolated glomeruli and proximal tubules. *Lab. Invest.* **52:** 93–102.
141. Anand-Srivastava, M. B., Vinay, P., Genest, J. and Cantin, M. (1986) Effect of atrial natriuretic factor on adenylate cyclase in various nephron segments. *Am. J. Physiol.* **251:** F417–F423.
142. Chamberlin, M. E., LeFurgey, A. and Mandel, L. J. (1984) Suspension of medullary thick ascending limb tubules from the rabbit kidney. *Am. J. Physiol.* **247:** F955–F964.
143. Koseki, C., Yamaguchi, Y., Furusawa, M. and Endou, H. (1988) Isolation by monoclonal antibody of intercalated cells of rabbit kidney. *Kidney Int.* **33:** 543–554.
144. Wilks, M. L. and Bach, P. H. (1992) Renal enzymes as the basis for alternative methods of safety screening *in vitro* and understanding the mechanism of nephrotoxicity. In Jung, K., Burchardt, U. and Matterheimer, H. (eds) *Urinary Enzymes in Clinical and Experimental Medicine*, pp. 299–317. Springer-Verlag, Heidelberg.
145. Jung, K. Y., Uchida, S. and Endou, H. (1989) Nephrotoxicity assessment by measuring cellular ATP content. I. Substrate specificities in the maintenance of ATP content in isolated rat nephron segments. *Toxicol. Appl. Pharmacol.* **100:** 369–382.
146. Jung, K. Y. and Endou, H. (1989) Nephrotoxicity assessment by measuring cellular ATP content. II. Intranephron site of ochratoxin A nephrotoxicity. *Toxicol. Appl. Pharmacol.* **100:** 383–390.
147. Ormstad, K., Jones, D. P. and Orrenius, S. (1981) Preparation and characterisation of isolated kidney cells. *Methods Enzymol.* **77:** 137–146.
148. Moldeus, P., Ormstad, M. and Reed, D. J. (1980) Turnover of cellular glutathione in isolated rat-kidney cells. *Eur. J. Biochem.* **116:** 13–16.
149. Kreisberg, J. I., Pitts, A. M. and Pretlow, T. G. (1977) Separation of proximal tubule cells from suspensions of rat kidney cells in density gradients of Ficoll in tissue culture medium. *Am. J. Pathol.* **86:** 591–602.
150. Cain, K. and Gurney, J. A. (1993) Isolation and purification of proximal kidney cells by centrifugal elutriation. *Toxicol. In Vitro* **7:** 117–127.
151. Cain, K. and Gurney, J. E. (1994) Immunomagnetic purification of rat proximal kidney cells. *Toxicol. In Vitro* **8:** 13–19.
152. Benns, S. E., Dixit, M., Ahmed, I., Ketley, C. P. and Bach, P. H. (1985) The use of cultured renal medullary cells as an alternative method to live animals for studying renal medullary toxicity. In Goldberg, A. (ed.) *Alternative Methods in Toxicology*, Vol. 3, pp. 435–447. M. A. Liebert, New York.
153. Rylander-Yueh, L.A., Gandolfi, A.J. and Brendel, K. (1985) Use of isolated rabbit renal tubules to examine inhibition of organic acid/base transport by toxins. In Bach, P. H. and Lock, E. A. (eds) *Renal Heterogeneity and Target Cell Toxicity*, pp. 531–534. Wiley, Chichester.
154. Ruegg, C. E. and Mandel, L. J. (1991) Bulk isolation of straight and convoluted proximal tubules from rabbit kidneys: differential glucose-dependent protection during anoxia. In Bach, P. H., Delacruz, L., Gregg, N. J and Wilks, M. F. (eds) *Nephrotoxicity: Early Diagnosis and Therapeutic Management*, pp. 459–465. Marcel Dekker, New York.
155. Edidin, M. (1970) Arapid quantitative fluorescence assay for cell damage by cytotoxic antibodies. *J. Immunol.*, **104**: 1303–1306.

156. Obatomi, D. K. and Plummer, D. T. (1991) Preparation of renal tubules from rat kidney for biochemical investigations *in vitro*. *Biosci. Res. Commun.* **3:** 59–67.
157. Kwizera, E. N., Wilks, M. F. and Bach, P. H. (1990) The effects of aminoglycosides on the incorporation of amino acids and fatty acid oxidation in freshly isolated rat renal proximal tubules. *Toxicol. In Vitro* **3:** 243–253.
158. Endou, H., Koseki, C., Yamada, H. and Obara, T. (1986) Evaluation of nephrotoxicity using isolated nephron segments. In Tanabe, T., Hook, I. B. and Endou, H. (eds) *Nephrotoxicity of Antibiotics and Immunosuppressants*, pp. 207–216. Elsevier Science Publishers BV, Amsterdam.
159. Obatomi, D. K. and Plummer, D. T. (1995) Renal damage caused by gentamicin: a study of the effect *in vitro* using isolated rat proximal tubular fragments. *Toxicol. Lett.* **75:** 75–83.
160. Holdsworth, S. R., Glasgow, E. F., Atkins, R. C. and Thomson, N. M. (1978) Cell characteristics of cultured glomeruli from different animal species. *Nephron* **22:** 454–459.
161. Meezan, E. and Brendel, K. (1973) Effect of ethacrynic acid on oxidative metabolism in isolated glomeruli. *J. Pharmacol. Exp. Ther.* **187:** 352–364.
162. Carlson, E. C. (1987) Morphology of isolated renal tubular and glomerular basement membranes. In Price, R. G. and Hudson, B. G. (eds) *Renal Basement Membranes in Health and Disease*, pp. 99–113. Academic Press, London.
163. Sraer, J. D., Baud, L., Sraer, J., Delarue, F. and Ardaillou, R. (1982) Stimulation of PGE_2 synthesis by mercuric chloride in rat glomeruli and glomerular cells *in vitro*. *Kidney Int.* **21:** S63–S68.
164. Skorecki, K. L., Ballermann, B. J., Rennke, H. G. and Brenner, B. M. (1983) Angiotensin II receptor regulation in isolated renal glomeruli. *Fed. Proc.* **42:** 3064–3071.
165. Barrio, V., De Arriba, G., Lopez-Novoa, J. M. and Rodriguez-Puyol, D. (1987) Atrial natriuretic peptide inhibits glomerular contraction induced by angiotensin II and platelet activating factor. *Eur. J. Pharmacol.* **135:** 93–96.
166. Striker, G. E., Killen, P. D. and Farin, F. M. (1980) Human glomerular cells *in vitro*: isolation and characterization. *Transplant. Proc.* **12:** 88–99.
167. Gordon, E. M., Whiting, P. H., Simpson, J. G. and Hawksworth, G. M. (1989) Isolated rat renal proximal tubular cells: a model to investigate drug induced nephrotoxicity. In Bach, P. H. and Lock, E. A. (eds) *Nephrotoxicity:* In Vitro *to* In Vivo, *Animals to Man*, pp. 725–730. Plenum Press, New York.
168. Lash, L. H. and Tokarz, J. J. (1989) Isolation of two distinct populations of cells from rat kidney cortex and their use in the study of chemical-induced toxicity. *Anal. Biochem.* **182:** 271–279.
169. Smith, W. L. and Garcia-Perez, A. (1985) Immunodissection: use of monoclonal antibodies to isolate specific types of renal cells. *Am. J. Physiol.* **248:** F1–F7.
170. Toutain, H., Fillastre, J.-P. and Morin, J.-P. (1989) Preparative free flow electrophoresis for the isolation of two populations of proximal cells from the rabbit kidney. *Eur. J. Cell Biol.* **49:** 274–280.
171. Chen, T. C., Curthoys, N. P., Langenaur, C. F. and Puschett, J. B (1989) Characterization of primary cell cultures derived from rat renal proximal tubules. *In Vitro Cell. Dev. Biol.* **25:** 714–722.
172. Fine, L. G. and Sakhrani, L. M. (1986) Proximal tubular cells in primary culture. *Mineral Electrol. Metab.* **12:** 51–57.
173. Grenier, F. C. (1986) Characteristics of renal collecting tubule cells in primary culture. *Mineral Electrol. Metab.* **12:** 58–63.
174. Toutain, H., Vauclin-Jaques, N., Fillastre, J. P. and Morin, J. P. (1991) Biochemical, functional, and morphological characterization of a primary culture of rabbit proximal tubule cells. *Exp. Cell Res.* **194:** 9–18.
175. Kreisberg, J. I., Hoover, R. L. and Karnovsky, M. J. (1978) Isolation and characterization of rat glomerular epithelial cells *in vitro*. *Kidney Int.* **14:** 21–30.
176. Kreisberg, J. I. and Hassid, A. (1986) Functional properties of glomerular cells in culture. *Mineral Electrol. Metab.* **12:** 25–31.
177. Foidart, J. B., Deckanne, C. A., Mahieu, P., Creutz, C. E. and DeMey, J. (1979) Tissue culture of normal rat glomeruli: isolation and morphological characterization of two homogeneous cell lines. *Invest. Cell Pathol.* **2:** 15–26.
178. Foidart, J. B., Dubois, C. H. and Foidart, J. M. (1980) Tissue culture of normal rat glomeruli: basement membrane biosynthesis by homogenous epithelial and mesangial cell lines. *Int. J. Biochem.* **12:** 197–202.

179. Foidart, J. B., Dechenne, C. A. and Mahieu, P. (1981) Tissue culture of normal rat glomeruli: characterization of collagenous and non-collagenous basement membrane antigens on the epithelial and mesangial cells. *Diagn. Histopathol.* **4:** 71–77.
180. Morita, T., Oite, T., Kihara, I. *et al.* (1980) Culture of isolated glomeruli from normal and nephritic rabbits. I. Characterization of outgrowing cells. *Acta Pathol. Jpn* **30:** 917–926.
181. Striker, G. E. and Striker, L. J. (1985) Biology of disease. Glomerular cell culture. *Lab. Invest.* **53:** 122–131.
182. Berman, J., Perantoni, A., Jackson, H. M. and Kingsbury, E. (1979) Primary epithelial cell cultures of adult rat kidney, enhancement of cell growth by ammonium acetate. *Exp. Cell Res.* **121:** 47–54.
183. Chatterjee, S., Trifillis, A. L. and Regec, A. L. (1985) Morphological and biochemical effects of gentamicin on cultured human renal tubular cells. In Bach, P. H. and Lock, E. A. (eds) *Renal Heterogeneity and Target Cell Toxicity*, pp. 549–552. Wiley, Chichester.
184. Trifillis, A. L., Regec, A. L., Hall-Graggs, M. and Trump, B. F. (1985) Effects of cyclosporin on cultured human renal tubular cells. In Bach, P. H. and Lock, E. A. (eds) *Renal Heterogeneity and Target Cell Toxicity*, pp. 545–548. Wiley, Chichester.
185. Trifillis, A. L., Regec, A. L. and Trump, B. F. (1985) Isolation, culture and characterization of human renal tubular cells. *J. Urol.* **133:** 324–329.
186. Green, N., Algren, A., Hoyer, J., Triche, T. and Burg, M. (1985) Differentiated lines of cells from rabbit renal medullary thick ascending limbs grown on amnion. *Am. J. Physiol.* **249:** C97–C104.
187. Valentich, J. D. and Stokols, M. F. (1986) An established cell line from mouse kidney medullary thick ascending limb. I. Cell culture techniques, morphology, and antigenic expression. *Am. J. Physiol.* **251:** C299–C311.
188. Allen, M. L., Nakao, A., Sonnenburg, W. K., Burnatowska-Hledin, M., Spielman, W. S. and Smith, W. L. (1988) Immunodissection of cortical and medullary thick ascending limb cells from rabbit kidney. *Am. J. Physiol.* **255:** F704–F710.
189. Drugge, E. D., Carroll, M. A. and McGiff, J. C. (1989) Cells in culture from rabbit medullary thick ascending limb of Henle's loop. *Am. J. Physiol.* **256:** C1070–C1081.
190. Trifillis, A. L. and Kahng, M. W. (1990) Characterization of an *in vitro* system of human renal papillary collecting duct cells. *In Vitro Cell. Dev. Biol.* **26:** 441–446.
191. Gonzalez, R., Redon, P., Lakhdar, B., Potaux, L., Cambar, J. and Aparicio, M. (1990) Cyclosporin nephrotoxicity assessed in isolated human glomeruli and cultured mesangial cells. *Toxicol. In Vitro* **4:** 391–395.
192. Sokol, P. P., Capodagli, L. C., Dixon, M. *et al.* (1990) Cyclosporin A and vehicle toxicity in primary cultures of rabbit renal proximal tubule cells. *Am. J. Physiol.* **259:** C897–C903.
193. Lash, L. H. and Anders, M. W. (1989) Uptake of nephrotoxic *S*-conjugates by isolated rat renal proximal tubular cells. *J. Pharmacol. Exp. Ther.* **248:** 531–537.
194. Lash, L. H. and Jones, D. P. (1985) Uptake of the glutathione conjugate *S*-(1,2-dichlorovinyl)glutathione by renal basal-lateral membrane vesicles and isolated kidney cells. *Mol. Pharmacol.* **28:** 278–282.
195. Cal, J. C., Merlet, D. and Cambar, J. (1989) *In vitro* and *in vivo* $HgCl_2$-induced nephrotoxicity assessed by tubular enzymes release. In Bach, P. H. and Lock, E. A. (eds) *Nephrotoxicity:* In Vitro *to* In Vivo, *Animals to Man*, pp. 99–106. Plenum Press, New York.
196. Toutain, H. and Morin, J. P. (1991) Separation of cells from the convoluted and straight portions of the proximal tubule from the rabbit kidney by free-flow electrophoresis. In Bach, P. H., Delacruz, L., Gregg, N. J. and Wilks, M. F. (eds) *Nephrotoxicity: Early Diagnosis and Therapeutic Management*, pp. 451–457. Marcel Dekker, New York.
197. Boogaard, P. J. (1992) Development of proximal tubular cell systems to study nephrotoxicity *in vitro*. *Pharm. Weekbl.* [*Sci.*] **14:** 203–204.
198. Blais, A., Morvan-Baleynaud, J., Friedlander, G. and Le-Grimellec, C. (1993) Primary culture of rabbit proximal tubules as a cellular model to study nephrotoxicity of xenobiotics. *Kidney. Int.* **44:** 13–18.
199. Handler, J. S. (1986) Studies of kidney cells in culture. *Kidney Int.* **30:** 208–215.
200. Morin, J. P., Toutain, H., Vauclin-Jacques, N. and Fillastre, J. P. (1991) Biochemical and functional characterization of a primary culture of rabbit proximal tubule cells: a time-course study. In Bach, P. H., Delacruz, L., Gregg, N. J. and Wilks, M. F. (eds) *Nephrotoxicity: Early Diagnosis and Therapeutic Management*, pp. 433–438. Marcel Dekker, New York.

201. Frick, H., Gstraunthaler, G. and Pfaller, W. (1989) Modification of membrane protein expression and protein secretion in LLC-PK_1 grown on different carbohydrates. *Renal Physiol. Biochem.* **12:** 393–399.
202. Richardson, J. C. W., Waterson, P. and Simmons, N. L. (1982) Isolation and culture of renal cortical tubules from neonate rabbit kidneys. *Quart. J. Exp. Physiol.* **67:** 287–301.
203. Pellet, O. L., Smith, M. L., Thoene, J. G., Schneider, J. A. and Jonas, A. J. (1984) Renal cell culture using autopsy material from children with cystinosis. *In Vitro* **20:** 53–58.
204. Regec, A., Trifillis, A. L. and Trump, B. F. (1986) The effect of gentamicin on human renal proximal tubular. *Toxicol. Pathol.* **14:** 238–241.
205. Aleo, M. D., Taub, M. L., Olson, J. R. and Kostyniak, P. J. (1990) Primary cultures of rabbit renal proximal tubule cells: II. Selected phase I and phase II metabolic capacities. *Toxicol. In Vitro* **4:** 727–733.
206. Scheinman, J. I. and Fish, A. (1978) Human glomerular cells in culture. Three subcultured cell types bearing glomerular antigens. *Am. J. Pathol.* **92:** 125–139.
207. Ardaillou, N., Nivez, M. P., Striker, G. and Ardaillou, R. (1983) Prostaglandin synthesis by human glomerular cells in culture. *Prostaglandins* **26:** 773–784.
208. Gregg, N. J., Elseviers, M. M., DeBroe, M. E. and Bach, P. H. (1989) The epidemiological and mechanistic basis of analgesic associated nephropathy. *Toxicol. Lett.* **46:** 141–152.
209. Gregg, N. J., Courtauld, E. A. and Bach, P. H. (1990) Enzyme histochemical changes in an acutely-induced renal papillary necrosis. *Toxicol. Pathol.* **18:** 39–46.
210. Gregg, N. J., Courtauld, E. A. and Bach, P. H. (1990) High resolution light microscopic morphological and microvascular changes in an acutely-induced renal papillary necrosis. *Toxicol. Pathol.* **18:** 47–55.
211. Bojsen, I. N. (1980) Fatty acid composition and depot function of lipid droplets triacylglycerols in renomedullary interstitial cells. In Mandal, A. K. and Bohman, S.-O. (eds) *The Renal Papilla and Hypertension*, pp. 121–147. Plenum, New York.
212. Taub, M. and Saier, M. H. (1981) Amiloride-resistant Madin-Darby canine kidney (MDCK) cells exhibit decreased cation transport. *J. Cell. Physiol.* **106:** 191–199.
213. Saier, M. H. (1981) Growth and differentiated properties of a kidney epithelial cell line (MDCK) *Am. J. Physiol.* **240:** C106–C109.
214. Boogaard, P. J., Commandeur, J. N. M., Mulder, G. J., Vermeulen, N. P. E. and Nagelkerke, J. F. (1989) Toxicity of the cysteine-*S*-conjugates and mercapturic acids of four structurally related difluoroethylenes in isolated proximal tubular cells from rat kidney. Uptake of the conjugates and activation to toxic metabolites. *Biochem. Pharmacol.* **38:** 3731–3741.
215. Boogaard, P. J., Nagelkerke, J. F. and Mulder, G. J. (1990) Renal proximal tubular cells in suspension or in primary culture as *in vitro* models to study nephrotoxicity. *Chem. Biol. Interact.* **76:** 251–292.
216. Boogard, P. J., Zoeteweij, J. P., van Berkel, T. J. C., van't Nordende, J. M., Mulder, G. J. and Nagelkerke, J. F. (1990) Primary culture of proximal tubular cells from normal rat kidney as an *in vitro* model to study mechanisms of nephrotoxicity. Toxicity of nephrotoxicants at low concentrations during prolonged exposure. *Biochem. Pharmacol.* **39:** 1335–1345.
217. Handler, J. S. (1983) Use of cultured epithelia to study transport and its regulation. *J. Exp. Biol.* **106:** 55–69.
218. Gstraunthaler, G. J. A. (1988) Epithelial cells in tissue culture. *Renal Physiol Biochem.* **11:** 1–42.
219. Troyer, D. A., Kreisberg, J. I. and Venkatachalam, M. A. (1986) Lipid alterations in LLC-PK_1 cells exposed to mercuric chloride. *Kidney Int.* **29:** 530–538.
220. Williams, P. D., Laska, D. A. and Hottendorf, G. H. (1986) Comparative toxicity of aminoglycoside antibiotics in cell cultures derived from human and pig kidney. *In Vitro Toxicol.* **1:** 23–32.
221. Casey, B., McGuinness, S., Pratt, I. *et al.* (1989) Uptake of cisplatin (^{195m}Pt) into LLCPK_1 cells in the presence of diethyldithiocarbamate (DDTC), mercaptoethanesulphate (MESNA) and amiloride. In Bach, P. H. and Lock, E. A. (eds) *Nephrotoxicity:* In Vitro *to* In Vivo, *Animals to Man*, pp. 353–356. Plenum Press, New York.
222. Vamvakas, S., Dekant, W., Schiffmann, D. and Henschler, D. (1989) Characterization of an unscheduled DNA synthesis assay with a cultured line of porcine kidney cells (LLC-PK_1) In Bach, P. H. and Lock, E. A. (eds) *Nephrotoxicity:* In Vitro *to* In Vivo, *From Animals to Man*, pp. 749–754. Plenum Press, New York.
223. Zimmermann, U. (1982) Electric field-mediated fusion and related electric phenomena. *Biochim. Biophys. Acta* **694:** 227–277.

224. Morin, J. P. and Fillastre, J. P. (1982) Aminoglycosides lysosomal dysfunctions in the kidney. In Whelton, A. and Neu, H. C. (eds) *Aminoglycosides, Microbiology, Clinical Use and Toxicology*, pp. 303–324. Marcel Dekker, New York.
225. Correll, I. G., Noorazar, S. and Plummer, D. T. (1982) The effect of gentamicin and cefuroxime in the stability of rat lysosomes *in vitro*. *Biochem. Soc. Trans.* **10:** 515–516.
226. Godson, C. and Ryan, M. P. (1989) Investigation of gentamicin nephrotoxicity using renal brush border membrane vesicles. In Bach, P. H. and Lock, E. A. (eds) *Nephrotoxicity:* In Vitro *to* In Vivo, *Animals to Man*, pp. 247–252. Plenum Press, New York.
227. Chakrabarti, S., Vu, D. D. and Cote, M. G. (1991) Effects of cysteine derivatives of styrene on the transport of *p*-aminohippurate ion in renal plasma membrane vesicles. *Arch. Toxicol.* **65:** 366–372.
228. Smith, J. H. and Hook, J. B. (1983) Mechanism of chloroform nephrotoxicity. II. *In vitro* evidence for renal metabolism of chloroform in mice. *Toxicol. Appl. Pharmacol.* **70:** 480–485.
229. Bailie, M. B., Smith, J. H., Newton, J. F. and Hook, J. B. (1984) Mechanism of chloroform nephrotoxicity. IV. Phenobarbital potentiation of *in vitro* chloroform metabolism and toxicity in rabbit kidneys. *Toxicol. Appl. Pharmacol.* **74:** 285–292.
230. Powell, J. H. and Reidenberg, M. M. (1982) *In vitro* response of rat and human kidney lysosomes to aminoglycosides. *Biochem. Pharmacol.* **31:** 3447–3453.
231. Carlier, M. B., Laurent, G. and Tulkens, P. (1984) *In vitro* inhibition of lysosomal phospholipases by aminoglycoside antibiotics: a comparative study. *Arch. Toxicol.* **7:** 282–285.
232. Aramaki, Y., Takahashi, M., Inaba, A., Ishii, Y. and Tsuchiya, S. (1986) Uptake of aminoglycoside antibiotics into brush-border membrane vesicles and inhibition of (Na^+-K^+)-ATPase activity of basolateral membrane. *Biochim. Biophys. Acta* **862:** 111–118.
233. Inselmann, G., Blank, M. and Baumann, K. (1989) Cyclosporine A-induced lipid peroxidation in rat renal microsomes and effect on glucose uptake by renal brush border membrane vesicles. In Bach, P. H. and Lock, E. A. (eds) *Nephrotoxicity:* In Vitro *to* In Vivo, *Animals to Man*, pp. 303–308. Plenum Press, New York.
234. Rush, G. F., Smith, J. H., Newton, J. F. and Hook, J. B. (1984) Chemically induced nephrotoxicity: role of metabolic activation. *Crit. Rev. Toxicol.* **13:** 99–160.
235. Bach, P. H. (1989) Detection of chemically induced renal injury: the cascade of degenerative morphological and functional changes that follow the primary nephrotoxic insult and evaluation of these changes by *in-vitro* methods. *Toxicol. Lett.* **46:** 237–249.
236. Wilks, M. F., Kwizera, E. N. and Bach, P. H. (1990) Assessment of heavy metal nephrotoxicity *in vitro* using isolated glomeruli and proximal tubular fragments. *Renal Physiol. Biochem.* **35:** 275–284.
237. Obatomi, D. K. and Bach, P. H. (1996) Selective cytotoxicity associated with *in vitro* exposure of fresh rat renal fragments and continuous cell lines to atractyloside *Archiv Toxicol*, In Press.
238. Obatomi, D. K. and Bach, P. H. (1996) Inhibition of mitochondrial respiration and oxygen uptake in isolated rat renal tubular fragments by atractyloside *Toxicol. Lett*, In Press.
239. Jeremy, J. Y. (1993) Meetings report: Human cells in *in vitro* pharmaco-toxicology testing – EC Symposium DG XII, Science, Research and Development, Brussels, Belgium, 23–24 September 1993. *J. Drug Dev.* **6:** 145–146.
240. Pohl, L. R., George, J. W. and Satoh, H. (1984) Strain and sex differences in chloroform-induced nephrotoxicity. Different rates of metabolism of chloroform to phosgene by the mouse kidney. *Drug. Metab. Dispos.*, **12:** 304–308.
241. Pohl, L. R. (1979) Biochemical toxicology of chloroform. *Rev. Biochem. Toxicol.* **1:** 79–107.
242. Smith, J. H. and Hook, J.B. (1984) Mechanism of chloroform nephrotoxicity. III. Renal and hepatic microsomal metabolism of chloroform in mice. *Toxicol. Appl. Pharmacol.* **73:** 511–524.
243. Berndt, W. O. and Mehendale, H. M. (1979) Effects of hexachlorobutadiene on renal function and renal organic ion transport in the rat. *Toxicology* **14:** 55–65.
244. Kluwe, W. M., Harrington, F. W. and Cooper, S. E. (1982) Toxic effects of organohalide compounds on renal tubular cells *in vivo* and *in vitro*. *J. Pharmacol. Exp. Ther.* **220:** 597–603.
245. Lock, E. A., Ishmael, J. and Hook, J. B. (1984) Nephrotoxicity of hexachloro-1:3-butadiene in the mouse: the effect of age, sex, strain, monooxygenase modifiers and the role of glutathione. *Toxicol. Appl. Pharmacol.* **72:** 484–494.
246. Nash, J. A., King, L. J., Lock, E. A,. and Green T. (1984) The metabolism and disposition of hexachloro-1:3-butadiene in the rat and its relevance to nephrotoxicity. *Toxicol. Appl. Pharmacol.* **73:** 124–137.

247. Wolf, C. R., Berry, P. N., Nash, J. A., Green, T. and Lock, E. A. (1984) The role of microsomal and cytosolic glutathione-*S*-transferases in the conjugation of hexachloro-1,3-butadiene and its possible relevance to toxicity. *J. Pharmacol. Exp. Ther.* **228:** 202–208.
248. Stevens, J. L. (1985) Cysteine conjugate *β*-lyase activities in rat kidney cortex: subcellular localisation and relationship to the hepatic enzyme. *Biochem. Biophys. Res. Commun.* **129:** 499–504.
249. Mertens, J. J. W. M., Weijnen, J. G. J., van Doorn, W. J., Spenkelink, B., Temmink, J. H. M. and van Bladeren, P. J. (1988) Differential toxicity as a result of apical and basolateral treatment of LLC-PK_1 with *S*-(1,2,3,4,4-pentachlorobutadienyl)glutathione and *N*-acetyl-*S*-(1,2,3,4,4-pentachlorobutadienyl)-L-cysteine. *Chem. Biol. Interact.* **65:** 283–293.
250. Mertens, J. J. W. M., Keukens, E. A. J., Appel, M., Spenkelink, B., Temmink, J. H. M. and van Bladeren, P. J. (1990) Cytotoxicity of *S*-(1,2,3,4,4-pentachlorobutadienyl)-L-cysteine after apical and basolateral exposure of LLC-PK_1 monolayers. Involvement of an amino acid transport system. *Chem. Biol. Interact.* **75:** 119–130.
251. Mertens, J. J. W. M., Sterck, J. G. H., Lau, S. S., Monks, T. J., van Bladeren, P. J. and Temmink, J. H. M. (1990) Cytotoxicity of nephrotoxic glutathione-conjugated halohydroquinones. *Toxicol. Lett.* **53:** 147–149.
252. Boogaard, P. J., Mulder, G. J. and Nagelkerke, J. F. (1989) Isolated proximal tubular cells from rat kidney as an *in vitro* model for studies on nephrotoxicity. I. An improved method for preparation of proximal tubular cells and their functional characterization by alpha-methylglucose uptake. *Toxicol. Appl. Pharmacol.* **101:** 135–143.
253. Boogaard, P. J., Mulder, G. J. and Nagelkerke, J. F. (1989) Isolated proximal tubular cells from rat kidney as an *in vitro* model for studies on nephrotoxicity. II. α-Methylglucose uptake as a sensitive parameter for mechanistic studies of acute toxicity by xenobiotics. *Toxicol. Appl. Pharmacol.* **101:** 144–157.
254. Vamvakas, S., Shrama, V. K., Sheu, S. S. and Anders, M. W. (1990) Perturbations of intracellular calcium distribution in kidney cells by nephrotoxic haloalkenyl cysteine *S*-conjugates. *Mol. Pharmacol.* **38:** 455–461.
255. Lock, E. A. (1989) Mechanism of nephrotoxic action due to organohalogenated compounds. *Toxicol. Lett.* **46:** 93–106.
256. MacFarlane M., Foster J. R., Gibson G. G., King L. J. and Lock E. A. (1989) Cysteine conjugate beta-lyase of rat kidney cytosol: characterization, immunocytochemical localization, and correlation with hexachlorobutadiene nephrotoxicity. *Toxicol. Appl. Pharmacol.* **98:** 185–197.
257. Dekant, W., Vamvakas, S. and Anders, M. W. (1990) Bioactivation of hexachlorobutadiene by glutathione conjugation. *Food Chem. Toxicol.* **28:** 285–293.
258. De Ceaurriz, J. and Ban, M. (1990) Role of gamma-glutamyltranspeptidase and beta-lyase in the nephrotoxicity of hexachloro-1:3-butadiene and methyl mercury in mice. *Toxicol. Lett.* **50:** 249–256.
259. Dohn, D. R. and Anders, M. W. (1982) Assay of cysteine conjugate *β*-lyase activity with *S*-(2-benzothiazolyl) cysteine as the substrate. *Anal. Biochem.* **120:** 379–386.
260. Jaffe, D. R., Hassall, C. D., Brendel, K. and Gandolfi, A. J. (1983) *In vivo* and *in vitro* nephrotoxicity of the cysteine conjugate of hexachlorobutadiene. *J. Toxicol. Environ. Health* **11:** 857–867.
261. Hwang, Y. and Elfarra, A. A. (1991) Kidney-selective prodrugs of 6-mercaptopurine: biochemical basis of the kidney selectivity of *S*-(6-purinyl)-L-cysteine and metabolism of new analogs in rats. *J. Pharmacol. Exp. Ther.* **258:** 171–177.
262. Finkelstein, M. B., Baggs, R. B. and Anders, M. W. (1992) Nephrotoxicity of the glutathione and cysteine conjugates of 2-bromo-2-chloro-1,1-difluoroethene. *J. Pharmacol. Exp. Ther.* **261:** 1248–1252.
263. Fisher, M. B., Hayden, P. J., Bruschi, S. A. *et al.* (1993) Formation, characterization, and immunoreactivity of lysine thioamide adducts from fluorinated nephrotoxic cysteine conjugates *in vitro* and *in vivo*. *Chem. Res. Toxicol.* **6:** 223–230.
264. Kays, S. E., Berdanier, C. D., Swagler, A. R., Lock, E. A. and Schnellmann, R. G. (1993) An *in vitro* model of renal proximal tubule cell regeneration. *J. Pharmacol. Toxicol. Methods* **29:** 211–215.
265. Ploemen, J. H. T. M., Van Ommen, B., De Haan, A., Schefferlie, J. G. and Van Bladeren, P. J. (1993) *In vitro* and *in vivo* reversible and irreversible inhibition of rat glutathione *S*-transferase isoenzymes by caffeic acid and its 2-*S*-glutathionyl conjugate. *Food Chem. Toxicol.* **31:** 475–482.

266. Lash, L. H., Sausen, P. J., Duescher, R. J., Cooley, A. J. and Elfarra, A. A. (1994) Roles of cysteine conjugate beta-lyase and *S*-oxidase in nephrotoxicity: studies with *S*-(1,2-dichlorovinyl)-L-cysteine and *S*-(1,2-dichlorovinyl)-L-cysteine sulfoxide. *J. Pharmacol. Exp. Ther.* **269:** 374–383.
267. Sastrasinh, M., Knauss, T. C., Weinberg, J. M. and Humes, H. D. (1982) Identification of the aminoglycoside binding site in rat renal brush border membranes. *J. Pharmacol. Exp. Ther.* **222:** 350–358.
268. Morin, J. P., Viotte, G., Vanderwalle, A., Van Hoof, F., Tulkens, P. and Fillastre, J. P. (1980) Gentamicin-induced nephrotoxicity: a cell biology approach. *Kidney Int.* **18:** 583–590.
269. Josepovitz, C., Farruggella, T., Levine, R., Lane, B. and Kaloyanides, G. J. (1985) Effect of netilmicin on the phospholipid composition of subcellular fractions of rat renal cortex. *J. Pharmacol. Exp. Ther.* **235:** 810–819.
270. Kaloyanides, G. J. (1984) Aminoglycoside-induced functional and biochemical defects in the renal cortex. *Fundament. Appl. Toxicol.* **4:** 930–943.
271. Carlier, M. B., Laurent, G., Claes, P. J., Vanderhaeghe, H. J. and Tulkens, P. M. (1983) Inhibition of lysosomal phospholipases by aminoglycoside antibiotics: *in vitro* comparative studies. *Antimicrob. Agents Chemother.* **23:** 440–449.
272. Ramsammy, L. S., Josepovitz, C., Lane, B. and Kaloyanides, G. J. (1989) Effect of gentamicin on phospholipid metabolism in cultured rabbit proximal tubular cells. *Am. J. Physiol.* **256:** C204–C213.
273. Schwertz, D. W., Kreisberg, J. I. and Venkatachalem, M. A. (1984) Effect of aminoglycosides on PTBBM phosphatidyl-inositol-specific phospholipase C. *J. Pharmacol. Exp. Ther.* **231:** 48–55.
274. Gilbert, D. N., Wood, C. A., Kohlhepp, S. J. *et al.* (1989) Polyaspartic acid prevents experimental aminoglycoside nephrotoxicity. *J. Infect. Dis.* **159:** 945–953.
275. Ramsammy, L. S., Josepovitz, C., Lane, B. P. and Kaloyanides, G. J. (1989) Polyaspartic acid protects against gentamicin nephrotoxicity in the rat. *J. Pharmacol. Exp. Ther.* **250:** 149–153.
276. Ramsammy, L. S., Josepovitz, C., Lane, B. and Kaloyanides, G. J. (1989) Effect of gentamicin on phospholipid metabolism in cultured rabbit proximal tubular cells. *Am. J. Physiol.* **256:** C204–C213.
277. Tulkens, P. M. (1989) Nephrotoxicity of aminoglycoside antibiotics. *Toxicol. Lett.* **46:** 107–123.
278. Giuliano, R. A., Paulus, G. J., Verpooten, R. A. *et al.* (1984) Recovery of cortical phospholipidosis and necrosis after acute gentamicin loading in rats. *Kidney Int.* **26:** 838–847.
279. Ramsammy, L. S., Josepovitz, C. and Kaloyanides, G. J. (1988) Gentamicin inhibits agonist stimulation of the phosphatidylinositol cascade in primary cultures of rabbit proximal tubular cells and in rat renal cortex. *J. Pharmacol. Exp. Ther.* **247:** 989–996.
280. Williams, P. D., Holohan, P. D. and Ross, C. R. (1981) Gentamicin nephrotoxicity. I. Acute biochemical correlates in rats. *Toxicol. Appl. Pharmacol.* **61:** 234–242.
281. Williams, P. D., Holohan, P. D. and Ross, C. R. (1981) Gentamicin nephrotoxicity. II. Plasma membrane changes. *Toxicol. Appl. Pharmacol.* **61:** 243–251.
282. Weinberg, J. M. and Humes, H. D. (1980) Mechanisms of gentamicin induced dysfunction of renal cortical mitochondria. I. Effects of mitochondrial respiration. *Arch. Biochem. Biophys.* **205:** 222–231.
283. Tune, B. M. and Fravert, D. (1980) Mechanism of cephalosporin nephrotoxicity: a comparison of cephaloridine and cephaloglycin. *Kidney Int.* **18:** 591–600.
284. Tune, B. M. and Hsu, C. Y. (1994) Toxicity of cephaloridine to carnitine transport and fatty acid metabolism in rabbit renal cortical mitochondria: structure–activity relationships. *J. Pharmacol. Exp. Ther.* **270:** 873–880.
285. Rush, G. F. and Ponsler, G. D. (1991) Cephaloridine-induced biochemical changes and cytotoxicity in suspensions of rabbit isolated proximal tubules. *Toxicol. Appl. Pharmacol.* **109:** 314–326.
286. Rush, G. F., Heim, R. A., Ponsler, G. D. and Engelhardt, J. (1992) Cephaloridine-induced renal pathological and biochemical changes in female rabbits and isolated proximal tubules in suspension. *Toxicol. Pathol.* **20:** 155–168.
287. Bertani, T., Poggi, A., Pozzoni, R. *et al.* (1982) Adriamycin-induced nephrotic syndrome in rats. Sequence of pathologic events. *Lab. Invest.* **46:** 16–23.
288. Hayashi, Y., Imaqawa, T., Kokubo,T., Kurokawa, Y. and Takahashi, M. (1984) Nuclear alterations of mycocardial cells and glomerular epithelial cells in rats after a single administration of Adriamycin. *Toxicol. Lett.* **20:** 105–110.
289. Burke, J. F. (1977) Doxorubicin hydrochloride-associated renal failure. *Arch. Int. Med.* **137:** 385–388.

290. O'Donnell, M. P. (1985) Adriamycin-induced chronic proteinuria: a structural and functional study. *J. Lab. Clin. Med.* **106:** 62–67.
291. Okuda S., Oh Y., Tsuruda H., Onoyama K., Fujimi S. and Fujishima, M. (1986) Adriamycin-induced nephropathy as a model of chronic progressive glomerular disease. *Kidney Int.* **29:** 502–510.
292. Frenk, S., Antonowicz, I., Craig, J. M. and Metcalf, J. (1955) Experimental nephrotic syndrome induced in rats by aminonucleoside: renal lesions and body electrolyte composition. *Proc. Soc. Exp. Biol. Med.* **89:** 424–427.
293. Calandra, S., Traugi, P., Ghisellini, M. and Gherardi, L. E. (1983) Plasma and urine lipoproteins during development of nephrotic syndrome induced in the rat by Adriamycin. *Exp. Mol. Pathol.* **39:** 282.
294. Bizzi, A. (1983) Adriamycin causes hyperlipemia as a consequence of nephrotoxicity. *Toxicol. Lett.* **18:** 291–300.
295. Ismail, A. A., Ramadan, A. M. and Amin, A. M. (1983) Morphological alterations induced by adriamycin. *Folia Morphol. (Warsz)* **42:** 283.
296. Kastner, S., Wilks, M. F., Gwinner, W., Soose, M., Bach, P. H. and Stolte, H. (1990) Metabolic heterogeneity of isolated cortical and juxtamedullary glomeruli in adriamycin nephropathy. *Renal Physiol. Biochem.* **14:** 48–54.
297. Soose, M., Haberstroh, U., Rovira-Halbach, G., Brunkhorst, R. and Stolte, H. (1988) Heterogeneity of glomerular barrier function in early adriamycin nephrosis of MWF rats. *Clin. Physiol. Biochem.* **6:** 310–315.
298. Andrews, P. M. and Coffey, A. K. (1983) Cytoplasmic contractile elements in glomerular cells. *Fed. Proc.* **42:** 3046–3051.
299. Zimmerhackl, B., Parekh, N., Kucherer, H. and Steinhausen, M. (1985) Influence of systemically applied angiotensin II on the microcirculation of glomerular capillaries in the rat. *Kidney Int.* **27:** 17–24.
300. Barros, E. J. G., Boim, M. A., Ajzen, H., Ramos, O. L. and Schor, N. (1987) Glomerular hemodynamics and hormonal participation on cyclosporine nephrotoxicity. *Kidney Int.* **32:** 19–25.
301. Cherian, M. G. (1985) Rat kidney epithelial cell culture for metal toxicity studies. *In Vitro Cell. Dev. Biol.* **21:** 505–508.
302. Wilks, M. F., Kwizera, E. N. and Bach, P. H. (1991) Effects of heavy metals on metabolic functions in isolated glomeruli and proximal tubule fragments. In Bach, P. H., Gregg, N. J., Wilks, M. W. and Delacruz, L. (eds) *Nephrotoxicity: Mechanisms, Early Diagnosis and Therapeutic Management*, pp. 363–366. Marcel Dekker, New York.
303. Templeton, D. M. and Chaitu, N. (1990) Effects of divalent metals on the isolated rat glomerulus. *Toxicology* **61:** 119–133.
304. Andreoli, S. P. and McAteer, J. A. (1990) Reactive oxygen molecule-mediated injury in endothelial and renal tubular epithelial cells *in vitro*. *Kidney Int.* **38:** 785–794.
305. Chen, Q. and Stevens, J. L. (1991) Inhibition of iodoacetamide and *t*-butylhydroperoxide toxicity in LLC-PK_1 cells by anti-oxidants: a role for lipid peroxidation in alkylation induced cytotoxicity. *Arch. Biochem. Biophys.* **284:** 422–430.
306. Lash, L. H. and Woods, E. B. (1991) Cytotoxicity of alkylating agents in isolated rat kidney proximal tubular and distal tubular cells. *Arch. Biochem. Biophys.* **286:** 46–56.
307. Kawaguchi, M., Yamada, M., Wada, H. and Okigaki, T. (1992) Roles of puromycin aminonucleoside. *Toxicology* **72:** 329–340.
308. Bertolatus, J. A., Klinzman, D., Bronsema, D. A., Ridnour, L. and Oberley, L. W. (1991) Evaluation of the role of reactive oxygen species in doxorubicin hydrochloride nephrosis. *J. Lab. Clin. Med.* **118:** 435–445.
309. Ghiggeri, G. M., Bertelli, R., Ginevri, F. *et al.* (1992) Multiple mechanisms for doxorubicin cytotoxicity on glomerular epithelial cells *in vitro*. *Eur. J. Pharmacol. Environ. Toxicol. Pharmacol.* **228:** 77–83.
310. Lund, B. O., Miller, D. M. and Woods, J. S. (1991) Mercury-induced H_2O_2 production and lipid peroxidation *in vitro* in rat kidney mitochondria. *Biochem. Pharmacol.* **Supplement 42:** S181–S187.
311. Lund, B. O., Miller, D. M. and Woods, J. S. (1993) Studies on Hg(II)-induced H_2O_2 formation and oxidative stress *in vivo* and *in vitro* in rat kidney mitochondria. *Biochem. Pharmacol.* **45:** 2017–2024.

312. Marnett, L. J. and Eling, T. E. (1983) Cooxidation during prostaglandin biosynthesis: a pathway for the metabolic activation of xenobiotics. In Hodgson E., Bend, J. R. and Philpot, R. M. (eds) *Reviews in Biochemical Toxicology*, Vol. 5, pp. 135–172. Elsevier, New York.
313. Bach, P. H. and Bridges, J. W. (1984) The role of prostaglandin synthase mediated metabolic activation of analgesics and non-steroidal anti-inflammatory drugs in the development of renal papillary necrosis and upper urothelial carcinoma. *Prostaglandins Leukot. Med.* **15:** 251–274.
314. Mohandas, J., Duggin, G. G., Horvath, J. S. and Tiller, D. J. (1981) Metabolic oxidation of acetaminophen (paracetamol) mediated by cytochrome P-450 mixed function oxidase and prostaglandin endoperoxide synthase in rabbit kidney. *Toxicol. Appl. Pharmacol.* **61:** 252–259.
315. Nelson, S. D., Dahlin, D. C., Rauckman, E. J. and Rosen, G. M. (1981) Peroxidase-mediated formation of reactive metabolites of acetaminophen. *Mol. Pharmacol.* **20:** 195–199.
316. Hull, R. N., Cherry, W. R. and Weaver, G. W. (1976) The origin and characteristics of a pig kidney cell strain, LLC-PK_1. *In Vitro* **12:** 670–677.
317. Hassid, A. (1983) Modulation of cyclic 3′5′-adenosine monophosphate in cultured renal (MDCK) cell by endogenous prostaglandins. *J. Cell. Physiol.* **116:** 297–307.
318. Homan-Muller, J. W. T., Weening, R. S. and Roos, D. (1975) Production of hydrogen peroxide by phagocytozing human granulocytes. *J. Lab. Clin. Med.* **85:** 198–207.
319. Greenspan, P., Mayer, E. P. and Fowler, S. D. (1985) Nile red: a selective stain for intracellular lipid droplets. *J. Cell. Biol.* **100:** 965–973.
320. Kaler, B., Morgan, W. A., Bomzon, A. and Bach, P. H. (1996) Effects of bile salts on freshly isolated rat glomerular and tubular fragments (submitted).
321. Kaler, B., Karram, T., Bomzon, A. and Bach, P. H. (1996) Effects of obstructive jaundice on renal function in rodents as shown by urinanalysis (submitted).
322. Hay, R. J. (1979) Cells for culture. In Reid, E. (ed.) *Cell Populations*, pp. 143–160. Ellis Horwood, Chichester.
323. Ash, S. R., Cuppage, F. E., Hodes, M. E. and Selkurt, E. E. (1975) Culture of isolated renal tubules: a method of assessing viability of normal and damaged cells. *Kidney Int.* **7:** 55–60.
324. Scholer, D. W. and Edelman, I. S. (1979) Isolation of rat kidney cortical tubules enriched in proximal and distal segments. *Am. J. Physiol.* **237:** F350–F359.
325. Barker, G. and Simmons, N. L. (1981) Identification of two strains of cultured canine renal epithelial cells (MDCK cells) which display entirely different physiological properties. *Quart. J. Exp. Physiol.* **66:** 61–72.

5

Experimental *In Vitro* Models to Evaluate Hepatotoxicity

ALISON E. M. VICKERS

I. Introduction 104
II. Hepatotoxicity 104
A. Liver cell types 104
B. Liver injury 104
C. Cytotoxicity 106
III. Hepatic models in drug development 107
IV. Adult rat hepatocytes 107
A. Hepatocyte isolation 107
B. Functional characterization 108
V. Fetal rat hepatocytes and slices 109
A. Fetal rat hepatocyte isolation 109
B. Fetal human hepatocyte isolation 110
C. Fetal liver slices 110
D. Characterization 110
VI. Liver slices 111
A. Liver slices as an *in vitro* model 111
B. Slice methodology 111
C. Incubation systems 114
D. Cytochrome P450 levels 115
VII. Application of slices 116
A. Tissue culture medium 116
B. Interactive toxicity 116
1. Ethanol potentiation of hepatotoxins 116
2. Cocaine 116
C. Ranking of compounds 117
D. Mechanistic studies 117
E. Surrogate markers 118
F. Induction and peroxisome proliferation 118
VIII. Application of hepatocytes 119
A. Comparing a series of compounds 119
B. Comparative transport 119
C. Mechanistic studies 119
D. DNA synthesis and adducts 120
IX. Conclusions 121
References 122

IN VITRO METHODS IN PHARMACEUTICAL RESEARCH
ISBN 0-12-163390-X

I. INTRODUCTION

The liver is the largest visceral organ in the body, representing about 2–5% of body-weight, and is the key processor of nutrients and xenobiotics coming from the intestinal tract into the body. Because of its location the liver receives a double blood supply. The portal vein provides about 80% of the afferent blood which is oxygen depleted from the intestinal tract, while the hepatic artery supplies 30–40% of the blood containing a high partial pressure of oxygen. The multifunctional capacity of the liver makes it central in providing sources of energy, carbohydrates, and amino acids to peripheral tissues, in synthesizing plasma proteins necessary for coagulation and renal blood flow, and in synthesizing lipoproteins and bile. The liver is also the major site of biotransformation and elimination, and is often a target organ for toxicity. In mammals, the liver has by far the greatest capacity to regenerate after injury of any organ.

II. HEPATOTOXICITY

A. Liver cell types

The liver parenchymal cells, hepatocytes, are the major cells of the liver, representing about 70% of liver cells and 60% of liver volume. The remaining non-parenchymal or liver sinusoidal cells (Kupffer cells, endothelial cells, fat storage cells, pit cells, bile duct epithelial cells) comprise 30–35% of liver cells and occupy 20% of liver volume. The remaining 20% of liver volume consists of extracellular spaces and extracellular matrix.[1]

In vivo hepatocytes and sinusoidal cells display both structural and functional differences within the various zones of the liver because of the gradient in oxygen and nutrients of the blood within the sinusoids: zone 1 is the most highly oxygenated region (periportal), zones 2 (mid-zonal) and 3 (centrolobular) the least oxygenated. Coordinate and reciprocal interactions exist between the different hepatocyte populations for maintaining glucose, ammonia and bicarbonate homeostasis. The differential activation of zonal metabolism between hepatocytes suggests that interactions between hepatocytes occur via humoral and nervous signals, and via interactions with the biomatrix.[2]

The biotransformation enzymes, cytochrome P450, are at higher levels in centrolobular hepatocytes, whereas periportal hepatocytes have higher levels of glutathione and a higher capacity for bile acid uptake and secrection into the canaliculi. In addition to hepatocytes, endothelial and Kupffer cells can biotransform compounds because of the presence of cytochrome P450 proteins and peroxidases.[3,4] These cells also release a variety of mediators which regulate the function of the hepatocytes and other non-parenchymal cells.[5]

B. Liver injury

Some of the clinical end-points currently used to assess liver injury include the measurement of liver-derived serum enzymes (alkaline phosphatase, aspartate and alanine aminotransferase), bilirubin (unconjugated and conjugated), albumin concentration, prothrombin time, clearance of indocyanine green, and the fibrinogenic peptides alipoprotein A_1 and type IV collagen.[6]

In general, the liver can recover from acute injury by hepatocellular regeneration with the production of new cells, which restore liver function and normal tissue architecture.[7,8] Chronic injury, however, often leads to fibrogenesis, scar formation, and distortion of normal tissue architecture. Presently acute injury is more easily studied *in vitro*, whereas multiple episodes of acute and chronic injury are difficult to reproduce.

Acute injury is often manifested as a depletion of cellular energy, ion deregulation, impaired cellular intermediary metabolism, an inhibition of transport functions, and an impaired stimulation of tissue repair (Table 5.1). These processes can be evaluated *in vitro* through the measurement of many liver, as well as general, parameters of cell function (Table 5.2). The sequence of events resulting in chronic injury are often not well defined, and the processes have been difficult to investigate *in vitro*. This, however, is improving because the technology now exists to detect earlier steps, such as messenger RNA levels for a particular event, which in turn will aid in the identification of underlying processes.

Table 5.1 Examples of mechanisms of hepatotoxicity.

Metabolic activation (free radical) and covalent binding
Metabolic activation, reduced glutathione, covalent binding
Metabolic activation, polypeptide antigen formation
Disruption of Ca^{2+} homeostasis
Disruption of tissue repair mechanisms
Inhibition of transport
Inhibition of cellular energy
Loss of cell volume homeostasis

Table 5.2 Current methods to evaluate hepatotoxicity.

Synthesis and secretion of albumin
Synthesis of cholesterol and lipoproteins
Transport of conjugated bile acids and bilirubin
Gluconeogenesis
Ureagenesis
CYP450 levels and activities
Glutathione levels
ATP, ADP, AMP
Intracellular K^+, Ca^{2+}
Membrane leakage of cytosolic enzymes (α-GST, LDH)
Release of nuclear matrix proteins or oligonucleosomes
DNA and protein synthesis
Morphologic changes

An important factor to consider is the key role the liver plays in the metabolic disposition of most drugs and xenobiotics. Hepatotoxicity is often linked with the biotransformation of the compound; therefore, the *in vitro* system should reproduce the *in vivo* biotransformation of compounds to be predictive for *in vivo* hepatotoxicity. It is becoming apparent that interpatient differences in the levels and catalytic activities of cytochrome P450 could account for the side-effects seen in the therapeutic range of the drug. For example, the increase of CYP2E1 levels in chronic alcoholics predisposes these people to acute acetaminophen toxicity, probably by producing more of the toxic metabolite at any given therapeutic dose.[9] It has also been proposed that the glutathione *S*-transferases, enzymes important in a metabolic and transport capacity, are polymorphic and may contribute to the variability in the intracellular transport of drugs and the activity of detoxification pathways with glutathione.[10]

Some drugs or xenobiotics may specifically injure liver cells other than hepatocytes. For example, injury to bile epithelial cells by such compounds as captopril, erythromycin, and ethinylestradiol is manifested as primary cholestasis without significant damage to the hepatocytes. Compounds could also affect the sinusoidal endothelial or Kupffer cells, such as the chemotherapeutic agents.[11]

A drug-induced immunologically mediated mechanism of hepatocyte injury has been identified for phenytoin, chlorpromazine, β-aminosalicylic acid, halothane, and tienilic acid.[9] For these compounds a reactive metabolite binds to a cellular membrane, rendering it antigenic. Sensitized lymphocytes are then produced and, upon re-exposure, a delayed hypersensitivity reaction triggers hepatocyte necrosis.

Cell death by apoptosis, a gene-directed activation of non-lysosomal endonucleases, results in the cleavage of double-stranded DNA into oligonucleosome length fragments. This cellular program of self-destruction is considered to be a very conserved process among cells, regardless of the mechanism by which it is induced, and may occur within a particular concentration range for a compound, while higher concentrations may cause necrosis. It may also be that cell ballooning and shrunken dead cells occur together in response to the same stimulus, indicating that some cells succumb to necrosis while others to apoptotic cell death. The DNA fragmentation seen in necrotic cells is induced by lysosomal enzymes.[13]

C. Cytotoxicity

Several cytotoxic mechanisms of cell death, induced by xenobiotics, have been identified and are applicable to liver cells, including cytoskeleton alterations, mitochondrial dysfunction and energy deprivation, loss of thiol status, and perturbation of intracellular Ca^{2+} homeostasis with subsequent activation of degradative enzymes. For instance, moderate damage to the cell could involve disruption of the cytoskeletal apparatus with associated changes in cell volume and plasma membrane protrusions known as blebs. Severe damage to either the plasma membrane or a block in ATP synthesis leads to an impaired energy-dependent ion pumping mechanism, the entry of sodium and calcium, and loss of K^+, producing a loss of plasma membrane volume control and acute cell swelling. Sustained increases of intracellular Ca^{2+} concentrations will lead to the disruption of the cytoskeleton and activation of degradative phospholipases and proteases, a switching to anaerobic glycolysis, a decreased intracellular pH, and a reduction of macromolecular synthesis, resulting in cell death with the rupture of organelles and plasma membrane.

A unifying mechanism in toxin-related cell injury is the disturbance of glutathione and calcium homeostasis.[13] Cellular glutathione pools are important in the regulation and maintenance of organelle function, in particular that of mitochondria, and in the maintenance of the cellular thio/disulphide status.[14] The liver is also the major source of glutathione for the rest of the body. Extraction of glutathione from the plasma pool by other organs, such as the kidney and lung, is replenished by the liver. Therefore, liver depletion of glutathione would have consequences for other organ toxicities.

III. HEPATIC MODELS IN DRUG DEVELOPMENT

Several *in vitro* systems have been developed to investigate the hepatic effects of compounds. Intact cellular systems including hepatocyte and slice cultures are particularly valuable. These *in vitro* models closely resemble the biotransformation and functional capacity of *in vivo* liver, allowing the investigator to make reliable predictions concerning the hepatic effects of compounds in development. Questions that can be addressed by the hepatocyte and slice culture systems include: species differences in biotransformation pathways and hepatotoxicity susceptibility, determining the concentrations at which toxicity occurs and the apparent risk for humans, and defining the mechanism of the hepatotoxicity for the purpose of circumventing or attenuating it *in vivo* or for the identification of surrogate markers to monitor a potential side-effect *in vivo* (Table 5.3). The *in vitro* technology, furthermore, provides a means, through the use of human tissue, for bridging the findings from the animal *in vivo* studies to the end-user human, and for identifying and assessing risk before human *in vivo* studies.

Table 5.3 Hepatotoxicity questions that could be addressed by *in vitro* liver systems.

Species (including human) differences and susceptibility
Investigate mechanism of adverse effects
Identify markers or surrogate markers for clinical use
Determine concentrations at which hepatotoxicity is reversible and irreversible
Address whether parent compound or metabolite(s) is responsible for toxicity
Cross-species comparison of compound biotransformation and metabolite ratios
Drug interactions, induction, peroxisome proliferation
Potential use of hepatoprotective agents to circumvent or attenuate toxicity
Investigate mechanisms and stimuli to induce liver regeneration
Aid in the design of further *in vivo* tests
Use results in combination with modeling to address risk assessment

IV. ADULT RAT HEPATOCYTES

A. Hepatocyte isolation

The two-step collagenase perfusion method, originally devised for the dissociation of rat liver, is now used for various species, including humans, and has recently been reviewed.[15,16] Hepatocytes cultured for at least 1 week as non-replicating cell monolayers were first reported by Bissel *et al.*[17] The primary culturing of hepatocytes provided an ideal way of increasing cell longevity, without losing any of the advantages this preparation offers: (1) cells from one liver can be divided over a large number of experimental units, which can be used for studying many different parameters with the same batch of cells; (2) the cell culture conditions are well defined and can be changed depending on the problem studied; and (3) the intact cells retain many biological functions, including uptake and intracellullar distribution of the substrate, generation of cofactors and cosubstrates, the interrelationship between metabolic pathways in drug metabolism, and competition between endogenous and exogenous substrates.[18,19]

The extracellular matrix of the liver is comprised largely of collagen, $1\,\mathrm{mg\,g^{-1}}$ wet liver weight in the rat and $5\,\mathrm{mg\,g^{-1}}$ in humans;[1] hence, the highest yields of viable hepatocytes are achieved by collagenase perfusion. Moreover, the biomatrix requires calcium for its maintenance, so the liver is initially perfused with a medium lacking calcium to aid in dissociation of the biomatrix. To perform the isolation of hepatocytes from rat liver, the portal vein is cannulated and perfused with a calcium-free oxygenated buffer (Krebs–Ringer bicarbonate buffer, Hanks' balanced salt solution (HBSS), or Dulbecco's phosphate-buffered saline), about 250 ml for 5–10 min, to clear the liver of blood. The perfusion buffer may also contain ethylene glycol-bis β-aminoethyl ether N,N,N,N-tetraacetic acid (EGTA) (0.1–1 mM), a calcium chelating agent, to favor the cleavage of hepatocyte desmosomes. The flow rate of the perfusate should be maintained within the range of $20\text{–}40\,\mathrm{ml\,min^{-1}}$ through an 8–10 g liver with a hydrostatic pressure of 20–25 $\mathrm{cmH_2O}$, since too low a perfusion rate could cause anoxia and too fast cell shearing.[20] Collagenase (0.025–0.1%) is then added to the reservoir and the liver perfused for an additional 10–15 min or until there is a visible softening. Collagenase lots vary in enzymatic activity and specificity, and are therefore often tested before their use. In the presence of collagenase, calcium (1–4 mM) is often included to facilitate its action. The perfusion can be carried out as either a single-pass or a recirculating perfusion. In the single-pass method the perfusate does not contain metabolic products released from the liver during the perfusion which would affect both the composition and the pH of the perfusate. To avoid pH adjustments during the perfusion, HEPES is generally included in the buffer for pH stabilization.

The liver cells are dissociated by disruption or removal of the liver capsule (Glisson's capsule) and gentle stroking of the cell mass. The resulting cell suspension is filtered through a double layer of sterile cotton gauze or nylon mesh of 50–250 μm. The cells are washed twice by centrifugation (70g for 2.5 min) in a swinging bucket rotor at room temperature, and the cloudy supernatant which contains residual collagenase, non-parenchymal cells, erythrocytes, non-viable hepatocytes, and cell debris is discarded. To obtain hepatocytes of the highest viability the cells are centrifuged through a density gradient of Percoll.[15,21] The cells are then suspended in a complete culture medium.

Variations in the hepatocyte isolation procedure allow for the isolation of periportal and centrolobular hepatocytes and hepatocyte couplets.[22,23] A technique for separating intact periportal and centrolobular hepatocytes uses digitonin during the perfusion via the portal vein or the inferior vena cava selectively to destroy one region of the acinus.[22] Additionally, processing techniques exist including centrifugal elutriation for obtaining enriched subpopulations (periportal and centrolobular) of hepatocytes and hepatocyte couplets following hepatocyte isolation.[24] Hepatocytes can also be isolated from slices by enzyme digestion. This may be particularly useful when working with liver from human or large animals. Hepatocytes isolated from rat liver slices were found to be comparable to slices prepared from the same liver for the biotransformation of biphenyl; however, for both dog and human hepatocytes, where the techniques are less refined, a decreased metabolizing activity was noted for hepatocytes compared with slices from the same animal.[25]

B. Functional characterization

A rapid method for assessing cellular integrity is to determine the percentage of trypan blue exclusion by the hepatocytes. This, however, is not confirmation that the hepatocytes are metabolically functional.[25] Other tests to check cell viability require an incubation period, such as the uptake of neutral red[26] or the reduction of the tetrazolium salt 3-[4,5-

dimethyltiazol-2-yl]-2,5-diphenyltetrazolium bromide (MTT) to 3-[4,5-dimethyltiazol-2-yl]-3,5-diphenylformazan (MTTF).[27] The method of choice for assessing damage during long-term incubation is the leakage of cellular enzymes such as lactate dehydrogenase.[28] Other means of determining cell integrity and function include the rate of oxygen uptake,[29] cellular ATP levels,[30] and cellular Ca^{2+} and K^{+} levels.[31,32] The measurement of liver-specific functions would include albumin synthesis,[33] gluconeogenesis,[34] ureogenesis,[35] and glutathione levels.[31]

Upon hepatocyte isolation there is a loss of cell polarity and organization of the tissue, a loss of cell–cell interactions, and a destruction of cell-surface receptors. These factors are important for the maintenance of differentiated hepatocyte functions. The proportion of periportal and centrilobular cells in the hepatocyte preparation is generally not defined and probably varies between preparations, suggesting that the enzymes regulating cellular metabolism and the cytochrome P450 content would also be variable between hepatocyte batches. Moreover, the technique for the further enrichment of the hepatocytes, centrifugation through Percoll, to obtain the most viable cells will also result in variations of hepatocyte subpopulations obtained between batches.

To establish hepatocytes that exhibit a stable differentiated phenotype in long-term culture, a number of conditions have to be considered. Firstly, it is essential to use a well-defined culture medium supplemented with various soluble factors including the hormones insulin and dihydrocortisone, growth factors, and extracellular matrix components.[36–38] The culturing of hepatocytes on fibronectin or a laminin-rich cell matrix like Matrigel, or maintained in co-culture with other epithelial cells, extends the viability and phenotypic stability of hepatocytes, and results in the production and deposition of extracellular matrix components.[36,39] The extracellular matrix is proving to be important in the control of hepatocyte differentiation, as a dynamic mesh that can bind cytokines and growth factors to trigger cellular responses. Recently, human hepatocyte cultures subcultured for 12 to 15 passages were shown to synthesize albumin and keratin 18, and to metabolize benzo[a]pyrene.[40]

The culturing of hepatocytes between two layers of a collagen matrix, as a sandwich configuration, has been shown to have a positive effect on the state of differentiation of the cells and formation of extensive canalicular networks.[41–43] Other methods employing a three-dimensional aspect to the culturing include cell aggregates. The culturing of rat and human hepatocytes as multicellular aggregates (spheroids) has been shown to form an organized structure of cuboidal cells in the interior and squamated cells on the outer layer, as well as bile canaliculi.[44] Cell aggregates as a suspension in three-dimensional collagen gels is also a possibility for maintaining hepatocyte viability and differentiated functions.[45]

V. FETAL RAT HEPATOCYTES AND SLICES

A. Fetal rat hepatocyte isolation

The isolation of hepatocytes from fetal rat livers is usually performed on days 15–21 of gestation. In general, the livers are excised, placed in a salt buffer such as HBSS or Dulbecco's phosphate-buffered saline at 1–2 g liver per isolation, minced, and shaken at 37°C in HBSS containing 5 mM ethylene diamine tetra-acetic acid (EDTA) for 5 min, followed by HBSS containing collagenase (0.8–2.5 mg ml^{-1}) for 5–20 min. Some studies report the addition of deoxyribonuclease (0.1 mg ml^{-1}) and $CaCl_2$ (5 mM) during the collagenase digestion.[46] Trypsin (0.2–0.25%) has also been used to digest the tissue enzymatically, followed by mechanical dissociation by stirring with small glass beads of 2 mm diameter.[47] The resulting cell suspension is poured through sterile cheese cloth or a nylon mesh and centrifuged twice at 20–50*g* for 1–2 min. The final cell pellet is resuspended in a tissue culture medium (MEM, Eagle's MEM, arginine-free MX-82 or arginine-free Eagle's MEM) with 5–10% fetal bovine serum or newborn calf serum. Cell viability is usually assessed by the exclusion of trypan blue. Cell yields are about 10×10^6 cells per fetal liver and cell viability is generally greater than 90%.

The rat fetal hepatocytes can be plated directly onto untreated tissue culture dishes or collagen-coated culture dishes at an initial density of 5.8×10^3 to 7.5×10^5 cells per ml culture medium per mm^2.[48–50] The cells are maintained in a humidified 5–10% carbon dioxide/90–95% air incubator at 37°C. After 2 h the medium is replaced with fresh medium containing epidermal growth factor (100 ng ml^{-1}), insulin (10 μg ml^{-1}), and hydrocortisone (1 μg ml^{-1}).[51]

B. Fetal human hepatocyte isolation

Fetal human liver (weeks 5–20 of gestation) is acquired following legal abortion. The liver is cut into pieces (0.5–0.7 mm thick and 100 mg wet weight) and incubated at 37°C in a calcium- and magnesium-free salt buffer, followed by enzymatic digestion with 0.05% collagenase and 5 mM $CaCl_2$ until the liver is well dissociated. The resulting suspension is filtered through a nylon mesh (100 μm), and the filtrate centrifuged (50*g*) for 10 min. The cells are resuspended and cultured in tissue culture medium such as Ham's F12 containing fetal calf serum (15%) or human serum (2%). The cell yield is about 9.83×10^6 cells per g liver and the purity is typically greater than 90%.[52–54]

C. Fetal liver slices

Precision-cut liver slices can also be prepared from rat neonates. The liver slices derived from the 4-, 6-, 8-, and 21-day-old neonate litters have the dimensions of 6 mm in diameter, 250 μm thickness, and a wet weight of 10–15 mg.[55] Several slices, about eight to attain approximately 100 mg of liver tissue, were pooled for culturing to obtain a sufficient detection level of the biotransformation pathways of interest. The slices were placed onto stainless steel mesh cylinders and transferred to roller culture vials containing Waymouth's media. The vials were gassed with 95% oxygen/5% carbon dioxide and maintained at 37°C.

D. Characterization

Expression of liver as well as fetal liver-specific functions, albumin and α-fetoprotein respectively, have been demonstrated by the presence of mRNAs and the protein product, both in the cytoplasm and secreted into the culture medium.[48,51,56]

In contrast to adult hepatocytes, fetal hepatocytes *in vivo* are growing cells. DNA synthesis, as measured by the rate of thymidine incorporation, has been demonstrated to be faster in rat fetal hepatocytes than in adult hepatocytes, and to be independent of serum or mitogens added to the cultures, distinguishing fetal from adult hepatocytes.[46] DNA synthesis in fetal hepatocytes can also be stimulated as in adult hepatocytes by the addition of various polypeptide growth factors, including epidermal growth factor and hepatocyte growth factor, whereas ethanol exposure can significantly inhibit DNA synthesis in fetal rat hepatocytes.[57]

Rat fetal hepatoyctes have exhibited biotransformation pathways including testosterone hydroxylation, ethoxycoumarin and ethoxyresorufin de-ethylation, and lauric acid hydroxylation. The biotransformation enzyme levels and activities are inducible by pretreatment of the cultures with dexamethasone, phenobarbital and clofibrate.[47,49,50] Furthermore, the induction of lauric acid hydroxylation by clofibrate was shown to be in a repressed dose-dependent manner by the addition of interleukin 1β.[50]

Both hepatocytes and slices derived from human fetuses can be regarded as fairly mature liver cells. The cells contain a fully developed rough endoplasmic reticulum, short sections of smooth endoplasmic reticulum, numerous matrix-rich mitochondria, many free ribosomes, and a well-developed Golgi apparatus.[52] The metabolism of benzodiazepine drugs in human fetal hepatocytes was inducible by phenobarbital and inhibitable by SKF 525A.[52] As in adult human hepatocytes, the fetal hepatocytes can produce an acute-phase response exhibited by the induced expression of C-reactive protein and α_1-antichymotrypsin upon treatment with the inflammatory mediator interleukin 6, exhibit a reduction of albumin synthesis in response to transforming growth factor β, and have the functional capacity to form bile.[54]

VI. LIVER SLICES

A. Liver slices as an *in vitro* model

A liver slice consists of all the cell types of the organ, and the cells maintain the normal liver architecture, acinar localization, and cell–cell communications (Fig. 5.1). The functional heterogeneity and biochemical capacity of the whole organ is therefore retained. Within the liver, various cell types can participate in the biotransformation of the compound and contribute to cell injury. The slice methodology provides a means to investigate selective toxicity (periportal versus pericentral) and interactive toxicity (where one cell type contributes to the toxicity of another). Furthermore, the slice *in vitro* system is flexible in that slices are prepared in a similar manner regardless of the species, providing a rapid means to investigate various species and various organs. The slice methodology is also an efficient use of tissue. Consequently, the slice system represents a complete and versatile *in vitro* model for its application of *in vivo* risk assessment.

B. Slice methodology

Improved methods for the preparation and culture of liver slices has led to the resurgence of this *in vitro* system: development of a mechanical slicer capable of rapidly producing minimally damaged uniform slices,[58] and development of culture conditions that provide adequate oxygen availability and nutrient exchange.[59]

Cylindrical cores of fresh laboratory animal or human liver are made by rotating, either manually or motor driven, a sharpened metal tube or biopsy punch (diameter 2–10 mm), wettened with medium into the tissue. The tissue cores are placed into a cylindrical tissue

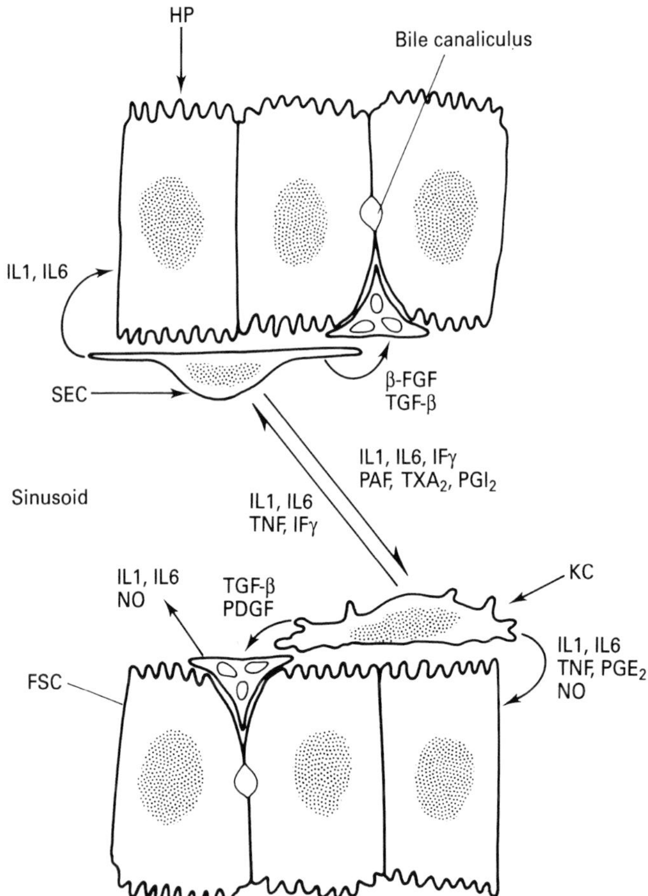

Fig. 5.1 Liver cell types and their interactions. In the adult mammalian liver, 65–70% of the cells are hepatocytes (HPs) and about 30–35% are non-parenchymal cells, including sinusoidal endothelial cells (SECs), Kupffer cells (KCs), and fat storage cells (FSCs). Most of these cell types can biotransform compounds, via cytochrome P450 and peroxidases, and the cells release a variety of mediators that regulate the function of other non-parenchymal cells or HPs. IF, interferon; IL, interleukin, FGF, fibroblast growth factor, NO, nitric oxide; PAF, platelet activating factor; PDGF, platelet-derived growth factor; PG, prostaglandin; TGF, transforming growth factor; TNF, tumor necrosis factor; TX, thromboxane.

compartment, matching the core diameter. A piston holding adjustable weights lightly compresses the tissue core. The tissue compartment is submerged in a preservation medium or an oxygenated buffer or tissue culture medium, to eliminate osmotic changes and dehydration. Slices are produced by moving the tissue compartment either manually or motor operated, across the rapidly motor-driven oscillating microtome blade. An internal current, supplied by a pump within the system, eliminates the adhesion of the tissue to the blade, such that the cut slice is rapidly removed from the blade and carried to a reservoir. Slice thickness is set by weights added to the piston and by adjusting the distance between the base plate, on which the tissue compartment stands, in relation to the microtome blade. The forces applied to the tissue during slicing are held constant and no manual pressure is required from the operator (Fig. 5.2).

To evaluate the conditions used during the slicing procedure on slice viability a rapid version of the reduction of the tetrazolium salt MTT (150 μg ml^{-1} EBSS, 15 min) to MTTF

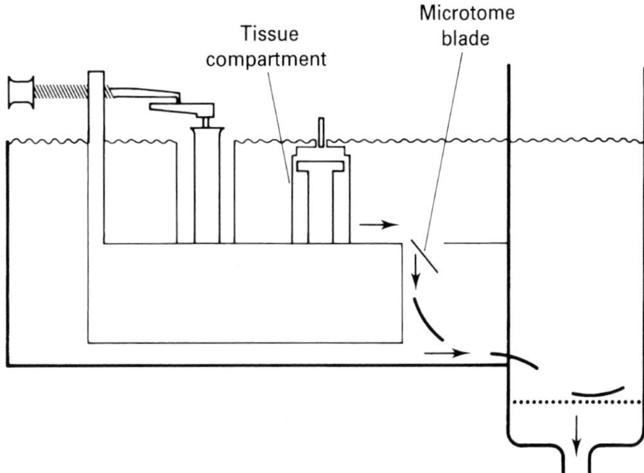

Fig. 5.2 Schematic of Krumdieck slicer. A tissue core is placed into a cylindrical tissue compartment which is submerged in medium. Slices are produced by moving the tissue compartment across the rapidly motor-driven oscillating microtome blade. An internal current rapidly removes the cut slice from the blade and carries it to a reservoir. Slice thickness is set by weights added to the piston and by adjusting the distance between the base plate, on which the tissue compartment stands, in relation to the microtome blade.

at 37°C is useful. The slice can be evaluated visually for the homogeneous or only peripheral distribution of MTTF.

It is also important to check and control slice thickness during slicing. Controlling slice thickness to within $200 \pm 25\,\mu m$ will affect both slice viability and its biotransformation capacity, particularly for long-term cultures. Slice thickness can be measured with a micrometer and determining the distance between two thin glass cover slips in the presence and absence of a slice. Another version of this method is to place the glass cover slips onto an electronic base plate and focus on a mark on the cover slip in the presence and absence of the slice (Fig. 5.3). The electronic readout of the difference between the two readings will be the slice thickness.

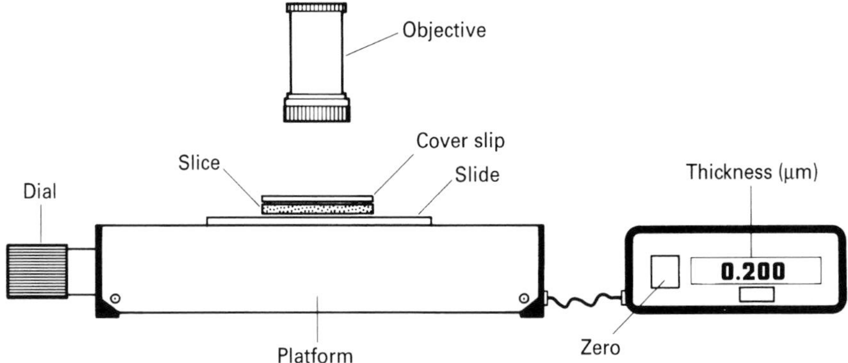

Fig. 5.3 Determination of slice thickness. A slice is placed between two cover slips or between a cover slip and a microscope slide, lying on top of an electronic base plate. The viewer focuses on a mark on the top cover slip in the presence and absence of the slice. The electronic readout of the difference between the two readings is the slice thickness.

Transfer of the slice to the culture insert (roller or plate) should be done carefully so as not to inflict mechanical damage to the slice. For example, the slice can be floated onto the insert, or lifted with a spatula, or transferred via manual aspiration of medium and slice through a seared wide-mouth sterile plastic pipette.

C. Incubation systems

The incubation systems are based on two types of principle: plate and roller cultures (Fig. 5.4). In plate cultures the slice is placed onto a platform so that it is just covered with medium. To facilitate gas and medium exchange with the slice, the medium is gently agitated by stirring the medium, or by rotating or rocking the plate. Culturing based on rotation of the slice through the gas and medium phases uses a roller insert placed into a glass scintillation vial containing enough medium to cover the slice as the vial is rotated. A small hole in the cap of the scintillation vial allows for gas exchange. The vials are rotated horizontally (about 2 r.p.m.) on a rotating rack in a controlled atmosphere or on rollers placed into a standard culturing incubator. The roller culture method for culturing the slices solved the problem of cell degeneration of the cells in the center of the slice and on the side of the tissue exposed to the medium.[60,61] The histological findings indicated that slices of thickness 250 μm cultured for 20 h were optimum in regard to morphology. Slices thinner than 100 μm were shown to have too large a ratio of cut to intact cells.[61]

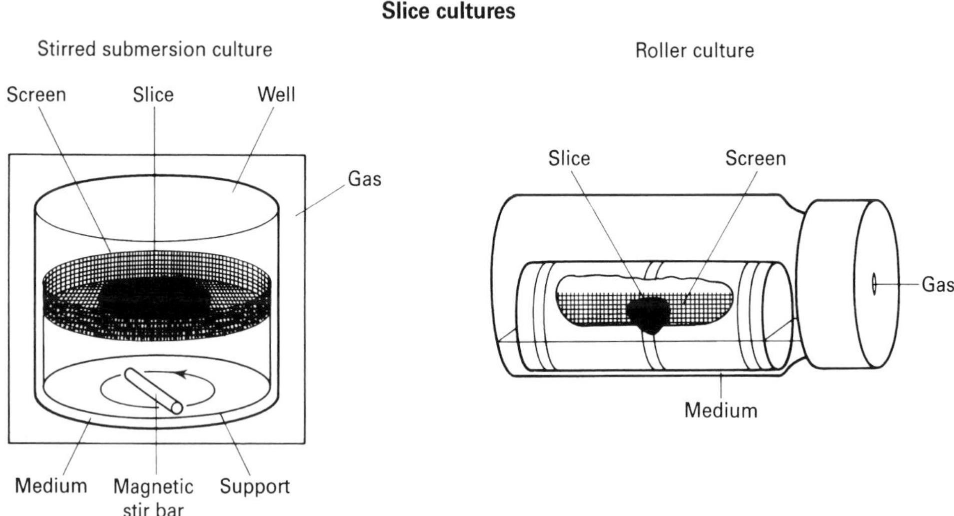

Fig. 5.4 Liver slice incubation systems. Slices are cultured either in plates as submersion cultures or in roller cultures. In plate cultures the slice is placed onto a platform, so that the slice is just covered with medium, and the medium is agitated by stirring or by rotating or rocking the plate to facilitate gas and nutrient exchange. For the roller culture method the slice is placed onto a roller insert and placed into a glass scintillation vial containing enough medium to cover the slice as the vial is rotated. A small hole in the cap of the scintillation vial allows for gas exchange. The vials are rotated horizontally (about 2 r.p.m.) on a rotating rack in a controlled atmosphere or on rollers placed into a standard culturing incubator.

Sensitive markers of viability, such as the leakage of α-glutathione *S*-transferases (α-GST) into the medium have been useful in optimizing culture conditions. The leakage of α-GST by human control liver slices generally exhibit medium α-GST levels of 20–30% after 24 h in roller cultures, depending on the organ quality and total organ preservation time. Control slices were more viable in roller cultures even up to 48 h of culture than slices from the same liver maintained in medium-stirred plate cultures.[62]

A preincubation period (90 min) of the slice in medium before addition of fresh medium and the compound allows the slices to recover from slicing and is critical for viability measurements.[59] Both human and rat liver slices are metabolically and functionally active when maintained in culture at 37°C (95% air/5% carbon dioxide) for 48–72 h.[62,63] With prolonged time in culture, cell clumps will continue to slough from the slice. The amount of sloughing is about 10% of the original slice protein within a 24 h period; this may, however, vary with compound treatment. The cells on the surface of the clumps often stain positively with trypan blue but the cell clumps can still be metabolically active. At various time points the slice and medium are separated and stored at − 80°C until analysis.

The viability and stability of rat liver slices has been assessed in the dynamic roller system. Intracellular levels of K^+, evidence for the intactness of liver cell membranes, activity of the sodium–potassium ion pump, and slice ATP levels were maintained for the 20 h of incubation. Markers of liver cell function including protein synthesis and secretion were linear over the culture period. The liver slices also synthesized glycogen in the presence of supplemental glucose and insulin, and responded to a glucagon challenge with glucose production.[61]

D. Cytochrome P450 levels

Some of the factors found to be beneficial for maintaining CYP450 levels in hepatocytes, including the culturing of hepatocytes on various substrata (floating collagen membranes, plastic plates coated with collagen or fibronectin) or co-culturing the hepatocytes with epithelial cells, should be an advantage for liver slices since tissue architecture and cell–cell interactions are maintained.[38,64] This, however, is not sufficient to maintain cytochrome P450 at *in vivo* levels.[63,65] The decline in cytochrome P450 content can in part be prevented by supplementation of the culture medium with hormones and ligands known to be beneficial for maintaining cytochrome P450 levels in hepatocyte cultures. Additionally, the compound to be tested could serve as a ligand for some of the cytochrome P450s, thereby maintaining their activity.[66]

The regulation of cytochrome P450 proteins is controlled in part locally in the liver, as well as by factors from outside the liver, i.e. the hypothalamopituitary axis, thyroid, and adrenals.[67,68] Thus, if these factors are lacking in the cultures, any liver *in vitro* system will not yield cytochrome P450 levels equal to those found *in vivo*. Furthermore, cytochrome P450 proteins and membrane phospholipids have half-lives of hours to days, a contributing factor to the loss observed.[69] Each *in vitro* system is also recovering from the trauma of slicing or the isolation procedure, such that, in the case of liver cell function, cells may be switching from pathways of homeostasis to a state of regeneration, thereby switching on some pathways and others off.

A validation that the liver slice preparation is metabolically competent is routinely to include an internal standard for which the biotransformation is well defined both *in vivo* and *in vitro*, and ideally a compound that is metabolized by several cytochrome P450 families. Such a validation procedure will also lead to optimization of the culture conditions, aid in judgment of the metabolic competence of the tissue, and increase the power of the prediction for an unknown compound. In general, biochemical activities measured in cultured hepatocytes can also be measured in slices, with appropriate adaptation of the technology.

VII. APPLICATION OF SLICES

A. Tissue culture medium

The composition of the culture medium affects liver cell viability and consequently the concentration and time of the toxicity profile. Rat liver slices maintained in a salt medium (Krebs–Henseleit buffer) exhibited toxicity to a series of chlorobenzenes at lower concentrations and earlier time–response curves than when the Krebs–Henseleit medium was supplemented with amino acids and vitamins.[70] Protection of oxidative damage to liver slice heme proteins has also been demonstrated by dietary supplementation of rats with vitamin E and selenium, in comparison to an antioxidant-deficient diet. Additionally, increasing the diversity of antioxidants in the diet was shown to provide significantly more protection.[71]

B. Interactive toxicity

1. *Ethanol potentiation of hepatotoxins*

Combination treatments of cocaine (0.5 mM) + ethanol (0.3%), and of cocaine (0.5 mM) + morphine (0.5 mM), have resulted in significant decreases in human liver slice viability compared with single treatments alone, demonstrating that the known potentiation of such hepatotoxins can be studied *in vitro*.[72] Combining ethanol (2%) with endotoxin, to mimic two toxins seen in trauma victims, has also been reported to produce an additive effect on toxicity in rat liver slices.[73]

2. *Cocaine*

A species and strain susceptibility to cocaine has been demonstrated *in vitro*. Liver slices derived from induced ICR mice and Sprague-Dawley rats displayed about three times more toxicity, assessed by slice K^+ and Ca^{2+} levels, to cocaine-mediated hepatotoxicity than liver slices derived from uninduced mice or rats, or pigs or humans.[74] Cocaine (1 mM)-mediated toxicity was reduced in rat liver slices through the irreversible inactivation of cytochrome P450 2B1 by chloramphenicol. A protection to the cocaine (0.5 mM) toxicity was shown by preincubating the liver slices with ρNO_2C1FA, a chloramphenicol analog and selective inactivator of 2B1/2, as well as in slices prepared from rats administered 200 mg kg^{-1} ρNO_2C1FA.[75]

Both chloroform ($CHCl_3$) and bromotrichloromethane ($BrCCl_3$) added to rat liver slices, irrespective of the order, resulted in a time-dependent loss of K^+ and cytochrome P450 levels. The cells most affected were the centrilobular hepatocytes, assessed by glucose-6-phosphate and isocitrate dehydrogenase activity, as opposed to the periportal cells, assessed by lactate dehydrogenase and alanine aminotransferase levels.[76]

C. Ranking of compounds

The toxicity ranking of a series of bromobenzene derivatives in rat liver slices paralleled the relative amount of covalent binding and correlated with the toxicity ranking noted from *in vivo* studies.[77,78] The hepatotoxicity of three dichlorobenzene isomers was also tested in human liver slices. Pretreatment of the human liver slices with the cytochrome P450 inhibitors SKF 525A and metyrapone inhibited the hepatotoxicity induced by 1,3- and 1,2-dichlorobenzene respectively, but had no effect on hepatotoxicity induced by 1,4-dichlorobenzene.[79]

The comparative toxic potential of cresol isomers (*o*-, *m*-, and *p*-methylphenol) was demonstrated in rat liver slices. The toxicity induced by *p*-methylphenol could be prevented by pretreatment of the slices with the thiol precursor *N*-acetylcysteine, and was enhanced with the glutathione-depleting agent diethyl maleate.[80]

The sensitivity of young children towards valproic acid-induced hepatotoxicity has been studied in liver slices from weanling and adult rats, and from a limited number of human livers. The rank order of toxicity by valproic acid and the metabolites, 2-propyl-2-pentenoic acid and 2-propyl-4-pentenoic acid, based on slice K^+ levels and protein synthesis was the same in both weanling and adult rat liver slices; however, the extent of toxicity was greater in the liver slices from weanling rats. Age-related differences toward the toxicity of valproic acid was evident in human liver slices. Liver slices from the donors less than 20 years of age exhibited more toxicity toward valproic acid than those from older donors.[81]

D. Mechanistic studies

The species susceptibility to acetaminophen toxicity known from *in vivo* studies has been demonstrated *in vitro*. Liver slices of hamster (sensitive species) exhibited a dose-dependent depletion of glutathione, and a greater extent of formation of the toxic metabolite, as determined by glutathione conjugate formation, than rat slices (insensitive species). A prediction of an 11-fold greater susceptibility of the hamster compared with the rat toward acetaminophen toxicity could be made. Rat liver slices had a greater capacity (35-fold) to form the non-toxic glucuronide and sulfate metabolites than to form the toxic metabolite, while in the hamster non-toxic pathways were only 2.25-fold greater than the toxic pathways. Damage to the centrilobular regions, loss of cellular architecture, and nuclear pyknosis, similar to the lesion found in the whole animal, were noted in the hamster liver slices but not rat.[12]

Following halothane exposure the major target of adduct formation in guinea-pig liver slices was to the cytosolic glutathione *S*-transferases (GSTs). Liver GSTs were also a target of adduct formation following the *in vivo* administration of halothane. Depletion of the liver glutathione levels by buthionine sulfoximine resulted in an increased covalent binding to cytosolic proteins only.[82]

The antioxidant *N*,*N*′-diphenyl-*p*-phenylenediamine has been shown to be effective in preventing the chemically induced oxidative stress induced by diquat dibromide. Both the amount of cellular lipid peroxidation and toxicity were reduced in the presence of the antioxidant.[83]

The cytotoxicity of allyl alcohol and bromobenzene in rat liver slices was inhibited by preincubation of the slices with the cytochrome P450 inhibitors, *β*-ethyl-2,2-diphenylvalerate hydrochloride (SKF 525 A) or pyrazole. The histopathology of the slices paralleled the biochemical changes – intracellular K^+ content, lactate dehydrogenase leakage, and protein synthesis – in the presence of toxicity; or lack of change in the absence of toxicity upon exposure of the slices to metabolic inhibitors.[84]

E. Surrogate markers

A goal in the use of *in vitro* models is to identify cellular markers that could be used *in vivo* to monitor the development or progression of a drug-induced side-effect or toxicity. For example, in liver transplant recipients the rate of decline of serum α-GST after operation, as well as the rate of increase of serum α-GST preceding rejection, exhibits significantly greater changes than the rate of change of other liver function measurements (transaminases, bilirubin). Following treatment for rejection, the median rate of decline of serum α-GST was about 30% per day, greater than twice the median rate of decline of all conventional biochemical liver function tests.[85] Hence, monitoring the serum α-GST levels provides a greater resolution of changes in hepatocellular integrity than conventional transaminase activities at a time when the risk of rejection and other complications is greatest. The measurement of α-GST levels can also serve as a marker *in vitro*, as has been demonstrated with human liver slice cultures to assess various culture conditions, as well as cell viability in the presence of cyclosporin derivatives.[62]

A marker for lipid disturbances as well as liver recovery post-transplantation may prove to be an increase in serum lipoprotein (a) (Lp(a)) levels.[86–88] Two recent studies demonstrate that cyclosporin A raises serum Lp(a) levels in renal transplant recipients.[89,90] Cyclosporin A is transported by plasma lipoproteins and perturbs the lipid profile of transplant recipients, raising plasma cholesterol, low density lipoprotein cholesterol, triglycerides, very low density lipoprotein triglycerides, and apolipoprotein B. The liver is a target in that it is the main site of lipoprotein synthesis and cyclosporin A metabolism. The usefulness of Lp(a) as a marker can be effectively studied only in those species where it has been detected: humans, apes, and non-human primates.[88] *In vitro* Lp(a) levels in human liver slices were increased by cyclosporin A (1 and 10 μM) within 24 h, about twofold over dimethyl sulfoxide (DMSO) control.[62] This *in vitro* finding mimicked the increased serum Lp(a) levels (1.8–3.6-fold) induced by cyclosporin A in renal transplant recipients.[89,90]

F. Induction and peroxisome proliferation

Rat liver slices exposed to the peroxisome proliferator compounds, nafenopin, ciprofibrate, and Wy-14,634, for 72 h exhibited a time- and concentration-dependent increase in palmitoyl coenzyme A oxidation and carnitine acetyl-transferase activities, with activities exceeding those of freshly cut slices at higher concentrations of the peroxisome proliferators. Morphologic investigations also revealed an increased number of peroxisomes in the liver slices exposed to ciprofibrate and Wy-14,634.[63,91]

Induction of several cytochrome P450s in rat liver slices has been demonstrated by the increased metabolism of 7-ethoxycoumarin, 7-benzoxyresorufin, and 7-ethoxyresorufin following phenobarbitone, β-naphthoflavone or Aroclor 1254 exposure. In general, induction was greater at 72 h of culture than at 48 h. CYP1A1 levels were detectable by immunoblotting in the β-naphthoflavone (25 μM) induced slices at 48 h, but not in the control slices.[91]

VIII. APPLICATION OF HEPATOCYTES

A. Comparing a series of compounds

Toxicity of three commonly used non-steroidal anti-inflammatory drugs of the aryl alkanoic acid group, ibuprofen, flurbiprofen, and butibufen, was demonstrated in rat hepatocytes at ten times the therapeutic plasma concentration. A marker of liver function, albumin synthesis, was inhibited at five times the therapeutic concentration.[35]

The potency ranking of five haloalkanes *in vitro* in rat hepatocytes and *in vivo* was the same except for one compound (1,1,2-trichloroethane; TCE) because of differences amongst the compounds in volatility and solubility in aqueous and lipid phases. The discepancy was solved by factoring the air : medium partition coefficient data into the EC_{50} values.[92]

Five anthracyclins (doxorubicin, daunorubicin, epirubicin, esorubicin, and idarubicin) were shown to be about twofold less toxic (LDH leakage and morphologic) to human than to rat hepatocytes. The species susceptibility could be explained by the more extensive biotransformation of the anthracyclins by human hepatocytes, including glucuronide formation, than by rat hepatocytes.[93]

B. Comparative transport

Both the uptake and transport of bile acids in rat and human hepatocytes has been demonstrated to be inhibited with increasing concentrations of the immunosuppressant cyclosporin A. These findings are the basis to understanding the hepatic dysfunction associated with cyclosporin A treatment, which is manifested as a rise in total serum bile acids and serum bilirubin with minor changes in serum transaminases.[94–96]

Hepatocyte couplets have been shown to retain much of their cell polarity during the isolation process, and represent a system for studying canalicular bile formation, including the secretion of compounds into the bile. Initially upon isolation of the couplets, the biliary canaliculus is collapsed and non-functional, but recovery is detected within 3–5 h. Differences in the amount of pericanalicular accumulation of F-actin has served as a marker for restoration of cell polarity and may prove to be a marker for an alteration of bile canalicular contractibility and cholestasis.[97]

C. Mechanistic studies

Pretreatment of human hepatocytes with ethanol (50–100 mM) decreased the half-maximal cytotoxic concentration of heroin by 70–55% and of methadone by 60–40%. Concomitant with the increased toxicity was a 40% increase in CYP2E levels in the hepatocytes.[98]

The toxicity of cocaine toward human hepatocytes was also enhanced by pretreatment of the cells with ethanol (50 mM). Cocaine concentrations (0.25 mM) which had no effect on hepatocyte function in the absence of ethanol caused a 20% inhibition in the rate of urea synthesis, and a reduction in glycogen stores (40%) and glutathione content (30%) after ethanol pretreatment. Ethanol increased the effects of cocaine on human hepatocytes by a factor of ten.[99]

Acetaminophen toxicity to centrilobular hepatoyctes has been demonstrated to be mediated by the higher expression of CYP2E1 and metabolism of acetaminophen in perivenous rather than periportal hepatocyte populations isolated from male rats. Following induction of CYP2E1 by ethanol pretreatment, the perivenous hepatocytes exhibited enhanced toxicity, increased covalent binding of acetaminophen intermediates, and depletion of glutathione. A CYP2E1 inhibitor, isoniazid, protected the cells against acetaminophen toxicity and glutathione depletion.[22]

An increased sensitivity of rat hepatoyctes to peroxisomal proliferators compared with human hepatocytes can be shown *in vitro*. Dose-related increases of peroxisomal fatty acid β-oxidation are correlated with an increased number of peroxisomes in rat hepatoyctes for several peroxisomal proliferating compounds, while hepatocytes derived from human, monkey, and guinea-pig show no effect at the same concentrations.[100–102]

The sensitivity of rat versus human hepatocytes to anoxia–reoxygenation injury was studied in hepatocytes maintained in a stationary phase with agarose and perfused under anoxic and reoxygenation conditions. During reoxygenation, after a 2.5-h period of anoxia, human hepatocytes were less sensitive, generated fewer oxygen-free radicals and lipoperoxides, and exhibited less cytotoxicity than rat hepatocytes.[103]

Hepatocytes have been used to demonstrate the formation of free radicals in intact liver cells. The formation of the nitrofurantoin radical anion from several nitrofuran and nitroimidazole compounds inside rat hepatocytes was observed by electron spin resonance (ESR) spectroscopy.[104]

The formation of trifluoroacetylated neoantigens occurs *in vitro* following exposure of human and rat hepatocytes to halothane.[105,106] Adduct formation was localized mainly to the endoplasmic reticulum, and in human hepatocytes to the plasma membrane. Adduct formation was also dependent on biotransformation of halothane to the reactive intermediate trifluoroacetyl halide, as demonstrated by the lack of adduct formation when hepatocytes were pretreated with the cytochrome P450 inhibitor SKF 525A.[106]

D. DNA synthesis and adducts

Both human and rat hepatocytes can undergo DNA synthesis in response to stimuli such as epidermal growth factor. Rat hepatocytes display an increased incorporation of [^{3}H]thymidine in response to compounds known to be liver tumor promoters in rodents, whereas human hepatocytes exhibit no compound-related effect.[107]

Chemically induced DNA repair, measured as unscheduled DNA synthesis, is routinely performed in rat hepatocytes to predict potential genotoxic effects in humans. When human hepatocytes are used, the interindividual variation is greater than for cultures derived from rat.[108]

A series of five *n*-alkanals was compared in rat and human hepatocytes to induce unscheduled DNA synthesis. Dose-dependent effects were seen in the rat hepatocytes, and no effects were picked up in human hepatoyctes. At the concentrations expected following ingestion of food or generated by lipid peroxidation, the five *n*-alkanals did not induce genotoxic effects in human liver.[109]

Evaluation of DNA adduct formation in rat versus human hepatocytes provides a means of assessing the carcinogenic risk for humans of some chemical carcinogens. For three chemical carcinogens, 2-acetyl-aminofluorene, 4-aminobiphenyl, and benzo[a]pyrene, the predominant DNA adducts were the same in rat and human hepatocytes. Some specific adducts were seen in the rat, or the converse. The extrapolation to humans *in vivo* is substantiated by the rat hepatocyte *in vitro* results, reflecting the predominant adducts found with rats exposed *in vivo*.[110] Adduct formation of ethylene bromide (EDB) was demonstrated to be dependent on the initial conjugation of EDB with glutathione to form an episulfonium ion which binds to DNA. Human hepatocytes displayed less adduct formation than rat hepatocytes at 0.5 mM EDB, but the genotoxic pathway of EDB metabolism in rats and humans is similar. Concurrent treatment of the hepatocytes with diethylmaleate to deplete intracellular glutathione inhibited EDB-induced unscheduled DNA synthesis.[111]

The induction of apoptosis in rat hepatoyctes has been demonstrated with transforming growth factor-β1 (TGF-β1). *In vivo* studies have revealed the presence of TGF-β1 in apoptotic liver cells. *In vitro* the exposure of hepatocytes to TGF-β1 induces cell rounding, condensation of the chromatin and nuclear fragmentation.[112]

An understanding toward the mechanism of increased cell volume, cell swelling, and proteolysis which can be induced by either culture conditions or compound exposure has been monitored in rat and human hepatocytes by the increased uptake of acridine orange, suggesting a role for alkalinization of acidic vesicles. However, the microtubule inhibitors colcemid and colchicine but not the inactive stereoisomer γ-lumicolchicine blocked the pH increase during osmotic swelling, indicating involvement of the microtubule network in controlling cell volume, lysosomal pH, and proteolysis.[113]

IX. CONCLUSIONS

The major contributions of *in vitro* systems, hepatocytes and slices, for studying hepatotoxicity include: the ranking of a series of compounds, the evaluation and comparison of species susceptibility, and investigation toward understanding the mechanism of the toxicity. A continuous goal for these systems is to demonstrate that the data obtained are predictive and can be used reliably in extrapolating from animals to humans for safety assessment. Further validation of the systems for risk assessment will increase the use of data obtained within companies and by regulatory authorities. Within companies the *in vitro* data could aid in the planning of investigational *in vivo* studies and the data could be used in combination with computer modeling to assess risk. In the future, *in vitro* data may change the type and number of *in vivo* studies performed, resulting in a further reduction in the total number of animals used.

A major impact of the hepatocyte and slice *in vitro* systems is in clearly defining species susceptibility, including human, to the side-effects or toxicity of the compound in question. This information could contribute to defining the safety margin or establishing the risk for humans. Furthermore, understanding the mechanism of toxicity may lead to the development of a compound with a wider safety margin or may result in a means of counteracting the effect *in vivo*. For example, the use of *S*-adenosylmethionine and *N*-acetylcysteine, glutathione precursors, has been beneficial in preventing experimentally induced paracetamol hepatotoxicity,[114] and *N*-acetylcysteine has reduced the mortality and worsening of encephalopathy in paracetamol-induced fulminant hepatic failure.[115]

Direct comparisons of hepatocyte functions normalized for the amount of cellular protein should not be made to slice protein values. Hepatocyte cultures are a selected, and often further enriched, population of liver cells containing more than 95% hepatocytes, whereas the slices contain all the cell types of the organ, of which 60% of the slice volume will be hepatocytes.

In future, cryopreservation of hepatocytes and slices will improve the availability of tissue and the application of these *in vitro* systems. Cyropreserved hepatocytes (from weeks to 4 years) from various species, including humans, are showing promising results.[116] Cold-preserved human liver slices (12–24 h) and kidney slices (4–6 days), as well as cryopreserved slices, are being used to optimize preservation solutions and methods. Following cryopreservation the viability of the liver slices is 65–90% and for kidney slices 70–90%. The viability parameters included intracellular K^+ levels, protein synthesis, gluconeogenesis, and urea synthesis (liver slices), and organic ion – anion and cation – transport (kidney slices).[117]

REFERENCES

1. Rojkind, M. (1994) The extracellular matrix of the liver. In Arias, I. M., Boyer, J. L., Fausto, N., Jakoby, W. B., Schachter, D. A. and Shafritz, D. A. (eds) *The Liver: Biology and Pathobiology*, 3rd edn, pp. 843–868. Raven Press, New York.
2. Desmet, V. J. (1994) Organizational principles. In Arias, I. M., Jakoby, W. B., Popper, H., Schachter, D. A. and Shafritz, D. A. (eds) *The Liver: Biology and Pathobiology*, 2nd edn, pp. 3–14. Raven Press, New York.
3. Steinberg, P., Lafranconi, W. M., Wolf, R. W., Waxman, D. J., Oesch, F. and Friedberg, T. (1987) Xenobiotic metabolizing enzymes are not restricted to parenchymal cells in rat liver. *Mol. Pharmacol.* **32:** 463–470.
4. Steinberg, P., Schramm, H., Schladt, L., Robertson, L. W., Thomas, H. and Oesch, F. (1989) The distribution, induction and isoenzyme profile of glutathione *S*-transferase and glutathione peroxidase in isolated rat liver parenchymal, Kupffer and endothelial cells. *Biochem. J.* **264:** 737–744.
5. Laskin, D. L. (1990) Nonparenchymal cells and hepatotoxicity. *Semin. Liver Dis.* **10:** 293–304.
6. Sallie, R., Tredger, J. M. and Williams, R. (1991) Drugs and the liver. Part 1: Testing liver function. *Biopharm. Drug Dispos.* **12:** 251–259.
7. Mehendale, H. M. (1991) Commentary: role of hepatocellular regeneration and hepatolobular healing in the final outcome of liver injury. A two stage model of toxicity. *Biochem. Pharmacol.* **42:** 1155–1161.
8. Mehendale, H. M., Roth, R. A., Gandolfi, A. E., Klaunig, J. E. Lemasters, J. J. and Curtis, L. R. (1994) Novel mechanisms in chemically induced hepatoxicity. *Faseb J.* **8:** 1285–1295.
9. Watkins, P. B. (1990) Role of cytochromes P450 in drug metabolism and hepatotoxicity. *Semin. Liver Dis.* **10:** 235–250.
10. Boyer, T. D. (1989) The glutathione *S*-transferases: an update. *Hepatology* **9:** 486–496.
11. Lee, W. M. (1993) Review article: drug-induced hepatoxicity. *Aliment. Pharmacol. Ther.* **7:** 477–485.
12. Miller, M. G., Beyer, J., Hall, G. L., DeGraffenried, L. A. and Adams, P. E. (1993) Predictive value of liver slices for metabolism and toxicity *in vivo*: use of acetaminophen as a model hepatotoxicant. *Toxicol. Appl. Pharmacol.* **122:** 108–116.
13. Reed, D. J. (1990) Status of calcium and thiols in hepatocellular injury by oxidative stress. *Semin. Liver Dis.* **10:** 285–292.
14. Deleve, L. D. and Kaplowitz, N. (1990) Importance and regulation of hepatic glutathione. *Semin. Liver Dis.* **10:** 251–266.
15. Berry, M. N., Halls, H. J. and Grivell, M. B. (1992) Techniques for pharmacological and toxicological studies with isolated hepatocyte suspensions. *Life Sci.* **51:** 1–16.
16. Blaauboer, B. J., Boobis, A. R., Castell, J. V. *et al.* (1994) The practical applicability of hepatocyte cultures in routine testing. *ATLA* **22:** 231–241.
17. Bissel, D. M., Hammaker, L. E. and Meyer, U. S. (1973) Parenchymal cells from adult rat liver in nonproliferating monolayer culture. *J. Cell. Biol.* **59:** 722–734.
18. Decad, G. M., Hsieh, D. P. H. and Byard, J. L. (1977) Maintenance of cytochrome P-450 and metabolism of aflatoxin B_1 in primary hepatocyte cultures. *Biochem. Biophys. Res. Commun.* **78:** 279–287.

19. Gomez-Lechon, M. J., Montoya, A., Lopez, P., Donato, M. T., Larrauri, A. and Castell, J. V. (1988) The potential use of cultured hepatocytes in predicting the hepatoxicity of xenobiotics. *Xenobiotica* **18:** 725–735.
20. Alpini, G., Phillips, J. O., Vroman, B. and LaRusso, N. F. (1994) Recent advances in the isolation of liver cells. *Hepatology* **20:** 494–514.
21. Guguen-Guillouzo, C. and Guillouzo, A. (1986) Methods for preparation of adult and fetal hepatocytes. In Guillouzo, A. and Guguen-Guillouzo, C. (eds) *Isolated and Cultured Hepatocytes*, pp. 1–12. Les Editions INSERM, Paris and John Libbey Eurotext, London.
22. Anundi, I., Lahteenmaki, T., Rundgren, M., Moldeus, P. and Lindros, K. O. (1993) Zonation of acetaminophen metabolism and cytochrome P450 2E1-mediated toxicity studied in isolated periportal and perivenous hepatocytes. *Biochem. Pharmacol.* **45:** 1251–1259.
23. Boyer, J. L., Phillips, J. M. and Graf, J. (1990) Preparation and specific applications of isolated hepatocyte couplets. *Methods Enzymol.* **192:** 501–516.
24. Wilton, J. C., Williams, D. E., Strain, A. J., Parslow, R. A., Chipman, J. K. and Coleman, R. (1991) Purification of hepatocyte couplets by centrifugal elutriation. *Hepatology* **14:** 180–183.
25. Powis, G., Melder, D. C. and Wilke, T. J. (1989) Human and dog, but not rat, isolated hepatocytes have decreased foreign compound-metabolizing activity compared to liver slices. *Drug Metab. Dispos.* **17:** 526–531.
26. Zhang, S.-Z., Lipsky, M. M., Trump, B. F. and Hsu, I.-C. (1990) Neutral red (nr) assay for cell viability and xenobiotic-induced cytotoxicity in primary cultures of human and rat hepatocytes. *Cell Biol. Toxicol.* **6:** 219–234.
27. Fry, J. R., Hammond, A. H., Atmaca, M., Dhanjal, P. and Wilkinson, D. J. (1995) Toxicity testing with hepatocytes: some methodological aspects. *ATLA* **23:** 91–96.
28. Ponsoda, X., Jover, R., Castell, J. V. and Gomez-Lechon, M. J. (1991) Measurement of intracellular LDH acticity in 96-well cultures: a rapid and automated assay for cytotoxicity studies. *J. Tissue Cult. Methods.* **13:** 21–24.
29. Schnellmann, R. G. (1994) Measurement of oxygen consumption. In *Methods in Toxicology*, Vol. 1B, pp. 128–139. Academic Press, New York.
30. Park, Y., Aw, T. Y. and Jones, D. P. (1994) ATP and other energetic parameters as indicators of cell injury. In *Methods in Toxicology*, Vol. 1B, pp. 140–151. Academic Press, New York.
31. Jover, R., Ponsoda, X., Gomez-Lechon, J. and Castell, J. V. (1993) Cocaine hepatotoxicity: two different toxicity mechanisms for phenobarbital – induced and non-induced rat hepatocytes. *Biochem. Pharmacol.* **46:** 1967–1974.
32. Kefalas, V. and Stacey, N. H. (1994) Cellular K^+. In *Methods in Toxicology*, Vol.1B, pp. 50–57. Academic Press, New York.
33. Castell, J. V., Montoya, A., Larrauri, A., Lopez, P. and Gomez-Lechon, M. J. (1985) Effects of benorylate and impacina on the metabolism of cultured hepatocytes. *Xenobiotica* **15:** 743–749.
34. Knowles, R. G. and Pogson, C. I. (1994) Gluconeogenesis in liver cells. In *Methods in toxicology*, Vol. 1B, pp. 248–257. Academic Press, New York.
35. Castell, J. V., Larrauri, A. and Gomez-Lechon, M. J. (1988) A study of the relative hepatotoxicity *in vitro* of the non-steroidal anti-inflammatory drugs ibuprofen, flurbiprofen and butibufen. *Xenobiotica* **18:** 737–745.
36. Bissel, D. M., Arenson, D. M., Maher, J. J. and Roll, F. J. (1987) Support of cultured hepatocytes by a laminin-rich gel. Evidence for a functionally significant subendothelial matrix in normal liver. *J. Clin. Invest.* **79:** 801–812.
37. Fujita, M., Spray, D. C., Chui, H. *et al.* (1987) Glycosaminoglycans and proteoglycans induce gap junction expression and restore transcription of tissue specific mRNAs in primary liver cultures. *Hepatology* **7:** 1–9.
38. Guillouzo, A., Morel, F., Ratanasavanh, D., Chesne, C. and Guguen-Guillouzo, C. (1990) Long-term culture of functional hepatocytes. *Toxicol. In Vitro* **4:** 415–427.
39. Guguen-Guillouzo, C., Clement, B., Baffet, G. *et al.* (1983) Maintenance and reversibility of active albumin secretion by adult rat hepatocytes co-cultured with another liver epithelial cell type. *Exp. Cell Res.* **143:** 47–54.
40. Gibson-D'Ambrosia, R. E., Crowe, D. L., Shuler, C. E. and D'Ambrosio, S. M. (1993) The establishment and continuous subculturing of normal human adult hepatocytes: expression of differentiated liver functions. *Cell Biol. Toxicol.* **9:** 385–403.
41. Dunn, J. C. Y., Tompkins, R. G. and Yarmush, M. L. (1991) Long-term *in vitro* function of adult hepatocytes in a collagen sandwich configuration. *Biotechnol. Prog.* **7:** 237–245.

42. Bader, A., Zech, K., Crome, O. *et al.* (1994) Use of organotypical cultures of primary hepatocytes to analyse drug biotransformation in man and animals. *Xenobiotica* **24:** 623–633.
43. LeCluyse, E. L., Audus, K. L. and Hochman, J. H. (1994) Formation of extensive canalicular networks by rat hepatocytes cultured in collagen-sandwich configuration. *Am. J. Physiol.* **266:** C1764–C1774.
44. Li, A. P., Colburn, S. M. and Beck, D. J. (1992) A simplified method for the culturing of primary adult rat and human hepatocytes as multicellular spheroids. *In Vitro Cell. Dev. Biol.* **28A:** 673–677.
45. Parsons-Wingerter, P. A. and Saltzman, W. M. (1993) Growth versus function in the three-dimensional culture of single and aggregated hepatocytes within collagen gels. *Biotechnol. Prog.* **9:** 600–607.
46. Curran, T. R., Bahner, R. I., Oh, W. and Gruppuso, P. A. (1993) Mitogen-independent DNA synthesis by fetal rat hepatocytes in primary culture. *Exp. Cell Res.* **209:** 53–57.
47. Kremer P., Roelandt, L., Stouvenakers, N., Goffinet, G. and Thome, J. P. (1994) Expression and induction of drug-metabolizing enzymes in cultured fetal rat hepatocytes. *Cell Biol. Toxicol.* **10:** 117–125.
48. Milward, E. A. and Yeoh, G. C. T (1990) Expression of alpha-fetoprotein by differentiating fetal rat hepatocytes *in vitro*. *Eur. J. Cell Biol.* **52:** 185–192.
49. Sherratt, A. J., Banet, D. E. and Prough, R. A. (1990) Glucocorticoid regulation of polycyclic aromatic hydrocarbon induction of cytochrome P450lA1, glutathione *s*-transferases, and NAD(P)H:quinone oxidoreductase in cultured fetal rat hepatocytes. *Mol. Pharmacol.* **37:** 198–205.
50. Parmentier, J.-H., Kremers, P., Ferrari, L., Batt, A.-M., Gielen, J. E. and Siest, G. (1993) Repression of cytochrome P450 by cytokines: IL-1β counteracts clofibric acid induction of cyp4A in cultured fetal rat hepatocytes. *Cell Biol. Toxicol.* **9:** 307–314.
51. Hoffmann, B., Piasecki, A. and Dieter, P. (1989) Proliferation of fetal rat hepatocytes in response to growth factors and hormones in primary culture. *J. Cell. Physiol.* **139:** 654–662.
52. Nau, H., Liddiard, C., Merker, H.-J. and Brendel, K. (1978) Preparation, morphology and drug metabolism of isolated hepatocyte and liver organ cultures from the human fetus. *Life Sci.* **23:** 2361–2372.
53. Liddiard, C., Mercker, H.-J. and Nau, H. (1980) An improved method for the preparation of human fetal and adult hepatocytes. *Toxicology* **44:** 107–112.
54. Bauer, J., Lengyel, G., Thung, S. N., Janas, U., Gerok, W. and Acs, G. (1990) Human fetal hepatocytes respond to inflammatory mediators and excrete bile. *Hepatology* **13:** 1131–1141.
55. Payne, A. K., Morgan, S. E., Gandolfi, A. J. and Brendel, K. (1995) Biotransformation of sevoflurane by rat neonate liver slices. *Drug Metab. Dispos.* **23:** 497–500.
56. De Juan, C., Benito, M. and Fabregat, I. (1992) Regulation of albumin expression in fetal rat hepatocytes cultured under proliferative conditions: role of epidermal growth factor and hormones. *J. Cell. Physiol.* **101:** 152–195.
57. Devi, B. G., Henderson, G. I., Frosto, T. A. and Schenker, S. (1993) Effect of ethanol on rat fetal hepatocytes: studies on cell replication lipid peroxidation and glutathione. *Hepatology* **18:** 648–659.
58. Krumdieck, C., Dos Santos, J. E. and Ho, K.-J. (1980) A new instrument for the rapid preparation of tissue slices. *Anal. Biochem.* **104:** 118–123.
59. Brendel, K., Fisher, R., Krumdieck, C. L. and Gandolfi, A. J. (1990) Precision-cut rat liver slices in dynamic organ culture for structure-toxicity studies. *J. Am. Coll. Toxicol.* **9:** 621–627.
60. Smith, P. F., Gandolfi, A. J., Krumdieck, C. L. *et al.* (1985) Dynamic organ culture of precision liver slices for *in vitro* toxicology. *Life Sci.* **36:** 1367–1375.
61. Smith, P. F., Drack, G., McKee, R. L. *et al.* (1986) Maintenance of adult rat liver slices in dynamic organ culture. *In Vitro Cell. Dev. Biol.* **22:** 706–712.
62. Vickers, A. E. M. (1994) Use of human organ slices to evaluate the biotransformation and drug-induced side-effects of pharmaceuticals. *Cell Biol. and Toxicol.* **10:** 407–414.
63. Beamand, J. A., Price, R. J., Cunninghame, M. E. and Lake, B. G. (1993) Culture of precision-cut liver slices: effect of some peroxisome proliferators. *Fd. Chem. Toxicol.* **31:** 137–147.
64. Michalopoulos, G., Sattler, G. L. and Pitot, H. C. (1976) Maintenance of microsomal cytochromes b5 and P-450 in primary cultures of parenchymal liver cells on collagen membranes. *Life Sci.* **18:** 1139–1144.
65. Wright, M. C. and Paine, A. J. (1992) Evidence that the loss of rat liver cytochrome P450 *in vitro* is not solely associated with the use of collagenase, the loss of cell–cell contacts and/or the absence of an extracellular matrix. *Biochem. Pharmacol.* **43:** 237–243.

66. Eliasson, E., Mkrtchian, S. and Ingelman-Sundberg, M. (1992) Hormone- and substrate-regulated intracellular degradation of cytochrome P450 (2E1) involving MgATP-activated rapid proteolysis in the endoplasmic reticulum membranes. *J. Biol. Chem.* **267:** 15 765–15 769.
67. Gustafsson, J. A., Eneroth, P., Hökfelt, T., Mode, A., Norstedt, G. and Skett, P. (1981) Role of the hypothalamo-pituitary–liver axis in sex differences in susceptibility of the liver to toxic agents. *Environ. Health Perspect.* **38:** 129–141.
68. Waxman, D. J., Morrissey, J. J and Leblanc, G. A. (1989) Hypophysectomy differentially alters P-450 protein levels and enzyme activities in rat liver: pituitary control of hepatic NADPH cyrochrome P-450 reductase. *Mol. Pharmacol.* **35:** 519–525.
69. Omura, T. (1989) Cytochrome P-450 linked mixed function oxidase turnover of microsomal components and effects of inducers on the turnover phospholipids, proteins and specific enzymes. *Pharmacol. Ther.* **8:** 489–499.
70. Fisher, R. L., Gandolfi, A. J., Sipes, I. G. and Brendel, K. (1993) Culture medium composition affects the relative toxicities of chlorobenzenes in rat liver slices and the isolated perfused liver. *Drug Chem. Toxicol.* **16:** 321–339.
71. Chen, H. and Tappal, Al. L. (1994) Protection by vitamin E, selenium, trolox C, ascorbic acid palmitate, acetylcysteine, coenzyme Q, beta-carotene, canthaxanthin, and (+)-catechin against oxidative damage to liver slices measured by oxidized heme proteins. *Free Radic. Biol. Med.* **16:** 437–444.
72. Connors, S., Rankin, D. R., Krumdieck, C. L. and Brendel, K. (1989) Interactive toxicity of cocaine with phenobarbital, morphine and ethanol in organ cultured human and rat liver slices. *Proc. West. Pharmacol. Soc.* **32:** 205–208.
73. Sawyer, J. S., Daller, J. A., Brendel, K., Yohem, K. and Putnam, C. W. (1994) The hepatoxicities of endotoxin and ethanol: comparisons *in vitro* using the precision-cut rat liver slice model. *Life Sci.* **55:** 1407–1417.
74. Connors, S., Rankin, D. R., Gandolfi, A. J., Krumdieck, C. L., Koep, L. J. and Brendel, K. (1990) Cocaine hepatotoxicity in cultured liver slices: a species comparison. *Toxicology* **61:** 171–183.
75. Poet, T. S., Brendel, K. and Halpert, J. R. (1994) Inactivation of cytochromes P450 2B protects against cocaine-mediated toxicity in rat liver slices. *Toxicol. Appl. Pharmacol.* **126:** 26–32.
76. Azri-Meehan, S., Mata, H. P., Gandolfi, A. J. and Brendel, K. (1994) The interactive toxicity of $CHCl_3$ and $BrCCl_3$ in precision cut rat liver slices. *Fundam. Appl. Toxicol.* **22:** 172–177.
77. Fisher, R., Hanzlik, H. P., Gandolfi, A. J. and Brendel, K. (1991) Toxicity of ortho-subsituted bromobenzenes in rat liver slices: a comparison to isolated hepatocytes and the whole animal. *In Vitro Toxicol.* **4:** 173–186.
78. Fisher, R., Brendel, K. and Hanzlik, R. P. (1993) Correlation of metabolism, covalent binding and toxicity for a series of bromobenzene derivatives using rat liver slices *in vitro*. *Chem. Biol. Interact.* **88:** 191–208.
79. Fisher, R., Barr, J., Zukoski, C. F. *et al.* (1991) *In vitro* hepatoxicity of three dichlorobenzene isomers in human liver slices. *Hum. Exp. Toxicol.* **10:** 357–363.
80. Thompson, D. C., Perera, K., Fisher, R. and Brendel, K. (1994) Cresol isomers: comparison to toxic potency in rat liver slices. *Toxicol. Appl. Pharmacol.* **125:** 51–58.
81. Fisher, R. L., Sanuik, J. T., Nau, H., Gandolfi, A. J. and Brendel, K. (1994) Comparative toxicity of valproic acid and its metabolites in liver slices from adult rats, weanling rats and humans. *Toxicol. In Vitro* **8:** 371–379.
82. Brown, A. P. and Gandolfi, A. J. (1994) Glutathione *S*-transferase is a target for covalent modification by a halothane reactive intermediate in the guinea pig liver. *Toxicology* **89:** 35–47.
83. Wolfgang, C. H., Jolly, R. A., Donarski, W. J. and Petry, T. W. (1991) Inhibition of diquat-induced lipid peroxidation and toxicity in precision-cut rat liver slices by novel antioxidants. *Toxicol. Appl. Pharmacol.* **108:** 321–329.
84. Smith, P. F., Fisher, R., Shubat, P., Gandolfi, A. J., Krumdieck, C. L. and Brendel, K. (1987) *In vitro* cytotoxicity of allyl alcohol and bromobenzene in a novel organ culture. *Toxicol. Appl. Pharmacol.* **87:** 509–522.
85. Trull, A. K., Facey, S. P., Rees, G. W. *et al.* (1994) Serum α-glutathione *S*-transferases – a sensitive marker of hepatocellular damage associated with acute liver allograft rejection. *Transplantation* **58:** 1345–1351.
86. Malmendier, C., Lontie, J., Mathe, D., Adam, R. and Bismuth, H. (1992) Lipid and apolipoprotein changes after orthotopic liver transplantation for end-stage liver diseases. *Clin. Chim. Acta.* **209:** 169–177.

87. Kostner, G. (1993) Interaction of Lp(a) and of Apo(a) with liver cells. *Arterioscler. Thromb.* **13:** 1101–1109.
88. Scanu, A. (1993) Structural basis for the presumptive atherothrombogenic action of lipoprotein (a) *Biochem. Pharmacol.* **46:** 1675–1680.
89. Brown, J., Anwar, N., Short, C. *et al.* (1993) Serum lipoprotein (a) in renal transplant recipients receiving cyclosporin monotherapy. *Nephrol. Dial. Transplant.* **8:** 863–867.
90. Webb, W., Reaveley, D., O'Donell, M., O'Connor, B., Seed, M. and Brown, E. (1993) Does cyclosporin increase lipoprotein(a) concentrations in renal transplant recipients? *Lancet* **341:** 268–270.
91. Lake, B. G., Beamand, J. A., Japenga, A. C., Renwick, A., Davies, S. and Price, R. J. (1993) Induction of cytochrome P-450 dependent enzyme activities in cultured rat liver slices. *Fd. Chem. Toxicol.* **31:** 377–386.
92. Tyson, C. A., Hawk-Prather, K., Story, D. L. and Gould, D. H. (1983) Correlations of *in vitro* and *in vivo* hepatoxicity for five haloalkanes. *Toxicol. Appl. Pharmacol.* **70:** 289–302.
93. Le Bot, M. A., Begue, J. M., Kernaleguen, D. *et al.* (1988) Different cytotoxicity and metabolism of doxorubicin, daunorubicin, epirubicin, esorubicin, and idarubicin in cultured human and rat hepatocytes. *Biochem. Pharmacol.* **37:** 3877–3887.
94. Kukongviriyapan, V. and Stacey, N. H. (1988) Inhibition of taurocholate transport by cyclosporin A in cultured rat hepatocytes. *J. Pharmacol. Exp. Ther.* **247:** 685–689.
95. Azer, S. A. and Stacey, N. H. (1993) Differential effects of cyclosporin A on the transport of bile acids by human hepatocytes. *Biochem. Pharmacol.* **46:** 813–819.
96. Azer, S. A. and Stacey, N. H. (1994) Differential effects of cyclosporin A on transport of bile acids by rat hepatocytes: relationship to individual serum bile acid levels. *Toxicol. Appl. Pharmacol.* **124:** 302–309.
97. Thibault, N., Claude, J. R. and Ballet, F. (1992) Actin filament alteration as a potential marker for cholestasis: a study in isolated rat hepatocyte couplets. *Toxicology* **73:** 269–279.
98. Jover, R., Ponsoda, X., Gomez-Lechon, M. J. and Castell, J. V. (1992): Potentiation of heroin and methadone hepatoxicity by ethanol: an *in vitro* study using cultured human hepatocytes. *Xenobiotica* **22:** 471–478.
99. Jover, R., Ponsoda, X., Gomez-Lechon, M. J., Herrero, C., del Pino, J. and Castell, J. V. (1991) Potentiation of cocaine hepatotoxicity by ethanol in human hepatocytes. *Toxicol. Appl. Pharmacol.* **107:** 526–534.
100. Elcombe, C. R. and Mitchell, A. M. (1986) Peroxisome proliferation due to di(2-ethylhexyl) phthalate (DEHP): species differences and possible mechanisms. *Environ. Health Perspect.* **70:** 211–219.
101. Bichet, N., Cahard, D., Fabre, G., Remandet, B., Gouy, D. and Cano, J. P. (1990) Toxicological studies on a benzofuran derivative. III. Comparison of peroxisome proliferation in rat and human hepatocytes in primary culture. *Toxicol. Appl. Pharmacol.* **106:** 509–517.
102. Blaauboer, B. J., van Holsteijn, C. W., Bleumink, R. *et al.* (1990) The effect of beclobric acid and clofibric acid on peroxisomal beta-oxidation and peroxisome proliferation in primary cultures of rat, monkey and human hepatocytes. *Biochem. Pharmacol.* **40:** 521–528.
103. Caraceni, P., Gasbarrini, A., Nussler, A., Di-Silvio, M., Bartoli, F. and Van Thiel, D. H. (1994) Human hepatocytes are more resistant than rat hepatocytes to anoxia–reoxygenation injury. *Hepatology* **20:** 1247–1254.
104. Rao, D. N. R., Jordan, S. and Mason, R. P. (1988) Generation of nitro radical anions of some 5-nitrofurans, and 2- and 5-nitroimidazoles by rat hepatocytes. *Biochem. Pharmacol.* **37:** 2907–2913.
105. Ilyin, G. P., Rissel, M., Malledant, Y., Tanguy, M. and Guillouzo, A. (1994) Human hepatocytes express trifluoroacetylated neoantigens after *in vitro* exposure to halothane. *Biochem. Pharmacol.* **48:** 561–567.
106. Van Pelt, F. N. A. M. and Kenna, J. G. (1994) Formation of trifluoroacetylated protein antigens in cultured rat hepatocytes exposed to halothane *in vitro. Biochem. Pharmacol.* **48:** 461–471.
107. Parzefall, W., Erber, E., Sedivy, R. and Schulte-Hermann, R. (1991) Testing for induction of DNA synthesis in human hepatocyte primary cultures by rat liver tumor promoters. *Cancer Res.* **51:** 1143–1147.
108. Butterworth, B. E., Smith-Oliver, T., Earle, L. *et al.* (1989) Use of primary cultures of hepatocytes in toxicology studies. *Cancer Res.* **49:** 1075–1084.

109. Martelli, A., Caonoero, R., Cavanna, M., Ceradelli, M. and Marinari, U. M. (1994) Cytotoxic and genotoxic effects of five *n*-alkanals in primary cultures of rat and human hepatocytes. *Mutat. Res.* **323:** 121–126.
110. Monteith, D. K. and Gupta, R. C. (1992) Carcinogen–DNA adducts in cultures of rat and human hepatocytes. *Cancer Lett.* **62:** 87–93.
111. Cmarik, J. L., Inskeep, P. B., Meredith, M. J., Meyer, D. J., Ketterer, B. and Guengerich, F. P. (1990) Selectivity of rat and human glutathione *S*-transferases in activation of ethylene dibromide by glutathione conjugation and DNA binding and induction of unscheduled DNA synthesis in human hepatocytes. *Cancer Res.* **50:** 2747–2752.
112. Oberhammer, F. A., Pavelka, M., Sharma, S. *et al.* (1992) Induction of apoptosis in cultured hepatocytes and in regressing liver by transforming growth factor-beta 1. *Proc. Natl Acad. Sci. U.S.A.* **89:** 5408–5412.
113. Busch, G. L., Schreiber, R., Dartsch, P. C. *et al.* (1994) Involvement of microtubules in the link between cell volume and pH of acidic cellular compartments in rat and human hepatoyctes. *Proc. Natl. Acad. Sci.* **91:** 9165–9169.
114. Tredger, J. M. and Davis, M. (1991) Drug metabolism and hepatoxicity. *Gut* **(suppl.)** S34–S39.
115. Harrison, P. M., Keays, R., Bray, G. P., Alexander, G. J. M. and Williams, R. (1990) Improved outcome of paracetamol-induced fulminant hepatic failure by late administration of acetylcysteine. *Lancet* **335:** 1572–1573.
116. Chesné, C., Guyomard, C., Fautrel, A. *et al.* (1993) Viability and function in primary culture of adult hepatocytes from various animal species and human beings after cryopreservation. *Hepatology* **18:** 406–414.
117. Fisher, R. L., Hasal, S. J., Sanuik, J. T., Scott, K. S., Gandolfi, A. J. and Brendel, K. (1993) Cold- and cryopreservation of human liver and kidney slices. *Cryobiology* **30:** 250–261.

6

Isolation, Culture and Use of Human Hepatocytes in Drug Research

MARÍA JOSÉ GÓMEZ-LECHÓN, TERESA DONATO, XAVIER PONSODA, RICARDO FABRA, RAMÓN TRULLENQUE AND JOSÉ V. CASTELL

I. Introduction 130
II. Isolation of human hepatocytes from liver biopsies 131
A. Equipment 131
B. Perfusion buffers 131
C. Choice of collagenase 133
D. Perfusion of the liver sample 133
E. Characterization of hepatocyte suspension 134
III. Culture of human hepatocytes in chemically defined medium 134
A. Culture medium 134
B. Culture of hepatocytes on plastic plates 134
1. Preparation of fibronectin-coated culture plates 134
2. Hepatocyte culture 135
C. Culture of hepatocytes on biomatrix and collagen gels 135
D. Co-cultures of hepatocytes 137
IV. Cryopreservation of human hepatocytes 137
V. Biochemical functionality in cultured human hepatocytes 138
VI. Biotransformation activities 139
A. Experimental procedures for measurement of drug-metabolizing activity in cultured human hepatocytes 140
1. 7-Ethoxycoumarin *O*-de-ethylase activity 140
2. Alkoxyresorufin *O*-de-alkylase activity 140
3. Coumarin 7-hydroxylase activity 141
4. *p*-Nitrophenol hydroxylase activity 141
5. Hydroxylation of testosterone 142
6. UDP-glucuronyltransferase activity 142
7. Glutathione *S*-transferase activity 142
B. Biotransformation activities in cultured human hepatocytes 143

IN VITRO METHODS IN PHARMACEUTICAL RESEARCH
ISBN 0-12-163390-X

VII. Use of human hepatocytes in drug research 144
A. Study of the hepatotoxicity of drugs 144
B. Drug metabolism 144
C. Investigation of the pharmacological effects of drugs and biomolecules on the liver 145
VIII. Future perspectives 147
Acknowledgements 148
References 148

I. INTRODUCTION

Human hepatocytes are a very attractive experimental model for studying the metabolic functions of the human liver. Early attempts to isolate viable human hepatocytes were made by enzymatic digestion of thin liver slices, needle, or edge biopsies.[1] The cell yields were, however, very low and this procedure is not used at present. The first successful and reproducible procedure to isolate human hepatocytes involved techniques similar to those used for isolating hepatocytes from other animal species (i.e. perfusion of the liver tissue with hydrolytic enzymes through blood vesels). The pioneering work of Strom *et al.*,[2] Guguen-Guillouzo *et al.*,[3] and Ballet *et al.*[4] laid the groundwork for obtaining high yields of viable hepatocytes suitable for primary culture. The enzymatic perfusion of liver through the blood vessels is, no doubt, the procedure of choice to obtain human hepatocytes from whole human liver or hepatic lobes. Another factor is the use of appropriate enzymes to weaken cell–cell junctions and liberate cells with minimal membrane damage.[2,5,6] Collagenase is the most widely used enzyme; however, its quality is of the utmost importance. Different grades of purity of this enzyme exist, containing minor amounts of other proteolytic enzymes which also contribute to cell–cell dissociation. Because of the variability of commercial collagenase preparations, previous testing to select the most appropriate one is strongly recommended.[7]

The availability of human tissue is a problem for most laboratories. Whole liver or large liver pieces from kidney donors have been until now the most common source of human hepatocytes.[4,8] These, however, are becoming less accessible for research purposes, as liver transplant programs increase in hospitals. National collection and distribution of liver preparations exists only in the United States (International Institute for the Advancement of Medicine, National Disease Research Interchange, Association of Human Tissue Users), but obtaining liver samples from human donors without liver damage or a previous history of intensive drug treatment, on a regular basis, is not easy.

We have explored the suitability of liver small surgical biopsies as a source of viable and metabolically competent human hepatocytes. Technical and ethical reasons make large samples of human liver hard to come by. In contrast, small tissue samples can be obtained in the course of liver surgery (i.e. trauma, tumor resection, cholecystectomy, etc.) or from tissue resected for pathological examination. These liver samples are available on a more regular basis and therefore constitute a more reliable source of viable human hepatocytes for research studies. In our laboratory a two-step microperfusion technique for the isolation of human hepatocytes has been successfully applied to very small samples of human liver (1–5 g).[8] These surgical biopsies must be obtained according to legal and ethical rules established by the ethical committee of the hospital.

II. ISOLATION OF HUMAN HEPATOCYTES FROM LIVER BIOPSIES

The key steps towards obtaining high yields of viable, minimally membrane-damaged, and metabolically competent cells are: (1) obtaining the biopsy, whenever possible, with a single cut surface and readily accessible blood vessels; (2) immediate cooling of the tissue to avoid warm ischemia, and processing of the tissue sample within the first 3 h; (3) adequate microcannulation of the small blood vessels to ensure efficient perfusion of the whole tissue sample; (4) use of tested collagenase; and (5) efficient oxygenation of the perfusion buffer during cell isolation.[8] Good yields and high viability cells can be reproducibly obtained with small sized surgical biopsies (Table 6.1).

Table 6.1 Isolation and culture of human hepatocytes from surgical biopsies ($n = 126$).

	Weight of biopsy (g)			
	1–3	3–5	5–8	14
No. of biopsies	39	67	19	1
Yield ($\times 10^{-6}$) (viable cells per g liver)	23.3 ± 4.8	22.4 ± 2.9	18.5 ± 4.9	6
Viability* (%)	95 ± 3	94 ± 5	92 ± 6	74
Attachment efficiency† (%)	70 ± 3	73 ± 4	71 ± 6	67
No. of successful cultures	37	65	17	1
Attachment after 24 h (μg cell protein per cm^2)	46.2 ± 13.4	48.0 ± 7.4	47.0 ± 11.3	44

* Mean ± s.d. percentage of cells excluding trypan blue.
† Expressed as the mean ± s.d. percentage of cells attached to the plate 1 h after cell seeding at an initial density of 8×10^4 cells per cm^2.

A. Equipment

The microperfusion equipment consists of a device for holding the liver specimen (i.e. glass funnel held over a flask); silicon catheters (0.75 mm diameter) introduced into the small blood vessels; a peristaltic pump for delivering perfusing solutions; a water bath to warm buffers to 37°C; a flask to collect perfusate; and a gas diffuser to oxygenate solutions. Warmed (37°C) and continuously gassed solutions (95% oxygen : 5% carbon dioxide) are gently pumped through microcatheters into the liver biopsy with the aid of a peristaltic pump. The effluent solution is drained off (Fig. 6.1A). Tube connections are changed in the course of perfusion (after addition of collagenase) to allow the solution coming from the liver sample to be gassed and recirculated back to the biopsy (Fig. 6.1B).

B. Perfusion buffers

Perfusion buffer 1 contains 137 mM NaCl, 2.68 mM KCl, 0.7 mM $Na_2PO_4 \cdot 12H_2O$, 10 mM HEPES, 10 mM glucose, 0.5 mM EGTA. The solution is made in double-distilled water and adjusted to pH 7.4 with 1 M HCl or NaOH as required. *Perfusion buffer 2* has the same composition as buffer 1 but without EGTA and with 5 mM $CaCl_2$. Collagenase (0.5 mg ml^{-1}; approximately 0.20 units ml^{-1}) is added to this buffer just before use.

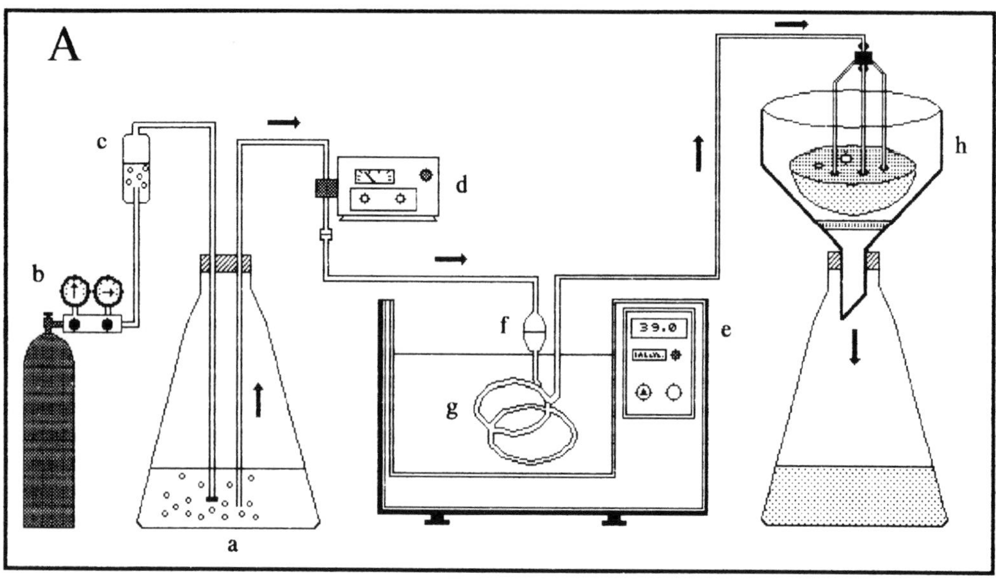

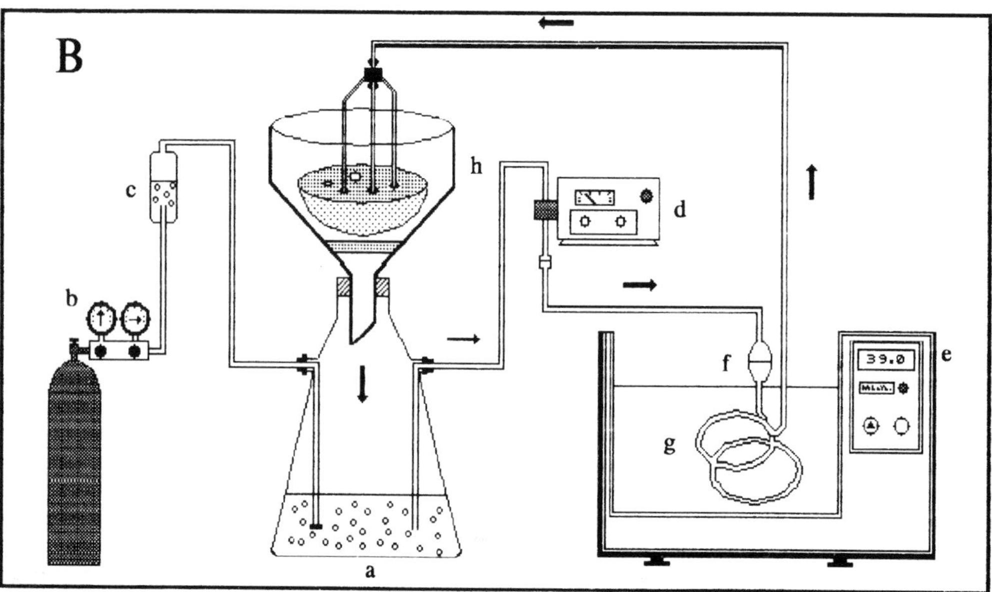

Fig. 6.1 Procedure and devices for liver biopsy perfusion. The microperfusion equipment consists of: (a) a flask containing perfusion solution; (b) carbogen; (c) a washing carbogen flask; (d) a peristaltic pump; (e) a water bath; (f) a bubble-trapping container; (g) a warming coil; (h) a funnel to hold the liver specimen; and (i) perfusing silicon catheters (0.75 mm in diameter). (A) During the first step the tissue is extensively washed by non-recirculating perfusion with a calcium-free buffer. The liver becomes pale brown, which indicates that the perfusion buffer is reaching all the tissue. (B) The second step is a recirculating perfusion with the same buffer, without EGTA but with calcium and collagenase. Perfusion is maintained at the same flow rate for about 30 min, until sufficient softening of the tissue is observed.

C. Choice of collagenase

Emphasis must be placed on the quality of collagenase. The specific activity of collagenase is a critical factor for assuring rapid and complete digestion of the biopsy without extensive cellular damage. Among the several lots of collagenase used in our laboratory, those with higher specific activity regularly produced higher yields of viable cells (Table 6.2). The use of collagenases with high specific activity helps to reduce perfusion time and increase the percentage of cell viability.[7]

Table 6.2 Isolation and culture of human hepatocytes after perfusion of liver biopsies with different collagenases.

	Specific activity of collagenase units mg^{-1}		
	0.35	0.29	0.19
No. of biopsies*	10	10	10
Yield ($\times 10^{-6}$) (viable cells per g liver)	22.3 ± 5.3	15.3 ± 5.7	9.8 ± 4.7
Viability† (%)	95 ± 3	90 ± 2	72 ± 7
Attachment efficiency‡ (%)	72 ± 3	66 ± 4	63 ± 5
No. of successful cultures	10	7	4

* Size of biopsy ranged between 1.5 and 5 g.
† Mean ± s.d. percentage of cells excluding trypan blue.
‡ Expressed as the mean ± s.d. percentage of cells attached to the plate 1 h after cell seeding at an initial density of 8×10^4 cells per cm^2.

D. Perfusion of the liver sample

Silicon catheters are carefully inserted into the lumen of the arterial orifices of the cut surface. It is essential to place several of these microcatheters inside blood vessels to ensure adequate perfusion of the biopsy.[8] The liver tissue sample is first extensively washed with 250 ml *perfusion buffer 1*. The optimal flow rate is close to 10 ml min^{-1} per catheter. Pressure greater than 20 cm H_2O should be avoided. The washing perfusate is allowed to drain off and is not recirculated. During this step the liver should gradually become pale brown, an indication that the buffer is reaching all the tissue. In a second stage, *buffer 2* containing 0.5 mg ml^{-1} collagenase is recirculated at the same flow for 30–45 min until sufficient softening of the tissue is observed. The perfusion buffers are continuously oxygenated with carbogen and warmed to reach the liver at 37°C.

Once the enzymatic digestion has been completed, the liver tissue is transferred to a Petri dish containing ice-cold *buffer 2* and cells are gently dispersed with a blunt tool. The cell suspension is filtered through gauze and there is no need for additional mechanical disruption of the tissue. The cellular suspension is centrifuged for 2 min at 100*g* and the pellet resuspended with ice-cold culture medium and again centrifuged. The pellet is finally resuspended in culture medium and cell viability determined. This cell preparation contains mostly hepatocytes (95–97%), but also a small percentage of Ito, endothelial, and few Kupffer cells. To obtain a pure hepatocyte suspension, gradient centrifugation through Ficoll or Percoll[1,9] or elutriation[5] is recommended. Typical yields are $23 \pm 3.5 \times 10^6$ viable hepatocytes per g liver, although this value depends greatly on the size of the biopsy, accessibility of vessels, and efficiency of perfusion.

E. Characterization of hepatocyte suspension

To provide information on the quality of the isolated hepatocytes, cell viability is currently assessed by means of a dye exclusion test (i.e. 0.4% trypan blue).[8] Cell viability should be around 85–95%. In addition, if hepatocytes are to be used for investigating the biotransformation of xenobiotics, data indicative of the biotransformation capability of hepatocytes should be obtained for each cell preparation. To this end, the metabolism of testosterone examined by high-performance liquid chromatography of culture medium or the de-ethylation of 7-ethoxycoumarin (fluorimetry), both assays involving several P450 isozyme activities, can be used for routine control.[7]

III. CULTURE OF HUMAN HEPATOCYTES IN CHEMICALLY DEFINED MEDIUM

A. Culture medium

In a recent European Centre for the Validation of Alternative Methods (ECVAM) workshop, William's E culture medium was recommended for primary culture of hepatocytes,[7] but other culture media are also currently used by researchers, i.e. DMEM/Lebovitz L-15 (1 : 1, v/v) and Ham's F12/Lebovitz L15 (1 : 1, v/v). For the experiments shown below, Ham's F12/ Lebovitz L15 (1 : 1, v/v) supplemented with 2% newborn calf serum, 0.2% bovine serum albumin, 10^{-8} M human insulin, 10 mM glucose, 50 units ml^{-1} penicillin and 50 $\mu g\,ml^{-1}$ streptomycin was used. After the first 24 h, hepatocytes are shifted to a serum-free medium containing 10^{-8} M dexamethasone.

B. Culture of hepatocytes on plastic plates

Culture on plastic plates is the simplest and more usual way to keep human hepatocytes in chemically defined primary culture. However, cell attachment of hepatocytes to plastic requires coating the surface of dishes with adhesive extracellular matrix components (i.e. fibronectin, laminin, collagen) to promote active attachment of cells.[8]

1. *Preparation of fibronectin-coated culture plates*

Commercial human or bovine fibronectin can be used to coat culture plates (0.5–1 $\mu g\,cm^{-2}$) before cell seeding. Alternatively, 5 $\mu l\,cm^{-2}$ of newborn calf serum can be spread on the plate under sterile conditions and allowed to adsorb for 30 min at room temperature. Fibronectin, one of the components of serum, binds rapidly and strongly to plastic without denaturation, building a layer that greatly facilitates the selective attachment of viable hepatocytes to culture plates.[8]

2. *Hepatocyte culture*

Currently a cell suspension of 5×10^5 viable cells per ml culture medium is seeded on fibronectin-coated culture plates (equivalent to 8×10^4 cells per cm^2). The attachment of human hepatocytes to fibronectin-coated plates is very efficient and rapid. One hour after seeding, plating efficiency (number of cells attached/number cells seeded) is typically 80%, and the Attachment Index (AI; number of cells attached/maximal number of attachable cells) reaches 90–100% (65×10^3 cells per cm^2). One hour after cell seeding the medium is aspirated to remove unattached cells and new medium is added. The spreading of human hepatocytes on plastic culture dishes takes about 18 h to complete. Twenty-four hours after cell plating, confluent monolayers of polygonal-shaped hepatocytes closely resembling cells *in vivo* are observed (Fig. 6.2), and cells are shifted to serum-free hormone-supplemented medium. Under these culture conditions cells survive up to 10–15 days but do not divide.[3,4,8,10,11]

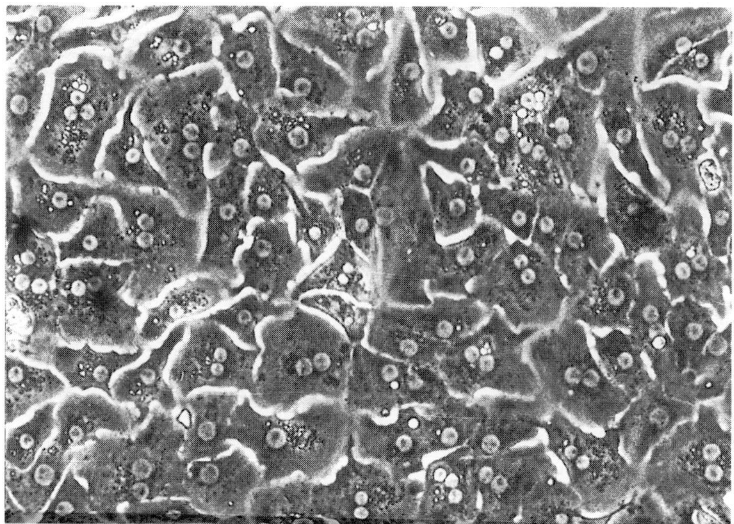

Fig. 6.2 Phase contrast microscopy of cultured human hepatocytes in 24-h confluent monolayer. (Original magnification × 250.)

Cultured human hepatocytes exhibit a cell surface completely covered with microvilli. Cells show a large number of glycogen particles forming rosettes spread throughout the cytoplasm, a well-defined rough endoplasmic reticulum and well-preserved Golgi with noticeable exocytotic vesicles. Lipid droplets of different sizes, lysosomes, and peroxisomes are also found evenly distributed in the cytoplasm. Once a confluent monolayer is formed, desmosomes, tight junctions, as well as intercellular structures covered with abundant microvilli and resembling bile canaliculi, are clearly observable (Fig. 6.3).

C. Culture of hepatocytes on biomatrix and collagen gels

A decrease in drug metabolizing capabilities preceding the gradual loss of cell functionality is a common finding in conventional serum-free cultures of hepatocytes. It has been

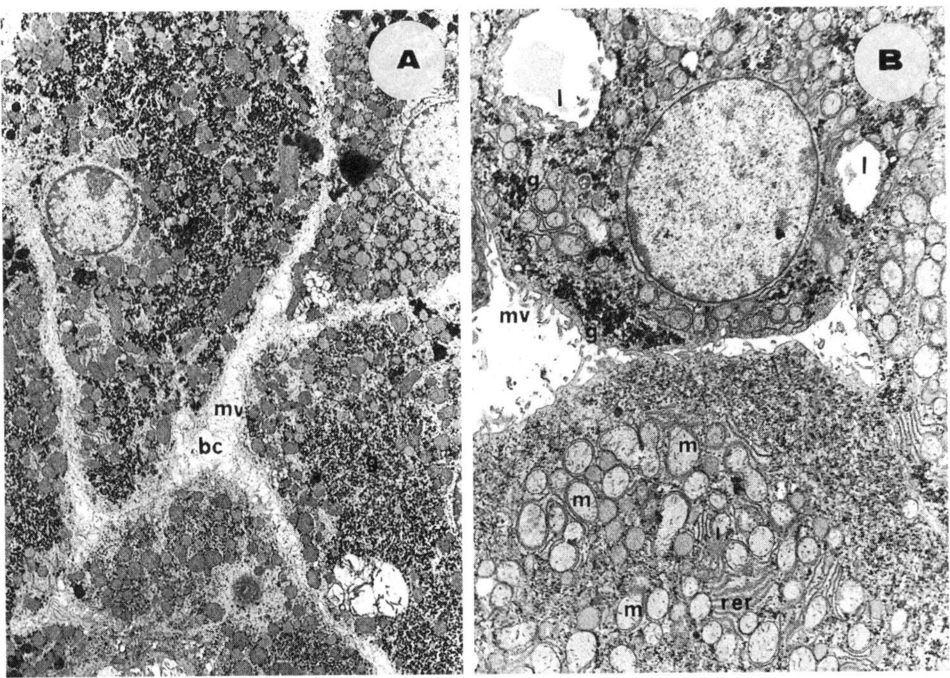

Fig. 6.3 Ultrastructure of cultured human hepatocytes. (A) Overview of a 24-h hepatocyte monolayer. Structures resembling bile canaliculus (bc) surrounded by microvilli (mv) are observed. (B) Glycogen particles (g), mitochondria (m), rough endoplasmic reticulum (rer), and lipid droplets (l) appear distributed in the cytoplasm.

hypothesized that this decrease could be the result of adaptive responses of hepatocytes to the new culture environment, or to the lack of critical elements in culture media essential to support the *in vivo* hepatocellular function.[12–14]

The key role of the extracellular matrix in the regulation of liver gene expression was recognized early in rat hepatocyte cultures,[15–19] and attempts were made to reproduce these complex cell–biomatrix interactions in culture in a practical way.

Liver-derived biomatrix[17,18] has been claimed to improve greatly the expression of differentiated functions of rat hepatocytes, including biotransformation activities. However, its poorly defined composition and the variability within biomatrix preparations have prevented its generalized use, and no data are available on human hepatocyte cultures. Matrigel, a solubilized preparation of basement membrane components derived from the mouse Engelbreth–Holm–Sarcoma (EHS), significantly improves the maintenance of specific functions in rat hepatocytes,[20] but has not been sufficiently explored with human hepatocytes to be recommended.

The use of collagen gels is a simplified alternative to more complex biomatrices. The culturing of hepatocytes in collagen gels represents an attempt to reproduce the *in vivo* three-dimensional microenvironment of hepatocytes in a more simple, reproducible, and technically feasible way. The collagen gel technique consists of setting hepatocytes in a sandwich configuration between two layers of collagen.[6,19,21] A fresh collagen solution (9 volumes of 1.11 mg ml^{-1} rat-tail collagen in 1 mM HCl and 1 volume of 10 × concentrated culture medium[22] is poured onto plates to form a 1–2 mm layer. Once the gel has formed, hepatocytes are seeded on top of the gel and, after cell attachment and medium removal, a second collagen layer is gently poured on the cell layer. Once this second layer has gelified, it is covered with fresh culture medium. By culturing cells in this fashion the situation in the liver (two-side exposure of hepatocytes within the space of Disse) can be better mimicked.

A simplification of the double gel method is the entrapping of hepatocytes within a homogeneous collagen gel.[23] This is done by gentle dispersion (1 : 1 v/v) of a hepatocyte suspension in rat-tail collagen solution. Collagen is immediately prepared before use by mixing 9 volumes of 1.5 mg ml^{-1} collagen in 1 mM HCl and 1 volume of 10 × concentrated culture medium. The cell suspension is poured onto plates and allowed to gelify (*c*.30 min). Fresh culture medium is finally added on top of the gel, and periodically renewed.

Human hepatocytes survived several weeks with a well-preserved morphology and high expression of hepatic-specific functions, in particular drug biotransformation activities.[23] However, certain drawbacks should be mentioned. First, the collagen gel influences the transport rate of drugs and metabolites to and from the cells. Second, it is hard to differentiate between live and dead cells. Third, entrapped cells need to be recovered from gel in order to express the experimental data accurately (i.e. in terms of cellular DNA). This can be done by digestion with collagenase (0.1 unit ml^{-1}).

D. Co-cultures of hepatocytes

Cell–cell contacts between hepatic cells are important in the expression of the cellular functions of hepatocytes. One way to reproduce this microenvironment *in vitro* is to bring hepatocytes into close contact with non-parenchymal cells. This idea, first described by Langenbach *et al.*[24] and Michalopoulos *et al.*[25] using fibroblasts as feeder layers, was later improved by Guguen-Guillouzo *et al.*,[26] who reported that, by co-culturing rat hepatocytes with rat liver epithelial cells, the hepatic adult phenotype was expressed for a much longer time than in conventional pure cultures.

The nature of the helping cells did not appear to be critical for their positive role in co-cultures[27,28] and, in fact, established cell lines of different origins have been used successfully to replace the epithelial cells in co-cultures of rat hepatocytes.[27,29,30–33] The suitability of a cell line for hepatocyte co-culturing depends on its ability to grow as a monolayer forming a stable support for hepatocyte attachment, its ability to survive in serum-free culture conditions, its metabolic compatibility with hepatocytes, and lack of drug-metabolizing enzymes.

Co-culturing human hepatocytes with rat epithelial cells had effects similar to those observed with rat hepatocytes: longer survival and expression of typical adult hepatocyte functions.[34,35] However, because of the greater stability of biotransformation enzymes in human hepatocytes, co-culturing is not an absolute requirement for drug metabolism studies in human hepatocytes.

IV. CRYOPRESERVATION OF HUMAN HEPATOCYTES

The irregular and limited availability of human liver has led to a need to develop techniques for cryopreserving freshly isolated human hepatocytes. Several protocols have been described, which basically consist of a freezing medium containing 10% dimethyl sulfoxide, propylene glycol, acetamide or polyethylene glycol as cryoprotectants, and a microcomputer-controlled freezing gradient.[36–39] Upon thawing, cell viability may be low (*c*.55–65%), but can be improved by Percoll centrifugation. Once attached to plastic, hepatocytes survive for several days, show typical ultrastructure and morphology, and express specific metabolic functions comparable with those observed in primary cultures.[36] Cytochrome P450 content and microsomal enzyme activities are reasonably well maintained (*c*.70% of fresh cell values). However, activities of the cytosolic enzymes glutathione *S*-transferase and glutathione reductase are not well preserved after storage of cells.[38]

V. BIOCHEMICAL FUNCTIONALITY OF CULTURED HUMAN HEPATOCYTES

Studies of the metabolism of cultured human hepatocytes have revealed interesting features. Hepatocytes maintain high levels of intracellular glycogen, similar to those reported for fed human liver *in vivo*. Basal unstimulated glycogenolysis is low, but insensitive to low levels of external glucose, and can be totally suppressed by insulin.[8,40] However, glycogen can be rapidly mobilized by glucagon: adding 10^{-8} M glucagon to culture medium results within 1–2 h in a 90% reduction in cellular glycogen, which renders glucose to the culture medium in about 85%. Synthesis and accumulation of glycogen in glycogen-depleted cells is stimulated by physiological concentrations of insulin, but is strongly dependent on the presence of lactate in the incubation media at postprandial portal concentrations.[41]

Table 6.3 Biochemical functions of human hepatocytes in primary culture.

Day of culture	Gluconeogenesis* (nmol glucose mg^{-1} min^{-1})	Glycolysis† (nmol lactate mg^{-1} min^{-1})	Ureogenesis‡ (nmol urea mg^{-1} min^{-1})
1	3.50 ± 0.17	15.51 ± 1.10	10.86 ± 0.49
2	1.70 ± 0.05	7.65 ± 0.37	4.82 ± 0.72
3	1.46 ± 0.19	10.36 ± 2.03	5.34 ± 0.89
4	1.17 ± 0.16	8.46 ± 0.30	4.70 ± 0.76
5	1.00 ± 0.03	11.10 ± 0.26	4.10 ± 0.20
Human liver[8]	2.0	4.0	1.2

* Gluconeogenesis was measured at different times in culture, after incubating hepatocytes with 10 mM lactate.[8]
† Basal glycolytic activity was evaluated daily in cultures incubated with 10 mM glucose. Lactate was enzymatically measured in culture medium.[8]
‡ Urea synthesis rate was evaluated daily in cultures stimulated to maximal production with 3 mM NH_4Cl.[8] Under non-stimulated conditions urea synthesis by human hepatocytes was 2.5–3.5 nmol mg^{-1} min^{-1}.

Hepatocytes efficiently convert lactate into glucose at rates similar to those estimated in the fasted human liver (Table 6.3). Gluconeogenesis from lactate can be stimulated by physiological concentrations of glucagon.[8] Basal glycolysis is somewhat higher than that estimated for liver cells *in vivo* (Table 6.3), and can be stimulated by physiological concentrations of insulin. Unlike rat hepatocytes, glucose is a more powerful modulator of fructose 2,6-bisphosphate, and hence glycolysis, than insulin itself in human hepatocytes.[41]

Human hepatocytes synthesize urea in culture (Table 6.3). When overloaded with ammonium ions, the rate of urea synthesis can be stimulated to a level five times that in human liver.[8]

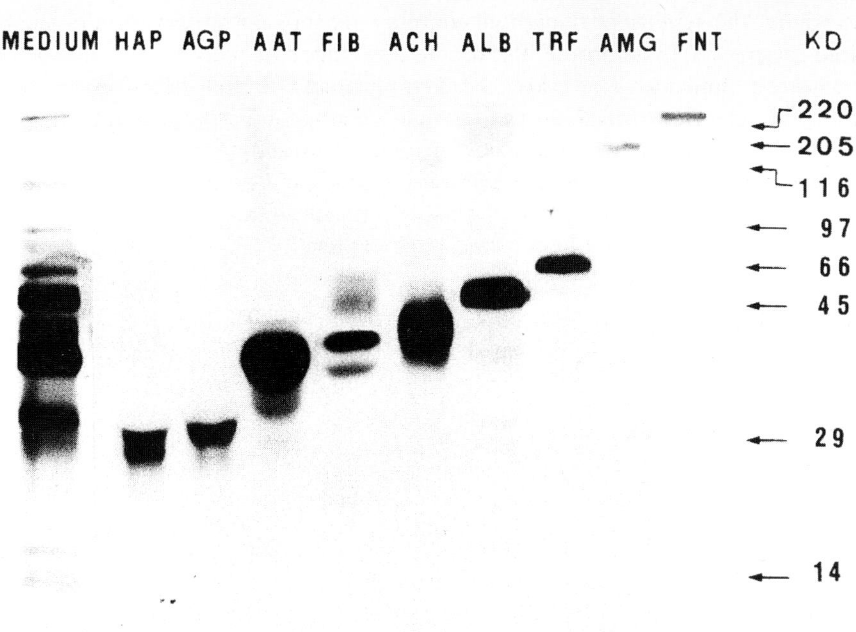

Fig. 6.4 Plasma protein synthesis by cultured human hepatocytes. Three-day cultured hepatocytes were shifted to methionine-free culture medium and ^{35}S-methionine was added to the cultures. Each protein was immunoprecipitated individually from the culture medium with specific antibodies, and separated by electrophoresis. The gel was subjected to fluorography and exposed to a photographic film. HAP, haptoglobin; AGP, α_1-acid glycoprotein; AAT, α_1- antitrypsin; FIB, fibrinogen; ACH, α_1-antichymotripsin; ALB, albumin; TRF, transferrin; AMG, α_2-macroglobulin; FNT, fibronectin.

Finally, human hepatocytes synthesize and secrete plasma proteins to culture medium (Fig. 6.4). Albumin, α_1-antitrypsin, α_1-antichymotrypsin, α_1-acid glycoprotein, C-reactive protein, serum amyloid A, fibronectin, fibrinogen, and α_2-macroglobulin are produced by cultured cells,[8,42,43] and their synthesis can be stimulated by inflammatory cytokines[44] as occurs *in vivo*.

VI. BIOTRANSFORMATION ACTIVITIES

Hepatic biotransformation of drugs involves mainly two types of reactions: redox reactions catalysed by the P450 mono-oxygenase complex, and conjugation with endogenous molecules. The mono-oxygenase system is an enzymatic complex formed by two functional units, a cytochrome P450 mono-oxygenase and a NADPH–cytochrome P450 reductase. The enzymes are integrated in the membrane of smooth endoplasmic reticulum, and when cells are homogenized they are found in the microsomal fraction. Since these enzymes are membrane bound, the activity of the whole complex depends on preservation of the bilayer phospholipid matrix.[45] Cytochrome P450, the key catalytic component of the monooxygenase system, constitutes a family of hemoproteins responsible for the oxidative metabolism of xenobiotics (drugs), as well as many endogenous compounds. The different cytochromes (CYP) present a characteristic, but often overlapping, substrate specificity. Of note, most of them are highly inducible by xenobiotics.[46–53] Cytochromes 1A2, 2A6, 2B6, 3A4, 2C9-11, 2D6, and 2E1 account for most of the biotransforming ability of human liver,[54,55] and have been detected in cultured hepatocytes.[56,57]

A. Experimental procedures for measurement of drug-metabolizing activity in cultured human hepatocytes

Determination of P450-dependent activity is crucial when assessing the drug-metabolizing capability of cells. This normally requires homogenization of cells, preparation of microsomes, and the use of specific substrates.[49–51,58] The number of cells needed to quantify these activities can be drastically reduced if enzymatic activity is measured in intact cells cultured in microwells. This basically depends on the availability of specific, non-cytotoxic, substrates with suitable optical properties. Whenever applicable, this approach allows the cells to be reused after enzyme measurement. Several procedures adapted in our laboratory are described here.

1. 7-Ethoxycoumarin O*-de-ethylase activity*

This reaction is catalyzed by several P450 isozymes (CYP1A2, CYP2A6, CYP2B6, CYP2C8-9, CYP2E1, CYP3A3-5)[59] and is an easy and rapid procedure for assessment of the biotransforming ability of a cell preparation.[7] The O-de-ethylation of 7-ethoxycoumarin results in the formation of 7-hydroxycoumarin, which is then readily estimated fluorimetrically.[60] This activity can be measured in subcellular fractions (microsomes or S-9 fraction), and also in intact monolayers with certain modifications.[61,62]

Measurement of activity in intact cells Plates are washed twice with warm phosphate-buffered saline and the assay is initiated by adding 800 μM 7-ethoxycoumarin to the culture medium. Cells are incubated for about 30 min at 37°C, and the reaction is stopped by aspirating the incubation medium from plates. To hydrolyze 7-hydroxycoumarin conjugates, if any, 1 ml of the medium sample is incubated with β-glucuronidase/arylsulfatase (200 Fishman units ml^{-1} 1200 Roy units ml^{-1}) for 2 h at 37°C. Hydrolysis is stopped by adding 125 μl 15% trichloroacetic acid and 2 ml chloroform and then shaking the mixture for 5–10 min at 37°C. After centrifugation (2000*g* for 10 min), the organic phase is extracted with 1 N NaOH and the fluorescence of the aqueous phase is measured (368 nm excitation, 456 nm emission) in a microplate fluorimeter. The activity is expressed as picomoles of 7-hydroxycoumarin formed per minute and per milligram of cell protein.

2. Alkoxyresorufin O*-de-alkylase activity*

7-Ethoxyresorufin O-de-ethylation is specific to CYP1A1/2 isozyme,[47] 7-pentoxyresorufin O-depenthylation and 7-benzyloxyresorufin O-debenzylation activities are linked to

CYP2B1 in rat[63] and probably to the same subfamily in humans.[59] The O-de-alkylation of alkoxyresorufin derivatives results in the production of resorufin, which is readily estimated fluorimetrically. The enzyme activities of cultured hepatocytes can be measured both in subcellular fractions[64,65] and in intact cells.[62,66]

Measurement of activity in intact cells Assays are initiated by adding an appropriate concentration of the substrate (8 μM ethoxyresorufin, 15 μM pentoxyresorufin and 15 μM benzyloxyresorufin) to the culture medium containing 10 μM dicoumarol.[65] After incubation for 30 min at 37°C, the medium is aspirated, and hydrolyzed with β-glucuronidase/arylsulphatase (165 Fishman units ml^{-1} and 1330 Roy units ml^{-1}, respectively) for 2 h at 37°C. Hydrolysis is stopped by adding 2.5 ml methanol. After centrifugation (2000*g* for 10 min), the fluorescence of the supernatant is measured at 530 nm excitation and 585 nm emission in a fluorimetric microplate reader. The activity is expressed as picomoles of resorufin formed per minute and per milligram of cell protein.[67]

3. *Coumarin 7-hydroxylase activity*

Coumarin 7-hydroxylation is the major pathway of coumarin metabolism by human liver microsomes.[68] Human CYP2A6 is largely or entirely responsible for catalyzing this hydroxylation.[69] The hydroxylation of coumarin results in the formation of a fluorescent 7-hydroxy derivative which is then readily quantified.[60,68,69]

Measurement of activity in intact cells Coumarin (100 μM in culture medium) is added to hepatocytes and incubated for 30 min at 37°C. The reaction is stopped by removing the medium from cells. To hydrolyze the hydroxycoumarin conjugates formed, culture supernatant is incubated with β-glucuronidase/arylsulfatase (200 Fishman units ml^{-1} 1200 Roy units ml^{-1}) in 250 μl 0.1 M sodium acetate buffer (pH 4.5). After 2 h at 37°C, samples are diluted (1 : 3) in 0.1 M Tris pH 9. The 7-hydroxycoumarin released is quantified fluorimetrically at 358 nm excitation and 368 nm emission. The activity is expressed as picomoles of 7-hydroxycoumarin formed per minute and per milligram of cell protein.

4. p-*Nitrophenol hydroxylase activity*

p-Nitrophenol is a suitable probe for measuring CYP2E1 activity in different species, including humans.[70,71] Hydroxylation of *p*-nitrophenol results in the formation of 4-nitrocatechol which, in alkaline medium, has a strong yellow color.[71–73]

Measurement of activity in intact cells Culture plates require extensive washing to remove phenol red present in conventional culture media which interferes in 4-nitrochatechol determination. Cells are incubated in Krebs-Ringer-HEPES buffer (pH 7.4) containing 20 mM sodium pyruvate, 1 mM ascorbic acid and 0.5 mM p-nitrophenol. After 30 min incubation at 37°C, aliquots of medium are alkalinized (10 μl of 10N NaOH per ml incubation media), centrifuged at 2000g for 5 min, transfered to 96-well microplates, the absorbance at 546 nm measured and refered to a standard curve of 4-nitrochatechol. Activity is expressed as picomoles formed per minute and per milligram of cell protein.[74]

5. *Hydroxylation of testosterone*

Testosterone is regio- and stereoselectively metabolized by human CYPs to several hydroxylated metabolites.[59,75] CYP isozymes involved in testoterone hydroxylation are 2B6 (16β)[76] and 3A3-5 (6β-, 2β-, and 15β).[59] Hydroxylation of testosterone can be measured in intact hepatocytes incubated with 250 μM testosterone.[77] Culture medium is transferred to Eppendorfs, and metabolites are extracted with ethylacetate and analyzed by HPLC (Spherisorb 5 μM, 20 cm $\times$ 4.5 mm, reverse-phase column). Samples are eluted with 40% methanol and 3.5% acetonitrile for 20 min, followed by a linear gradient to 40% methanol and 20% acetonitrile for 30 min, at a flow rate of 0.8 ml min^{-1}. Column effluents are monitored at 254 nm. 11β-Hydroxytestosterone is used as internal standard.[77]

6. *UDP-glucuronyltransferase activity*

Conjugation with glucuronic acid, a process catalyzed by the UDP-glucuronyltransferase, is quantitatively the most important phase II reaction in the human liver. UDP-glucuronyltransferases are a multigene family in which individual isozymes show certain differences in terms of regulation and substrate specificity.[78,79] The enzyme is involved in the conjugation of drugs yielding *O*-, *N*-, *S*- and *C*-glucuronides.[80] 4-Methylumbellipherone is a suitable and very sensitive substrate for the quantification of at least two isozymes, HLUGP1 and HLUG4.[79]

Measurement of activity in intact cells The assay is started by addition of 100 μM 4-methylumbellipherone in culture medium. After 60 min incubation, aliquots of culture supernatant are taken. Samples are diluted (1 : 20) in 10 mM NaOH and the remaining 4-methylumbellipherone is quantified fluorimetrically (376 nm excitation, 460 nm emission). The activity is expressed as nanomoles of 4-methylumbellipherone conjugated per minute and per milligram of cell protein.

7. *Glutathione* S*-transferase activity*

The glutathione *S*-transferases (GSHTs) are a family of isozymes that catalyze the conjugation of reduced glutathione (GSH) to electrophilic compounds. The multiplicity of GSHTs has been a feature in most species studied,[81] and several major isozymes (α, μ, π, θ) have been identified so far.[82] In general, GSHTs show broad substrate specificities, although certain isozymes are very specific.[83] A convenient and sensitive spectrophotometric method for analyzing GSH-transferase activity is conjugation of GSH with 1-chloro-2,4-dinitrobenzene reaction catalyzed by α, μ, and π isoenzymes. The product formed (2,4-dinitrophenyl-glutathione) shows a characteristic absorption at 340 nm which is absent in the reagent, and GSHT activity can be assayed by recording the increase in absorbance at 340 nm as a function of time.

Assays are carried out in spectrophotometer cuvettes at 25°C. The reaction mixture contains 10–25 μg S-9 fraction protein and 1 μmol substrate (added as 2% ethanolic solution) in 1 ml 0.1 M potassium phosphate buffer (pH 6.5). The reaction is started by adding 1 μmol GSH, and the conjugation rate is measured directly by the increase in absorbance at 340 nm. The extinction coefficient of the product is known[84] to be 9.6×10^3 M^{-1} cm^{-1}. The activity is expressed as nanomoles of conjugate formed per minute and per milligram of protein.

B. Biotransformation activities in cultured human hepatocytes

Human hepatocytes cultured for 24 h show significant variability in individual enzyme activities (Table 6.4). This variability has also been reported by other authors,[85,86] and does not seem to be attributable to differences in the quality of the culture.[77,87] Rather, it may reflect the known interindividual variability of mono-oxygenase activities in humans, which is associated not only with intrinsic factors (sex, age, pathologic state, genetic variability[68,88,89]) but also to life habits (diet, drug intake, smoking habit, alcohol consumption, life-style[90]). In general, mono-oxygenase levels found in human hepatocytes are qualitatively similar to those obtained in microsomes prepared from human liver.[86]

Table 6.4 Drug metabolizing activities in 24-h primary cultured human hepatocytes.

Isozyme	Reaction	Activity*	
P450†		65 ± 8	($n = 10$)
NADPH-Cc‡	Cytochrome *c* oxidation	23 ± 2	($n = 10$)
CYP1A1/2d§	Aryl hydrocarbon hydroxylation	2.93 ± 0.99	($n = 7$)
	7-Ethoxyresorufin *O*-de-ethylation	3.09 ± 2.52	($n = 14$)
CYP2A6§	Coumarin 7-hydroxylation	137 ± 42	($n = 6$)
CYP2B6§	7-Pentoxyresorufin *O*-depentylation	3.28 ± 1.76	($n = 10$)
	7-Benzoxyresorufin *O*-debenzylation	1.38 ± 0.33	($n = 5$)
CYP2C9§	4′-Diclofenac hydroxylation	317 ± 73	($n = 9$)
CYP2E1§	*p*-Nitrophenol hydroxylation	89 ± 42	($n = 6$)
	Chlorzoxazone 6-hydroxylation	27 ± 3	($n = 3$)
CYP3A3-5§	Testosterone 6β-hydroxylation	195 ± 122	($n = 7$)
	Testosterone 2β-hydroxylation	61 ± 16	($n = 7$)
	Testosterone 15β-hydroxylation	12.4 ± 8.6	($n = 7$)
mEH§	Benzo(a)pyrene 7,8-oxide hydration	180 ± 72	($n = 10$)
UDPG-t‡	4-Methylumbelliferone conjugation	3.6 ± 0.4	($n = 5$)
GSH-t‡	1-Chloro-2,4-dinitrobenzene conjugation	301 ± 112	($n = 8$)

* Mean ± s.d. enzymatic activity determined in 24-h cultured human hepatocytes.
† Cytochrome P450 content is expressed as picomoles per milligram of cellular protein.
‡ NADPH-C, UDPG-t and GSH-t activities are expressed as nanomoles per milligram per minute.
§ CYP enzymatic activities are expressed as picomoles per milligram per minute.

The conjugation enzymes glucuronyl transferases and glutathione transferases are also expressed in cultured cells at levels as high as those measured in isolated hepatocytes.[8,91,92] Finally, although the level of intracellular glutathione transiently decreases during isolation and the first hours in culture, it later returns to levels similar to those measured in human liver.[8]

A gradual decrease in total cytochrome P450 activity, and in individual isoenzymes, is observed with time in culture. Compared with rat hepatocytes, human CYP activities decrease more slowly, and by 5–6 days they are ca. 50% of those measured during the first day of culture. The associated cytochrome *c* reductase activity remains fairly constant, which indicates that the loss of cytochrome P450 isozymes is mainly responsible for the reduced biotransforming capability of cultured cells.[8,31,92] The stability of glucuronyl transferases and glutathione transferases seems to be greater than that of the mono-oxygenases.

In practical terms, human hepatocytes in pure culture can be used for up to 1–2 days for drug metabolism studies. Experience in preventing cytochrome P450 decay has been gained mostly from rat hepatocyte studies. Of the different strategies explored to minimize (delay) this decay, co-culture with rat epithelial cells and hepatocyte entrapment in collagen gels have shown significant advantages over pure cultures. Co-cultures prolong not only cell survival but also the expression of mono-oxygenases and conjugation activities. As reported by Ratanasavanh *et al.*,[93] higher levels of P450 isozymes, NADPH cytochrome *c* reductase, and epoxide hydrolase were found in co-cultures of human hepatocytes than in pure cultures. Collagen-cultured cells, as described by Koebe *et al.*,[23] showed the ability to metabolize paracetamol after 16 days and maintenance of *p*-nitroanisole demethylation over 24 days.

VII. USE OF HUMAN HEPATOCYTES IN DRUG RESEARCH

The primary culture of human hepatocytes is a simplified model of the more complex human liver. Despite its limitations, cultured hepatocytes express many of the biochemical hepatic functions of hepatocytes *in vivo*, and they provide an attractive and unique experimental model for investigating drug metabolism and the effects of drugs on specific metabolic functions of the human liver.[94,95] As the closest model to human liver, primary culture can be used to examine the potential effects on the liver of drugs under development, which for obvious ethical reasons cannot be administered to human volunteers.

A. Study of the hepatotoxicity of drugs

This constitutes one interesting application of human hepatocytes. The cytotoxicity of a new compound can be monitored by incubating cells with increasing concentrations of the drug and examining cell viability. For this purpose, both primary cultures and hepatic-derived cell lines can be used. However, cell lines are able to detect only those drugs that are *directly* toxic to the cell: compounds that must be biotransformed to elicit their toxic potential are not accurately predicted with cell lines. Since primary cultured hepatocytes retain many of the critical functions, they are a more appropriate model for investigating liver-specific toxicity.[94,96]

The short-term effects (acute effects) of a drug can be investigated satisfactorily in primary cultures of hepatocytes (see Chapter 16). However, the suitability of a culture type for investigating the long-term effects of xenobiotics is strongly dependent on maintenance of the adult phenotype in culture and, in particular, the biotransformation and defence mechanisms.

B. Drug metabolism

Drug metabolism often shows significant species differences. In the case of pharmaceuticals, the relevance of such differences may be very important in terms of drug pharmacokinetics and the risk–benefit balance of a particular drug. Unfortunately, no animal model can accurately predict the human metabolism of drugs, and differences may become evident only after the drug has been administered for the first time to human volunteers. The use of human hepatocytes[95,97] can help to anticipate more accurately the metabolic profile of a new drug in humans and can be of great value in selecting the most appropriate animal model to investigate its effects. Early knowledge of the human metabolism of a new drug is desirable for two main reasons: (1) drug metabolism is the major determinant of the pharmacokinetics and interactions with other compounds; and (2) species differences in metabolism are often responsible for the difficulties in extrapolating from laboratory animals to humans.[98,99]

C. Investigation of the pharmacological effects of drugs and biomolecules on the liver

Cultured hepatocytes also offer the possibility of testing the pharmacological effects of drugs and biomolecules (interferons, cytokines, hepatotrophic factors, etc.) on the growth, metabolism, and functionality of human liver, and to examine their potential side-effects.

Interferons are natural body defenses against viral infection. Their present clinical use includes treatment of hepatic viral infections B and C. Some previous clinical evidence pointed to interferons as compounds that might influence drug metabolizing activities in human liver, as had been observed in laboratory animals.[100] The direct effects of interferon (IFN) -α and -γ on the expression of specific cytochrome P450 isozymes in adult human hepatocytes have been investigated in human hepatocytes[101,102] and the results evidenced a transient decrease in the activity of CYP1A and 2B subfamilies, and moderate inhibition of CYP3A. Moreover, interferon partially prevented the typical induction of the CYP1A2 by methylcholanthrene (Fig. 6.5). Experimental evidence in human hepatocytes suggests that interferon can impair mono-oxygenase activity by two different mechanisms, one associated with increased production of nitric oxide, and subsequent inhibition of the enzyme, and the other involving regulation of gene expression.

Cytokines are intercellular pleiotropic factors acting on many different cells and influencing specific cell functions.[103] They are now being considered as promising therapeutic agents. The use of cultured hepatocytes can allow anticipation of potential hepatic side-effects in humans. Tumor necrosis factor (TNF) α, for instance, has potent tumoricidal activity. However, it influences the expression of human hepatic genes (plasma protein genes[104]) as well as CYP1A2 and the CYP3A subfamily.[102,105] Interleukin 6 is a potent growth factor for differentiated B cells, but also a potent inflammatory signal for human hepatocytes. When added to cultured human hepatocytes it acts on many hepatic genes, stimulating the synthesis of acute-phase plasma proteins as occurs in the course of acute inflammation in humans.[44,104]

Hepatic growth factor (HGF), a potent signal for initiating DNA synthesis in human hepatocytes, is involved in the control of liver regeneration and has potential therapeutic use in degenerative liver disease. HGF can stimulate DNA synthesis in primary cultures of human hepatocytes.[10,11] Cell cycle analysis by flow cytometry revealed that after 48 h incubation with the factor, most quiescent 2c cells had left G0/G1 and entered the cell cycle. Human recombinant HGF was a much more potent mitogen for human hepatocytes than

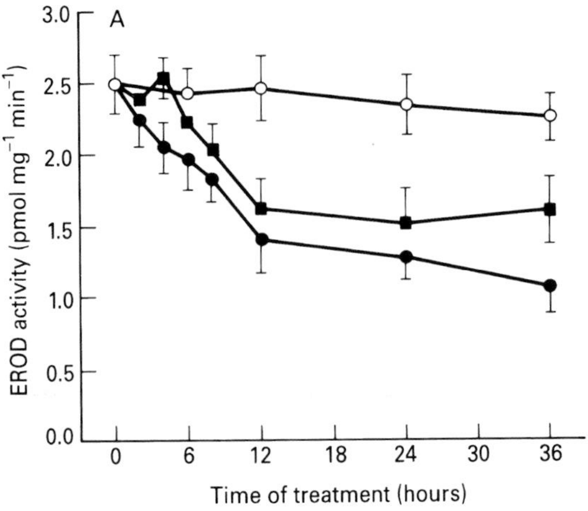

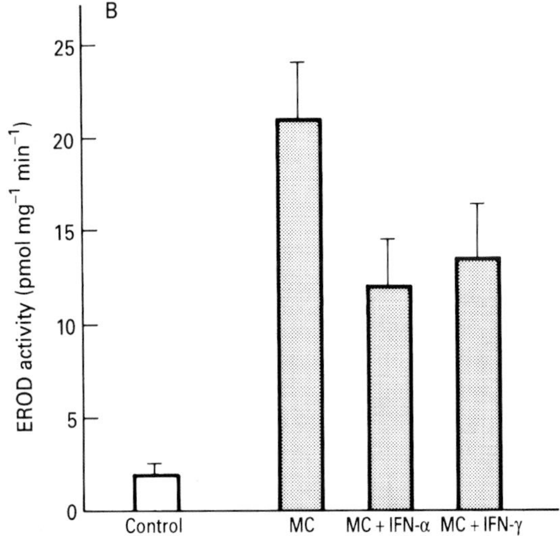

Fig. 6.5 Effect of interferon on basal and induced CYP1A2 (7-ethoxyresorufin-O-de-ethylase; EROD) activity in 24-h cultured human hepatocytes. (A) Human hepatocytes were exposed to 300 units ml^{-1} interferon (IFN)-α (●) or IFN-γ (■); EROD activity was measured at the indicated times and compared with that of untreated cultures (○). (B) Hepatocytes were exposed to 2 μM 3-methylcholanthrene (MC) and 300 units ml^{-1} IFN-α or IFN-γ, and EROD activity was determined 24 h later.

other growth factors (epidermal growth factor, insulin, glucagon; Fig. 6.6), and its effects on DNA synthesis could be inhibited by transforming growth factor β.[11] But, interestingly, HGF influenced the expression of many other hepatic genes not involved in cell growth. For instance, it stimulated the synthesis of albumin, transferrin, and fibronectin, decreased that of α_1-antichymotrypsin and haptoglobin, and stimulated that of α_2-macroglobulin. Of note, these effects were divergent from those elicited by interleukin 6.[106]

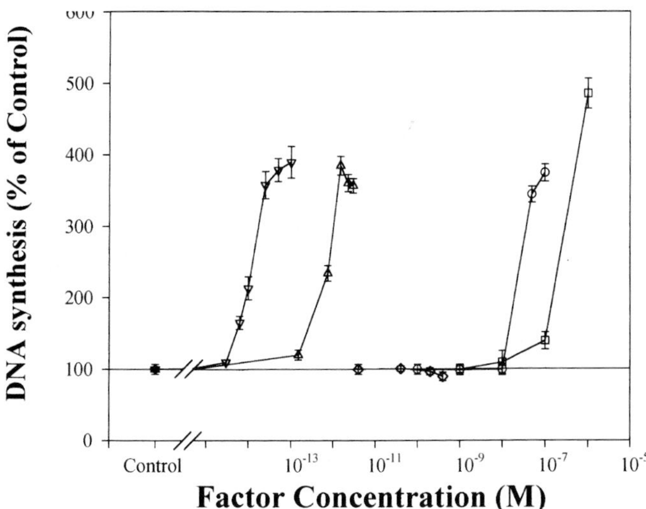

Fig. 6.6 Stimulation of DNA synthesis by growth factors in human hepatocytes. Human hepatocytes were stimulated for 96 h with increasing concentrations of HGF (▽), EGF (△), TGF-β (◇), insulin (○), and glucagon (□). Twenty-four hours before the end of the assay, 5 μCi ml^{-1} [^{3}H]thymidine was added to wells, together with the change of medium. After pulse labeling, hepatocytes were harvested and analysed for DNA synthesis. Data are expressed as the mean ± s.d. percentage of [^{3}H]thymidine incorporated compared with unstimulated hepatocytes.

VIII. FUTURE PERSPECTIVES

The interest of human hepatic cells in pharmacotoxicological research relies on the fact that this is the closest experimental model to human liver. However, use of primary cultures of human hepatocytes is severely restricted by the availability of human tissue and by the fact that hepatocyte growth in culture is very limited. Both facts constitute serious drawbacks to the widespread use of primary cultures of human hepatocytes.

There are several approaches to overcome this problem: (a) immortalization of human hepatocytes by means of appropriate viral vectors; (b) obtaining hybrids of hepatocytes and hepatoma cells; and (c) use of cell lines, genetically manipulated to express hepatic genes.

Several strategies have been explored to immortalize adult human hepatocytes. The most frequently used has been transformation with retroviral vectors.[107–110] The results, however, have not been completely satisfactory. Human cells are very refractory to transformation and, in addition, this process is frequently accompanied by loss of differentiated metabolic functions (i.e. biotransforming activities).

A further possibility is the use of stem cells isolated from human liver. These cells show the ability to proliferate in culture and, upon adequate stimulus, can differentiate into mature hepatocytes.[111] By co-culturing human hepatocytes with rat epithelial cells in a highly enriched medium, spontaneous immortalization of human hepatocytes has been reported.[112] These immortalized cells show, in addition to other typical hepatic functions (plasma protein synthesis), measurable aryl hydrocarbon hydroxylase, 7-ethoxyresorufin-O-de-ethylase, and 7-methoxyresorufin-O-demethylase activities.

It is also conceivable that, by fusing human hepatomas with human hepatocytes, the resulting hybrids may share properties of both cell types, i.e. continuously growing but also expression of drug biotransforming enzymes. The first attempts with rat hepatoma–hepatocytes have been promising.[113,114] The rat–rat hybrids divided readily, were phenotypically stable, and shared biochemical characteristics of both cell types. Although this strategy should be applicable to human hybrids, no positive results have yet been reported.

By using expression vectors encoding full-length human cytochrome genes, several groups have succeeded in expressing fully active cytochrome P450 isozymes in hepatic and non-hepatic cells (see Chapter 18). These cells express CYP activities under the control of a strong promoter. The utility of such manipulated cells for establishing the role of a particular P450 isozyme in the metabolism of a drug is starting to be appreciated.[109,115,116] However, its value in the accurate prediction of the human metabolic profile of a new drug remains to be demonstrated.

ACKNOWLEDGEMENTS

The authors acknowledge the financial support of the European Union (Biomed I, Project Nr. BMH1-1097 and AIR, Project Nr. CT93-0860), the Spanish Fondo de Investigaciones Sanitarias (Project Nr. 94/1084) and The ALIVE Foundation.

REFERENCES

1. Tulp, A., Welagen, J. J. and Emmelot, P. (1976) Separation of intact rat hepatocytes and rat liver nuclei into ploidy classes by velocity sedimentation at unit gravity. *Biochem. Biophys. Acta* **451:** 576–582.
2. Strom, S. C., Jirtle, R. L., Jones, R. S. *et al.* (1982) Isolation, culture, and transplantation of human hepatocytes. *J. Natl Cancer Inst.* **68:** 771–778.
3. Guguen-Guillouzo, C., Campion, J. P., Brissot, D. *et al.* (1982) High yield preparation of isolated human adult hepatocytes by enzymatic perfusion of the liver. *Cell Biol. Int. Rep.* **6:** 625–628.
4. Ballet, F., Bouma, M. E., Wang, S. R. *et al.* (1984) Isolation, culture and characterization of adult human hepatocytes from surgical liver biopsies. *Hepatology* **4:** 849–854.
5. Le Rumeur, E., Guguen-Guillouzo, Ch., Beaumont, C., Saunier, A. and Guillouzo, A. (1983) Albumin secretion and protein synthesis by cultured diploid and tetraploid rat hepatocytes separated by elutriation. *Exp. Cell Res.* **157:** 247–254.
6. Ryan, C. M., Carter, E. A., Jenkins, R. L., Sterling, L. M., Yarmush, M. L. and Matl, R. A. (1993) Isolation and long-term culture of human hepatocytes. *Surgery* **113:** 48–54.
7. Blaauboer, B. J., Boobis, A. R., Castell, J. V. *et al.* (1994) The practical applicability of hepatocyte cultures in routine testing. The report and recommendations of ECVAM Workshop 1. *ATLA* **22:** 231–241.
8. Gómez-Lechón, M. J., López, P., Donato, T. *et al.* (1990) Culture of human hepatocytes from small surgical liver biopsies. Biochemical characterization and comparison with *in vivo*. *In Vitro Cell. Dev. Biol.* **26:** 67–74.
9. Kreamer, B. L., Staecker, J. L., Sawada, N., Sattler, G. L., Hsia, M. T. S. and Pitot, H. C. (1986) Use of a low-speed, iso-density percoll centrifugation method to increase the viability of isolated rat hepatocyte preparations. *In Vitro Cell. Dev. Biol.* **22:** 201–211.
10. Strain, A. J., Ismail, T., Tsubouchi, H. *et al.* (1991) Native and recombinant human hepatocyte growth factors are highly potent promoters of DNA synthesis in both human and rat hepatocytes. *Clin. Invest.* **87:** 1853–1857.
11. Gómez-Lechón, M. J., Castell, J. V., Guillen, I. *et al.* (1995) Effects of hepatocyte growth factor on the growth and metabolism of human hepatocytes in primary culture. *Hepatology* **21:** 1248–1254.

12. Suolinna, E. M. (1982) Isolation and culture of liver cells and their use in the biochemical research of xenobiotics. *Med. Biol.* **60:** 237–254.
13. Holme, J. A. (1985) Xenobiotic metabolism and toxicity in primary monolayer cultures of hepatocytes. *NIPH Ann.* **8:** 49–63.
14. Guillouzo, A. (1986) Use of isolated and cultured hepatocytes for xenobiotic metabolism and cytotoxicity studies. In Guillouzo, A. and Guguen-Guillouzo, C. (eds) *Research in Isolated and Culture Hepatocytes*, pp. 313–332. Les Editions INSERM/John Libbey Eurotext, London.
15. Michalopoulos, G. and Pitot, H. C. (1975) Primary culture of parenchymal liver cells on collagen membranes. *Exp Cell Res.* **94:** 70–78.
16. Michalopoulos, G., Sattler, G. L. and Pitot, H. C. (1976) Maintenance of microsomal cytochrome b5 and P-450 in primary cultures of parenchymal liver cells on collagen membranes. *Life Sci.* **18:** 1139–1144.
17. Rojkind, M., Gatmaitan, Z., MacKensen, S., Giambrone, M. A., Ponce, P. and Reid, L. M. (1980) Connective tisue biomatrix: Its isolation and utilization for long-term cultures of normal rat hepatocytes. *J. Cell Biol.* **87:** 255–263.
18. Reid, L. M., Narita, M., Fujita, M., , Murray, Z., Liverpool, C. and Rosenberg, L. (1986) Matrix and hormonal regulation of differentiation in liver cultures. In Guillouzo, A. and Guguen-Guillouzo, Ch. (eds) *Isolated and Cultured Hepatocytes*, pp. 225–258. Les Editions INSERM/John Libbey Eurotext, London.
19. Dunn, J. C., Yarmush, M. K. L., Koebe, H. G. and Tomkins, R. G. (1989) Hepatocyte function and extracellular matrix geometry: long-term culture in a sandwich configuration. *FASEB J.* **3:** 174–177.
20. Guzelian, P. S., Li, D., Schuetz, E. G. *et al.* (1988) Sex change in cytochrome P-450 phenotype by growth hormone treatment of adult rat hepatocytes maintained in a culture system on matrigel. *Proc. Natl Acad. Sci. U.S.A.* **85:** 9783–9788.
21. Bader, A., Zech, K., Crome, O., Christians, U., Ringe, B., Pichlmayr, R. and Sewing, K. (1994) Use of organotypical cultures of primary hepatocytes to analyse drug biotransformation in man and animals. *Xenobiotica* **24:** 623–633.
22. Dunn, J. C. Y., Tompkins, R. G. and Yarmush, M. L. (1992) Hepatocytes in collagen sandwich: evidence for transcriptional and translational regulation. *J. Cell Biol.* **116:** 1043–1053.
23. Koebe, H. G., Pahernik, S., Eyer, P. and Schildberg, F. W. (1994) Collagen gell immobilization: a useful cell culture technique for long-term metabolic studies on human hepatocytes. *Xenobiotica* **24:** 95–107.
24. Langenbach, R., Malick, L., Tompa, A., Kuszynski, C., Freed, H. and Huberman, E. (1979) Maintenance of adult rat hepatocytes on C3H/10T1/2 cells. *Cancer Res.* **39:** 3509–3514.
25. Michalopoulos, G., Rusell, F. and Biles, C. (1979) Primary cultures of hepatocytes on human fibroblasts. *In Vitro* **15:** 796–806.
26. Guguen-Guillouzo, C., Clement, B., Baffet, G. *et al.* (1983) Maintenance and reversibility of active albumin secretion by adult rat hepatocytes co-cultured with another liver epithelial cell type. *Exp. Cell Res.* **143:** 47–54.
27. Morin, O. and Norman, C. (1986) Long-term maintenance of hepatocyte functional activity in co-culture: requirements for sinusoidal endothelial cells and dexamethasone. *J. Cell. Physiol.* **129:** 103–110.
28. Goulet, F., Normand, C. and Morin, O. (1988) Cellular interactions promote tissue-specific function, biomatrix deposition and junctional communication of primary cultured hepatocytes. *Hepatology* **8:** 1010–1018.
29. Kuri-Harcuch, W. and Mendoza-Figueroa, T. (1989) Cultivation of adult rat hepatocytes on 3T3 cells: expression of various liver differentiated functions. *Differentiation* **41:** 148–157.
30. Donato, M. T., Castell, J. V. and Gómez-Lechón, M. J. (1990) Prolonged expression of biotransformation activities of rat hepatocytes co-cultured with established cell lines. *Toxicol. In Vitro* **4:** 461–466.
31. Donato, M. T., Gómez-Lechón, M. J. and Castell, J. V. (1990) Drug metabolizing enzymes in rat hepatocytes co-cultured with cell lines. *In Vitro Cell. Dev. Biol.* **26:** 1057–1062.
32. Donato, M. T., Castell, J. V. and Gómez-Lechón, M. J. (1991) Co-cultures of hepatocytes with epithelial-like cell lines: expression of drug-biotransformation activities by hepatocytes. *Cell Biol. Toxicol.* **7:** 1–14.
33. Donato, M. T., Gómez-Lechón, M. J. and Castell, J. V. (1991) Rat hepatocytes cultured on a monkey kidney cell line: expression of biotransformation and hepatic metabolic activities. *Toxicol. In Vitro* **5:** 435–438.

34. Begué J., Guguen-Guillouzo, C., Pasdeloup, N. and Guillouzo, A. (1984) Prolonged maintenance of active cytochrome P-450 in adult rat hepatocyte co-cultured with another liver cell type. *Hepatology* **4:** 839–842.
35. Clement, B., Guguen-Guillouzo, Ch., Campion, J. P., Glaise, D., Bourel, M. and Guillouzo, A. (1984) Long-term co-cultures of adult human hepatocytes with rat liver epithelial cells: modulation of albumin secretion and accumulation of extracellular material. *Hepatology* **4:** 373–380.
36. Rijntjes, P. J. M., Moshage, H. J., Van Gemert, P. J. L., De Waal, R. and Yap, S. H. (1986) Cryopreservation of adult human hepatocytes. The influence of deep freezing storage on the viability, cell seeding, survival, fine structures and albumin synthesis in primary cultures. *J. Hepatology.* **3:** 7–18.
37. de Sousa, G., Dou, M., Barbe, D., Lacarelle, B., Placidi, M. and Rahmani, R. (1991) Freshly isolated or cryopreseved human hepatocytes in primary culture: influence of drug metabolism on hepatotoxicity. *Toxicol. In Vitro* **5:** 483–486.
38. Coundouris, J. A., Grant, M. H., Engest, J., Petrie, J. C. and Hawksworth, G. M. (1993) Cryopreservation of human adult hepatocytes for use in drug metabolism and toxicity studies. *Xenobiotica* **23:** 1399–1409.
39. Chesne, C., Guyomard, C., Fautrel, C. *et al.* (1993) Viability and function in primary culture of adult hepatocytes from various animal species and human beings after cryopreservation. *Hepatology* **18:** 406–414.
40. López, M. P., Gómez-Lechón, M. J. and Castell, J. V. (1991) Role of glucose, insulin and glucagon in glycogen mobilization in human hepatocytes. *Diabetes* **40:** 263–268.
41. López, M. P., Gómez-Lechón, M. J. and Castell, J. V. (1991) Glucose: a more powerful modulator of fructose 2,6-bisphosphate levels than insulin in human hepatocytes. *Biochim. Biophys. Acta* **1094:** 200–206.
42. Munk Petersen, C., Christiansen, B. S., Heickendorff, L. and Ingerslev, J. (1988) Synthesis and secretion of α_2-macroglobulin by human hepatocytes in culture. *Eur. J. Clin. Invest.* **18:** 543–548.
43. Christiansen, B. S., Ingerslev, J., Heickendorff, L. and Petersen, C. M. (1988) Human hepatocytes in culture synthesize and secrete fibronectin. *Scand. J. Clin. Lab. Invest.* **48:** 685–690.
44. Castell, J. V., Gómez-Lechón, M. J., David, M., Fabra, R., Trullenque, R. and Heinrich, P. (1990) Acute-response of human hepatocytes, regulation of acute-phase protein synthesis by interleukin-6. *Hepatology* **12:** 1179–1186.
45. Ingelman-Sundeberg, M. (1986) Cytochrome P450 organization and membrane interaction. In Ortiz de Montellano, P. R. (ed.) *Cytochrome P-450: Structure, Mechanisms, and Biochemistry*, pp. 119–160. Plenum Press, London.
46. Gonzalez, F. J. (1989) The molecular biology of cytochrome P450s. *Pharmacol. Rev.* **40:** 243–288.
47. Gonzalez, F. J. (1990) Molecular genetics of the P-450 superfamily. *Pharmacol. Ther.* **45:** 1–38.
48. Okey, A. B. (1990) Enzyme induction in the cytochrome P-450 system. *Pharmacol. Ther.* **45:** 241–298.
49. Gonzalez, F. J. and Gelboin, H. V. (1991) Human cytochromes P450: evolution, catalytic activities and interindividual variations in expression. In *New Horizons in Biological Dosimetry*, pp. 11–20. Wiley–Liss, London.
50. Guengerich, F. P. (1992) Human cytochrome P450 enzymes. *Life Sci.* **50:** 1471–1478.
51. Guengerich, F. P. (1992) Characterization of human cytochrome P450 enzymes. *FASEB J.* **6:** 745–748.
52. Nelson, D. R,. Kamataki, T., Waxman, D. J. *et al.* (1993) The P450 superfamily: update on new sequences, gene expression, accession numbers, early trivial names of enzymes and nomenclature. *DNA Cell Biol.* **12:** 1–51.
53. Paine, A. (1995) Heterogeneity of cytochrome P450 and its toxicological significance. *Hum. Exp. Toxicol.* **4:** 1–7.
54. Hakkola, J., Pasanen, M., Purkunen, R. *et al.* (1994) Expression of xenobiotic-metabolizing cytochrome P450 forms in human adult and fetal liver. *Biochem. Pharmacol.* **48:** 59–64.
55. Lucas, D. L., Berthou, F., Dreano, Y., Lozach, P., Volant, A. and Menez, J. F. (1993) Comparison of levels of cytochromes P-450, CYP1A2, CYP2E1, and their related monooxygenase activities in human surgical liver samples. *Alcohol Clin. Exp. Res.* **17:** 900–905.
56. Morel, F., Beaune, P.H., Ratanasavanh, D. *et al.* (1990) Expression of cytochrome P-450 isozymes in cultured human hepatocytes. *Eur. J. Biochem.* **191:** 437–444.
57. Pichard, L., Fabre, I., Daujat, M., Domergue, J., Joyeux, H. and Maurel, P. (1992) Effect of corticosteroids on the expression of cytochromes P450 and on cyclosporin A oxidase activity in primary cultures of human hepatocytes. *Mol. Pharmacol.* **41:** 1047–1055.

58. Guengerich, F. P. (1994) Catalytic selectivity of human cytochrome P450 enzymes: relevance to drug metabolism and toxicity. *Toxicol. Lett.* **70:** 133–138.
59. Waxman, D. J., Lapenson, D. P., Aoyama, T., Gelboin, H. V., Gonzalez, F. J. and Korzekwa, K. (1991) Steroid hormone hydroxylase specificities of eleven cDNA-expressed human cytochrome P450s. *Arch. Biochem. Biophys.* **290:** 160–166.
60. Greenlee, W. F. and Poland, A. (1978) An improved assay of 7-ethoxycoumarin-O-deethylase activity: induction of hepatic enzyme activity in C57 BL/6J and DBA/2J mice by phenobarbital, 3-methylcholanthrene and 2,3,7,8-tetrachlorobenzo-*p*-dioxin. *J. Pharmacol. Exp. Ther.* **205:** 569–605.
61. Rogiers, V., Adriaenssens, L., Vandenberghe, Y., Gepts, E., Callaerts, A. and Vercruysse, A. (1986) Critical evaluation of 7-ethoxycoumarin O-deethylase activity measurement in intact isolated rat hepatocytes. *Xenobiotica* **16:** 817–826.
62. Kremers, P., Negro, L. and Gielen, J. (1990) Rat fetal hepatocytes in cultures: a model for metabolic and toxicological studies. *Acta Pharmacol. Jugosl.* **40:** 383–393.
63. Burke, M. D., Thompson, S., Elcombe, C. R., Halpert, J., Haaparanta, T. and Mayer, R. T. (1985) Ethoxy-, pentoxy-, and benzyloxyphenoxazones and homologues, a series of substrates to distinguish between different induced cytochromes P-450. *Biochem. Pharmacol.* **34:** 3337–3345.
64. Grant, M. H., Melvin, M. A. L., Shaw, P., Melvin, W. T. and Burke, M. D. (1985) Studies on the maintenance of cytochromes P-450 and b5, monooxygenases and cytochrome reductases in primary cultures of rat hepatocytes. *FEBS Lett.* **190:** 99–103.
65. Lubet, R. A., Nims, R. W., Mayer, R. T., Cameron, J. W. and Schechtman, L. M. (1985) Measurement of cytochrome P-450 dependent dealkylation of alkoxyphenoxazones in hepatic S9s and hepatocyte homogenates: effects of dicumarol. *Mutat. Res.* **142:** 127–131.
66. Wortelboer, H. M., de Kruif, C. A., van Iersel, A. A. J., Falke, H. E., Noordhoek, J. and Blaauboer, B. J. (1990) The isozyme pattern of cytochrome P450 in rat hepatocytes in primary culture, comparing different enzyme activities in microsomal incubations and in intact monolayers. *Biochem. Pharmacol.* **40:** 2525–2534.
67. Donato, M. T., Gómez-Lechón, M. J. and Castell, J. V. (1993) A microassay for measuring cytochrome P450IA1 and P450IIB1 activities in intact human and rat hepatocytes cultured on 96-well plates. *Anal Biochem.* **213:** 20–33.
68. Pearce, R., Greenway, D. and Parkinson, A. (1992) Species differences in interindividual variation in liver microsomal citochrome p450 2A enzymes: effects on coumarin, dicumarol, and testosterone oxidation. *Arch. Biochem. Biophys.* **298:** 211–225.
69. Yun, C. H., Shimada, T. and Guengerich, F.P. (1991) Purification and characterization of human liver microsomal cytochrome P-450 2A6. *Mol. Pharmacol.* **40:** 679–685.
70. Tassaneeyakul, W., Veronese, M. E., Birkett, D. J., Gonzalez, F. J. and Miners, J. O. (1993) Validation of 4-nitrophenol as an *in vitro* substrate probe for human liver CYP2E1 using cDNA expression and microsomal kinetic techniques. *Biochem. Pharmacol.* **46:** 1975–1981.
71. Patten, C. J., Ishizaki, H., Aoyama, T. *et al.* (1992) Catalytic properties of the human cytochrome P450 2E1 produced by cDNA expression in mammalian cells. *Arch. Biochem. Biophys.* **299:** 163–171.
72. Reinke, L. A. and Moyer, M. J. (1985) A microsomal oxidation which is highly inducible by ethanol. *Drug Metab. Disp.* **13:** 548–552.
73. Thummel, K. E., Kharasch, E. D., Podoll, T. and Kunze, K. (1993) Human liver microsomal enflurane defluoration catalyzed by cytochrome P-450 2E1. *Drug Metab. Disp.* **21:** 350–357.
74. Dicker, E, McHugh, T. and Cederbaum, A. J. (1990) Increased oxidation of *p*-nitrophenol and aniline by intact hepatocytes isolated from pyrazole-treated rats. *Biochim. Biophys. Acta* **1035:** 249–256.
75. Maenpaa, J., Syngelma, T., Honkakoski, P., Lang, M. A. and Pelkonen, O. (1991) Comparative studies on coumarin and testosterone metabolism in mouse and human livers. Differential inhibitions by the anti-P450Coh antibody and metyrapone. *Biochem. Pharmacol.* **42:** 1229–1235.
76. Ohmori, S., Shirakawa, C., Motohashi, K. *et al.* (1993) Purification from liver microsomes from untreated cynomolgus monkeys of cytochrome P450 closely related to human cytochrome P450 2B6. *Mol. Pharmacol.* **43:** 183–190.
77. Donato, M. T., Castell, J. V. and Gómez-Lechón, M. J. (1995) Effect of model inducers on cytochrome P450 activities of human hepatocytes in primary cultures. *Drug Metab. Dispos.* **23:** 553–558.
78. Burchell, B., Nebert, D. W., Nelson, D. R. *et al.* (1991) The UDP glucuronosyl transferase gene

superfamily, suggested nomenclature based on evolutionary divergence. *DNA Cell Biol.* **10:** 487–494.
79. Miners, J. O. and Mackenzie, P. I. (1991) Drug glucuronidation in humans. *Pharmacol. Ther.* **51:** 347–369.
80. Bock, K. W., Clausbruch, U. C., Kaufmann, R. *et al.* (1980) Functional heterogeneity of UDP-glucuronyltransferase in rat tissues. *Biochem. Pharmacol.* **29:** 495–500.
81. Jakoby, W. B. and Habig, W. H. (1980) Glutathione transferases. In Jakoby, W. J. (ed.) *Enzymatic Basis of Detoxication*, Vol. I, pp. 63–94. Academic Press, New York.
82. Missiaen, L., Taylor, C. W. and Berridge, M. J. (1992) Nomenclature for human glutathione transferases. *Biochem. J.* **282:** 305–308.
83. Board, P., Coggan, M., Johnston, P., Ross, V., Suzuki, T. and Webb, G. (1991) Genetic heterogeneity of the human glutathione transferases, a complex of gene families. *Pharmacol. Ther.* **48:** 357–369.
84. Habig, W. H. and Jakoby, W. B. (1981) Assays for differentiation of glutathione *S*-transferases. *Methods Enzymol.* **77:** 398–405.
85. Berthou, F., Ratanasavanh, D., Riche, C., Picart, D., Voirin, T. and Guillouzo, A. (1989) Comparison of caffeine metabolism by slices, microsomes and hepatocyte cultures from adult human liver. *Xenobiotica* **19:** 401–417.
86. Stevens, J. C., Shipley, L. A., Cashman, J. R., Vandenbranden, M. and Wrighton, S. A. (1993) Comparison of human and rhesus monkey *in vitro* phase I and phase II hepatic drug metabolism activities. *Drug Metab. Dispos.* **21:** 753–760.
87. Donato, M. T., Gómez-Lechón, M. J. and Castell, J. V. (1990) Effect of xenobiotics on monooxygenase activities in cultured human hepatocytes. *Biochem. Pharmacol.* **39:** 1320–1326.
88. Schmucker, D. L., Woodhouse, K. W., Wang, R. K. *et al.* (1990) Effects of age and gender on *in vitro* properties of human liver microsomal monooxygenases. *Clin. Pharmacol. Ther.* **48:** 365–374.
89. Shimada, T., Yamazaki, H., Mimura, M., Inui, Y. and Guengerich, F. P. (1994) Interindividual variations in human liver cytochrome P450 enzymes involved in the oxidation of drugs, carcinogens and toxic chemicals: studies with liver microsomes of 30 Japaneses and 30 Caucasians. *J. Pharmacol. Exp. Ther.* **270:** 414–423.
90. Guengerich, F. P. (1995) Influence of nutrients and other dietary materials on cytochrome P450 enzymes. *Am. J. Clin. Nutr.* **61:** 651S–658S.
91. Grant, M. H., Burke, M. D., Hawksworth, G. M., Duthie, S. J., Engeset, J. and Petrie, J. C. (1987) Human adult hepatocytes in primary monolayer culture. Maintenance of mixed function oxidase and conjugation pathways of drug metabolism. *Biochem. Pharmacol.* **36:** 2311–2316.
92. Donato, M. T., Castell, J. V. and Gómez-Lechón, M. J. (1992) Biotransformation of drugs by cultured hepatocytes. In Castell, J. V. and Gómez-Lechón, M. J. (eds) In Vitro *Alternatives to Animal Pharmaco-toxicology*, pp. 149–178. Farmaindustria, Madrid.
93. Ratanasavanh, D., Beaune, Ph., Baffet, G. *et al.* (1986) Immunocytochemical evidence for the maintenance of cytochrome P450 isozymes, NADPH cytochrome *c* reductase, and epoxide hydrolase in pure and mixed primary cultures of adult human hepatocytes. *J. Histochem. Cytochem.* **34:** 527–533.
94. Hawksworth, G. M. (1995) Advantages and disadvantages of using human cells for pharmacological and toxicological studies. *Hum. Exp. Toxicol.* **13:** 568–573.
95. Ball, S. E., Scatina, J. Z. A., Sisenwine, S. F. and Fisher, G. L. (1995) The application of *in vitro* models of drug metabolism and toxicity in drug discovery and drug development. *Drug Chem. Toxicol.* **18:** 1–28.
96. Castell, J. V. and Gómez-Lechón, M. J. (1992) The *in vitro* evaluation of the potential risk of hepatotoxicity of drugs. In Castell, J. V. and Gómez-Lechón, M. J. (eds) In Vitro *Alternatives to Animal Pharmaco-toxicology*, pp. 179–204. Farmaindustria, Madrid.
97. Guillouzo, A., Morel, F., Fardel, O. and Meunier, B. (1993) Use of human hepatocyte cultures for drug metabolism studies. *Toxicology* **82:** 209–219.
98. Sandker, G. W., Vos, R. M., Delbressine, L. P., Slooff, M. J., Meijer, D. K. and Groothuis, G. M. (1994) Metabolism of three pharmacologically active drugs in isolated human and rat hepatocytes: analysis of interspecies variability and comparison with metabolism *in vivo*. *Xenobiotica* **24:** 143–155.
99. de Sousa, G., Florence, N., Valles, B., Coassolo, P. and Rahmani, R. (1995) Relationship between *in vitro* and *in vivo* biotransformation of drugs in humans and animals: pharmatoxicological consequences. *Cell Biol. Toxicol.* **11:** 147–153.

100. Singh, G. and Renton, K. W. (1982) Homogeneous interferon from *E. coli* depresses hepatic cytochrome P450 and drug biotransformation. *Biochem. Biophys. Res. Commun.* **106:** 1256–1261.
101. Donato, M. T., Herrero, E., Gómez-Lechón, M. J. and Castell, J. V. (1993) Inhibition of monooxygenase activities in human hepatocytes by interferons. *Toxicol. In Vitro* **7:** 481–485.
102. Abdel-Razzak, Z., Loyer, P., Fautrel, A. *et al.* (1993) Cytokines downregulate expression of major cytochrome P-450 enzymes in adult human hepatocytes in primary culture. *Mol. Pharmacol.* **44:** 707–715.
103. Braulen, M. E. and Wahl, S. M. (1994) Inflammatory cytokines: an overview. In Schook, L. B. and Caskin, D. L. (eds) *Xenobiotics and Inflammation*, pp. 33–70. Academic Press, London.
104. Castell, J. V., Gómez-Lechón, M. J., David, M. *et al.* (1989) Interleukin-6 is the major regulator of acute phase protein synthesis in adult human hepatocytes. *FEBS Lett.* **242:** 237–239.
105. Abdel-Razzak, Z., Corcos, K. L., Fautrel, A., Campion, J. P and Guillouzo, A. (1994) Transforming growth factor-β1 downregulates basal and polycyclic aromatic hydrocarbon induced cytochromes P-4501A1 and 1A2 in adult human hepatocytes in primary culture. *Mol. Pharmacol.* **46:** 1100–1110.
106. Guillen, I., Gómez-Lechón, M. J., Nakamura, T. and Castell, J. V. (1996) The hepatocyte growth factor regulates the synthesis of acute-phase proteins in human hepatocytes. Divergent effect on IL6-stimulated genes. *Hepatology* **23**: 1345–1352.
107. Wu, G. S. (1993) Establishment and mechanistic characterization of SV40 T antigen immortalized human fetal hepatocytes. *Chung Hua Chung Liu Tsa Chih* **15:** 415–418.
108. Ueno, T., Miyamura, T., Saito, I. and Mizuno, K. (1993) Immortalization of differentiated human hepatocytes by a combination of a viral vector and collagen gel culture. *Hum. Cell* **6:** 126–136.
109. Pfeifer, A. M., Cole, K. E., Simoot, D. T. *et al.* (1993) Simian virus 40 large tumor antigen-immortalized normal human liver epithelial cells express hepatocyte characteristics and metabolize chemical carcinogens. *Proc. Natl Acad. Sci. U.S.A.* **90:** 5123–5127.
110. Pfeifer, A. M. A., Mace, K., Tromvoukis, Y. and Lipsky, M. M. (1995) Highly efficient establishment of immortalized cells from human liver. *Methods Cell Sci.* **17:** 83–89.
111. Gibson-D'Ambrosio, R. E., Crowe, D. L., Shuler, C.E. and D'Ambrosio, S. M. (1993) The establishment and continous subculturing of normal human adult hepatocytes: expression of differentiated liver functions. *Cell. Biol. Toxicol.* **9:** 385–403.
112. Roberts, E. A., Furuya, K. N., Tang, B. K. and Kalow, W. (1994) Caffeine biotransformation in human hepatocyte lines derived from normal liver tissue. *Biochem. Biophys. Res. Commun.* **201:** 559–566.
113. Katz, N., Immenschue, S., Gerbracht, U., Eigenbrodt, E., Follmann, W. and Petzinger, E. (1992) Hormone-sensitive carbohydrate metabolism in rat hepatocyte–hepatoma hybrid cells. *Eur. J. Cell Biol.* **57:** 117–124.
114. Petzinger, E., Follmann, W., Blumrich, M. *et al.* (1994) Immortalization of rat hepatocytes by fusion with hepatoma cells. I. Cloning of a hepatocytoma cell line with bile canaliculi. *Eur. J. Cell Biol.* **64:** 328–338.
115. Crespi, C. L, Gonzalez, F. J., Steimel, D. T. *et al.* (1991) A metabolically competent human cells line expressing five cDNAs encoding procarcinogen and promutagen-activating enzymes: application to mutagenicity testing. *Chem. Res. Toxicol.* **4:** 566–572.
116. Guengerich, F. P., Gillam, E. M., Ohmori, S. *et al.* (1993) Expression of human cytocrome P450 enzymes in yeast and bacteria and relevance to studies on catalytic activity. *Toxicology* **82:** 21–37.

7

Studies of Neurotoxicity in Cellular Models

ELIZABETH McFARLANE ABDULLA AND
IAIN C. CAMPBELL

I. General introduction 156
A. Neurotoxicity 156
B. Neuronal vulnerability 157
1. Limitations of *in vitro* studies 157
C. Differentiation, apoptosis and susceptibility to toxicity 157
D. Neurotrophic factors 158
II. Primary dissociated neuronal cell culture 159
A. Advantages and disadvantages of primary dissociated neuronal culture . . . 159
B. CNS cell culture methods 159
1. Cerebral cortical and hippocampal neurones: studies of the basis of excitotoxicity 160
2. Cerebellar granule cells: developmental aspects of vulnerability 161
3. Chick embryo neuronal cultures: use in studies of organophosphates . . 161
4. Embryonic rat hippocampal, septal and cortical neurones: studies of neuroprotection by growth factors and neurotrophic factors 161
5. Embryonic rat cortical neurones: studies of oxidative stress and apoptosis 162
6. Dopamine- or 5-hydroxytryptamine-containing neurones cultured from mesencephalon or raphe nuclei of rat fetuses: studies on the toxicity of pharmacological agents 162
III. Neuronal cell lines 162
A. Immortalized cell lines 162
1. Human SHSY5Y neuroblastoma cell line: studies of differential specificity to organophosphates 163
2. Murine septal (SN56) lines, motor neurone (NSC19) lines and human neuroblastoma (LA-N-2) cells: use of differentiated cholinergic cells for evaluating acetylcholinesterase inhibitors 163
3. Human SKNSH and mouse NB41A3 neuroblastoma cell line: inhibition of neuronal differentiation as a measure of toxicity 164
IV. Transfected cells and cell lines 166
V. Transformed and transfected cells based on disease models 166
VI. Hybrid cell line cultures 167
1. Glioma × neuroblastoma hybrid cell (NG108-15) lines: studies of developmental toxicity 167

IN VITRO METHODS IN PHARMACEUTICAL RESEARCH
ISBN 0-12-163390-X

VII. Co-culture . . . 167
1. Primary models for reactive and type-1-like astrocytes: studies of EAA toxicity . . . 168
2. Mixed cultures of spinal cord neurones and muscle cells from *Xenopus laevis* embryos: use in developmental studies . . . 168
VIII. Complex primary culture systems . . . 168
1. Hippocampal slice culture: use in studies of EAA-induced toxicity . . . 168
2. Organotypic cultures: studies of neurotoxicity associated with β-amyloid protein, cytochemical changes and apoptotic cell death . . . 169
3. Reaggregate cultures: use in the study of developmental neurotoxicity. 169
4. Cultured spinal neurones and hippocampal brain slices: studies of calcium chelation as a neuroprotective strategy . . . 169
5. Micromass culture: use in teratogenicity testing and in studies of axonal transport for assessment of toxicity . . . 170
IX. Parameters for assessing neurotoxicity *in vitro* . . . 170
A. Mitochondrial function . . . 170
B. Mitochondrial potential . . . 170
C. Pinocytosis and transcellular traffic of solutes . . . 171
D. Plasma membrane integrity . . . 171
E. Cellular oxidation . . . 171
F. Cellular ATP levels . . . 171
G. Assessment of change along the growth–differentiation axis . . . 171
1. Cytoskeletal components . . . 171
2. Synaptogenesis . . . 172
3. Nitric oxide synthetase and nitric oxide . . . 172
H. Assessment of intracellular free calcium . . . 172
I. Assessing intracellular pH change . . . 172
J. Proto-oncogenes and transcription factors . . . 172
K. Stress response genes . . . 173
L. Ubiquitin . . . 173
M. Measures of apoptosis . . . 173
N. Receptor binding and neurotransmitter release . . . 174
X. Conclusions . . . 174
References . . . 176

This chapter reviews the use of *in vitro* culture systems in neurotoxicology and, following a General Introduction, there are seven major sections and a Conclusion. The sections describe and discuss a range of selected experimental models used in *in vitro* neurotoxicology; emphasis is placed on the advantages and limitations of these and on some specific methodological details.

I. GENERAL INTRODUCTION

A. Neurotoxicity

The biological mechanism of action of many neurotoxic substances is ill-defined and their toxicity is described largely on the basis of clinical data. The issue is complicated by the fact that, in the nervous system, there are several compensatory mechanisms: thus, a toxic insult may be overcome by the plasticity of the nervous system or by the fact that, in a specific neuronal system (CNS), there is a large degree of functional redundancy. This can make the interpretation of mechanistic data complex and *in vivo* it may mask the effects of toxic insult. It is also important to accept that toxic effects are dose dependent and, because *in vitro* testing may involve measurement of normal physiological parameters and responses, two major questions must always be considered: (a) at what point is an effect toxic? and (b) when is a substance to be considered toxic?

B. Neuronal vulnerability

Neurones do not divide. They are diverse in structure and function, are excitable, and are the most metabolically active cells in the body. They are highly ramified and thus have a large surface to volume ratio, diverse functional intracellular regions and a complex cytoskeleton.[1] They also exhibit plasticity and, under normal circumstances, their sole source of energy is glucose. In addition, the excitability of neurones and the presence of both voltage- and receptor-sensitive ion channels make them vulnerable to ionic imbalance which can result in osmotic- or enzyme-induced damage or to alterations in conduction. Hence, there is considerable potential for aberrant effects, e.g. in response to pharmacological compounds and to heavy metals and other noxious agents.

1. *Limitations of* in vitro *studies*

The CNS is a dynamic integrated system in which neurones are involved in complex electrical events and are subject to feedback from other cells and from soluble neurotrophic and/or other factors, which control synaptic plasticity, neuronal survival and responsivity. It is arguable, therefore, that the complexity of the nervous system is such that no single cell, or even multicellular complex culture, can be particularly relevant to its study. The most difficult part of *in vitro* investigations is thus the extrapolation of results to the whole animal. While this is acknowledged, it is noteworthy that our current understanding of neurobiology is derived substantially from a ‘reductionist’ approach.

Glia (astroglia, oligodendroglia and microglia) are a major cellular component of the nervous system. They participate in formation of the blood–brain barrier, exchange of materials between capillaries and neurones, biochemical modulation of synaptic activity, guidance of neuronal processes during development and repair, and immunological activity. They are also a reservoir for potassium, water and some neurotransmitters, e.g. glutamate. Therefore, studies of glial cultures and complex systems such as reaggregate culture (with ratios of neurones to glia resembling many areas in the brain) have been increasingly used in neurotoxicology.[2]

C. Differentiation, apoptosis and susceptibility to toxicity

In addition to having a complex structure and relationship with other cells, neurones undergo a series of differentiation stages to their terminal state, which in some cases can be apoptosis. Both differentiation and apoptosis are of interest to toxicologists; differentiation presents a period of particular vulnerability to toxic insult, and apoptosis provides a natural system for studying cell death. In addition, cell division and differentiation are mutually exclusive phenomena and the 'switch' process between them is important because it appears that low doses of some neurotoxicants move cells from a differentiating to a dividing state (dedifferentiation to mitosis). The question therefore arises: can the induction of such a switch be used as an acceptable measure of neurotoxicity? It has been shown that apoptosis can occur when differentiated cells are exposed to a range of adverse stimuli including nerve growth factor (NGF)-deprivation.[3] Apoptosis can be precipitated when the neurones attempt to re-enter the cell cycle while levels of expression of growth-associated proteins are low. The greater the degree of differentiation, the lower the levels of growth-associated proteins.[3]

Under some circumstances, neurotoxic effects that inhibit differentiation can lead to a quiescent state in the neurones, which persists until the appropriate conditions for differentiation are present (e.g. neurotrophic factors, cell-surface adhesion molecules and/or corticosteroids). For example, when neurones of the midbrain raphé–hippocampal axis cease to differentiate following adrenalectomy, they do not apoptose but become quiescent forming 'neurospores' (in many ways similar to developmental neuronal progenitor cells); however, they redifferentiate when exposed to dexamethasone.[4]

Differentiating neuronal cells extend processes that are difficult to define as axon or dendrite, and are usually termed neurites. The main physiological cues (i.e. both facilitatory and inhibitory signals) for neurite outgrowth are: (1) growth or neurotrophic factors, in particular NGF (via a tyrosine kinase receptor, trkA); (2) extracellular matrix (ECM) proteins, e.g. laminin (via integrin receptors); and (3) the immunoglobulin superfamily of cell adhesion molecules (CAMs), i.e. the Ca^{2+}-dependent N-cadherin (via N-cadherin and catenins) and Ca^{2+}-independent N-CAM, L1 and F11/F3 (via other NCAM receptors and vinculin, for example).[5] NGF, ECM proteins and N-cadherin (N-CAM) apparently facilitate neurite outgrowth by distinct pathways;[6] this provides an experimental means of establishing distinct targets of damage. The CAMs are expressed on (and are often secreted from) the surface of neurones and glial cells, and provide spatial and temporal cues which guide and control neurites. They can be trophic (nutritional) and/or tropic (directional) and/or inhibitory; in this last case, they may sometimes be capable of mediating growth cone collapse or paralysis of growth cone mobility (e.g. chick brain collapsin[7]).

Organotypic, micromass and reaggregate cultures are excellent systems for examining differentiation and neurite outgrowth and, in the case of reaggregate cultures, synaptogenesis. Differentiation can also be achieved using co-culture of neurones with glia or muscle cells and combinations of growth or neurotrophic factors with ECM^- (e.g. laminin) coating of culture dishes. Laminin β_2 or s-laminin, a differentially spliced variant of laminin, has been shown to act as a 'stop' signal for growing neurites and regulates the formation of motor nerve terminals.[8]

Neuronal health and susceptibility to toxic insult may be a function of the degree of cellular differentiation. The *bcl*-2 gene (a cell-death prevention gene), when transfected into PC12 cells, prevents apoptotic cell death when NGF is withdrawn (or when oxygen levels are high); however, it also facilitates differentiation.[9] Similarly, cycloheximide prevents oxidative stress-induced apoptosis[10] *and* stimulates neurite outgrowth in embryonic and newborn cortical neurones in culture, respectively.[11]

D. Neurotrophic factors

Neuronal loss can be reduced by neurotrophic factors such as NGF, insulin-like growth factor insulin-like growth factor 2 (IGF-2), ciliary neurotrophic factor (CNTF), brain-derived neurotrophic factor (BDNF) and neurotrophins (NT-3 and NT-4, is also known as

NT-5).[12] The recently discovered NT-6 (from the teleost fish Xiphophorus) remains attached to the neuronal membrane or to the ECM proteins and requires heparin to become soluble; it has approximately similar neurotrophic activity to NGF with a lower potency, although its neuroprotective capacity has not yet been established.[13] Recent studies indicate that glial cell line-derived neurotrophic factor (GDNF) can prevent neuronal loss in amyotrophic lateral sclerosis and Parkinson's disease.[14–16] There is also evidence in mice of the efficacy of intraparenchymal injection of GDNF *after* administration of the specific dopaminergic neurotoxic agent methyl-4-phenylpyridinium (MPP^+).[17] In addition, NGF has been shown to attenuate taxol-induced neurotoxicity in rat dorsal root ganglion and spinal cord cultures[18] and taxol-induced neuropathy in mice.[19] Thus, there is considerable therapeutic potential for neurotrophic molecules, particularly in amyotrophic lateral sclerosis, for the protection of dopaminergic neurones in Parkinson's disease, and also in combination with antimitotic drugs in cancer therapy to alleviate the neuropathy that is induced by many of these compounds. These findings are important in the present context as neurotoxic effects are partially dependent on the culture conditions and to some extent on growth or neurotrophic factors that are present.

II. PRIMARY DISSOCIATED NEURONAL CELL CULTURE

A. Advantages and disadvantages of primary dissociated neuronal culture

Neurotoxicology aims to predict the effects a substance will have on a neurone *in vivo* and, for this reason, effects on primary cells seem more reliable than effects on cell lines, which are essentially abnormal 'tumour cells'. Primary culture also allows tissue to be selected from areas of special interest or which contain neuronal populations with properties that make them susceptible to specific neurotoxic substances. For example, primary hippocampal neurones will respond differently from cerebellar granule cells as their receptor populations, their calcium channels, etc., at least partially, will govern their susceptibility. In addition, primary culture allows neurones to be chosen at any developmental stage from progenitor cell to fully differentiated neurone.

The main disadvantages of primary dissociated neuronal cultures are: (a) the difficulty of obtaining sufficient cells of a specific type for the investigation; (b) their finite life span *in vitro*; and (c) the problem of obtaining reproducible pure cultures without the use of mitogen inhibitors such as cytosine arabinoside, which prevent the division of glial cells. In addition, the *in vivo* phenotype changes with time in culture, even if the culture conditions provide a combination of neurotrophic factors and ECM proteins. Finally, the electrical activity of neurones is gradually reduced in culture and this results in subtle changes in phenotype. Examples of the use of primary culture systems in *in vitro* neurotoxicology are presented below; as will be seen, their use has been extensive in studies of excitotoxicity.[20]

B. CNS cell culture methods

The methodology described below has been used successfully for preparation of both rat and human brain dissociated cell cultures. Although the methods were initially developed for hippocampal cells, they have now been used for preparing cells from other brain regions.[21]

Positively charged substrates are used to precoat plastic dishes or plates, or glass coverslips, for primary neuronal culture. This may be poly-L-lysine (10 μg ml^{-1} for plastic and 1 mg ml^{-1} for glass). The culture surface is covered for 1 h with the poly-L-lysine and washed twice with phosphate-buffered saline (PBS). Recent studies conducted on glass surfaces, especially those involving long-term cultures, have employed polyethyleneimine (50% solution, 1 in 1000) in borate buffer overnight, followed by four washes with PBS.

Brains are removed from rat embryos (17 or 18 days of gestation) and placed in 60 mm Petri dishes containing cold HEPES-buffered (10 mM) Hanks' balanced saline solution (HBSS) without Ca^{2+} or Mg^{2+} and containing gentamicin sulphate (10 μg ml^{-1}). Removal of meninges and manipulation and dissection of specific brain regions is performed with a magnifying lamp or dissecting microscope. Brain tissues from the embryos are pooled (rats: 10–16 per pregnant rat) into 35 mm Petri dishes; cerebral hemispheres are cut into 1 mm^3 pieces and hippocampi are left intact. Both these tissues are transferred to 15 ml tubes containing 3–5 ml 0.2% trypsin in HBSS for 15–20 min. After digestion, the tissue is rinsed in fresh HBSS and then incubated for 5 min in 0.1% soybean trypsin inhibitor. A further wash in HBSS is followed by trituration of tissue (without bubbling) through the narrowed bore of a fire-polished pasteur pipette to achieve a monodisperse suspension of cells. Dissociation solution volumes are as follows: eight rat hippocampi, 1 ml; six to eight rat cerebral hemispheres, 1 ml; one human fetal cerebral hemisphere, 30 ml. Aliquots of the cell suspensions, 20–100 μl per 35 mm diameter Petri dish or 200–300 μl per 60 mm Petri dish, are added to culture dishes containing the following medium: Gibco MEM, sodium bicarbonate (10 mM), L-glutamine (2 mM), pyruvate (1 mM), KCl (20 mM) and 10% heat-inactivated (30 min at 56°C) fetal calf serum (FCS). This medium maintains dissociated neuronal cultures of embryonic rat hippocampus, cerebral cortex or septal area for up to 3 weeks and human fetal cerebral cortical neurones for up to 2 months. Serum encourages growth of glial cells and thus the necessary addition of cytosine arabinoside (10 μM) (used to limit glial cell growth) may eventually compromise long-term survival of neurones; serum substitute, Neurobasal with B27 supplements (Gibco), can be used to limit the growth of glial cells without use of antimitotics. Cryopreservation of fetal rat or human brain can be achieved using Gibco MEM plus 8% dimethylsulphoxide (DMSO).[21]

1. *Cerebral cortical and hippocampal neurones: studies of the basis of excitotoxicity*

Human fetal cerebral cortical and hippocampal neurones have been successfully used after cryopreservation to study the neurotoxicity of excitatory amino acids (EAAs) and calcium influx.[22,23]

Wang and Thayer[24] explored the possibility that glutamate-induced increases in intracellular Ca^{2+} concentration are: (a) sequestered by mitochondria; (b) uncouple respiration; and (c) produce metabolic acidosis. Treatment of hippocampal neurones in culture with the mitochondrial uncoupling agent carbonylcyanid-p-trifluoromethoxyphenyl-hydrazone (FCCP) has little effect on the basal intracellular free Ca^{2+} concentration ($[Ca^{2+}]_i$). However, during glutamate-induced Ca^{2+} influx, FCCP increases the amplitude of the $[Ca^{2+}]_i$ transiently, suggesting that mitochondria are an important Ca^{2+} buffer. Thus, these data are consistent with this hypothesis.

Furthermore, activation of *N*-methyl-D-aspartate (NMDA) receptors produces a Ca-dependent intracellular acidification in single hippocampal neurones, and it is possible that this is part of the toxicological process. The metabolic inhibitor 2-deoxyglucose (2DG) prevents this glutamate-induced acidification. Ba^{2+}, which carries charge through Ca^{2+}

channels, including the Ca^{2+} uniporter on the inner mitochondrial membrane, substitutes for Ca^{2+} in mediating glutamate-induced cytoplasmic acidification. Microinjection of ruthenium red, which blocks mitochondrial Ca^{2+} sequestration, reduces glutamate-induced acidification. Addition of glutamate plus FCCP synergistically elicits morphological degeneration and neuronal death, even when cytoplasmic pH remains neutral. Thus, from these various studies, it has been possible to conclude that acidification is not the cause of toxicity, although it is symptomatic of metabolic stress.[24]

2. *Cerebellar granule cells: developmental aspects of vulnerability*

Cultures established from human 14-week fetuses become increasingly sensitive to glutamate (acting at NMDA and kainate receptors) after 30 days *in vitro*. Development of glutamate-induced rises in $[Ca^{2+}]_i$ precedes sensitivity to excitotoxicity by several weeks in human neurones, whereas glutamate-induced rises in $[Ca^{2+}]_i$ and susceptibility develop more rapidly and are more closely related in rat neurones. This difference apparently exists because human neurones have a greater capacity to buffer a calcium load than rat neurones.[22,23] Thus, the ability of neurones to buffer a calcium load and vulnerability to EAAs is species specific and developmental stage specific. Human cortical neurones become sensitive to EAAs during the prenatal period, suggesting that they have a role in development as well as in neurodegenerative processes; it has been shown that glutamate regulates neurite outgrowth in developing rodent neurones.[24,25] Studies of cultured embryonic rat hippocampal neurones reveal that, for several days after differentiation, pyramidal neurones are insensitive to EAAs. The neurones then express glutamate receptors of the kainate/quisqualate type and subsequently NMDA receptors.[23] This temporal expression of different glutamate receptors, and the development of vulnerability, has been extensively corroborated.[26,27]

3. *Chick embryo neuronal cultures: use in studies of organophosphates*

Chick embryo neuronal cultures provide a convenient and economical system for studying a variety of toxicants. These cultures are resilient to treatment manipulation, and Sawyer[28] has used them to assess the cytotoxicity of diverse compounds. They are highly sensitive to agents that inhibit acetylcholinesterase (AChE), and the potencies of organophosphate neuroactive compounds and of organophosphate and carbamate insecticides as inhibitors of this enzyme *in vitro* correlate with their reported *in vivo* toxicities.

4. *Embryonic rat hippocampal, septal and cortical neurones: studies of neuroprotection by growth factors and neurotrophic factors*

Cheng *et al.*[12] demonstrated that pretreatment with tumour necrosis factor (TNF) α and β provides neuroprotection against glucose deprivation, exposure to glutamate, NMDA or α-amino-3-hydroxy-5-methyl-4-isoxazole (AMPA) in cultured embryonic rat hippocampal, septal and cortical neurones. TNFs stabilize $[Ca^{2+}]_i$, partly by increasing the expression of the calcium binding protein calbindin-D28k in hippocampal neurones, in common with neurotrophic factor 3 (NT-3), BDNF and fibroblast growth factor (FGF), but not NGF. However, NGF also reduces the calcium current induced by glucose deprivation in hippocampal neurones and alters the expression of calcium channels and calcium binding proteins in PC12 cells. Therefore, the control of $[Ca^{2+}]_i$, at least in part, mediates the neuroprotective mechanism of these neurotrophic factors.

5. *Embryonic rat cortical neurones: studies of oxidative stress and apoptosis*

Immature embryonic rat cortical neurones are reported to be susceptible to glutamate-induced neurotoxicity via a non-receptor-mediated mechanism involving cystine transport inhibition, glutathione depletion and oxidative stress.[29,30] This model of neuronal oxidative stress has been used to assess mechanisms by which free radicals induce death: it has been found that glutathione depletion leads to hypercondensation and fragmentation of chromatin, a morphological signature of apoptosis.[10] These changes, which are accompanied by DNA 'laddering', can be prevented by antioxidants and by inhibitors of macromolecular synthesis.[31] Protection by these agents is derived from shunting of the amino acid cysteine from protein synthesis into the formation of glutathione. Overall, these results suggest that oxidative stress can induce apoptosis in neurones and that protein synthesis inhibitors protect by augmenting antioxidant defences. Therefore, this system provides a useful model for studying neuronal apoptosis induced by reactive oxygen species.

6. *Dopamine- or 5-hydroxytryptamine-containing neurones cultured from mesencephalon or raphe nuclei of rat fetuses: studies on the toxicity of pharmacological agents*

Primary neuronal cultures can be used to answer specific neurotoxicological questions. For example, what is the nature of the toxic effect of metamphetamine on dopaminergic (DA) cells and of methylene dioxymetamphetamine (MDMA, 'Ecstasy') on serotonergic (5-hydroxytryptamine; 5-HT) cells? These drugs of abuse cause an acute release of the neurotransmitters *in vivo* and *in vitro*, and their use is associated with long-term monoamine depletion.[32] Although their toxic effects are well documented, the mechanism by which they destroy DA and 5-HT terminals (and subsequently neurones) is unclear. Cerruti *et al.*[33] used DA and 5-HT cells cultured from mesencephalon or raphe nuclei of rat fetuses and showed that MDMA causes dose-dependent cytototoxicity which is attenuated by the nitric oxide synthetase (NOS) inhibitors, nitro-L-arginine and L-nitro-methylarginine, which block constitutive and inducible nitric oxide formation respectively. Metamphetamine decreases the number of cells immunostained with an antibody against tyrosine hydroxylase, and also increases cells immunostained with anti-GFAP (glial fibrillary acidic protein) antibody; nitro-L-arginine and benzodiazepine attenuate these effects. Overall, the data suggest that both metamphetamine- and MDMA-induced neurotoxicity involves excessive nitric oxide formation.[33]

III. NEURONAL CELL LINES

A. Immortalized cell lines

Neuronal cell lines can be derived from any species including human and from every type of neurone including those of central origin. Perhaps the most commonly used neuronal cell lines are neuroblastomas, e.g. the mouse C-1300 subclone, from which NB41A3 is derived, and the human SKNSH (and SHSY5Y) neuroblastomas. Primary brain cells have also been fused to neuroblastoma cell lines to obtain post-mitotic cell products expressing highly differentiated neuronal phenotypes.[34] For example, the dopaminergic (DA) cell line MN9D requires 10^{-6} M MPP^+ to reduce DA by 40%, while the parent N18 neuroblastoma requires 10^{-4} M MPP^+ (in common with the rat phaeochromocytoma PC12 cells which contain dopamine). The overriding disadvantage of neuronal tumour or virally transformed cell lines is that they are capable of dividing and are therefore abnormal. This may fundamentally alter their pharmacological and neurotoxicological responses. However, their ability to proliferate (in high serum conditions) provides large numbers of a homogeneous population of cells. Characteristics and karyotypes of transformed cells will eventually change at different rates depending on the particular cell line, and thus they should be studied using stringently controlled culture conditions (e.g. avoiding glucose deprivation) and between a given and limited number of passages.

1. *Human SHSY5Y neuroblastoma cell line: studies of differential specificity to organophosphates*

Organophosphates are widely used as insecticides, lubricants and plasticizers and may cause acute toxicity and/or delayed neuropathy. The acute toxicity is (partly) due to, and concomitant with, inhibition of AChE; organophosphate-induced delayed neuropathy (OPIDN) follows inhibition of neuropathy target esterase (NTE) in humans and susceptible animal species. These enzyme markers for organophosphate toxicity are expressed in the human SKNSH (and the subclone SHSY5Y) neuroblastoma cell lines, and thus provide an opportunity to study susceptibility to the organophosphates that cause both acute toxicity and/or OPIDN. The SKNSH human neuroblastoma cell line isolated from bone marrow metastasis is a mixture of neuronal (SHSY5Y) cells and neuroepithelial cells.[35] Both the SHSKN and SHSY5Y cell lines can be induced to differentiate and grow neurites; the SHSY5Y cell line reaches a higher resting membrane potential than SKNSH[36] and forms functional synaptic contacts with appropriate target cells.[37]

When incubated for 1 h at 10^{-5} M with the SHSY5Y cell line, five of five active toxicants capable of causing OPIDN inhibit NTE: none of the active toxicants that do not cause OPIDN inhibit the esterase, although they inhibit AChE.[38] Protoxicants (before metabolic conversion) do not cause significant inhibition of either AChE or NTE. Therefore, this *in vitro* system can apparently differentiate between the two types of direct-acting organophosphates.

2. *Murine septal (SN56) lines, motor neurone (NSC19) lines and human neuroblastoma (LA-N-2) cells: use of differentiated cholinergic cells for evaluating acetylcholinesterase inhibitors*

Cell lines (e.g. SN56 and NSC19) have also been developed to identify and/or characterize compounds that cause OPIDN.[39] SN56 cells are derived from the septal nucleus and closely resemble brain cholinergic neurones. They develop neurites when treated with agents that increase intracellular cyclic AMP levels and, concomitantly, their acetylcholine (ACh) synthesis and release are enhanced. Retinoic acid causes a several-fold stimulation of ACh synthesis in these cells and this effect is additive to that of forskolin. NSC19 cells and LA-N-2 cells are similarly capable of synthesizing ACh.[39] These three cell lines have proved very useful in examining, for example, the effects of organophosphates (using diisopropyl phosphorofluoridate (DFP), a prototypical OPIDN-causing compound, and (paraoxon) an organophosphate that does not cause delayed neurotoxicity). The examination of several types of cholinergic cell line has identified cells that are particularly vulnerable to AChE inhibition, and the use of human and murine cell lines has allowed assessment of the importance for OPIDN.

3. *Human SKNSH and mouse NB41A3 neuroblastoma cell lines: inhibition of neuronal differentiation as a measure of toxicity*

Studies in human SKNSH cells have examined inhibition of neurite outgrowth (neuronal differentiation) *in vitro* as a measure of potential neurotoxicity.[40] Neurite outgrowth can be estimated indirectly using an enzyme-lined immunosorbent assay (ELISA) for neurofilament subunit proteins; L (light, 68 kD), M (medium, 160 kD) and H (heavy, 200 kD), which are major components of the neurites. Neurotoxic compounds, for instance the glutamate analogue L-β-N-methylamino-L-alanine (L-BMAA) and also acrylamide, alter levels of neurofilament proteins in culture (mouse NB41A3 neuroblastoma plus L-BMAA [Fig. 7.1a]; mouse NB41A3 neuroblastoma plus acrylamide [Fig. 7.1b]). The cultures for neurofilament ELISA are fixed in 4% paraformaldehyde and permeabilized with Triton-X100 before the addition of specific neurofilament protein subunit antibodies. As can be seen, a 65–75% relative *decrease* in the net level of neurofilament M and L subunits is present after 6 days of exposure to acrylamide (10^{-11} M; $n = 3$, $P < 0.0001$; L 75.0%, M 75.3%) or to L-BMAA (10^{-11} M; $n = 5$, $P < 0.0001$; L 65.4%, M 71.2%) compared with unexposed control cultures. The cytotoxic dose (IC_{50}) for L-BMAA is $> 10^{-4}$ M and for acrylamide 10^{-6} M, demonstrated by an MTT (3-(4,5-dimethylthiazol-2-yl)-2,5-diphenyl terazolium bromide) assay performed on unfixed parallel cultures of cells. The decrease in neurofilament protein subunits at concentrations much lower than the cytotoxic dose could be due to the occurrence of a neurotoxic 'de-differentiation', i.e. a shift towards the cell division cycle. If this occurs, it may also contribute to the eventual doubling in the cell content of neurofilament protein subunits seen at high concentrations of L-BMAA. Whether exposure to low non-cytotoxic doses of neurotoxic substances produces a shift in the growth–differentiation axis can be studied by measuring proliferating cell nuclear antigen (PCNA), a protein that is required during new DNA synthesis and which increases threefold during mitosis.[41] It can also be examined by measuring changes in incorporation of [^{3}H]thymidine or bromodeoxyuridine. Such measurements of cell proliferation will establish whether the observed changes in neurofilament proteins reflect mitosis or accumulation of aberrant neurofilament M. Similar biphasic changes in neurofilament protein subunits have been observed following 6 days' exposure to kainate.[42]

Human SKNSH neuroblastoma cells can be fully differentiated from neuronal cells plus neuroepithelial cells to neuronal cells using retinoic acid or the protein kinase C (PKC) activator phorbol ester, whereas the mouse NB41A3 neuroblastoma cell line, established by cloning the C1300 neuroblastoma cell line,[43] appears as mature neurones expressing both choline acetylase and tyrosine hydroxylase, in culture conditions optimal for differentiation. Thus, if, for example, the objective of a study is to examine whether the toxic insult prevents initiation of differentiation rather than the actual process of neurite outgrowth *per se*, then the human line that requires retinoic acid stimulation is probably the best option. The demonstration of inhibition of neurite outgrowth by neurotoxic substances, in the two cell lines, helps to establish the generality of the phenomenon and supports its use as a screening test to predict the potential of a compound to cause neurotoxic damage *in vivo*.

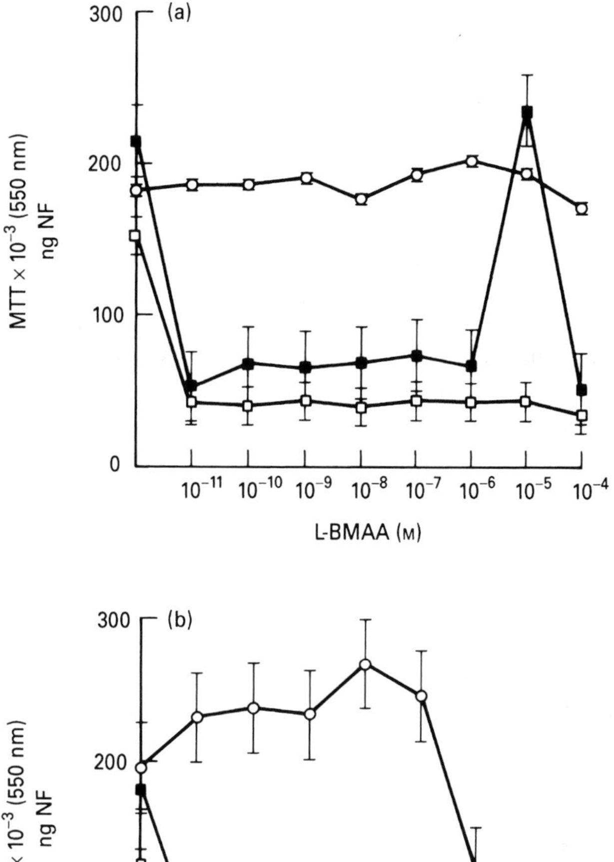

Fig. 7.1 (a) Mouse NB41A3 neuroblastoma plus L-BMAA. (b) Mouse NB41A3 neuroblastoma plus acrylamide. Neurofilament (NF) ELISAs show a 65–75% relative decrease in the net level of NF M and L subunit after 6 days of exposure to 10^{-11} M acrylamide ($n = 3$, $P < 0.0001$; NFL, 75.0% below control, NFM, 75.3% below control) or to 10^{-11} M L-BMAA ($n = 5$, $P < 0.0001$; NFL, 65.4% below the control, NFM, 71.2% below the control). Control cultures were not exposed to drugs. The IC_{50}, measured by MTT assay, was less than 10^{-4} M for L-BMAA and 10^{-6} M for acrylamide. ○, Control; □, NFL; ■, NFM.

IV. TRANSFECTED CELLS AND CELL LINES

Neuronal cells and neuronal cell lines can be transfected with a variety of genetic constructs. Using this approach it has been possible to demonstrate, for example, that DA receptor pharmacology and function is dependent on cell lineage: transfected D_4 receptors are linked to the modulation of adenylate cyclase when expressed in the N18–mesencephalic neurone hybrid MN9D cell, but not when expressed in a fibroblast cell line.[44]

In addition to studies with neuronal cells, extensive use has been made of *Xenopus* oocytes by transfection of a variety of receptors which mediate neuropharmacological and toxicological effects, e.g. studies of excitatory amino acids (EAA) $[Ca^{2+}]_i$ and the metabotropic glutamate receptors[45] and of the effects of Pb^{2+} on different ACh receptor subtypes.[46]

Prion protein biosynthesis has been studied in scrapie-infected and non-infected neuroblastoma cells.[47] These studies have revealed that the scrapie-associated form of prion, PrP^{Sc} (which is partially protease resistant, unlike normal PrP), is made from a cell-surface precursor that is both protease- and phospholipase-sensitive.[48] The normal cellular prion PrP^{c}, which is synthesized and degraded rapidly, is transported within secretory vesicles to the cell surface where it is anchored by glycosyl phosphatidylinositol. PrP^{Sc} is synthesized slowly and is post-translationally modified (by an unknown mechanism) and accumulates inside the cell.[49] However, the aetiology of prion disease remains elusive.

V. TRANSFORMED AND TRANSFECTED CELLS BASED ON DISEASE MODELS

Exposure to toxic agents in the environment may contribute to neurodegenerative diseases. With the identification of genetic mutations linked to familial forms of neurodegenerative diseases, it is possible to study the interaction between expression of a predisposing gene and exposure to specific neurotoxic chemicals, using quantifiable end-points in laboratory experiments. These *in vitro* models have been used in the risk assessment process and in the testing of candidate therapies.[50]

Various methods of introducing foreign genes into cell lines and primary neurones have been used: liposome-mediated transfection, adenoviral transduction, and culture of nervous tissue from transgenic animals. Such models have been established for two diseases in which specific mutations have been identified in several affected families: (1) familial amyotrophic lateral sclerosis (ALS) linked to mutations in the gene encoding Cu–Zn superoxide dismutase;[50] and (2) familial Alzheimer's diseases linked to mutations in the gene encoding β-amyloid precursor protein (β-APP).[51]

VI. HYBRID CELL LINE CULTURES

1. *Glioma × neuroblastoma hybrid cell (NG108-15) lines: studies of developmental toxicity*

Maternal chemical dependency may cause changes in the fetal brain that persist into adulthood. Thus, prenatal exposure to drugs such as methamphetamine may permanently modify the synaptic organization of the brain. *In utero*, methamphetamine results in a dose-related change in monoamine content and uptake sites in many regions of rat brain, 30 days postnatally. However, at high doses ($10\,\mathrm{mg\,kg^{-1}}$ $\mathrm{day^{-1}}$), there is evidence that metamphetamine is not only neurotoxic to some neuronal populations, but can also stimulate growth of axonal terminals.[52] These observations are consistent with both the known neurotoxic effects of amphetamines on monoamine function and the ability of the immature nervous system to compensate partially for fetal insult.

In vitro drug exposure in neuronally derived cell lines has been used in modelling the *in vivo* developmental changes caused by methamphetamine exposure.[52] Studies have also been done using neuronal fusion cell lines displaying a combination of neuronal and glial features. A neuroblastoma × glioma hybrid was formed by Sendai virus-induced fusion of the mouse neuroblastoma clone N18TG-2 and the rat glioma clone C6 BV-1, and therefore contains some of the characteristics of both parental cell types.[53] In separate studies treatment of rat neuroblastoma and primary neuronal cells also produced a dose-related effect on growth and differentiation patterns.

VII. CO-CULTURE

Co-culture systems are used to simulate some of the *in vivo* conditions and cues which induce neuronal differentiation. It can, however, be difficult to maintain and reproduce a culture system of two different cell types as each have different growth rates. In addition, the background 'noise' for the chosen signal, e.g. leakage of lactate dehydrogenase as a measure of cell death, is likely to be higher in such systems. Thus, co-cultures are sometimes even more difficult to standardize than complex culture systems, which contain most of the representative components of the CNS. Another problem that can arise with co-culture is that the neuronal phenotype is modulated. For example, the DA cell line MN9D suffers a marked reduction in its DA phenotype when co-aggregated with non-dopaminergic cells of the optic tectum or thalamus.[54] This response of cells to their milieu is also seen when sensory neurones are co-cultured with Chinese Hamster Ovary (CHO) cells transfected with the mouse neural cell adhesion molecule F3 (of the immunoglobulin superfamily),[55] where a marked stimulation of neurite outgrowth is observed. Given these limitations, it is also important to note that for studies of glutamate toxicity, for example, the presence of glial cells in a neuronal culture will provide a much closer measure of the *in vivo* excitotoxicity because of the presence of the glial glutamate transporter.

1. *Primary models for reactive and type-1-like astrocytes: studies of EAA toxicity*

Glutamate-induced excitotoxicity is a major cause of damage following stroke. Astrocytes are important in regulating synaptic levels of glutamate, and the processes for disposing of glutamate have been examined. Such studies have shown, for example, that a reduction in the astrocytic membrane potential can cause inhibition of glutamate uptake and non-vesicular release of the transmitter. The reduction in the astrocytic membrane potential may be due to ion channel changes (inhibition or activation) caused by alterations in different extracellular ion concentrations; an alternative explanation is that there is depletion of cellular energy.[56]

Using primary culture models for reactive and type-1-like astrocytes and a continuous glioma cell line, have shown that uptake of glutamate at a neurotoxic concentration requires the presence of excess oxygen. Thus the neurotoxic action of organic solvents and heavy metals, which inhibit respiration, may be related to reduced glutamate inactivation.

Astrocyte cultures have also been used for studying the membrane-mediated CNS-depressing effect of organic solvents.[57] By regulating the ionic balance, astrocytes maintain the proper environment for neurones and it has been shown that, in organic solvent toxicity, the activities of the membrane-bound total ATPase and Mg^{2+} ATPase are decreased after exposure to cyclohexane, *n*-hexane, 2-hexanone, 2-hexanol and 2,5-hexanedione. The inhibitory effect on ATPase is greater in cultured astrocytes than in whole-brain reaggregate cultures or in synaptosomes.

2. *Mixed cultures of spinal cord neurones and muscle cells from* Xenopus laevis *embryos: use in developmental studies*

Dissociated cell cultures of *Xenopus laevis* embryo spinal cord have been used to study the developmental temporal expression of neural ionic channels and to examine the role of microtubules in developing neurones.[58] A correlation has been found between the *in vivo* development of neurofilament subunit protein expression and these *in vitro* neurones, especially for neurofilament L and M.[58] They therefore provide a useful *in vitro* model system for studying the developmental effects of different neurotoxic agents and the mechanism of action of neurotoxic substances that affect the cytoskeleton, particularly neurofilaments.

VIII. COMPLEX PRIMARY CULTURE SYSTEMS

1. *Hippocampal slice culture: use in studies of EAA-induced toxicity*

Complex culture systems commonly contain most of the cellular components of the CNS *in vivo* and, for example, hippocampal slice culture, which retains many of its *in situ* properties such as cytoarchitecture and neural circuitry. This slice preparation has provided a valuable experimental system for studies of EAA-induced toxicity, as there is a high level of these receptors in the hippocampus. The toxicity of glutamate analogues has been extensively studied in this system, as the glial cells are present in the correct topology and their protective effects can be assessed. In addition, the system is valuable because neither the glutamate receptors nor the glutamate transporters are damaged or removed by trypsin treatment, which is routinely used in the preparation of primary neuronal cultures.

Brain slices have also been used to study the neurotoxicity of a wide range of compounds including acrylamide, trimethyl and ethyl tin, lead (Pb^{2+}) and mercury.[59]

2. Organotypic cultures: studies of neurotoxicity associated with β-amyloid protein, cytochemical changes and apoptotic cell death

It is widely accepted that β-amyloid protein may play an integral role in the pathogenesis of Alzheimer's disease.[60] Many studies have demonstrated the neurotoxicity of this protein in dissociated neuronal cultures,[61] but replicating these effects either *in vivo* or in organotypic cultures has proved difficult. Whether this is a methodological problem, or is a truly discrepant response of intact tissue to β-amyloid protein, has been examined by Allen *et al.*[62] They used a range of organotypic culturing systems to investigate cytochemical changes after β-amyloid protein exposure: immunochemical methods were used to measure levels of proteins such as the molecular chaperonin ubiquitin and the mictrotubule-associated protein tau. The results show that β-amyloid protein induces neurodegenerative changes in organotypic cultures, including apoptosis, and that the dentate gyrus (in this *in vitro* system) is particularly vulnerable.

3. Reaggregate cultures: use in the study of developmental neurotoxicity

Examination of the sensitivity of the developing CNS to therapeutic agents or to drugs of abuse requires the study of dose–effect relationships over time as well as an assessment of the ability of the CNS to recover from such exposure. These experimental requirements can be difficult to achieve in intact animals, but can be accomplished by the application of *in vitro* tissue culture systems. Reaggregate cultures, formed from all the dissociated component cells of a CNS region, form synapses and can be maintained *in vitro* for up to 1 year.[2,63,64]

Such reaggregates can be monitored for transmitter release, and serial neurochemical and morphological measurements can be made using standard methods. As an example, the developmental effects of a series of amphetamine derivatives on the central DA and serotonergic projections have been determined.[65] As in intact brain, the monoamine levels increase with developmental time in the cultures and dose-dependent reductions in monoamine levels of these developing neurones have been observed with metamphetamine, methylene dioxyamphetamine and fenfluramine. Following removal of the drug, the monoaminergic neurones in such cultures resume their normal developmental increases in transmitter level, although the initial decrements in monoamine levels produced by exposure to the drug are maintained throughout the remainder of the normal developmental period.[65]

4. Cultured spinal neurones and hippocampal brain slices: studies of calcium chelation as a neuroprotective strategy

Using cultured spinal neurones and hippocampal brain slices, Tymianski *et al.*[66] have studied the effects of calcium chelating 1,2-bis(O-aminophenoxy)ethane-N,N,N′,N′tetra acetic acid tetra-[acetoxymethyl]-ester (BAPTA) analogues on glutamate-dependent neurotoxicity, Ca^{2+} dependent currents and excitatory neurotransmission. Interestingly, the protective effects of BAPTA analogues correlate poorly with the chelator's affinity for Ca^{2+} within a wide K_D (dissociation constant) range. The *in vitro* data suggest that glutamate-dependent neurotoxicity requires high, localized Ca^{2+} increases within the cell, i.e. exceeding several μM, and that permeant Ca^{2+} chelators may attenuate excitotoxicity by both presynaptic and postsynaptic mechanisms which depend on the compound's ability rapidly to dissipate localized $[Ca^{2+}]_i$ increases from critical subplasma membrane areas.[66]

5. Micromass culture: use in teratogenicity testing and in studies of axonal transport for assessment of toxicity

The micromass culture procedure, developed and extensively characterized by Oliver Flint,[67,68] is a well-established short-term test for teratogens. The midbrain CNS cells used in this system undergo differentiation processes, which closely resemble those occurring *in vivo*. Immunochemical analysis[69] reveals the presence of differentiated neurones containing GQ ganglioside, neural cell adhesion molecule (NCAM), microtubule-associated protein 2 (MAP-2), MAP-5 (also known as MAP-1b), neurone-specific enolase (NSE) and acetylated tubulin. The system has also been used to study subteratogenic effects on brain development of, for example, retinoids, where functional rather than morphological changes are seen. Using differentiation-related expression of neurofilament and proto-oncogene *src* protein in micromass culture, dose-dependent decreases in protein expression have been demonstrated.[70,71]

Micromass culture has also been used to develop a method for measuring changes in the rate of axonal transport.[72] In these studies, individual mitochondria are rendered visible inside the neurites of a fascicle, using a fluorescent mitochondrial label, rhodamine 123. A fixed area of neurite is fluorescence bleached and the time taken for the bleached rhodamine 123 to return to normal provides a measure of transport impairment after toxic treatment. While this system is not suitable as a simple screening procedure, it has potential use in mechanistic studies of neurotoxicity, which involve impaired transport.

IX. PARAMETERS FOR ASSESSING NEUROTOXICITY *IN VITRO*

Overall strategies for assessing neurotoxicity *in vitro* have been reviewed recently.[73] The following section provides a brief overview of several of the most commonly used techniques for assessing neuronal cell health.

A. Mitochondrial function

There are various methods for assessing cell health and viability. Incubation of MTT [$1\,\mathrm{mg\,ml^{-1}}$ solution in phenol red-free Dulbecco's minimum essential medium (DMEM)] with cells for 2 h at 37°C leads to the formation of formazan by mitochondrial dehydrogenases; the resultant colour is therefore proportional to mitochondrial function.[74]

Mitochondrial function (measured by MTT), may be perturbed by adverse stimuli and is not only influenced by cell proliferation/differentiation or cell number, but is a more complex reflection of diverse energy-dependent metabolic changes and calcium buffering capacity.[75]

B. Mitochondrial potential

Rhodamine 123 ($5\,\mu\mathrm{M}$ for 10 min at 37°C) is a stain for live cells and detects a mitochondrial potential that is not present in dead cells.[21]

C. Pinocytosis and transcellular traffic of solutes

Neutral red dye is taken up by pinocytic vesicles and lysosomes of the cell during the normal transcellular traffic of solutes. When the cells are compromised, transcellular traffic is slower and the dye is less intense. Dead cells do not take up the dye.[76]

D. Plasma membrane integrity

Trypan blue (0.4%) is excluded from healthy cells. After 5–10 min incubation cells are washed with saline solution and visualized microscopically; dead cells appear blue, live cells are bright with no colour.

E. Cellular oxidation

Several methods measure levels of oxygen free radicals in living cells; oxidation-sensitive compounds are converted to a fluorescent product by peroxides. For example, 2,7-dichlorofluorescin diacetate (DCF) (50 μM) is incubated for 50 min at 37°C and converted to 2,7-dichlorofluorescein.[21]

F. Cellular ATP levels

Decrease in cellular ATP levels can be conveniently assessed using the decrease in light absorbance at 340 nm. The effect is due to decreases in NADH concentration and is based on the fact that 3-phosphoglycerate is converted to 1,3-diphosphoglycerate by phosphoglycerate phosphokinase, and conversion of this with NADH to glyceraldehyde-3-phosphate plus NAD plus phosphate by glyceraldehyde phosphate dehydrogenase.

G. Assessment of change along the growth–differentiation axis

Several proteins that indicate the degree of differentiation of neurones can be assessed by ELISAs; some of these are described briefly below.

1. Cytoskeletal components

Cytoskeletal proteins that increase with neurite outgrowth include neurofilament protein subunits L (light, 68 kD), M (medium, 160 kD) and H (heavy, 200 kD); tubulin;[77] tau;[78] and MAP-2.[79]

2. *Synaptogenesis*

Growth associated protein (GAP)-43, synaptophysin and phosphotyrosine phosphatase[80] are among the proteins specifically increased during synaptogenesis; they can be measured by ELISA.

3. *Nitric oxide synthetase and nitric oxide*

The level of nitric oxide synthetase inducible (iNOS) increases during NGF-induced differentiation of PC12 neurones[81] and possibly also during NO-mediated, activity dependent synaptic suppression at developing synapses.[82] Various different NOS isoenzymes have been isolated and the tissue in which they were first described has conferred three separate names: endothelial eNOS, macrophage mNOS or neuronal nNOS.[83] The nomenclature is unfortunate because all three types can be found in neurones. There is increasing evidence that some toxic effects on neurones are manifest as de-differentiation or as a re-entry into the cell cycle. In some cells, this is abortive, particularly in terminally differentiated neurones when growth-associated genes have been downregulated: the end result is apoptosis.[84] Measures of cell proliferative capacity such as PCNA, the level of which increases threefold during division, can therefore be used, particularly in studies of neuroblastoma cells.[41] PCNA can also be used in fluorescence-activated cell sorting (FACS) analysis, which is more informative than the ELISA method as the exact proportion of cells expressing PCNA can be measured. Other measures of cell division that are widely used are [^{3}H]thymidine uptake[85] or bromodeoxyuridine uptake.[86]

H. Assessment of intracellular free calcium

The use of *in vitro* systems for the investigation of calcium homoeostasis and calcium-induced cell damage has been recently reviewed.[87] Calcium indicator dyes, Fura-2 and Indo-1, can be used to assess changes in intracellular free calcium levels during and following a neurotoxic insult. Fluo-3 can be used in combination with carboxyseminapthorhodofluor-1 (SNARF-1), which assesses intracellular pH fluctuation to obtain a $[Ca^{2+}]_i$ pH ratio.[21]

I. Assessing intracellular pH change

As mentioned above, the fluorescent indicator SNARF can be used to assess intracellular pH change. An efficient (though costly) alternative is the 'microphysiometer', a pH electrode which detects minute changes in intracellular pH. Intracellular pH is known to change in response to a wide range of extracellularly mediated signal transduction events. The microphysiometer has to date been exploited most effectively for the study of the binding to tissues or receptors of neuroactive and neurotoxic agents.[88]

J. Proto-oncogenes and transcription factors

Cellular stress causes alterations in gene expression; within 1 h of the stress event (exposure to 42°C or 33°C, heat shock; redox stress; high concentrations of oxygen free radicals or low levels of oxygen) the 'immediate early genes' (IEGs) are switched on. These include c-*fos* and c-*jun*, and are rapidly increased in response to a diverse array of adverse stimuli. The protein products of these genes are transcription factors which form homodimers or heterodimers and thus activate a range of other proteins.[89] Because the induction of these IEGs occurs in response to physiological change, and to many different minor insults, their use as predictors of toxicity may be limited.

Xenometrix (Colorado, USA) is currently developing various *in vitro* neurotoxicity methods (S. E. Beard, personal communication). For example, the human NT2 teratoma cell line (Layton Biosciences[90]) is terminally differentiated by retinoic acid (and expresses glutamate receptors) and is used in the CAT-Tox(N) ELISA assays. These are based on the use of chloramphenicol acetyltransferase (CAT) reporter gene fused to various different promoters or response elements for genes which are transcriptionally activated by DNA damage, oxidative stress, protein damage, heavy metal toxicity, apoptosis and neurotransmitter signals. These include heat shock protein (hsp 72), c-*fos*, iNOS, gadd153, DNA polymerase β, quinone reductase, NT-3 and proencephalon, and also the response elements NfkB, p53 and the cyclic AMP response element.

There are some genes, such as *NfkB*, which are increased by oxidative stress; it is not known whether the accompanying activation of the protein itself leads to the increase in the *NFkB* gene expression or whether the gene is separately activated. NFkB is a member of a family of proteins including RelA, RelB and RelC. The Rel–NFkB proteins are usually kept inactive in the cytosol by IkB. Activation can be triggered in response to various toxic stimuli (including inflammatory mediators interleukin-1 (IL-1), TNF, the phorbol myristate ester (PMA) which activates PKC, ultraviolet light, viruses, redox stress, ceramide, okadaic acid and pervanadate). When activation occurs, DNA binding regions are exposed on the Rel–NfkB dimers, which are translocated from the cytosol to the nucleus, where they act as transcription factor for various other 'defence' genes (adhesion molecules, cytokines, immunoreceptors, acute phase proteins and NOS).[91]

K. Stress response genes

The chaperonins (e.g. hsp90,[92] hsp72[93] and hsp27[94]) are induced during the stress response. They can be detected with antibodies in ELISA methods.

L. Ubiquitin

Ubiquitin, a chaperonin (and a heat shock protein), is required to degrade protein inside the cell[95] and is increased in response to many types of neurotoxic insult, including ischaemia.[96] The lesions found in several neurodegenerative diseases, including amyotrophic lateral sclerosis[97] and Alzheimer's disease,[98] have ubiquitin associated with them. Antibody to ubiquitin can thus be used to detect neurotoxic damage in neurones.

M. Measures of apoptosis

Necrotic cell death is characterized by inflammation accompanied by release of chemotactic and inflammatory mediators (e.g. IL-1 and TNF), and leads to polymorphonuclear cell recruitment into the area. Apoptotic cell death of neurones is an integral part of the development of the CNS, where it is hypothesized that limited supplies of neurotrophic factors allow the survival of only a fraction of the total neurones. Neurones that do not receive adequate neurotrophic factors shrink; the cell nucleus is degraded by endonucleases and proteases causing DNA 'laddering' (i.e. the DNA is cleaved into fragments that homogeneously span the molecular weight range and separate as a ladder on polyacrylamide gel electrophoresis). Apoptosing neurones are characteristically difficult to identify by normal light microscopy but there are several alternative means of assessment; translation of uridine end-labelling (TUNEL) measures DNA fragmentation. Proteins that characterize and distinguish apoptosing cells (from necrosing cells), and which can be measured by ELISA, include Fas/Apo-1,[99] IL-1β converting enzyme (ICE)[100] and p53.[101] Annexin V (part of the lipocortin, calpactin family of proteins) can be used to detect phosphatidylserine released from apoptosing cells whose membrane integrity is not yet disrupted; the appearance of phosphatidylserine on the extracellular surface of the cell membrane indicates a change concomitant with apoptosis.[102] The bcl-2 protein is implicated in the prevention of cell death and resides in the inner mitochondrial membrane. Bak and bax are part of the bcl-2 family of proteins which, when expressed in a sufficiently high level in the cell, will counteract the effect of bcl-2 and cause apoptosis. Measurement of the ratio and hetero- and homodimerisation of bcl-2 : bax provides an indication of the likelihood of apoptosis.[103]

N. Receptor binding and neurotransmitter release

Brain slice preparations and astrocytes have been used to study γ-aminobutyric acid (GABA) A and B receptor binding, antagonist and neurotoxic agent effects, benzodiazepine and glutamate analogue effects, and neurotransmitter release, e.g. noradrenaline.

Table 7.1 lists many of the parameters that have been discussed for neurotoxicity assessment *in vitro*.

X. CONCLUSIONS

Within the last 25 years there has been a parallel synergistic advance of technology and knowledge which has facilitated our ability to manipulate cells and organs *ex vivo*. However, the creation of *in vitro* systems that reproduce *in vivo* conditions remains an ambitious undertaking, particularly for studies of the CNS. In addition to the task of accruing sufficient knowledge of the factors, substrates and conditions to optimize systems, there are complications that arise from exposing the tissues and cells to the environment outside the whole organism. For such reasons, the role of *in vitro* studies in neuropharmacology and neurotoxicology is always likely to remain an adjunct to *in vivo* studies. However, once *in vitro* observations have been supported by *in vivo* data, there is immense scope for studies of, for example, the effects of endogenous components of the nervous system, including growth and/or neurotrophic factors, and also of differentiation cues such as NCAMs and N-cadherin, and myelin-associated neurite inhibitory molecules [antibody to inhibitor neutralizing (IN-1) has recently been shown to enhance spinal neurone regeneration in adult rats[104]].

Table 7.1 *In vitro* neurotoxicity assessment.

Cellular system	Assay	Parameter
Neuronal culture	MTT Alamar blue, rhodamine 123, JC-1 Propidium iodide	Mitochondrial function Mitochondrial potential Dead cells, DNA stain
Neuronal culture	2,7-Dichlorofluorescin diacetate → 2,7-dichlorofluoresein	Cellular oxidation (indicates intracellular level of reactive oxygen species)
Neuronal culture	3-Phosphoglycerate → 1,3-diphosphoglycerate NADH → glyceraldehyde-3-phosphate + NAD + P	Cellular ATP levels
Neuronal culture	Fura-2, Indo-1 Fluo-3 Fluo-3/SNARF Microphysiometer or SNARF	Calcium indicator dyes (CID) Signal tranduction studies CID/pH-organelle localization of $[Ca^{2+}]_i$, longer-term studies Intracellular pH change
Neuronal, neuronal–glial and reaggregate cultures	Neurofilament and PCNA, MAP-2, tau, spectrin, tubulin, phosphotyrosine phosphatase, GAP-43, synaptophysin, nitric oxide synthetase	ELISAs: differentiation or mitosis, degeneration, development, synaptogenesis and plasticity, growth arrest preceding neurite outgrowth
Brain slices	$GABA_A$, $GABA_B$, GluRs	Receptor binding
Astrocytes	Benzodiazepine	Chloride ion uptake
Brain slices	Neurotransmitter	Release (noradrenaline), uptake
Neuronal culture	*c-fos*/*c-jun* mRNA NFkB hsp90, hsp72, hsp27 bcl-2/bak(x) ratio, Apo-1, p53	Proto-oncogenes Transcription factor Stress response Apoptosis/differentiation

Characterization of the *in vitro* system is perhaps both the most onorous and the most essential part of the reductionist approach. How long can the cultured cells retain their *in vivo* phenotype? Which of their *in vivo* properties cannot be consistently retained, and which of those that are lost can be manipulated and re-induced by co-culture and/or the addition of extrinsic or intrinsic factors? How abnormal is a tumour cell or transformed cell line, and how relevant are the results obtained from these mutants? This makes the development of organotypic, complex and single cell culture systems protracted, expensive and, sometimes, frustrating. Thus, although this difficult and reiterative process, which is part of the *in vitro*:*in vivo* investigation paradigm, will continue to be central to the advance of neurobiology, attempts should be made to remove the common misconception that *in vitro* experimental systems provide inexpensive, simple alternatives to *in vivo* (neuro)toxicological assessment.

REFERENCES

1. Lin, C. H. and Forscher, P. (1993) Cytoskeletal remodelling during growth cone-target interactions. *J. Cell Biol.* **121:** 1369–1383.
2. Atterwill, C. K. (1987) Brain reaggregate cultures in neurotoxicological investigations. In Atterwill, C. K. and Steele, C. E. (eds) In Vitro *Methods in Toxicology*, pp. 133–164. Cambridge University Press, Cambridge.
3. Ferrari, G. and Greene, L. A. (1994) Proliferation inhibition by dominant-negative Ras rescues naive and neuronally differentiated PC12 cells from apoptotic cell death. *EMBO J.* **13:** 5922–5928.
4. Azmitia, E. C. and Liao, B. (1994) Dexamethasone reverses adrenalectomy-induced neuronal de-differentiation in midbrain raphe–hippocampus axis. *Ann. N.Y. Acad. Sci.* **746:** 180–193.
5. Walsh, F. and Doherty, P. (1991) Glycosylphosphatidyl inositol anchored recognition molecules that function in axonal fasciculation: growth and guidance in the nervous system. *Cell Biol. Int. Rep.* **15:** 1151–1166.
6. Bixby, J. L. and Jhabvala, P. (1990) Extracellular matrix molecules and cell adhesion molecules induce neurites through different mechanisms. *J. Cell Biol.* **111:** 2725–2732.
7. Luo, Y., Raible, D. and Raper, J. A. (1993) Collapsin: a protein in brain that induces the collapse and paralysis of neuronal growth cones. *Cell* **75:** 217–227.
8. Noakes, P. G., Gautam, M., Mudd, J., Sanes, J. R. and Merlie, J. P. (1996) Aberrant differentiation of neuromuscular junctions in mice lacking s-laminin/laminin $\beta 2$. *Nature* **374:** 258–262.
9. Sato, N., Hotta, K., Waguri, S. *et al.* (1994) Neuronal differentiation of PC12 cells as a result of prevention of cell death by bcl-2. *J. Neurobiol.* **25:** 1227–1234.
10. Ratan, R. R., Murphy, T. H. and Baraban, J. M. (1994) Oxidative stress induces apoptosis in embryonic cortical neurons. *J. Neurochem.* **62:** 376–379.
11. Louis, J.-C., Burnham, P. and Varon, S. (1993) Neurite outgrowth from cultured CNS neurons is promoted by inhibitors of protein and RNA synthesis. *J. Neurobiol.* **25:** 209–217.
12. Cheng, B., Christakos, S. and Mattson, M. P. (1994) Tumor necrosis factors protect neurons against metabolic–excitotoxic insults and promotes maintenance of calcium homeostasis. *Neuron* **12:** 139–153.
13. Götz, R., Köster, R., Winkler, C., Raulf, F., Lottspeich, F., Schartl, M. and Thoenen, H. (1995) Neurotrophin-6 is a new member of the nerve growth factor family. *Nature* **372:** 266–269.
14. Beck, K. D., Valverde, J., Alexi, T. *et al.* (1995) Mesencephalic dopaminergic neurons protected by GDNF from axotomy-induced degeneration in the adult brain. *Nature* **373:** 339–341.
15. Yan, Q., Matheson, C. and Lopez, O. T. (1995) *In vivo* neurotrophic effects of GDNF on neonatal and adult facial motor neurons. *Nature* **373:** 341–344.
16. Oppenheim, R. W., Houenou, L. J., Johnson, J. E. *et al.* (1995) Developing motor neurons rescued from programmed and axotomy-induced cell death by GDNF. *Nature* **373:** 344–347.
17. Tomac, A., Lindqvist, E., Lin, L.-F. H. *et al.* (1995) Protection and repair of the nigrostriatal dopaminergic system by GDNF *in vivo*. *Nature* **373:** 335–339.
18. Peterson, E. R. and Crain, S. M. (1982) Nerve growth factor attenuates neurotoxic effects of taxol on spinal cord–ganglion explants from fetal mice. *Science* **217:** 377–379.
19. Apfel, S. C., Lipton, R. B., Arrezzo, J. C. and Kessler, J. A. (1991) Nerve growth factor prevents toxic neuropathy in mice. *Ann. Neurol.* **29:** 87–90.
20. Hartley, D. M., Kurth, M. C., Bjerkness, L., Weiss, J. H. and Choi, D. W. (1993) Glutamate receptor-induced $^{45}Ca^{2+}$ accumulation in cortical cell culture correlates with subsequent neuronal degeneration. *J. Neurosci.* **13:** 1993–2000.
21. Mattson, M. P., Barger, S. W., Begley, J. G. and Mark, R. J. (1995) Calcium, free radical and excitotoxic neuronal death in primary cell culture. *Methods Cell Biol.* **46:** 187–216.
22. Mattson, M. P., Rychlik, B., You, J.-S. and Sisken, J. E. (1991) Sensitivity of cultured embryonic cerebral cortical neurons to excitatory amino acid-induced calcium influx and neurotoxicity. *Brain Res.* **542:** 97–106.
23. Mattson, M. P., Lee, R. E., Adama, M. E., Guthrie, P. B. and Kater, S. B. (1988) Interactions between entorhinal axons and target hippocampal neurons: a role for glutamate in the development of hippocampal circuitry. *Neuron* **1:** 865–876.

24. Wang, G. J. and Thayer, S. A. (1994) Glutamate-induced intracellular acidification of hippocampal neurons demonstrates altered energy metabolism resulting from Ca^{2+} loads. *J. Neurophysiol.* (in press).
25. Balazs, R., Hack, N. and Jorgensen, O. S. (1988) Stimulation of the *n*-methyl-D-aspartate receptor has a tropic effect on differentiating cerebellar granule cells. *Neurosci. Lett.* **87:** 80–86.
26. Hamon, B. and Heinemann, U. (1988) Developmental changes in neuronal sensitivity to excitatory amino acids in area CA1 of the rat hippocampus. *Dev. Brain Res.* **38:** 286–290.
27. Repressa, A., Tremblay, E. and Ben-Ari, Y. (1989) Transient increase of NMDA-binding sites in human hippocampus during development. *Neurosci. Lett.* **99:** 61–66.
28. Sawyer, T. (1995) Practical applications of neuronal tissue culture in *in vitro* toxicology. *Clin. Exp. Pharmacol. Physiol.* **22:** 295–296.
29. Ratan, R. R., Murphy, T. H. and Baraban, J. M. (1990) Immature cortical neurons are uniquely sensitive to glutamate toxicity by inhibition of cystine uptake. *FASEB J.* **4:** 1624–1633.
30. Murphy, T. H., Schnaar, R. L. and Cole, J. T. (1990) Immature cortical neurons are uniquely sensitive to glutamate toxicity by inhibition of glutamate uptake. *FASEB J.* **4:** 1624–1633.
31. Ratan, R. R., Murphy, T. H. and Baraban, J. M. (1994) Macromolecular synthesis inhibitors prevent oxidative stress-induced apoptosis in embryonic cortical neurons by shunting cysteine from protein synthesis to glutathione. *J. Neurosci.* **14:** 4385–4392.
32. Brodkin, J., Malyala, A. and Nash, J. F. (1993) Effect of monoamine depletion on 3,4-methylenedioxymethamphetamine-induced neurotoxicity. *Pharmacol. Biochem. Behav.* **45:** 647–653.
33. Cerruti, C., Sheng, P., Epstein, C. J. and Cadet, J.-L. (1995) Involvement of oxidative and L-arginine-NO pathways in the neurotoxicity of drugs of abuse *in vitro*. *Clin. Exp. Pharmacol. Physiol.* **22:** 381–382.
34. Wainer, B. H. and Heller, A. (1992) Neuronal cell line: Generation, characterization and utility. In Wood, J. N. (ed.) *Cell Lines in Neurobiology*, pp. 1–26. Oxford University Press, New York.
35. Abemayor, E. and Sidell, N. (1989) Human neuroblastoma cell lines as models for the *in vitro* study of neoplastic and neuronal cell differentiation. *Environ. Health Perspect.* **80:** 3–15.
36. Pålman, S., Mamaeva, S., Meyerson, G. *et al.* (1990) Human neuroblastoma cells in culture: a model for neuronal cell differentiation and function. *Acta Physiol. Scand. Suppl.* **140:** 25–37.
37. Adem, A., Mattson, M. E. K., Norberg, A. and Pålman, S. (1987) Muscarinic receptors in human SK-SY5Y neuroblastoma cell line: regulation by phorbol ester and retinoic acid-induced differentiation. *Dev. Brain Res.* **33:** 235–242.
38. Ehrich, M. and Veronesi, B. (1995) Esterase comparison in neuroblastoma cells of human and rodent origin. *Clin. Exp. Pharmacol. Physiol.* **22:** 385–386.
39. Blusztajn, J. K. and Davis, R. O. (1995) Use of differentiated cholinergic and second messenger endpoints to evaluate cholinesterase inhibitors. *Clin. Exp. Pharmacol. Physiol.* **22:** 368–369.
40. Abdulla, E. M., Calaminici, M.-R. and Campbell, I. C. (1995) Comparison of neurite outgrowth with neurofilament protein subunit levels in neuroblastoma cells following mercuric chloride exposure. *Clin. Exp. Pharmacol. Physiol* **22:** 362–363.
41. Suzuki, I., Daidoji, H., Matsuoka, M. *et al.* (1989) Gene for proliferating cell nuclear antigen (DNA polymerase delta auxillary protein) is present in both mammalian and higher plant genomes. *Proc. Natl Acad. Sci. U.S.A.* **86:** 3189–3193.
42. Abdulla, E. M. and Campbell, I. C. (1993) L-BMAA and kainate-induced modulation of neurofilament concentrations as a measure of neurite outgrowth: implications for an *in vitro* test of neurotoxicity. *Toxicol. In Vitro* **7:** 341–344.
43. Augusti-Tocco, G. and Sato, G. (1969) Establishment of functional clonal cell lines of neurons from mouse neuroblastoma. *Proc. Natl Acad. Sci. U.S.A.* **64:** 311–315.
44. Tang, L., Todd, R. L., Heller, A. and O'Malley, K. L. (1994) Pharmacological and functional characterization of D_2, D_3 and D_4 dopamine receptors in fibroblast and dopaminergic cell lines. *J. Pharmacol. Exp. Ther.* **268:** 495–502.
45. Pin, J. P., Waeber, C., Prezeau, L. *et al.* (1992) Alternative splicing generates metabotropic glutamate receptors inducing different patterns of calcium release in *Xenopus* oocytes. *Proc. Natl Acad. Sci. U.S.A.* **89:** 10 331–10 335.
46. Oortgiesen, M., Zwaart, R., van Kleef, R. G. D. M and Vijverberg, H. P. M. (1995) Subunit-dependent action of lead on neuronal nicotinic acetylcholine receptors expressed in *Xenopus* oocytes. *Clin. Exp. Pharmacol. Physiol.* **22:** 364–365.
47. Caughey, B., Race, R. E., Ernst, D. *et al.* (1989) Prion protein biosynthesis in scrapie-infected and uninfected neuroblastoma cells. *J. Virol.* **63:** 175–181.

48. Caughey, B. and Raymond, G. J. (1991) The scrapie-associated form of PrP is made from a cell surface precursor that is both protease and phospholipase-sensitive. *J. Biol. Chem.* **266:** 18 217–18 223.
49. Prusiner, S. B. and DeArmond, S. J. (1994) Prion disease and neurodegeneration. *Ann. Rev. Neurosci.* **17:** 311–339.
50. Durham, H. D., O'Brien, C., Nalbantoglu, J. and Figlewicz, D. A. (1995) Introduction of mutant genes associated with neurodegenerative disease into primary cultured neurones and cell lines to study environmental–genetic interactions. *Clin. Exp. Pharmacol. Physiol.* **22:** 366–367.
51. Chartier-Harlin, M. C. (1991) Segregation of a missense mutation in the amyloid precursor protein gene with familial Alzheimer's disease. *Nature* **353:** 704.
52. Weissman, A. D. and Caldecott-Hazard, S. (1995) Developmental neurotoxicity to metamphetamines. *Clin. Exp. Pharmacol. Physiol.* **22:** 372–374.
53. Hamprecht, B. (1977) Structural, electrophysiological, biochemical and pharmacological properties of neuroblastoma–glioma cell hybrids in culture. *Int. Rev. Cytol.* **49:** 99–170.
54. Choi, H. K., Won, L., Roback, J. D., Wainer, B. H. and Heller, A. (1992 Specific modulation of dopamine expression in neuronal hybrid cells by primary cells from different brain regions. *Proc. Natl Acad. Sci. U.S.A.* **89:** 8943–8947.
55. Gennarini, G., Durbec, P., Boned, A., Rougon, G. and Goridis, C. (1991) Transfected F3/F11 neuronal cell surface protein mediates intercellular adhesion and promotes neurite outgrowth. *Neuron* **6:** 595–606.
56. Walum, E., Eriksson, G., Peterson, A., Holme, E., Larsson, N. G., Eriksson, C. and El-Shamy, W. (1995) Use of primary cultures and continuous cell lines to study effects on astrocytic regulatory functions. *Clin. Exp. Pharmacol. Physiol.* **22:** 284–287.
57. Vaalavirta, L. and Tahti, H. (1995) Effects of selected organic solvents on the astrocyte membrane ATPase *in vitro*. *Clin. Exp. Pharmacol. Physiol.* **22:** 293–294.
58. Weichun, L. and Szaro, B. G. (1994) Maturation of neurites in mixed cultures of spinal cord neurons and muscle cells from *Xenopus laevis* embryos followed with antibodies to neurofilament proteins. *J. Neurobiol.* **25:** 1235–1248.
59. Tyler, T. J. and Fountain, S. B. (1995) Brain slice techniques. In Chang, L. W. and Slikker, W. M. Jr. (eds) *Neurotoxicology: Approaches and Methods*, pp. 517–536. Academic Press, New York.
60. Wisniewski, H. M., Iqbal, K., Baucher, C., Miller, D. and Currie, J. (1989) Cytoskeletal pathology and formation of beta amyloid fibres in Alzheimer's disease. *Neurobiol. Aging* **10:** 409–412.
61. Rabizadeh, S., Bitler, C. M., Butcher, L. L. and Bredescer, D. E. (1994) Expression of the low affinity NGF receptor enhances beta amyloid peptide toxicity. *Proc. Natl Acad. Sci.* **91:** 10 703–10 706.
62. Allen, Y. S., Devanathan, P. H. and Owen, G. P. (1995) Neurotoxicity of beta-amyloid protein: cytochemical changes and apoptotic cell death investigated in organotypic cultures. *Clin. Exp. Pharmacol. Phsyiol.* **22:** 370–371.
63. Atterwill, C. K., Johnson, H. and Thomas, S. M. (1992) Models for the *in vitro* assessment of neurotoxicity in the nervous system in relation to xenobiotic and neurotrophic factor-mediated events. *Neurotoxicology* **13:** 39–54.
64. Heller, A., Won, L., Choi, H., Heller, B. and Hoffman, P. C. (1993) Reaggregate cultures. In Tyson, C. A. and Frazier, J. M. (eds) In Vitro *Biological Systems: Preparation and Maintenance, Methods in Toxicology*, Vol. 1, pp. 27–45. Academic Press, New York.
65. Heller, A., Won, L., Heller, B. and Hoffman, P. C. (1995) Examination of developmental neurotoxicity by the use of tissue culture model systems. *Clin. Exp. Pharmacol. Physiol.* **22:** 375–378.
66. Tymianski, M., Charlton, M. P., Carlen, P. L. and Tato, C. H. (1994) Properties of neuroprotective cell-permeant Ca^{2+} chelators: effects on $[Ca^{2+}]_i$ and glutamate neurotoxicity *in vitro*. *J. Neurophysiol.* **267:** 1973–1992.
67. Flint, O. P. (1983) A micromass culture method for rat embryonic neural cells. *J. Cell Sci.* **61:** 247–262.
68. Flint, O. P. (1987) An *in vitro* test for teratogens using cultures of rat embryo cells. In Atterwill, C. K. and Steele, C. E. (eds) In Vitro *Methods in Toxicology*, pp. 339–363. Cambridge University Press, Cambridge.
69. Whittaker, S. G., Wroble, J. T., Silbernagel, S. M. and Faustman, E. M. (1993) Characterization of differentiation-specific and cytoskeletal markers in micromass cultures of embryonic rat midbrain cells. *Cell Biol. Toxicol.* **9:** 359–375.

70. Sweeney, C. and Faustman, E. M. (1990) Differentiation-related expression of proto-oncogene *src* in CNS micromass cultures: effects of chemical exposure. *Toxicology* **1:** 28–35.
71. Sweeney, C. and Faustman, E. M. (1990) Expression of differentiated characteristics in rodent embryo central nervous system cell cultures: effect of teratogen exposure. *Teratology* **3:** 484–490.
72. Chute, S. K., Flint, O. P. and Durham, S. K. (1995) An analysis of the steady-state dynamics of organelle motion in cultured neurites: putative indicator of neurotoxic effect. *Clin. Exp. Pharmacol. Physiol.* **22:** 360–361.
73. Campbell, I. C. and Abdulla, E. M. (1995) Strategic approaches to *in vitro* neurotoxicology. In Chang, L. W. and Slikker, W. M. Jr. (eds) *Neurotoxicology: Approaches and Methods*, pp. 495–504. Academic Press, New York.
74. Denizot, F. and Lang, R. (1986) Rapid colorimetric assay for cell growth and survival. Modification of the tetrazolium dye procedure giving improved sensitivity and reliability. *J. Immunol. Methods* **89:** 271–277.
75. Kiedrowski, L. and Costa, E. (1995) Glutamate-induced destabilization of intracellular calcium concentration homeostasis in cultured cerebellar granule cells: role of mitochondria in calcium buffering. *Mol. Pharmacol.* **47:** 140–147.
76. Babich, H. and Borenfreund, E. (1990) Applications of the neutral red cytotoxicity assay to toxicology. *ATLA* **18:** 129–144.
77. Hoffman, P. N. (1988) Distinct roles of neurofilament and tubulin gene expression in axonal growth. *Ciba Found. Symp.* **138:** 192–204.
78. Viereck, C., Tucker, R. P. and Matus, A. (1989) The adult rat olfactory system expresses microtubule associated proteins found in developing brain. *J. Neurosci.* **9:** 3547–3557.
79. Caceres, A., Banker, G. A. and Binder, L. (1986) Immunocytochemical localization of tubulin and MAP2 during the development of hippocampal neurons in culture. *J. Neurosci.* **6:** 712–714.
80. Sahin, M., Dowling, J. J. and Hockfield, S. (1995) Seven protein tyrosine phosphatases are differentially expressed in the developing rat brain. *J. Comp. Neurol.* **351:** 617–631.
81. Peunova, N. and Enikolopov, G. (1995) Nitric oxide triggers the switch to growth arrest during differentiation of neuronal cells. *Nature* **375:** 68–73.
82. Wang, T., Xie, Z. and Lu, B. (1995) Nitric oxide mediates activity dependent synaptic suppression at developing synapses. *Nature* **374:** 262–266.
83. Griffiths, O. W. and Stuehr, D. J. (1995) Nitric oxide synthases: properties and catalytic mechanism. *Ann. Rev. Physiol.* **57:** 707–736.
84. Pandey, S. and Wang, E. (1995) Cells *en route* to apoptosis are characterised by the up-regulation of c-fos, c-myc, c-jun, cdc2 and RB phosphorylation, resembling events of early cell cycle traverse. *J. Cell. Biochem.* **58:** 135–150.
85. Valverde, F., Lopez-Mascaraque, L., Santacana, M. and De Carlos, J. A. (1995) Persistence of early-generated neurons in the rodent subplate: assessment of cell death in neocortex during the early postnatal period. *J. Neurosci.* **15:** 5014–5024.
86. Memberg, S. P. and Hall, A. K. (1995) Dividing neuron precursors express neuron specific tubulin. *J. Neurobiol.* **27:** 26–43.
87. Campbell, I. C. and Abdulla, E. M. (1995) *In vitro* systems for the investigation of calcium homeostasis and calcium-induced cell damage. In Chang, L. W. and Slikker, W. M. Jr. (eds) *Neurotoxicology: Approaches and Methods*, pp. 595–602. Academic Press, New York.
88. Baxter, G. T., Young, M. C., Miller, D. L. and Owicki, J. C. (1994) Using the microphysiometer to study the pharmacology of exogenously expressed m_1 and m_3 muscarinic receptors. *Life Sci.* **55:** 573–583.
89. Andersson, G., Pahlman, S., Parrow, V., Johansson, I. and Haammerling, U. (1994) Activation of the human NPY gene during neuroblastoma cell differentiation – induced transcriptional activities of AP-1 and AP-2. *Cell Growth Differ.* **5:** 27–36.
90. Younkin, D. P., Tang, C.-M., Hardy, M. *et al.* (1993) Inducible expression of neuronal glutamate receptor channels in the human NT2 human cell line. *Neurobiology* **90:** 2174–2178.
91. Seibenlist, U., Franzoso, G. and Brown, K. (1994) Structure, regulation and function of NF-kB. *Ann. Rev. Cell Biol.* **10:** 405–455.
92. Satoh, K., Wakui, H., Komatsuda, A. *et al.* (1994) Induction and altered localization of 90kD heat shock protein in rat kidneys with cisplatin-induced acute renal failure. *Ren. Fail.* **16:** 313–323.
93. Geddes, J. W., Schwab, C., Craddock, S., Wilson, J. L. and Pettigrew, L. C. (1994) Alterations in tau immunostaining in the rat hippocampus following transient cerebral ischaemia. *J. Cereb. Blood Flow Metab.* **14:** 554–564.

94. Ungar, D. R., Hailat, N., Strahler, J. R. *et al.* (1994) Hsp27 expression in neuroblastoma: correlation with disease stage. *J. Natl Cancer Inst.* **86:** 780–784.
95. Jennissen, H. P. (1995) Ubiquitin and the enigma of intracellular protein degradation. *Eur. J. Biochem.* **231:** 1–30.
96. Vidal, A., Blanco, R. and Ferrer, I. (1994) Ubiquinated structures in the white matter of the gerbil following chronic cerebral hyberfusion. *Neuroreport* **5:** 2606–2608.
97. Garofolo, O., Kennedy, P. G. E., Swash, M. *et al.* (1991) Ubiquitin and heat shock protein expression in amyotrophic lateral sclerosis. *Neuropathol. Appl. Neurobiol.* **17:** 39–45.
98. Cruz-Sanchez, F. F. (1994) Antigenic determinant properties of neurofibrillary tangles: relevance to progressive supra nuclear palsy. *J. Neural Transm. Suppl.* **42:** 165–178.
99. Schulze-Ostoff, K., Krammer, P. H. and Droge, W. (1994) Divergent signalling via Apo-1, Fas and the TNF receptor, two homologous molecules involved in cell death. *EMBO J.* **13:** 4587–4596.
100. Wilson, K. P., Black, J. A., Thomson, J. A. *et al.* (1994) Structure and mechanism of IL-1 beta converting enzyme. *Nature* **370:** 270–275.
101. Yonish-Rouach, E., Ernwald, D., Wilder, S. *et al.* (1993) p53 mediated cell death: relationship to cell cycle control. *Mol. Cell. Biol.* **13:** 1415–1423.
102. Eberhard, D. A., Brown M. D. and Vandenberg, S. R. (1994) Alterations of annexin expression in pathological neuronal and glial reactions: immunochemical localisation of annexins I, II (p36 and p11). *Am. J. Pathol.* **145:** 640–649.
103. Hainaut, P. (1995) The tumour suppressor p53, a receptor to genotoxic stress that controls cell growth and survival. *Curr. Opin. Oncol.* **7:** 76–82.
104. Bregman, B. S., Kunkel-Bagden, E., Schnell, L., Dai, H. N., Gao, D. and Schwab, M. E. (1995) Recovery from spinal cord injury mediated by antibodies to neurite growth inhibitors. *Nature* **378:** 498–501.

8

Chondrocyte Culture: A Target System to Evaluate Pharmacotoxicological Effects of Drugs

MONIQUE ADOLPHE, SOPHIE THENET-GAUCI AND SYLVIE DEMIGNOT

I. Introduction 182
II. Various models of cultured chondrocytes. 185
A. Cartilage slices. 186
B. Monolayer culture 186
C. Three-dimensional culture 188
D. Immortalized chondrocytes. 189
III. Tests for chondrocyte-specific functions. 190
A. Study of proteoglycans. 191
1. Alcian blue staining 191
2. Proteoglycan synthesis (^{35}S incorporation into GAGs) 191
3. Proteoglycan analysis 192
4. Expression of specific proteoglycan genes 192
B. Study of collagen 192
1. Global collagen synthesis 193
2. Analysis of synthesized collagen chains 193
3. Immunological methods (immunofluorescence, ELISA) 194
4. Study of different collagen gene expression 195
C. Alkaline phosphatase 196
IV. Use of chondrocyte culture to evaluate pharmacotoxicological effects of drugs 196
A. Growth factors and hormones 196
B. Cytokines 197
C. Vitamins 197
D. Anti-inflammatory drugs 198
E. Anti-osteoarthritic drugs. 198
F. Various toxic drugs for cartilaginous tissue 198
V. Conclusion 199
Acknowledgements 199
References. 199

IN VITRO METHODS IN PHARMACEUTICAL RESEARCH
ISBN 0-12-163390-X

I. INTRODUCTION

Cartilaginous diseases constitute a growing major medical problem as a result of increased life expectancy. The main diseases are rheumatoid arthritis (RA) and osteoarthritis (OA). These diseases are extremely common and no really effective treatment has been able to cure them.

Also, cartilage has been established as a target of some drugs used in therapy, such as anti-inflammatory drugs. Finally, it is important to evaluate the teratogenic effects of agents on limb development because, at the beginning of fetal life, cartilage temporarily constitutes the main part of the cytoskeleton. All these justify the development of *in vitro* tests to evaluate the pharmacotoxicological effects of drugs on chondrocytes.

The cartilage, of mesodermic origin, plays an important role in skeletal protection by withstanding pressure and absorbing shock. It is mainly composed of an extracellular matrix which is continuously synthesized and degraded by the unique cell type of this tissue: the chondrocyte. However, cartilage is not a homogeneous tissue. Its structure and morphology differ depending on age (immature or adult) and localization (extraskeletal, as for larynx, nose and Eustachian tube, for example, or articular in the movable joints). However, at the molecular level, there are gross similarities in molecular composition, although some tissue-specific composition differences may exist.[1]

Although a few sparse blood vessels actually penetrate the cartilage, the cartilage can be considered mostly as a non-vascularized tissue. Hence, chondrocytes are exposed to low oxygen tensions and the major source of nutrients come only by diffusion (e.g. from the tissue fluid and from the synovium in articular cartilage).[2] However, the cartilaginous tissue is always in a complex environment in direct or indirect contact with other types of cells (e.g. osteoblasts and synoviocytes). This leads to complex regulatory mechanisms mediated by factors derived from chondrocytes themselves, their different matrix components, and from neighbouring cells. This situation becomes more complicated in pathology (i.e. rheumatoid arthritis) because of the interaction of lymphocytes and macrophages.

The structure and organization of the different zones of cartilage is particularly well defined in the primary growth plates of developing mammalian long bones (Fig. 8.1). The growth plate can be divided, from the surface of the joint to the deep zone, into four zones. The reserve zone contains approximately spherical cells which exhibit little or no cell division.[3] In the proliferative zone, where oxygen tension is the highest,[4] cells divide to give rise to long columns of flattened cells. In the zone of maturation, in which chondrocytes mature into hypertrophic chondrocytes, cells enlarge and round up. Finally, the hypertrophic zone can be subdivided into two zones:[5] the upper hypertrophic zone where hypertrophic cells enlarge five- to tenfold, and the lower hypertrophic zone where mineralization takes place. In the lowermost layer of the hypertrophic zone, it is usually admitted that the hypertrophic cells eventually die as a result of extensive mineralization of matrix around them, leading to loss of nutrition.[6] However, the event of cell death is an issue that has recently been reopened.[7]

Even though cell proliferation is important in the early stages of growth of all cartilage, normal adult cartilage cell growth is infrequent.[8] However, Kunz *et al.*[9] showed proliferation of articular cartilage cells in the course of repair after damage.

The matrix of cartilage, consisting of 95–98% of tissue volume, is a mixture of collagen fibrils and proteoglycan aggregates. The collagen fibrils provide elements of high tensile strength, while proteoglycan aggregates exert an internal swelling pressure due to their hydrophilic character. Articular cartilage is not uniform in composition but varies within a single joint from the surface to the deep zone. The proportions of its major constituents are

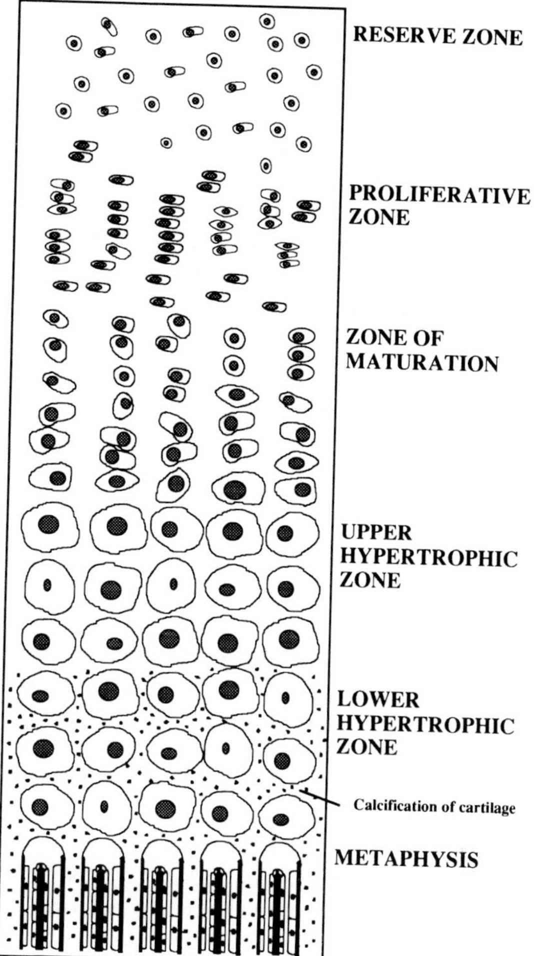

Fig. 8.1 Schematic organization of a primary mammalian growth plate (proximal fetal bovine tibia).

also known to vary between different types of cartilage, with ageing and disease.[1,10–12] On a net weight basis, the water content may lie in the range 65–80%, collagen in the range 15–25% and proteoglycans in the range 3–10%.[13] The majority of matrix biosynthesis takes place in the proliferative, maturing and upper hypertrophic zone.[14,15] The collagen fibrils contain type II collagen as the major component and smaller amounts of type IX and XI collagen.[16–18] Type XI collagen accounts for 8–10% of cartilage collagen, while type IX collagen accounts for about 5%. Type XI collagen participates in regulating the size of the collagen fibrils and stabilizing the fibril network.[19] Type IX collagen molecules are located at the surface of collagen fibrils.[20] Type X collagen, which is not found in cartilage that is not committed to calcification, is synthesized only by cells of the hypertrophic and maturing zone.[21,22]

There are three major types of proteoglycans that are synthesized by chondrocytes: (1) large cartilage-specific aggregating proteoglycans (aggrecan); (2) small proteoglycans (decorin, biglycan and fibromodulin); and (3) cell-associated proteoglycans.[23–25] The two latter types of proteoglycans are not specific to cartilage.

The large cartilage-specific aggregating proteoglycans, major proteoglycans of cartilage, consist of a central core protein (aggrecan) along which chondroitin sulfate and keratan sulfate are situated. These subunits interact with hyaluronic acid to form aggregates stabilized by link proteins. The size of the aggregates decreases markedly with age.[26,27]

The small proteoglycans of cartilage are ubiquitous to extracellular matrices of all connective tissues. In mature cartilage, these proteoglycans constitute approximately 5% of total proteoglycans and are substituted with chondroitin/dermatan sulfate or keratan sulfate glycosaminoglycans (GAGs) chains. The core protein of decorin is substituted with one chondroitin/dermatan sulfate chain, whereas biglycan contains two similar GAG chains. The core protein of fibromodulin is substituted with keratan sulfate chains.

In addition to these macromolecules, a number of other proteins have been described in cartilage matrix:[28] anchorin CII, a specific type II collagen binding protein; cartilage matrix protein (CMP); chondrocalcin, the C-propeptide of type II collagen; collagen binding protein (CBP); cartilage matrix glycoprotein (CMGP) and cartilage oligomeric matrix protein (COMP); Ch21 protein; chondronectin; fibronectin and tenascin.

Alkaline phosphatase, an enzyme with the capacity to liberate inorganic phosphate from organic or inorganic substrates, is mainly localized in the hypertrophic zone where matrix mineralization takes place.[29,30] It is primarily localized in the plasma membranes of chondrocytes and in matrix vesicles.

Chondrocytes are remarkable in their capacity to synthesize, organize and regulate the deposition of their complex surrounding matrix in a highly ordered and efficient manner. At each stage of growth or development, the relative rates of synthesis and degradation are adjusted to achieve net growth, remodelling, or a balanced equilibrium. Many proteinases that can degrade matrix components have been identified in connective tissue and inflammatory cells. The synthesis of these enzymes has been shown to be altered by a variety of cytokines, growth factors and hormones. All are produced as inactive proforms which are later converted to active proteinases, which are in turn subject to inhibition by a range of protein inhibitors. The availability of proteolytic activity is therefore carefully regulated at several stages.

Articular chondrocytes can synthesize and secrete at least four different types of neutral proteinases.[31] Three of them – collagenase (MMP-1), gelatinase (MMP-2) and stromelysin (MMP-3) – are matrix metalloproteases, while the fourth, plasminogen activator, is a serine protease. Between them, these enzymes can degrade the entire extracellular macromolecular matrix of cartilage. The inhibitors of these neutral metalloproteases are the tissue inhibitors of metalloproteinases (TIMPs), which are synthesized by chondrocytes. Other proteases, such as lysosomal cysteine proteinases (cathepsin B and L), may be involved in extracellular matrix destruction in pathology.

Upon ageing, articular cartilage takes a xanthous appearance, as opposed to the white colour of young cartilage; cartilage has reduced thickness, and areas that are exposed to mechanical stress are frequently denuded. A high number of samples show fibrillations and softening of the articular surface. Fibrillated areas are characterized by a loss of proteoglycans and a discontinuity in the collagen network. Many of these cases can be classified as ostheoarthritis (OA; osteoarthrosis), although these may not be symptomatic yet.

Ageing of cartilage is associated with alteration in extracellular matrix, increased deposition of calcium crystals and decreased cellularity.[32] The age-related changes may be related to regulatory imbalances. Chondrocytes in adult cartilage express a low level of replicative and biosynthetic activity, which leads to reduced repair capacity of older cells and may account for persistent tissue damage.

The most striking difference between fetal and adult cartilage is the decrease in cartilage cellularity. Osteoarthritic joints contain even fewer cells per gram of tissue, suggesting a predisposition to matrix degeneration as a consequence of loss of chondrocytes.

Proteoglycans in ageing cartilage are smaller in size.[26,27,33] The total glycosaminoglycan content in human articular cartilage may not change significantly with ageing. However, there is a decrease in the size and number of chondroitin sulfate chains, a decrease in the chondroitin sulfate 4/6 ratio, and an increase in the size and number of keratan sulfate chains. The changes in chondroitin sulfate are thought to account for the decreased water content in aged cartilage. Ageing cartilage also contains increased quantities of hyaluronic acid binding protein, which is generated by proteolysis of the proteoglycan core protein. The size of hyaluronic acid is reduced and link proteins show increased heterogeneity and fragmentation in human ageing.

The failure of the chondrocyte to maintain the balance between synthesis and degradation of the extracellular matrix leads to OA, which is very common in those aged over 50 years.[34] Inflammation, when present, is thought to be a late and transient event, arising probably from products of cartilage degradation inducing secondary synovitis in the adjacent tissue.

One of the earliest changes reported to occur in osteoarthritic cartilage is an increase in collagen synthesis as well as an increased synthesis of proteoglycans. In OA, proteoglycans are lost from the tissue at a rate exceeding the deposition of newly synthesized proteoglycans. Depletion of proteoglycans is a common feature, despite increased DNA and matrix synthesis indicating that degradation of the matrix is markedly accelerated.[35] This is consistent with the identification of increased proteolytic activity in osteoarthritic cartilage. A close correlation was found with enzyme activity and severity of the lesions. Levels of neutral metalloproteinases are significantly raised in osteoarthritic human cartilage compared with normal cartilage.

The identity of the mediators involved in the initiation and/or progression of this disease have not been clearly established. However, interleukin (IL) 1 and tumour necrosis factor (TNF) have been detected in the synovial fluid of patients with OA, even when there are no overt signs of local or systemic inflammation.

Rheumatoid arthritis (RA) is a systemic inflammatory disease characterized by primary synovitis in the joints. This disorder has a world-wide distribution, affecting approximately 1% of the population. In RA, synovial fluids and tissues contain high concentrations of cytokines derived primarily from synovial macrophages, especially IL-1, TNF-α and IL-6.[31,36,37] These cytokines are proinflammatory, affecting fibroblasts, chondrocytes and lymphocytes, all of which are found in inflammed synovial tissues. IL-1 and TNF-α induce proteoglycan depletion in cartilage by increasing the rate of degradation and decreasing synthesis. The proteoglycan and collagen degradation are due to increased proteolytic activity. Thus, products of activated macrophages appear to be capable of producing many of the features of RA.

The pharmacotoxicological effect of drugs on cartilaginous tissue can be studied on various animal models or on *in vitro* cell culture models, the latter being detailed in the next section. The main pertinent end-points for assessing drug effects on chondrocytes will be developed in the following section (proteoglycans, collagens and alkaline phosphatase). Finally, the last section deals with various examples of pharmacotoxicological studies of drugs.

II. VARIOUS MODELS OF CULTURED CHONDROCYTES

Whatever the cartilaginous origin, different types of culture can be used: cartilage slices, monolayer culture, three-dimensional culture and cell lines derived either from chondrosarcoma or from normal chondrocytes immortalized by viral infection or oncogene transfection. The common point between all these types of culture is the use of a rich synthetic medium. Indeed, chondrocytes have high nutritional requirements for the production of matrix components. The media used are HAM F-12 or DMEM supplemented with fetal calf serum (10%) or serum substitutes. Recently, it appeared that the addition of an insulin-containing serum substitute was permissive for expression of type II collagen.[38] However, chondrocyte culture in defined medium had also been attempted.[39–41]

A. Cartilage slices

The articular tissue is dissected, cut into slices 1–2 mm thick and placed in tissue culture dishes containing medium. The medium level is adjusted to cover the tissue, to allow efficient gas exchange. Cultures are generally fed every 1–2 days with fresh medium. Another technique consists in cultivating tissue at the interface of air–medium using 0.45 μm millipore filters cemented on to stainless steel grids.

The use of cartilage slices allows chondrocytes to be studied in the presence of normal cell–matrix interactions as the tissue remains intact. This type of culture permits maintenance of the chondrocyte phenotype, as demonstrated by the fact that cells continue to synthesize cartilage-specific proteoglycans.[42]

This method presents, for the moment, a renewed interest, but the limits are related to the variability in the sampling of cartilage explants and difficulty in performing biochemical and molecular biology techniques on slices.

B. Monolayer culture

Monolayer culture is the type of chondrocyte culture most frequently referred to in the literature. Release of cartilaginous cells from joint tissue is usually achieved using the technique of Green[43] (Fig. 8.2), which is based on serial enzymatic digestions with hyaluronidase, trypsin and finally collagenase in order to degrade the collagenous matrix. Benya has proposed a modification of this technique using a short collagenase step (0.3%) followed by overnight treatment with collagenase at a lower concentration (0.06%) in the presence of 10% of fetal calf serum (FCS). This procedure permits the release of approximatively 90% of the chondrocytes present in rabbit cartilage slices (P. D. Benya, personal communication).

Monolayer culture is characterized by a high proliferative capacity. Ronot *et al.*[44] showed that rabbit articular chondrocytes cultivated in Ham's F12 and 10% FCS remain in suspension for the first 48–72 h. The growth curve contains a lag period until day 3 and an exponential growth phase from day 3 to day 5. In contrast, subcultured cells multiply exponentially until day 3 following a very short lag period. The length of the cell cycle and the doubling time are 19 and 20 h, respectively. However, the time required to form a monolayer depends on cellular density. A cell culture is referred to as a 'monolayer culture' when cell density varies between 5 and 16 $\times$ 10^3 per cm^2. Beyond this cell concentration, the culture can be defined as high-density culture, which has characteristics very different from those of a monolayer.

When cells derived from articular cartilage are subcultured, chondrocytes undergo *in vitro* senescence similar to that described for other mesodermic diploid cells. Moskalewski *et al.*[45] demonstrated that chondrocytes isolated from rabbit articular cartilage exhibited the onset of phase III senescence after 10 to 14 population doublings. Evans and Georgescu[46]

① Sampling of cartilaginous tissue

② Dissection in 1-2 mm explants

③ Serially enzymatic digestion

- Hyaluronidase (not very useful)
- Trypsine 0.1% HamF-12 - 30 min.
  (supernatant discarded)
- Collagenase 0.2% in HamF-12 - 45 min x 3

④ Centrifugation followed by numeration and seeding

Fig. 8.2 Method for obtaining isolated chondrocytes from cartilaginous tissue.[43]

established that the population-doubling capacity of rabbit, dog and human chondrocytes in culture is related to the life span of the donor and inversely related to the age of the donor. Using rabbit articular chondrocytes subcultured several-fold, Dominice *et al.*[47] described a slowing down of the proliferative capacity at the fourth passage, followed by a complete loss of division after 8 ± 1 passages. Chondrocytes at the fourth passage subculture can be considered as senescent and are characterized by a decrease in proliferative capacity, a reduction in the proportion of cells in S and G2 + M phases of the cell cycle, and a concomitant enhancement in protein content related to the increase in cell size. Immunocytochemistry revealed a rigid cytoarchitecture with an increase in the quantity and organization of three cytoskeletal components: actin, tubulin and vimentin.

The main disadvantage of monolayer culture is that the matrix produced in culture is quite different from that produced *in vivo*. The chondrocyte phenotype is labile with respect to collagen synthesis. It has been shown in rabbit chondrocytes culture that a switch from type II to type I collagen occurs.[48,49] This phenomenon, which appears as soon as the end of the primary culture, is particularly evident in the first and subsequent subcultures. With regard to proteoglycan synthesis, it has been shown that decreasing proportions of proteoglycans and increasing proportions of hyaluronan are synthesized when the number of passages in culture increases. The proteoglycans have a lower avidity for hyaluronan. Consequently, relatively fewer proteoglycan aggregates are formed. Furthermore, chondroitin sulfate is replaced in the proteoglycans by dermatan sulfate and the glycosaminoglycans in the proteoglycan macromolecule are less sulfated.

However, this de-differentiation is reversible. De-differentiated chondrocytes can re-express the differentiated phenotype in various conditions, such as the use of dihydrocytochalasin B,[50] staurosporine[51] or in three-dimensional culture.[52]

C. Three-dimensional culture

Three-dimensional cell culture may be divided in two main types: one consists of embedding the chondrocytes in a gel (collagen, agarose or alginate), and the other one is the result of particular culture conditions (suspension or high-density culture) in which chondrocytes themselves produce their three-dimensional environment.

The first report of chondrocytes embedded in a gel was from Horwitz and Dorfman;[53] however, it was not until 1982 that several studies were published regarding chondrocyte culture in collagen or agarose. Gibson *et al.*[54] and Yasui *et al.*[55] isolated chondrocytes from sternal embryonic cartilage and embedded them in collagen gels. Under these conditions, evidence for cell viability, growth and deposition of extracellular matrix has been reported. Benya and Shaffer[52] also observed that chondrocytes de-differentiated by serial monolayer culture can re-express their differentiated phenotype during suspension culture in firm gels of 0.5% low melting agarose. Proteoglycan and collagen synthesis rates returned to those that existed in primary culture.

Guo *et al.*[56] described chondrocyte culture in alginate beads. Within such gels, chondrocytes present a rounded morphology (Fig. 8.3). This methodology, applied to chondrocytes cultured within a gel or more frequently in single beads, was shown to be able to maintain the differentiative phenotype[57–59] and to permit re-expression of this phenotype after de-differentiation.[60]

The major drawback of this culture system is the low rate of cell proliferation, which limits its suitability.

Chondrocyte culture in suspension has also been successful. Deshmukh and Kline[61] demonstrated that, upon transfer from monolayer to suspension culture, the cells synthezise type II collagen in a medium devoid of $CaCl_2$. On the other hand, Wiebkin and Muir[62] found that chondrocytes isolated from the larynx of adult pigs and cultured in suspension synthesized cartilage-specific proteoglycans. The transfer of de-differentiated chicken chondrocytes to suspension culture was used to demonstrate that the resultant cellular accumulation of type II collagen mRNA is regulated not only at the transcriptional level, but also through stabilization of the RNA transcripts.[63]

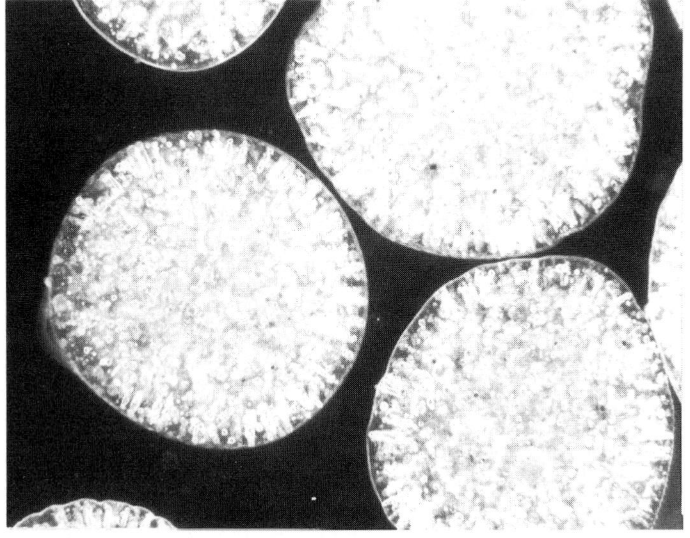

Fig. 8.3 Three-dimensional culture of chondrocytes in alginate beads (original magnification × 44).

High-density cultures are obtained by seeding chondrocytes at a concentration greater than 10^5 cells per cm^2. After a few days, cells re-establish a territorial matrix which is rich in collagen fibrils and proteoglycans.[64]

Aggregate suspension culture and high-density culture appear more suitable for large numbers of cells than cells suspended in gel. However, in most cases, cellular proliferation and extracellular matrix deposition are rapidly initiated and then decline substantially. On the other hand, embryo limb-bud cells, cultured at a high density, proliferate and differentiate into a number of cell types including cartilage. This technique in micromass was originally described by Umansky[65] and has been developed by Flint and Orton[66] to perform short-term *in vitro* assays for teratogens.

D. Immortalized chondrocytes

Studies on cultured chondrocytes are limited by their relative short life span and the frequent instability of their differentiated properties. The dream of obtaining a chondrocyte cell line possessing both the capacity for infinite proliferation and maintenance of specific functions has stimulated research in this field. An immortalized chondrocyte cell line would be particulary interesting because there are few continuous cell lines of this type. The most famous one is a tumorigenic cell line, the swarm rat chondrosarcoma. Takigawa *et al.*[67] have also established a cell line from human chondrosarcoma. However, these cell lines are cancerous and present a low growth capacity.

Gionti *et al.*[68] used infection by the avian myelocytomatosis virus (MC29) carrying the *myc* oncogene to obtain immortalized quail embryo chondrocytes which still expressed type II collagen and cartilage proteoglycans. Primary fetal rat costal chondrocytes infected with a recombinant retrovirus carrying *myc* and *raf* oncogenes produced an immortalized cell line which synthesized high levels of cartilage proteoglycan, but showed weak type II collagen expression.[69] Gionti *et al.*[70] generated a continuous cell line of chicken embryo cells from a culture of chondrocytes infected with Rous sarcoma virus. These cells exhibited reduced serum requirements, were able to grow in a semisolid medium and were not tumorigenic. However, this cell line did not synthesize type II or X collagen, which are the differentiation markers of normal chicken chondrocytes in culture. Immortalized rabbit articular chondrocytes were obtained by transfection with SV40 large T and little t encoding genes.[71] These cells have been maintained in culture for 2 years. Growth curves of normal and SV40-transfected chondrocytes were compared and displayed similar doubling times (approximately 20 h). They retained polygonal morphology, but the synthesis of alcian blue stainable matrix was reduced about 20-fold. Northern blot analysis of RNAs from these immortalized chondrocytes cultured in monolayer did not detect any type II procollagen mRNAs. Two-dimensional cyanogen bromide peptide maps of labelled collagens from these cultures showed that the major collagen synthesized was type I collagen. No type II collagen was detectable. Several attempts to stimulate re-expression of collagen type II after culturing these immortalized cells in collagen gel or after treatment with dihydrocytochalasin B have been unsuccessful.

More recently, Mallein-Gerin and Olsen[72] infected primary embryonic mouse limb chondrocytes with a retrovirus carrying the simian virus 40 early region and obtained a chondrocyte cell line expressing type II, IX and XI collagens as well as cartilage aggrecan and link protein. Goldring *et al.*[38] described how they obtained immortalized human chondrocytes, established by transfection of primary cultures of juvenile costal chondrocytes with vectors encoding SV40 large T antigen and by selection in suspension culture over agarose. Stable cell lines were generated that exhibited chondrocyte morphology, continuous proliferative capacity during 80 passages and expression of mRNAs encoding chondrocyte-specific collagens II, IX, X and XI as well as proteoglycans in a culture medium supplemented with insulin-rich serum substitute.

Whatever the model of cultured chondrocytes, all these types of culture can be established from healthy or pathological cartilages such as arthritic or osteoarthritic tissues (*vivo–vitro* or *ex vivo* experiments). However, some pathological models can be obtained from healthy chondrocytes modified *in vitro* by several drugs (*vivo–vitro* experiments). For example, after treatment with IL-1, chondrocytes produce degradative enzymes which could be responsible for the matrix perturbation observed in several rheumatoid arthritic diseases. This model appears useful for the investigation of degradative enzyme inhibitors.

As oxygen free radicals play a prominent part in the process of cartilage degradation, a model has been developed by treating monolayer culture of chondrocytes with oxygen free radicals generated by the enzymatic action of xanthine oxidase upon hypoxanthine. Various perturbations concerning proliferation and oncogene expression were observed.[73,74] Thus, this model could be useful for the study of oxygen free radical scavengers.

III. TESTS FOR CHONDROCYTE-SPECIFIC FUNCTIONS

The indicators commonly used in *in vitro* cytotoxicity testing can be classified as non-specific or organ-specific criteria. Non-specific criteria concern general cell functions such as membrane integrity, subcellular perturbations, cell growth, protein synthesis and metabolic activities. A large variety of tests (most of them can be miniaturized) have been used and are described in a previous chapter. Chondrocyte-specific criteria are related to the quantity and quality of the cartilaginous matrix. This section focuses on its main components, the collagens and proteoglycans.

Roughly, one can distinguish two kinds of analysis. The first are able to measure, in a quantitative but global manner the expression or synthesis of one matrix component (e.g. collagens or proteoglycans). Such techniques are suitable for the analysis of a large number of samples but are unable to differentiate the cartilage-specific collagen chains or proteoglycans. To study these cartilage-specific macromolecules, techniques with greater resolution have to be performed, which are generally long and tricky, and thus poorly adapted to large screening studies. These aspects are summarized in Table 8.1. As a general guide, global techniques might be used for a first screening study, performing more specific investigations on a restricted number of samples.

Many agents or drugs are able to induce cartilage matrix degradation, which is performed by a variety of proteinases produced by the chondrocytes themselves. Evaluation of degradation activity can be assessed by measuring degradation products or by assaying degradative enzymes. The former methods are long and difficult as they consist of measuring the release of radiolabelled components into the medium over several days and evaluating their half-lives. However, interpretation of the data obtained from the latter methods is difficult because the regulation of proteinase activity is complex (production of inactive proforms and inhibitors; see introductory section). These methods will not be developed in this chapter, but valuable information can be found in Tyler.[31]

Table 8.1 Methods of analysis.

	Quantitative*	Suitable for a large number of samples†	Specificity‡	Use of radioelements
Collagen				
Global synthesis	Yes	Yes	No	Yes
Collagen analysis	Semi	No	Yes	Yes
Transcript analysis	Semi	No	Yes	Yes
ELISA (type II)	Yes	Yes	Yes	No
Proteoglycans				
Alcian blue staining	Yes	Yes	No	No
^{35}S incorporation	Yes	Yes	No	Yes
Separation of aggregates	No	No	Yes	Yes
Transcript analysis	Semi	No	Yes	Yes
Alkaline phosphatase	Yes	Yes	No	No

* Indicates whether the data obtained are quantitative, semiquantitative or qualitative.
† Includes the aspects of rapidity and the possibility of miniaturization.
‡ Indicates whether the method can differentiate cartilage-specific molecules from those of the same family which are not cartilage-specific (e.g. type II versus type I collagen).

A. Study of proteoglycans

As described in the introductory section, there are three types of proteoglycans in cartilage. Alcian blue staining or measure of ^{35}S incorporation reflect respectively the quantity and the synthesis of glycosaminoglycans (GAGs), and thus of global proteoglycans. The large aggregating proteoglycan which ensures the functionality of cartilage can be analysed only by chromatographic methods. Its specific core protein (aggrecan) can be studied at the transcriptional level.

1. *Alcian blue staining*

Alcian blue staining at acidic pH is widely used as an indicator of the presence of sulfated GAGs.[75,76] This method of proteoglycan evaluation has been especially used for the evaluation of teratogenic effects on micromass cultures of limb-bud mesenchymal cells[66] and has been miniaturized.[77]

The cultures are rinsed twice with PBS and fixed in 2% glacial acetic acid in ethanol, then rehydrated through 95% and 70% ethanol. Fixed cultures are stained overnight with 0.5% Alcian blue in 0.1 N HCl and rinsed twice with 0.1 N HCl to remove any unbound dye. A final rinse with distilled water is aspirated to near dryness. Alcian blue is then extracted by 4 M guanidine HCl overnight at 4°C. Absorbance values are read at 600 nm after temperature equilibration. Wells are rinsed twice with distilled water and the same volume of 4 M guanidine HCl is added to obtain the blank values, which are subtracted from the gross values.

2. *Proteoglycan synthesis (^{35}S incorporation into GAGs)*

For studying proteoglycans synthesis, ^{35}S-sulfate is the radioisotope of choice as it is incorporated preferentially (>90%) into chondroitin sulfate and keratan sulfate of the newly synthesized proteoglycans. This can be performed both on cartilage in explant culture or on isolated chondrocytes in monolayer or three-dimensional culture.[57,78] The general protocol is as follows.

Cultures are incubated for 4–24 h in presence of ^{35}S (20 μCi ml^{-1}). Slices, monolayer or gels are then rinsed and extracted at 4°C with 4 M guanidine HCl, 0.05 M sodium acetate, pH 6.0, containing protease inhibitors. Extracted samples and/or culture medium are subjected to sieve chromatography on Sephadex G25 (PD 10 columns) equilibrated and eluted with 4 M guanidine HCl, 0.05 M sodium acetate, 0.1 M sodium sulfate, 0.5% Triton X-100, pH 7.5. Radioactivity in the excluded peak, representing newly synthesized proteoglycan, is measured by scintillation counting.

A rapid filtration assay for the quantification of ^{35}S-labelled proteoglycan or ^{35}S-labelled GAGs in a large number of samples has been recently described.[79] In this assay, separation of ^{35}S-labelled proteoglycan and ^{35}S-labelled GAGs from unincorporated ^{35}S is effected by forming insoluble complexes between alcian blue and the GAG moieties of the proteoglycan and then filtering the solutions through Durapore membrane discs (0.45 μM pore size) fitted in a 96-well plate. Following brief rinsing steps, the discs are punched out and ^{35}S-labelled macromolecules are then quantified by scintillation counting.

3. *Proteoglycan analysis*

To learn more about the sizes of the synthesized monomeric proteoglycan, 4 M guanidine HCl extracts can be subjected to chromatography on Sepharose CL-2B, which separates large from small proteoglycan.[80] This step is generally preceded by a preliminary step of proteoglycan purification either by caesium chloride gradient centrifugation,[81,82] sieve chromatography on Sephadex G50[78] or on Biogel P-6 in urea buffer followed by Sephacel ion-exchange chromatography.[57,80] Aggregates of proteoglycans with hyaluronate and link protein can be shown after reassociation by dialysis with 0.4 M guanidine HCl and elution in the void volume of a Sepharose CL-2B column eluted with a non-dissociative buffer.[57,83] The ability of synthesized proteoglycans to form large aggregates can also be studied after extraction under dissociative conditions and reassociation assays with hyaluronic acid[80,83–85] or bovine nasal proteoglycan aggregates.[57]

4. *Expression of specific proteoglycan genes*

Expression of the chondrocyte-specific aggrecan and link protein can be analysed at the transcriptional level (by Northern blot, for example) using conventional transfer and hybridization techniques.[86] The preparation of total RNAs from chondrocyte cultures does not present any difficulty using classical methods such as those employing guanidine HCl[86] or commercial kits, for example RNA[B] (from Bioprobe Systems, Montreuil sous Bois, France). Several complementary DNA probes for aggrecan[87–90] and link protein[91,92] from rat, human, mouse or chick have been characterized.

B. Study of collagen

Type II collagen represents 85–90% of total collagen synthesized by chondrocytes in cartilage or primary culture. It is very specific of this cell type and is considered to be its main differentiation marker. In most studies of phenotypic modulation, type II collagen synthesis is reduced or suppressed and non-equivalently replaced by synthesis of type I, type III and/or type I trimer collagen.[48] Thus, global collagen synthesis can be determined as a rough indicator of chondrocyte damage. However, for a precise evaluation of chondrocyte function, the synthesis of at least type II, and eventually the cartilage-specific minor collagens, should be assessed.

1. *Global collagen synthesis*

An assay procedure in which radioactive collagen may be measured quantitatively even in the presence of large amounts of other proteins was developed by Peterkofsky and Diegelmann.[93] It is based on the digestion of radiolabelled proteins by bacterial collagenase, and quantification of trichloroacetic acid-precipitated proteins by scintillation counting. Cells are incubated for 24 h in presence of 2 μCi ml^{-1} [^{3}H]proline, 25 μg ml^{-1} ascorbate and 62.5 μg ml^{-1} β-aminopropionitrile in culture medium. For each sample, two 400 μl aliquots of medium are sampled, one of which is incubated in presence of 5 units/ml^{-1} bacterial collagenase (form III, Advance Biofactures Corporation, Lynbrook, USA) for 24 h at 37°C. The tubes are then chilled to 4°C for 15 min and proteins are precipitated by the addition of 100 μl 25% TCA containing 1.25% tannic acid for 2 h at 4°C, then centrifuged at 5000*g* for 10 min at 4°C. Pellets are washed in 1 ml 5% TCA, 0.25% tannic acid and centrifuged again; this step is repeated twice to ensure complete removal of unincorporated [^{3}H]proline. Pellets are resuspended in 100 μl 1 N NaOH, samples are bleached and finally quantified by scintillation counting. Synthesis of collagen proteins is evaluated by the difference of radioactivity incorporated in total proteins and in non-digested proteins (non-collagen proteins) for each sample. Using the same principle, a microassay to quantitate collagen synthesis and DNA in 24-well plates has been proposed more recently.[94] In another microassay performed on 96-well plates, [^{3}H]proline-labelled collagen is simply extracted with pepsin in 0.5 N acetic acid and precipitated by the addition of 5% NaCl.[95]

2. *Analysis of synthesized collagen chains*

For a precise analysis of the collagen phenotype, sodium dodecyl sulfate polyacrylamide gel electrophoresis (SDS-PAGE) of purified collagen after [^{3}H]proline incorporation, and SDS-PAGE and two-dimensional electrophoresis of CNBr peptides have to be performed.

With regard to major collagens, 5% SDS-PAGE analysis of pepsinized collagen chains can reveal the presence of type III collagen and of the α_2(I) chain of collagen I (Fig. 8.4). However, it cannot separate the α_1 chain of types I and II, i.e. make a distinction between type II and type I trimer collagen. Collagen chains can be cleaved by cyanogen bromide and the resulting peptides are analysed by 16% SDS-PAGE, which resolves a single major band for each of the chains in collagen types I, II and III.[48] The characteristic peptide derived from α_1(I) chains is α_1(I)-CB6; from α_1(II), α_1(II)-CB10,5; and from α_1(III), the mixture of peptides α_1(III)-CB5 + 9 (Fig. 8.5). In some cases, some labelled proteins may co-migrate with the peptide CB10. That is why two-dimensional CNBr peptide mapping[48] is sometimes necessary to confirm type II collagen expression.

With regard to minor collagens, types IX, X and XI can be separated by SDS-PAGE,[18,96] although type XI chains are not separated from type V chains, which are not cartilage specific.

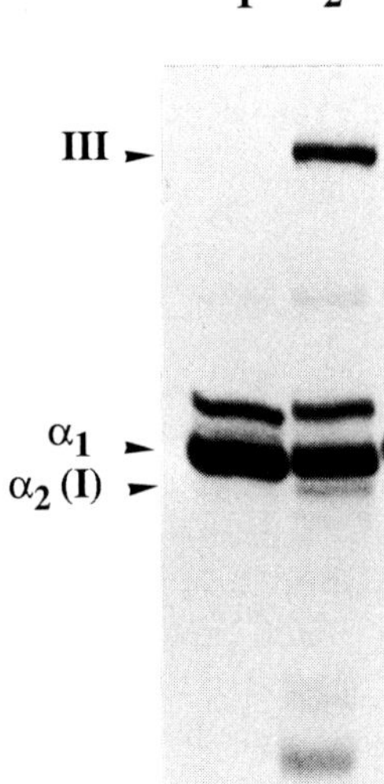

Fig. 8.4 Six per cent SDS-PAGE of [^{3}H]proline-labelled collagens purified from confluent monolayer primary cultures. Control chondrocytes (lane 1); chondrocytes treated for 48 h with 1 μg ml^{-1} retinoic acid (lane 2). Positions of type III collagen, α_1 and α_2(I) collagen chains are indicated by arrowheads.

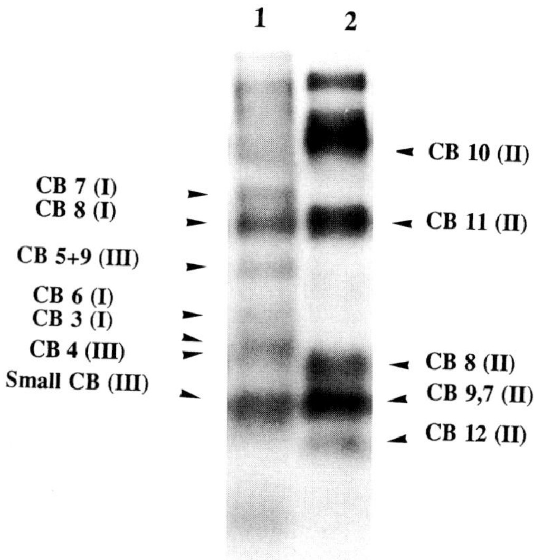

Fig. 8.5 Sixteen per cent SDS-PAGE of CNBr peptides from collagens purified from confluent cultures of chondrocytes. Passage 2 cells treated for 48 h with 1 μg ml^{-1} retinoic acid (lane 1); primary cultures (lane 2). Type II collagen CNBr peptides (CB_n(II)), indicated on the right of the figure, are present in cells expressing a differentiated phenotype. Type I and III collagen CNBr peptides (CB_n(I) and CB_n(III), respectively), indicated on the left of the figure, are present when cells express a de-differentiated phenotype.

3. *Immunological methods (immunofluorescence, ELISA)*

Type II collagen-specific antibodies can be used for indirect immunofluorescent staining or enzyme-linked immunoadsorbent assay (ELISA). Only the latter methods can be quantitative and are thus suitable for pharmacotoxicological studies. Several ELISAs have been developed. In inhibition assays,[97,98] plastic microtiter wells are coated with type II collagen, then antibodies are allowed to bind to the insolubilized antigen in each well. The amount of bound antibody is determined by incubation with a second antibody, which is covalently linked to alkaline phosphatase or horseradish peroxidase, and subsequent addition of an appropriate substrate. The level of type II collagen in the culture supernatant is estimated from its ability to inhibit the binding of the first antibody to the antigen-coated well. Such assays have also been adapted for other cartilage matrix components, in particular type I collagen.[98] In a direct ELISA,[99] proteins from cultures to be assayed are precipitated by the addition of ethanol (final concentration 85%) and centrifugation. Precipitates are dissolved in 0.05 M sodium carbonate buffer, pH 9.6 and adsorbed on to the wells of a 24-well microtiter plate. Fixation of type II collagen to the wells is assayed by incubating the wells sequentially with anti-type II collagen antibody, alkaline phosphatase-conjugated second antibody and alkaline phosphatase substrate solution.

4. *Study of different collagen gene expression*

The expression of these genetically distinct collagens can also be analysed at the transcriptional level (Northern blot) with conventional transfer and hybridization techniques (Fig. 8.6).[86] Probes for pro-α_1(II),[100,101] pro-α_1(I),[101,102] α_1(IX)[101] and pro-α_1(X)[103] have been published. Because of sequence homology between different collagen genes, hybridization and washing conditions must be tested and must be stringent enough to avoid cross-hybridization. However, to avoid such problems the most recent probes[101] cover mainly sequences in the 3′ untranslated region of the gene, where homology is considerably lower, and detect only the specific mRNAs under normal hybridization and washing conditions.

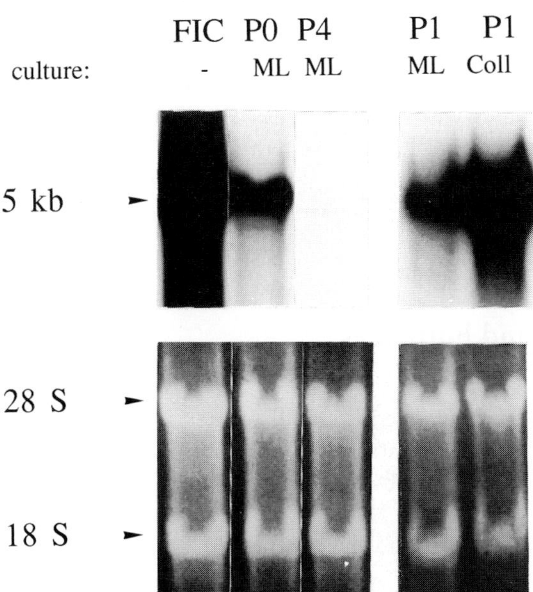

Fig. 8.6 Northern blot analysis of pro-α_1 (II) mRNAs (5 kb) in freshly isolated chondrocytes (FIC), in chondrocytes in primary culture (P0) or at the fourth passage (P4) in monolayer (ML), and in chondrocytes at the first passage (P1) cultured either in monolayer or within collagen gels for 12 days (Coll). The probe used was from Elima *et al.*[100] rRNAs 28S and 18S were stained with ethidium bromide.

C. Alkaline phosphatase

Alkaline phosphatase is preferentially produced by hypertrophic chondrocytes from mineralizing zones (see Introduction). Alkaline phosphatase levels can be determined with a fluorometric substrate, 4-methylumbelliferyl phosphate.[104] The substrate is incubated with cell lysates in 40 mM glycine buffer, pH 10 at 37°C. The reaction is stopped by the addition of several volumes of 320 mM glycine, 200 mM $NaCO_3$, 1 mM ethylene diamine tetra-acetic acid (EDTA), pH 10.5. The fluorescence of the 4-methylumbelliferone formed by action of the alkaline phosphatase is measured at 450 nm after excitation at 370 nm. Another assay measures the hydrolysis by alkaline phosphatase of *p*-nitro-phenylphosphate (pNP), which can be monitored by change of absorbance at 410 nm.[105,106] Briefly, cell lysates are incubated with 1 volume of 1 M Tris–HCl, pH 9 containing 1 mM pNP and 1 mM $MgCl_2$. The reaction is stopped by addition of 0.25 volumes of 1 N NaOH. This latter assay can be performed with a kit purchased from Sigma (catalogue no. 104 LL).[107]

IV. USE OF CHONDROCYTE CULTURE TO EVALUATE PHARMACOTOXICOLOGICAL EFFECTS OF DRUGS

Chondrocyte culture has been used particularly for physiological studies of growth factors, hormones, cytokines and vitamins. The knowledge of biological regulations of chondrocytes should result in important progress in the pharmacology of cartilaginous tissue.

According to the close relation between physiological regulation and the future of pharmacotoxicology, we will describe several points concerning the main factors of regulation: insulin-like growth factor (IGF), fibroblast growth factor (FGF), transforming growth factor (TGF) β, IL-1, TNF-α and vitamins C, D_3 and A.

Among the pharmacotoxicological studies, anti-inflammatory and antiosteoarthritic drugs are the most important, as well as several drugs exhibiting a toxic effect on cartilage.

The main end-points studied are: proliferation and DNA synthesis; production of proteoglycan and collagen by biochemical or molecular biology techniques; production of various enzymes such as collagenase, stromelysin, proteoglycanase and alkaline phosphatase.

A. Growth factors and hormones

The mitogenic effect of FGF was clearly demonstrated in cultured chondrocytes. However, its effect on matrix production is not clear. FGF stimulated radiosulfate incorporation in proteoglycan, but this action was observed only when FGF was present during exponential growth of the cells.[108] In contrast, Nataf *et al.*[109] showed a decrease in proteoglycan and collagen synthesis in prepubertal rabbit epyphysal chondrocytes grown in high-density culture.

IGF-1 has been described as mitogenic for various types of cultured chondrocytes[110,111] and appears as a major regulator of cartilage proteoglycan.[112,113]

Many reports have described the effects of TGF-β on various models of cultured chondrocytes. With respect to cell proliferation, the results obtained appear complex: a stimulating or inhibiting effect can be observed depending on the presence or absence of serum[114–116] and on the type of cartilage.[117] Its action on cartilage phenotype seems less variable: TGF-β stimulates the proteoglycan synthesis of explants from human articulations[118] but its effect depends on culture conditions.[119] Collagen synthesis is also stimulated[120] and under serum-free culture conditions[50] TGF-β leads to re-expression of the differentiated phenotype after de-differentiation by retinoic acid.

Among the hormones, the more recent papers concern parathyroid hormone (PTH). PTH enhances the proliferation of chick growth plate chondrocyte and stimulates proteoglycan synthesis, but collagen synthesis and alkaline phosphatase activity are decreased.[121]

B. Cytokines

Many papers have reported on the effects of IL-1 and TNF-α on various models of cultured chondrocytes. IL-1 and TNF-α are potent stimulators of collagenase and stromelysine at the transcriptional as well as at the traductional level.[122–125] These data suggest that these cytokines may be implicated in cartilage degradation. In parallel, IL-1 and TNF-α inhibit proteoglycan synthesis,[126,127] collagen synthesis,[128,129] collagen type X and alkaline phosphatase activity on growth-plate chondrocytes.

C. Vitamins

Three vitamins have been studied in cultured chondrocytes: vitamins C, D_3 and A. Krystal *et al.*[130] showed that ascorbic acid increases the incorporation of [^{3}H]thymidine in monolayer and organ culture of rabbit chondrocytes. McDevitt *et al.*[82] found that ascorbic acid increases the amount of radiosulfate incorporated into GAGs. Ascorbic acid is, in general, an essential co-factor for matrix synthesis and is required for collagen secretion.

In chick limb buds plated in micromass culture, ascorbic acid mediates mineralization.[114] This phenomenon was confirmed on chick embryo sternal chondrocytes, where the cells required ascorbate for the induction of alkaline phosphatase and type X collagen.

Many studies have looked at vitamin D_3 and its physiological metabolites (24,25$(OH)_2$-D_3 and 1,25$(OH)_2$-D_3). The latter increased the content of DNA in growth-plate chondrocytes.[131] The effects of vitamin D metabolites on the growth of various types of chondrocytes have been confirmed by several authors.[132,133] In fact this action is dose dependent: stimulatory at low concentrations (10^{-12} M) and inhibitory at high (10^{-8} M) concentrations.[134] Vitamin D_3 metabolites stimulated proteoglycan synthesis by rabbit chondrocytes[131,135] but decreased alkaline phosphatase activity.[131,136]

It is well known that vitamin A inhibits chondrogenesis.[137,138] As vitamin A is the most important of the retinoids, its study led to the study of these drugs. Retinoids inhibit the proliferation of chondrocytes; however, biphasic dose-dependent effects of retinoic acid were observed.[139,140] The effects of vitamin A and retinoids on matrix molecules are important. Sternal chondrocytes cultured in the presence of vitamin A produce smaller proteoglycans, which are released and degraded more rapidly.[141, 142] The profile of GAGs produced by chondrocytes from rat cartilage, when grown in the presence of retinoids, resembles that of fibroblasts.[143]

Retinoic acid treatment of rabbit articular chondrocytes leads to the complete loss of type II collagen synthesis and the induction of type I trimer collagen, in parallel with an eightfold decrease in collagen and proteoglycan synthesis.[144] Modulation of the phenotype is dose dependent and is correlated with an alteration in cell morphology. Such cells have been described as 'fibroblast-like' in appearance. In summary, retinoids appear to contribute to cartilage destruction by increasing the turnover of matrix molecules and provoking the synthesis of abnormal matrix components.

D. Anti-inflammatory drugs

Most of the papers on anti-inflammatory drugs concern the action of non-steroidal agents. Indomethacin, acetylsalicylate and naproxen reduce the proliferation of articular chondrocytes in monolayer or three-dimensional culture.[145–150] In contrast, at concentrations similar to those found in plasma, clear inhibition of proteoglycan synthesis is observed.[151,152] However, a stimulatory action on proteoglycan synthesis has been described for benoxaprofen,[153] piroxicam, niflumic acid[154,155] and ketoprofen, but only on explant from young human articular cartilage.

High concentrations of non-steroidal drugs inhibit collagen synthesis[156–158] and type II collagen gene expression.[159] More recent studies have examined the effects of non-steroidal anti-inflammatory drugs on both proteoglycan matrix breakdown and on metalloprotease synthesis.[160] In comparison, more and more reports have investigated the effects of new antirheumatic agents on chondrocytes in primary culture (monolayer or three-dimensional culture) which have been stimulated by human recombinant IL-1, which induces proteoglycans depletion.[161]

E. Anti-osteoarthritic drugs

Bassleer *et al.*,[162] using cultures of aggregated cells, demonstrated that a peptidic glycosaminoglycan (PGAG) complex, isolated from calf cartilage and bone marrow, stimulated proliferation and production of matrix components (type II collagen and proteoglycans). On high-density culture of human chondrocytes originating from osteoarthritic articulations, Harmand *et al.*[163] showed that adenosylmethionine induced a higher rate of synthesis of proteins and proteoglycans. These drugs may thus have chondroprotective properties.

A derivative of hyaluronic acid (Hylan) reduces proteoglycan depletion in isolated chondrocytes exposed to IL-1.[164] It has also been shown that hyaluronan decreases the production of prostaglandin E_2.[165]

Extracts of avocado and soya bean seem to limit the deleterious effects of IL-1 in osteoarticular diseases[166] and stimulate matrix synthesis.[167]

F. Various toxic drugs for cartilaginous tissue

Among antibacterial drugs, quinolones appear to damage the articular cartilage of immature animals. Several experiments have been performed on various types of limb-bud culture.[168] Ofloxacin inhibited proteoglycan and collagen type II synthesis in murine cartilage organoid culture.[169] The mechanism of this toxic action is not understood. Recently, Thuong-Guyot *et al.*[170] demonstrated that various fluoroquinolones induce an early stimulation of oxidative metabolism in immature rabbit cultured articular chondrocytes.

In contrast, the effect of gallium nitrate on alkaline phosphatase activity was studied in a differentiating chick limb-bud mesenchymal cell culture. Cultures maintained in media containing gallium nitrate showed drastically decreased alkaline phophatase activity.[171]

Finally, the anticonvulsant drug, valproic acid, which is known to be teratogenic in humans, decreased mitotic activity and extracellular matrix production in human chondrocytes cultured in a three-dimensional agarose gel.[172]

V. CONCLUSION

Chondrocyte culture is an efficient target system for evaluation of the pharmacological and toxicological effects of drugs acting on cartilaginous tissue. Many types of culture exist and have their own advantages and drawbacks. For example, in monolayer culture chondrocytes do not retain all of their specific functions. Cartilage slices and three-dimensional culture maintain chondrocytes in a differentiated state but without noticeable cell division. Therefore, it is necessary to choose the type of culture relevant to the pharmacological and toxicological end-point being considered.

Anti-inflammatory and antiosteoarthritic drugs have been especially studied on cultured chondrocytes. Moreover, several toxic drugs for cartilaginous tissue have been explored in these *in vitro* models. Study of the interactions of growth factors, cytokines and vitamins with cartilage should permit an increase in our knowledge of the complex regulations of chondrocytes and open the way to the development of new antirheumatic drugs. It appears obvious that chondrocyte culture already belongs to the group of specialized cultures for use in a complete toxicological study.

ACKNOWLEDGEMENTS

The authors wish to thank Evelyne Derguy for typing the manuscript. Laurence Borge, Christiane Hecquet, Carine Nizard, Laurent Pascual Le Tallec and Patrice Penfornis are also warmly acknowledged for their contribution to the preparation of this chapter.

REFERENCES

1. Heinegard, D. and Paulsson, M. (1987) Cartilage. *Methods Enzymol.* **145:** 336–363.
2. Greenwald, A. S. and Haynes, D. W. (1979) A pathway for nutriments from the medullary cavity to articular of the femoral head. *J. Bone Joint Surg.* **51B:** 747–753.
3. Kember, N. F. (1960) Cell division in endochondral ossification: a study of cell proliferation in rat bones by the method of tritiated thymidine autoradiography. *J. Bone Joint Surg. [Br.]* **42:** 824–839.
4. Brighton, C. T. and Heppenstall, R. B. (1971) Oxygen tension in zones of the epiphyseal plate, the metaphysis, and diaphysis. An *in vitro* and *in vivo* study in rabbits. *J. Bone Joint Surg.* **53:** 719–728.
5. Buckwalter, J. A., Mower, D., Ungar, R., Scheaffer, J. and Ginsberg, B. (1986) Morphometric analysis of chondrocyte hypertrophy. *J. Bone Joint Surg.* **68:** 243–255.

6. Farnum, C. E. and Wilsman, N. J. (1987) Morphologic stages of the terminal hyperthrophic chondrocytes of growth plate cartilage. *Anat. Rec.* **219:** 221–232.
7. Roach, H. I. (1992) Trans-differentiation of hypertrophic chondrocytes into cells capable of producing a mineralized bone matrix. *Bone Miner.* **19:** 1–20.
8. Mankin, H. J. (1963) Localization of tritiated thymidine in articular cartilage of rabbits. III. Mature articular cartilage. *J. Bone Joint Surg.* **45:** 529–540.
9. Kunz, J., Welmitz, G., Paul, U. and Fuhrmann, I. (1979) Histoautoradiographic studies on chondrocyte proliferation in healing of experimental cartilage injuries. *Zentralbl. Allg. Pathol.* **123:** 539–549.
10. Mayne, R. and Irwin, M. H. (1986) Collagen types in cartilage. In Kuettner, K. E., Scheyerback, R. and Hascall, V. C. (eds) *Articular Cartilage Biochemistry*, pp. 23–35. Raven Press, New York.
11. Carney, S. L. and Muir, H. (1988) The structure and function of cartilage proteoglycans. *Physiol. Rev.* **68:** 858–910.
12. Scott, J. E. (1988) Proteoglycan-fibrillar collagen interactions. *Biochem. J.* **252:** 313–323.
13. Maroudas, A. (1979) Physico-chemical properties of articular cartilage. In Freeman, M. A. R. (ed.) *Adult Articular Cartilage*, pp. 215–290. Pitman Medical, Tunbridge Wells, UK.
14. Greulich, R. C. and Leblond, C. P. (1953) Radioautographic visualisation of radiocarbon in the organs and tissues of newborn rats following administration of ^{14}C labeled bicarbonate. *Anat. Rec.* **115:** 559–585.
15. Bélanger, L. F. (1954) Autoradiographic visualization of the entry and transit of 35S in cartilage, bone, and dentine of young rats and the effect of hyaluronidase *in vitro*. *Can. J. Physiol. Biochem.* **32:** 161–169.
16. Mayne, R. (1989) Cartilage collagens. What is their function, and are they involved in articular disease? *Arthritis Rheum.* **32:** 241–246.
17. Mendler, M., Eich-Bender, S. G., Vaughan, L., Winterhalter, K. H. and Bruckner, P. (1989) Cartilage contains mixed fibrils of collagen types II, IX and XI. *J. Cell Biol.* **108:** 191–197.
18. Petit, B., Freyria, A. M., Van Der Rest, M. and Herbage, D. (1992) Cartilage Collagens. In Adolphe, M. (ed.) *Biological Regulation of the Chondrocytes*, pp. 33–84. CRC Press, Boca Raton, FL.
19. Eikenberry, E. F., Mendler, M., Burgin, R., Winterhalter, K. H. and Bruckner, P. (1992) Fibrillar organization in cartilage. In Kuettner, K. E., Schleyerbach, R., Peyron, J. G. and Hascall, V. C. (eds) *Articular Cartilage and Osteoarthritis*, pp. 133–149. Raven Press, New York.
20. Vaughan, L., Mendler, M., Bruckner, P., Winterhalter, K. H., Irwin, M. H. and Mayne, R. (1988) D-Periodic distribution of collagen type IX along cartilage fibrils. *J. Cell Biol.* **106:** 991–997.
21. Schmid, T. M. and Linsenmayer, T. F. (1985) Immunohistochemical localization of short-chain cartilage collagen (type X) in avian tissues. *J. Cell Biol.* **100:** 598–605.
22. Schmid, T. M. and Linsenmayer, T. F. (1987) Type X collagen. In Mayne, R. and Burgeson, R. E. (eds) *Structure and Function of Collagen Types*, pp. 223–259. Academic Press, New York.
23. Hardingham, T. E., Beardmore-Grey, M., Dunham, D. G. and Ratcliffe, A. (1986) Cartilage proteoglycans. *Ciba Found. Symp.* **124:** 30–46.
24. Heinegard, D. and Oldberg, A. (1989) Structure and biology of cartilage and bone matrix noncollagenous macromolecules. *FASEB J.* **3:** 2042–2051.
25. Hardingham, T. E. and Fosang, A. J. (1992) Proteoglycans: many forms and many functions. *FASEB J.* **6:** 861–870.
26. Buckwalter, J. A. and Rosenburg, L. C. (1983) Structural changes during development in bovine fetal epiphyseal cartilage. *Coll. Relat. Res.* **3:** 489–504.
27. Hardingham, T. E. and Bayliss, M. (1990) Proteoglycans of articular cartilage: changes in aging and joint disease *Sem. Arthritis Rheum.* **20:** 12–33.
28. Thomas, J. T., Ayad, S. and Grant, M. E. (1994) Cartilage collagens: strategies for the study of their organisation and expression in the extracellular matrix. *Ann. Rheum. Dis.* **53:** 488–496.
29. Väänänan, H. K. (1980) Immunohistochemical localization of alkaline phosphatase in the chicken epiphyseal growth cartilage. *Histochemistry* **65:** 143–148.
30. De Bernard, B., Bianco, P., Bonucci, E. *et al.* (1986) Biochemical and immunohistochemical evidence that in cartilage an alkaline phosphatase is a Ca^{2+}-binding glycoprotein. *J. Cell Biol.* **103:** 1615–1623.
31. Tyler, J. A. (1991) Cartilage degradation. In Hall, B. and Newman, S. (eds) *Cartilage: Molecular Aspects*, pp. 213–256. CRC Press, Boca Raton, FL.
32. Lotz, M. (1992) Regulation of chondrocytes in aging. In Adolphe, M. (ed.) *Biological Regulation of the Chondrocytes*, pp. 237–274. CRC Press, Boca Raton, FL.

33. Thonar, J. M. A., Bjornsson, S. and Kuettner, K. E. (1986) Age-related changes in cartilage proteoglycans. In Kuettner, K. E., Scheyerback, R. and Hascall, V. C. (eds) *Articular Cartilage Biochemistry*, pp. 273–288. Raven Press, New York.
34. Malemud, C. J. and Hering, T. M. (1992) Regulation of chondrocytes in osteoarthrosis. In Adolphe, M. (ed.) *Biological Regulation of the Chondrocyte*, pp. 295–319. CRC Press, Boca Raton, FL.
35. Bayliss, M. T. (1986) Proteoglycan structure in normal and osteoarthritic human cartilage. In Kuettner, K. E., Scheyerback, R. and Hascall, V. C. (eds) *Articular Cartilage Biochemistry*, pp. 295–310. Raven Press, New York.
36. Aydelotte, M. B., Raiss, R. X., Caterson, B. and Kuettner, K. E. (1992) Influence of interleukin-1 on the morphology and proteoglycan metabolism of cultured bovine articular chondrocytes. *Connect. Tissue Res.* **28:** 143–159.
37. Martel-Pelletier, J., Pelletier, J. P., Cloutier, J. M., Rebert, N. and Malemud, C. J. (1992) Proteoglycan structural changes in rheumatoid articular cartilage. *Clin. Exp. Rheumatol.* **10:** 151–159.
38. Goldring, M. B., Birkhead, J. R., Suen, L. F. *et al.* (1994) Interleukin-1 beta-modulated gene expression in immortalized human chondrocytes. *J. Clin. Invest.* **94:** 2307–2316.
39. Jennings, S. D. and Ham, R. G. (1983) Clonal growth of primary culture of rabbit ear chondrocytes in a lipid-supplemented defined medium. *Exp. Cell Res.* **145:** 415–423.
40. Adolphe, M., Froger, B., Ronot, X., Corvol, M. T. and Forest, N. (1984) Cell multiplication and type II collagen production by rabbit articular chondrocytes cultivated in a defined medium. *Exp. Cell Res.* **155:** 527–536.
41. Kato, Y. and Gospodarowicz, D. (1985) Effects of exogenous extracellular matrices on proteoglycan synthesis by cultured rabbit costal chondrocytes. *J. Cell Biol.* **100:** 486–495.
42. Handley, C. J., Ng, C. K. and Curtis, A. J. (1990) Short and long-term explant culture of cartilage. In Kuettner, K. and Maroudas, A. (eds) *Methods in Cartilage Research*, pp. 105–110. Academic Press, London.
43. Green, W. T. (1971) Behavior of articular chondrocytes in cell culture. *Clin. Orthop.* **75:** 248–260.
44. Ronot, X., Hecquet, C., Jaffray, P. *et al.* (1983) Proliferation kinetics of rabbit articular chondrocytes in primary culture and at the first passage. *Cell Tissue Kinet.* **16:** 531–537.
45. Moskalewski, S., Adamiec, I. and Golaszewska, A. (1979) Maturation of rabbit articular chondrocytes grown *in vitro* in monolayer culture. *Am. J. Anat.* **155:** 339–348.
46. Evans, C. H. and Georgescu, H. I. (1983) Observations on the senescence of cells derived from articular cartilage. *Mech. Ageing Dev.* **22:** 179–191.
47. Dominice, J., Levasseur, C., Larno, S., Ronot, X. and Adolphe, M. (1986) Age-related changes in rabbit articular chondrocytes. *Mech. Ageing Dev.* **37:** 231–240.
48. Benya, P. D., Padilla, S. R. and Nimni, M. E. (1977) The progeny of rabbit articular chondrocytes synthesize collagen types I and III and type I trimer, but not type II. Verifications by cyanogen bromide peptide analysis. *Biochemistry* **16:** 865–872.
49. Von Der Mark, K., Gauss, V., Von Der Mark, H. and Muller, P. (1977) Relationship between cell shape and type of collagen synthesized as chondrocytes lose their cartilage phenotype in culture. *Nature* **267:** 531–532.
50. Benya, P. D. and Padilla, S. R. (1993) Dihydrocytochalasin B enhances transforming growth factor-beta-induced reexpression of the differentiated chondrocytes phenotype without stimulation of collagen synthesis. *Exp. Cell Res.* **204:** 268–277.
51. Benya, P. D. and Padilla, S. R. (1990) Staurosporine, an inhibitor of protein kinase C, enhances reexpression of the differentiated chondrocyte collagen phenotype. *Trans. Orthop. Res. Soc.* **15:** 183.
52. Benya, P. D. and Shaffer, J. D. (1982) Dedifferentiated chondrocytes reexpress the differentiated collagen phenotype when cultured in agarose gels. *Cell* **30:** 215–224.
53. Horwitz, A. I. and Dorfman, A. (1970) The growth of cartilage cells in soft agar and liquid suspension. *J. Cell Biol.* **45:** 434–439.
54. Gibson, G. J., Schor, S. L. and Grant, M. E. (1982) Effects of matrix macromolecules on chondrocyte gene expression: synthesis of a low molecular weight collagen species by cells cultured within collagen gels. *J. Cell Biol.* **93:** 767–774.
55. Yasui, N., Osawa, S., Ochi, T., Nakashima, H. and Ono, K. (1982) Primary culture of chondrocytes embedded in collagen gels. *Exp. Cell Biol.* **50:** 92–100.
56. Guo, J., Jourdian, G. W. and MacCallum, D. K. (1989) Culture and growth characteristics of chondrocytes encapsulated in alginate beads. *Connect. Tissue Res.* **19:** 277–297.

57. Häuselmann, H. J., Aydelotte, M. B., Schumacher, B. L., Kuettner, K. E., Gitelis, S. H. and Thonar, J.-M. A. (1992) Synthesis and turnover of proteoglycans by human and bovine adult articular chondrocytes cultured in alginate beads. *Matrix* **12:** 116–129.
58. Häuselmann, H. J., Fernandes, R. J., Mok, S. S. *et al.* (1994) Phenotype stability of bovine articular chondrocytes after long-term culture in alginate beads. *J. Cell Sci.* **107:** 17–27.
59. Grandolfo, M., D'Andra, P., Paoletti, S. *et al.* (1993) Culture and differentiation of chondrocytes entrapped in alginate gels. *Calcif. Tissue Int.* **52:** 42–48.
60. Bonaventure, J., Kakhom, N., Cohen-Solal, L. *et al.* (1994) Reexpression of cartilage-specific genes by dedifferentiated human articular chondrocytes cultured in alginate beads. *Exp. Cell Res.* **212:** 97–104.
61. Deshmukh, K. and Kline, W.H. (1976) Characterization of collagen and its precursors synthesized by rabbit articular cartilage cells in various culture systems. *Eur. J. Biochem.* **69:** 117–123.
62. Wiebkin, O.W. and Muir, H. (1977) Synthesis of cartilage specific proteoglycan by suspension culture of adult chondrocytes. *Biochem. J.* **164:** 269–272.
63. Dozin, B., Quarto, R., Rossi, F. and Cancedda, R. (1990) Stabilization of the mRNA follows transcriptional activation of type II collagen in differentiating chicken chondrocytes. *J. Biol. Chem.* **265:** 7216–7220.
64. Handley, C. J. and Lowther, D. A. (1979) Extracellular matrix metabolism by chondrocytes. V. The proteoglycans and the glycosaminoglycans synthesized by chondrocytes in high-density cultures. *Biochim. Biophys. Acta* **582:** 234–239.
65. Umansky, R. (1966) The effects of cell population density on the developmental fate of reaggregating mouse limb bud mesenchyme. *Dev. Biol.* **13:** 31–56.
66. Flint, O. P. and Orton, T. C. (1984) An *in vitro* assay for teratogens with cultures of rat embryo mid-brain and limb bud cells. *Toxicol. Appl. Pharmacol.* **76:** 383–385.
67. Takigawa, M., Tajima, K., Pan, H. O. *et al.* (1989) Establishment of a clonal human chondrosarcoma cell line with cartilage phenotypes. *Cancer Res.* **49:** 3996–4002.
68. Gionti, E., Pontarelli, G. and Cancedda, R. (1985) Avian myelocytomatosis virus immortalizes differentiated quail chondrocytes. *Proc. Natl Acad. Sci. U.S.A.* **82:** 2756–2760.
69. Horton, W. E., Cleveland, J., Rapp, U. *et al.* (1988) An established rat cell line expressing chondrocyte properties. *Exp. Cell Res.* **178:** 457–468.
70. Gionti, E., Julien, P., Pontarelli, G. and Sanchez, M. (1989) A continuous cell line of chicken embryo cells derived from a chondrocyte culture infected with RSV. *Cell Differ.* **27:** 215–223.
71. Thenet, S., Benya, P. D., Demignot, S., Feunteun, J. and Adolphe, M. (1992) SV40-immortalization of rabbit articular chondrocytes. Alteration of differentiated functions. *J. Cell. Physiol.* **150:** 158–167.
72. Mallein-Gerin, F. and Olsen, B. R. (1993) Expression of simian virus 40 large T (tumor) oncogene in mouse chondrocytes induces cell proliferation without loss of the differentiated phenotype. *Proc. Natl Acad. Sci. U.S.A.* **90:** 3289–3293.
73. Vincent, F., Brun, H., Clain, E., Ronot, X. and Adolphe, M. (1989) Effects of oxygen-free radicals on proliferation kinetics of cultured rabbit articular chondrocytes. *J. Cell. Physiol.* **141:** 262–266.
74. Vincent, F., Corral, M., Defer, N. and Adolphe, M. (1991) Effects of oxygen-free radicals on articular chondrocytes in culture: C-*myc* and C-Ha-*ras* messenger RNAs and proliferation kinetics. *Exp. Cell Res.* **192:** 333–339.
75. Lev, R. and Spicer, S. S. (1964) Specific staining of sulfate groups with alcian blue at low pH. *J. Histochem. Cytochem.* **12:** 309.
76. Ahrens, P. B., Solursh, M. and Reiter, R. S. (1977) Stage-related capacity for limb chondrogenesis in cell culture. *Dev. Biol.* **60:** 69–82.
77. Paulsen, D. F. and Solurch, M. (1988) Microtiter micromass cultures of limb-bud mesenchymal cells. *In Vitro Cell. Dev. Biol.* **24:** 138–147.
78. Aydelotte, M. B., Greenhill, R. R. and Kuettner, K. E. (1988) Differences between sub-populations of cultured bovine articular chondrocytes. II. Proteoglycan metabolism. *Connect. Tissue Res.* **18:** 223–234.
79. Masuda, K., Shirota, H. and Thonar, E. J.-M. A. (1994) Quantification of ^{35}S-labeled proteoglycan complexed to alcian blue by rapid filtration in multiwell plates. *Anal. Biochem.* **217:** 167–175.
80. Heinegard, D. and Sommarin, Y. (1987) Isolation and characterization of proteoglycans. *Methods Enzymol.* **144:** 319–372.
81. Campbell, M. A., Handley, C. J., Hascall, V. C., Campbell, R. A. and Lowther, D. A. (1984) Turnover of proteoglycans in cultures of bovine articular cartilage. *Arch. Biochem. Biophys.* **234:** 275–289.

82. McDevitt, C. A., Lipman, J. M., Ruemer, R. J. and Sokoloff, L. (1988) Stimulation of matrix formation in rabbit chondrocyte cultures by ascorbate. II. Characterization of proteoglycan. *J. Orthop. Res.* **6:** 518–523.
83. Kimura, J. H., Shinomura, T. and Thonar, J.-M. A. (1987) Biosynthesis of cartilage proteoglycan and link protein. *Methods Enzymol.* **144:** 372–393.
84. Kimura, J. H. and Kuettner, K. E. (1986) Studies on the synthesis and assembly of cartilage proteoglycan. In Kuettner, K. E., Schleyerbach, R. and Hascall, V. C. (eds) *Articular Cartilage Biochemistry*, pp. 113–124. Raven Press, New York.
85. Kimura, J. H., Hardingham, T. E. and Hascall, V. C. (1980) Assembly of newly synthesized proteoglycan and link protein into aggregates in cultures of chondrosarcoma chondrocytes. *J. Biol. Chem.* **255:** 7134–7143.
86. Sambrook, J., Fritsch, E. F. and Maniatis, T. (1989) *Molecular Cloning: A Laboratory Manual*, 2nd edn. Cold Spring Harbor Laboratory Press, Cold Spring Harbor.
87. Doege, K., Fernandez, P., Hassel, J. R., Sazaki, M. and Yamada, Y. (1986) Partial cDNA sequence encoding a glomerular domain at the C terminus of the rat cartilage proteoglycan. *J. Biol. Chem.* **261:** 8108–8111.
88. Doege, K. J., Sasaki, M., Kimura, T. and Yamada, Y. (1991) Complete coding sequence and deduced primary structure of the human cartilage large aggregating proteoglycan, aggrecan. *J. Biol. Chem.* **266:** 894–902.
89. Li, H., Schwartz, N. B. and Vertel, B. M. (1993) cDNA cloning of chick cartilage chondroitin sulfate (Aggrecan) core protein and identification of a stop codon in the aggrecan gene associated with the chondrodystrophy, nanomelia. *J. Biol. Chem.* **268:** 23 504–23 511.
90. Glumoff, V., Savontaus, M., Vehanen, J. and Vuorio, E. (1994) Analysis of aggrecan and tenascin gene expression in mouse skeletal tissues by Northern and *in situ* hybridization using species specific cDNA probes. *Biochim. Biophys. Acta* **1219:** 613–622.
91. Doege, K., Hassel, J. R., Caterson, B. and Yamada, Y. (1986) Link protein cDNA sequence reveals a tandemly repeated protein structure. *Proc. Natl Acad. Sci. U.S.A.* **83:** 3761–3765.
92. Dudhia, J., Bayliss, M. T. and Hardingham, T. E. (1994) Human link protein gene: structure and transcription pattern in chondrocytes. *Biochem. J.* **303:** 329–333.
93. Peterkofsky, B. and Diegelmann, R. (1971) Use of a mixture of proteinase-free collagenases for the specific assay of radioactive collagen in the presence of other proteins. *Biochemistry* **10:** 988–994.
94. Diegelmann, R. F., Bryson, G. R., Flood, L. C. and Graham, M. F. (1990) A microassay to quantitate collagen synthesis by cells in culture. *Anal. Biochem.* **186:** 296–300.
95. Scutt, A., Berg, A. and Mayer, H. (1992) A semiautomated, 96-well plate assay for collagen synthesis. *Anal. Biochem.* **203:** 290–294.
96. Ricard-Blum, S., Ville, G. and Hartmann, D. J. (1988) Use of the Pharmacia Phast System for sodium dodecyl sulfate polyacrylamide gel electrophoresis of non-globular proteins: application to collagens. *J. Chromatogr.* **431:** 474–476.
97. Rennard, S. I., Berg, R., Martin, G. R., Foidart, J. M. and Gehron Robey, P. (1980) Enzyme-linked immunoassay (ELISA) for connective tissue components. *Anal. Biochem.* **104:** 205–214.
98. Zlabinger, G. J., Menzel, J. E. and Steffen, C. (1988) Determination of collagen in culture supernatants of human chondrocytes. *Agents Actions* **23:** 45–47.
99. Harrison, E. T., Luyten, F. P. and Reddi, A. H. (1992) Transforming growth factor-beta: its effect on phenotype reexpression by dedifferentiated chondrocytes in the presence and absence of osteogenin. *In Vitro Cell. Dev. Biol.* **28A:** 445–448.
100. Elima, K., Mäkelä, J. K., Vuorio, T., Kauppinen, S., Knowles, J. and Vuorio, E. (1985) Construction and identification of a cDNA clone for human type II procollagen mRNA. *Biochem. J.* **229:** 183–188.
101. Metsäranta, M., Toman, D., De Combrugghe, B. and Vuorio, E. (1991) Specific hybridization probes for mouse type I, II, III and IX collagen mRNAs. *Biochim. Biophys. Acta* **1089:** 241–243.
102. Mäkelä, J. K., Raassina, M., Virta, A. and Vuorio, E. (1988) Human proα_1(I) collagen: cDNA sequence for the C-propeptide domain. *Nucl. Acids Res.* **16:** 349.
103. Apte, S. S., Seldin, M. F., Hayashi, M. and Olsen, B. R. (1992) Cloning of the human and mouse type X collagen genes and mapping of the mouse type X collagen gene to chromosome 10. *Eur. J. Biochem.* **206:** 217–224.
104. Habuchi, H., Conrad, H. E. and Glaser, J. H. (1985) Coordinate regulation of collagen and alkaline phosphatase levels in chick embryo chondrocytes. *J. Biol. Chem.* **260:** 13 029–13 034.

105. Pacifici, M., Golden, E. B., Iwamoto, M. and Adams, S. L. (1991) Retinoic acid treatment induces type X collagen gene expression in cultured chick chondrocytes. *Exp. Cell Res.* **195:** 38–46.
106. Iwamoto, M., Golden, E. B., Adams, S. L., Noji, S. and Pacifici, M. (1993) Responsiveness to retinoic acid changes during chondrocyte maturation. *Exp. Cell Res.* **205:** 213–224.
107. Tacchetti, C., Quarto, R., Campanile, G. and Cancedda, R. (1989) Calcification of *in vitro* developed hypertrophic cartilage. *Dev. Biol.* **132:** 442–447.
108. Kato, Y. and Gospodarowicz, D. (1985) Sulfated proteoglycan synthesis by confluent cultures of rabbit costal chondrocytes grown in the presence of fibroblast growth factor. *J. Cell Biol.* **100:** 477–485.
109. Nataf, V., Tsagris, L., Dumontier, M. F., Bonaventure, J. and Corvol, M. (1990) Modulation of sulfated proteoglycan synthesis and collagen gene expression by chondrocytes grown in the presence of bFGF alone or combined with IGF1. *Reprod. Nutr. Dev.* **30:** 331–342.
110. Trippel, S. B., Corvol, M. T., Dumontier, M. F., Rappaport, R., Hung, H. H. and Mankin, H. J. (1989) Effect of somatomedin-C/insulin-like growth factor 1 and growth hormone on cultured growth plate and articular chondrocytes. *Pediatr. Res.* **25:** 76–82.
111. Guerne, P. A., Sublet, A. and Lotz, M. (1994) Growth factor responsiveness of human articular chondrocytes: distinct profiles in primary chondrocytes, subcultured chondrocytes, and fibroblasts. *J. Cell. Physiol.* **158:** 476–484.
112. Luyten, F. P., Hascall, V. C., Nissley, S. P., Morales, T. I. and Reddi, A. H. (1988) Insulin-like growth factors maintain steady-state metabolism of proteoglycans in bovine articular cartilage explants. *Arch. Biochem. Biophys.* **267:** 416–425.
113. Schalkwijk, J., Joosten, L. A., Van der Berg, W. B., Van Wyk, J. J. and Van de Putte, L. B. (1989) Insulin-like growth factor stimulation of chondrocyte proteoglycan synthesis by human synovial fluid. *Arthritis Rheum.* **32:** 66–71.
114. Boskey, A. L., Stiner, D., Doty, S. B. and Binderman, I. (1991) Requirement of vitamin C for cartilage calcification in a differentiating chick limb-bud mesenchymal cell culture. *Bone* **12:** 277–282.
115. Frazer, A., Bunning, R. A. and Russel, R. G. (1994) Effects of transforming growth factor beta and interleukin-1 beta on ^{3}H thymidine incorporation by human articular chondrocyte *in vitro*. *Biochim. Biophys. Acta* **1226:** 193–200.
116. Vivien, D., Galéra, P., Lebrun, E., Loyau, G. and Pujol, J. P. (1990) Differential effects of transforming growth factor-beta and epidermal growth factor on the cell cycle of cultured rabbit articular chondrocytes. *J. Cell. Physiol.* **143:** 534–545.
117. Brenner, R. E., Nerlich, A., Heinze, E., Vetter, U. and Teller, W. M. (1993) Different regulation of clonal growth by transforming growth factor-beta 1 in human fetal articular and costal chondrocytes. *Pediatr. Res.* **33:** 390–393.
118. Lafeber, F. P., Van der Kraan, P. M., Huber-Bruning, O., Van den Berg, W. B. and Bijlsma, J. W. (1993) Osteoarthritic human cartilage is more sensitive to transforming growth factor beta than in normal cartilage. *Br. J. Rheumatol.* **32:** 281–286.
119. Glansbeek, H. L., Van Der Kraan, P. M., Vitters, E. L. and Van Den Berg, W. B. (1993) Correlation of the size of type II transforming growth factor beta (TGF-beta) receptor with TGF-beta responses of isolated bovine articular chondrocytes. *Ann. Rheum. Dis.* **52:** 812–816.
120. Galéra, P., Viven, D., Pronost, S. *et al.* (1992) Transforming growth factor-beta 1 (TGF-beta 1) up-regulation of collagen type II in primary cultures of rabbit articular chondrocytes (RAC) involves increased mRNA levels without affecting mRNA stability and procollagen processing. *J. Cell. Physiol.* **153:** 596–606.
121. Loveys, L. S., Gelb, D., Hurwitz, S. R., Puzas, J. E. and Rosier, R. N. (1993) Effects of parathyroid hormone-related peptide on chick growth plate chondrocytes. *J. Orthop. Res.* **11:** 884–891.
122. Mitchell, P. G. and Cheung, H. S. (1991) Tumor necrosis factor alpha and epidermal growth factor regulation of collagenase and stromelysin in adult porcine articular chondrocytes. *J. Cell. Physiol.* **149:** 132–140.
123. Mitchell, P. G. and Cheung, H. S. (1993) Protein kinase regulation of tumor necrosis factor alpha stimulated collagenase and stromelysin message levels in chondrocytes. *Biochem. Biophys. Res. Commun.* **196:** 1133–1142.
124. Ogata, Y., Pratta, M. A., Nagase, H. and Arner, E. C. (1992) Matrix metalloproteinase 9 (92-kDa gelatinase/type IV collagenase) is induced in rabbit articular chondrocytes by cotreatment with interleukin 1 beta and a protein kinase C activator. *Exp. Cell Res.* **201:** 245–249.

125. Smith, R. J., Justen, J. M., Ulrich, R. G., Lund, J. E. and Sam, L. M. (1992) Induction of neutral proteinase and prostanoid production in bovine nasal chondrocytes by interleukin-1 and tumor necrosis factor alpha: modulation of these cellular responses by interleukin-6 and platelet-derived growth factor. *Clin. Immunol. Immunopathol.* **64:** 135–144.
126. Enomoto, M., Pan, H. O., Kinoshita, A., Yutani, Y., Suzuki, F. and Takigawa, M. (1990) Effects of tumor necrosis factor alpha on proliferation and expression of differentiated phenotypes in rabbit costal chondrocytes in culture. *Calcif. Tissue Int.* **47:** 145–151.
127. Malfait, A. M., Verbruggen, G., Veys, E. M., Lambert, J., De Ridder, L. and Cornelissen, M. (1994) Comparative and combined effects of interleukin 6, interleukin 1 beta, and tumor necrosis factor alpha on proteoglycan metabolism of human articular chondrocytes cultured in agarose. *J. Rheumatol.* **21:** 314–320.
128. Chandrasekhar, S., Harvey, A. K., Higginbotham, J. D. and Horton, W. E. (1990) Interleukin-1-induced suppression of type II collagen gene transcription involves DNA regulatory elements. *Exp. Cell Res.* **191:** 105–114.
129. Lefevre, V., Peeters-Joris, C. and Vaes, G. (1990) Modulation by interleukin 1 and tumor necrosis factor alpha of production of collagenase, tissue inhibitor of metalloproteinase and collagen types in differentiated and dedifferentiated articular chondrocytes. *Biochim. Biophys. Acta* **1052:** 366–378.
130. Krystal, G., Morris, C. M. and Sokoloff, L. (1982) Stimulation of DNA synthesis by ascorbate in cultures of articular chondrocytes. *Arthritis Rheum.* **25:** 318–325.
131. Kato, Y., Shimazu, A., Iwamoto, M. *et al.* (1990) Role of 1,25-dihydroxycholecalciferol in growth-plate cartilage: inhibition of terminal differentiation of chondrocytes *in vitro* and *in vivo*. *Proc. Natl Acad. Sci. U.S.A.* **87:** 6522–6526.
132. Sato, K., Iwamoto, M., Nakashima, K., Suzuki, F. and Kato, Y. (1990) 1 alpha, 25-dihydroxyvitamin D_3 stimulates colony formation of chick embryo chondrocytes in soft agar. *Exp. Cell Res.* **187:** 335–338.
133. Takano-Yamamoto, T., Soma, S., Kyung, H. M., Nakagawa, K., Yamashiro, T. and Sakuda, M. (1992) Differential effects of 1 alpha, 25-dihydroxycholecalciferol and 24R, 25-dihydroxycholecalciferol on the proliferation and the differentiated phenotype of rabbit craniofacial chondrocytes in primary culture. *J. Osaka Univ. Dent. Sch.* **32:** 51–59.
134. Klaus, G., Konig, B., Hügel, U., Ritz, E. and Mehls, O. (1993) Intermittent and continuous exposure to $1,25(OH)_2D_3$ have different effects on growth plate chondrocytes. *Kidney Int.* **44:** 708–715.
135. Corvol, M. T., Dumontier, M. F., Tsagris, L., Lang, F. and Bourgignon, J. (1981) Cartilage and vitamin D *in vitro*. *Ann. Endocrinol.* **42:** 482–485.
136. Kyung, H. M., Takano-Yamamoto, T., Soma, S. and Sakuda, M. (1992) Stimulation of alkaline phosphatase activity by ascorbic acid and suppression by 1,25-dihydroxycholecalciferol in rabbit craniofacial chondrocytes in culture. *J. Osaka Univ. Dent. Sch.* **32:** 60–67.
137. Hassel, J. R., Pennypacker, J. P. and Lewis, O. A. (1978) Chondrogenesis and cell proliferation in limb bud cell cultures treated with cytosine arabinoside and vitamin A. *Exp. Cell Res.* **112:** 409–417.
138. Pacifici, M., Cossu, G., Molinaro, M. and Tato, F. (1980) Vitamin A inhibits chondrogenesis but not myogenesis. *Exp. Cell Res.* **129:** 469–474.
139. Ronot, X., Nafziger, J., Hecquet, C. *et al.* (1985) Retinoic acid: modulating effects on the proliferation kinetics of mastocytes and chondrocytes. *Biol. Cell.* **55:** 5–9.
140. Enomoto, M., Pan, H., Suzuki, F. and Takigawa, M. (1990) Physiological role of vitamin A in growth cartilage cells: low concentrations of retinoic acid strongly promote the proliferation of rabbit costal growth cartilage cells in culture. *J. Biochem.* **107:** 743–748.
141. Vasan, N. S. (1981) Proteoglycan synthesis by sternal chondrocytes perturbed with vitamin A. *J. Embryol. Exp. Morphol.* **63:** 181–191.
142. Lau, W. F., Tertinegg, I. and Heersche, J. N. (1993) Effects of retinoic acid on cartilage differentiation in a chondrogenic cell line. *Teratology.* **47:** 555–563.
143. Shapiro, S. S., Mott, D. J. and Nutley, N. J. (1981) Modulation of glycosaminoglycan biosynthesis by retinoids. *Ann. N.Y. Acad. Sci.* **359:** 306–312.
144. Benya, P. D. and Padilla, S. R. (1986) Modulation of the rabbit chondrocyte phenotype by retinoic acid terminates type II collagen synthesis without inducing type I collagen: the modulated phenotype differs from that produced by subculture. *Dev. Biol.* **118:** 296–305.
145. Kirkpatrick, C. J., Mohr, W., Wildfeuer, A. and Haferkamp, O. (1983) Influence of non steroidal anti-inflammatory agents on lapine articular chondrocyte growth *in vitro*. *J. Rheumatol.* **42:** 58–65.

146. Kato, Y., Iwamoto, M., Nakashima, K., Sato, K., Yan, W. and Koike, T. (1988) Rabbit articular chondrocytes in soft agar are useful to test the effects of non-steroidal anti-inflammatory drugs on chondrocyte replication. *Scand. J. Rheumatol.* **77**: 3–6.
147. Bassleer, C., Henrotin, Y. and Franchimont, P. (1990) *In vitro* assays of chondrocyte functions: the influence of drugs and hormones. *Scand. J. Rheumatol.* **81**: 13–20.
148. Bassleer, C. T., Henrotin, Y. E., Reginster, J. L. and Franchimont, P. P. (1992) Effects of tiaprofenic acid and acetylsalicylic acid on human articular chondrocytes in 3-dimensional culture. *J. Rheumatol.* **19**: 1433–1438.
149. Redini, F., Mauviel, A., Loyau, G. and Pujol, J. P. (1990) Modulation of extracellular matrix metabolism in rabbit articular chondrocytes and human rheumatoid synovial cells by the non-steroidal anti-inflammatory drug etodolac II: glycosaminoglycan synthesis. *Agents Actions* **31**: 358–367.
150. Collier, S. and Ghosh, P. (1991) Comparison of the effects of non-steroidal anti-inflammatory drugs (NSAIDs) on proteoglycan synthesis by articular cartilage explant and chondrocyte monolayer cultures. *Biochem. Pharmacol.* **41**: 1375–1384.
151. Palmoski, M. J. and Brandt, K. D. (1979) Effect of salicylate on proteoglycan metabolism in normal canine articular cartilage *in vitro*. *Arthritis Rheum.* **22**: 746–754.
152. Palmoski, M. J. and Brandt, K. D. (1983) Relationship between matrix proteoglycan content and the effects of salicylate and indomethacin on articular cartilage. *Arthritis Rheum.* **26**: 528–531.
153. Palmoski, M. J. and Brandt, K. D. (1983) Benoxaprofen stimulates proteoglycan synthesis in normal canine knee cartilage *in vitro*. *Arthritis Rheum.* **26**: 771–774.
154. Verbruggen, G., Veys, E. M., Malfait, A. M. *et al.* (1989) Proteoglycan metabolism in isolated chondrocytes from human cartilage and in short-term tissue-cultured human articular cartilage. *Clin. Exp. Rheumatol.* **7**: 13–17.
155. Verbruggen, G., Veys, E. M., Malfait, A. M. *et al.* (1990) Proteoglycan metabolism in isolated chondrocytes from human cartilage. Influence of niflumic acid. *Clin. Rheumatol.* **9**: 32–41.
156. Lowther, D. A., Handley, C. J. and Gundalach, A. (1978) Effect of salicylic acid on articular cartilage in organ culture. *Pharmacology* **17**: 50–55.
157. Fontagne, J., Loizeau, M., Adolphe, M. and Lechat, P. (1984) Effect of indomethacin on collagen biosynthesis by rabbit articular chondrocytes in monolayer cultures. *Int. J. Tissue React.* **6**: 233–241.
158. Kato, Y., Nakashima, K., Iwamoto, M. *et al.* (1993) Effects of interleukin-1 on syntheses of alkaline phosphatase, type X collagen, and 1,25-dihydroxyvitamin D_3 receptor, and matrix calcification in rabbit chondrocyte cultures. *J. Clin. Invest.* **92**: 2323–2330.
159. Fujii, K., Tajiri, K., Sai, S., Tanaka, T. and Murota, K. (1989) Effects of non steroidal anti-inflammatory drugs on collagen biosynthesis of cultured chondrocytes. *Semin. Arthritis Rheum.* **18**: 16–18.
160. Pelletier, J. P. and Martel-Pelletier, J. (1993) Effects of nimesulide and naproxen on the degradation and metalloprotease synthesis of human osteoarthritic cartilage. *Drugs* **46**: 34–39.
161. Watanabe, K., Hayashi, H. and Mori, Y. (1994) Effect of a benzilidene derivative, novel antirheumatic agent, on the production of tissue inhibitor of metalloproteinases. *Biol. Pharm. Bull.* **17**: 58–61.
162. Bassleer, C., Gysen, P., Bassleer, R. and Franchimont, P. (1988) Effects of peptidic glycosaminoglycans complex on human chondrocytes cultivated in three dimensions. *Biochem. Pharmacol.* **37**: 1939–1945.
163. Harmand, M. F., Vilamitjana, J., Maloche, E., Duphil, R. and Ducassou, D. (1987) Effects of *S*-adenosylmethionine on human articular chondrocyte differentiation. An *in vitro* study. *Am. J. Med.* **83**: 48–54.
164. Larsen, N. E., Lombard, K. M., Parent, E. G. and Balazs, E. A. (1992) Effects of hylan on cartilage and chondrocyte cultures. *J. Orthop. Res.* **10**: 23–32.
165. Akatsuka, M., Yamamoto, Y., Tobetto, K., Yasui, T. and Ando, T. (1993) *In vitro* effects of hyaluronan on prostaglandin E_2 induction by interleukin-1 in rabbit articular chondrocytes. *Agents Actions* **38**: 122–125.
166. Mauviel, A., Loyau, G. and Pujol, J. P. (1991) Effect of unsaponifiable extracts of avocado and soybean (Piasclédine) on the collagenolytic action of cultures of human rheumatoid synoviocytes and rabbit articular chondrocytes treated with interleukin-1. *Rev. Rhum. Mal. Osteoartic.* **58**: 241–245.
167. Harmand, M. F., Rodriguez, V., Savineau, C. and Gonfrier, P. (1994) *In vitro* pharmacological

evidence of a protective effect of IAS (Soja and Avocado unsaponifiables) on cartilage. *Osteoarthritis and Cartilage* **2** (**Suppl 1**): 20.

168. Amacher, D. E., Schomaker, S. J., Gootz, T. D. and McGuirk, P. R. (1989) Proteoglycan and procollagen synthesis in rat embryo limb bud cultures treated with quinolone antibacterials. Presented to the Johns Hopkins Center of Alternative to Animal Testing Symposium, Baltimore, USA, 4–5 April 1989.
169. Schroter-Kermani, C., Hinz, N., Risse, P., Stahlman, R. and Merker, H. J. (1992) Effects of ofloxacin on chondrogenesis in murine cartilage organoid culture. *Toxicol. In Vitro* **6:** 465–474.
170. Thuong-Guyot, M., Domarle, O., Pocidalo, J. J. and Hayem, G. (1994) Effects of fluoroquinolones on cultured articular chondrocytes flow cytometric analysis of free radical production. *J. Pharmacol. Exp. Ther.* **271:** 1544–1549.
171. Boskey, A. L., Ziecheck, W., Guidon, P. and Doty, S. B. (1993) Gallium nitrate inhibits alkaline phosphatase activity in a differentiating mesenchymal cell culture. *Bone Miner.* **20:** 179–192.
172. Aulthouse, A. L. and Hitt, D. C. (1994) The teratogenic effects of valproic acid in human chondrogenesis *in vitro*. *Teratology* **49:** 208–217.

9

Primary Cultures of Cardiac Myocytes as *In Vitro* Models for Pharmacological and Toxicological Assessments

ENRIQUE CHACON, DANIEL ACOSTA AND JOHN J. LEMASTERS

I. Introduction 210
II. Primary cultures of cardiac myocytes 211
  A. Neonatal rat cardiac myocyte cultures 211
    1. Preparation of neonatal rat cardiac myocyte cultures using trypsin dissociation with purification by rate of attachment 211
    2. Preparation of neonatal rat cardiac myocyte cultures using collagenase and pancreatin dissociation with purification by elutriation 212
  B. Adult cardiac myocytes 213
    1. Preparation of adult rabbit cardiac myocyte cultures 214
III. End-point assays 215
  A. Cell death assays 215
    1. Propidium iodide dye exclusion assay 216
    2. Cytosolic enzyme release 216
  B. Functional assays 217
    1. Contractile activity 217
    2. Intracellular reactive oxygen species 217
    3. Cellular energy capacity 218
    4. Succinate dehydrogenase activity (MTT assay) 218
    5. Mitochondrial membrane potential 218
    6. Proton motive force 220
    7. Calcium homeostasis 221
IV. Conclusion 221
  References 222

IN VITRO METHODS IN PHARMACEUTICAL RESEARCH
ISBN 0-12-163390-X

I. INTRODUCTION

A number of pharmaceutical companies have prompted the development of *in vitro* research methods for rapid pharmacological and toxicological screening. Pharmaceutical companies are directing research efforts at developing a series of *in vitro* assays that could serve as reliable, reproducible, and inexpensive alternatives to *in vivo* animal testing. In this review, we present ideas and methodologies which may aid in assisting the effectiveness and efficiency of *in vitro* methods for pharmacological and toxicological assessments of cardioactive compounds.

In vitro end-point assays may be summarized as those that measure cellular functions and those that measure cell death. Cell death assays, often referred to as permeability assays, evaluate irreversible changes such as breakdown of the sarcolemma. Permeability assays estimate failure of the plasma membrane permeability barrier, which represents irreversible cell injury. Functional assays typically evaluate reversible events that reflect a state of impairment (toxicity) or pharmacological response (efficacy). Fig. 9.1 illustrates a matrix of

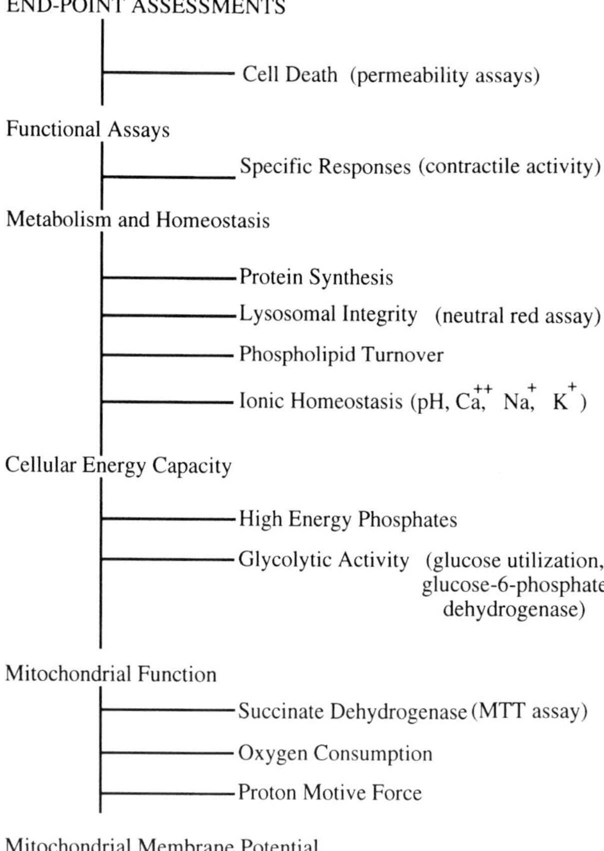

Fig. 9.1 Cardiac events and respective end-points that can be assessed using *in vitro* assays. Breakdown of the plasma membrane is associated with loss of cellular viability (cell death). Assessment of specific functional parameters associated with cellular functions can be studied with *in vitro* assays that reflect mechanism of action. Functional assays are too narrowly focused to make generalized cytotoxicity assessments.

cardiac cellular events and characteristic end-points that can be measured to assess pharmacological and/or toxicological responses. In this chapter we describe methodologies for the preparation of primary cultures of neonatal rat cardiac myocytes, adult rabbit cardiac myocytes, and several end-point assays that can be used to assess pharmacological and toxicological responses of cardioactive compounds. In addition, we describe new technologies in fluorescence microscopy that provide powerful tools to investigate mechanisms of actions.

II. PRIMARY CULTURES OF CARDIAC MYOCYTES

Cell culture systems permit assessment of cellular responses that are technically difficult *in vivo*. In particular, primary cell cultures of cardiac cells have served to further our understanding of the cellular and molecular basis of myocardial cell injury.[1–3] Several heart cell culture systems are routinely used. Nearly all primary cultures of cardiac myocytes are derived from the hearts of the chick, rat, or rabbit. It has been argued that cardiac myocytes in culture change from β-oxidation (characteristic of muscle cells *in vivo*) to glycolysis as their main energy supply. However, experience from our laboratories with cultured heart cells indicates that mitochondrial metabolism is preserved in cultured myocytes and serves as a vital source of energy. Cardiac cells in culture will utilize β-oxidation as a major energy source provided that appropriate substrates are present.[4,5] The ability of myocardial cell cultures to maintain these *in vivo* characteristics makes them appropriate models for pharmacological and toxicological assessments. Furthermore, myocardial cell cultures provide informative data with minimal investment of time and expense in comparison with models utilizing whole organs or live animals. Two methods are presented to culture neonatal rat cardiac myocytes and a single method to culture adult rabbit cardiac myocytes. These methods provide high yields of cardiac cells.

A. Neonatal rat cardiac myocyte cultures

Various methods are available for the isolation of neonatal rat cardiac myocytes. In general, hearts are separated into a heterogeneous suspension of muscle and non-muscle cells. To prevent overgrowth of fibroblasts and other cells, myocytes should be purified before culturing. We present two methods that our laboratories use routinely to obtain relatively pure myocyte preparations. One method is based on the rapid rate of attachment of non-muscle cells to plastic culture dishes.[6] Non-attached myocytes are then decanted into separate culture dishes. Another technique to separate cardiac muscle cells from non-muscle cells is centrifugal elutriation,[7] which separates cells based on size. Heart digests are infused into a rotating chamber against a centrifugal field. Cells remain trapped in the chamber until flow is increased or rotor speed decreased. As the force of flow begins to exceed the force of gravity, the smallest cells are eluted first.

1. Preparation of neonatal rat cardiac myocyte cultures using trypsin dissociation with purification by rate of attachment

Neonatal primary myocardial cell cultures are prepared by modification of the procedure described by Wenzel *et al.*[6] Postnatal Sprague-Dawley rats aged 2–4 days are euthanized by decapitation. The hearts are removed and placed in a cold Hanks' balanced salt solution (BSS) (136 mM NaCl, 5 mM KCl, 0.2 mM Na_2HPO_4, 0.5 mM KH_2PO_4, 5.5 mM glucose, 4 mM $NaHCO_3$, and 16 μM phenol red at pH 7.4). The hearts are finely minced and rinsed twice with cold Hanks' BSS. The minced hearts are transferred to a 50-ml dissociation flask containing a 1 inch sterilized stirring bar and 18 ml warm (37°C) Hanks' BSS. An 0.8 ml aliquot of Difbaco 1:250 trypsin (10 ml vial) that has been reconstituted with 9 ml cold Hanks' BSS is added to digest the heart tissue. Decreases in pH of the digestion buffer are monitored by the appearance of an orange to yellow color from the pH indicator phenol red. The pH is adjusted to 7.4 and maintained during digestion with 1 mM $NaHCO_3$.

The dissociation is maintained, in a 37°C water bath with gentle stirring. The flask is kept covered with sterile aluminum foil during the dissociation. This initial digestion is carried out for 10 min. The supernatant of first dissociation contains mainly cellular debris and is discarded. After the initial dissociation, three more digestions are performed for 15 min each. After each 15 min digestion, the heart tissue is allowed to settle. The supernatant containing cells is decanted and centrifuged at 400*g* for 5 min. The resultant cell pellet is rinsed of contaminating trypsin by resuspending the cells with 5 ml Eagle's minimal essential medium (MEM) supplemented with 5% newborn calf serum and antibiotics (1 unit ml^{-1} penicillin G potassium, 0.1 mg ml^{-1} streptomycin sulfate, and 1 μg ml^{-1} amphotericin B). The cell suspension is again centrifuged at 400*g* for 5 min and the resulting cell pellet is resuspended in 2 ml Eagle's MEM and placed in a 37°C incubator with 5% carbon dioxide. Subsequent digestions of the remaining heart tissue are accomplished by replenishing the heart mince with 18 ml Hanks' BSS and 0.8 ml trypsin. Three digestions are pooled, resuspended, and counted on a hemocytometer. The cells are diluted to a final concentration of 500 000 cells per ml and plated in 75 ml culture flasks in 10 ml aliquots.

Muscle cells are separated from non-muscle cells by a pour-off technique based on the differential rate of attachment of the cells to the culture flasks. After 3 h, the culture flasks are shaken to resuspend non-attached myocytes and the medium is poured into a sterile Erlenmeyer flask. The resultant 95% myocyte cell suspension is used to plate culture dishes (10^6 cells per 35 mm dish), 96-well microtiter plates (75 000 cells per well), or glass coverslips (placed in a 35 mm dish). Myocyte cultures are maintained in Eagle's MEM supplemented with 5% newborn calf serum and antibiotics. Media is replaced after 24 h and every other day afterwards. Medium should be changed 24 h before the experiments. Cells are grown in a humidified atmosphere (37°C) of 5% carbon dioxide and 95% air. Experiments can be conducted 3–4 days after the initial plating of the myocytes. The procedure yields approximately 40 million cells. Typically, about 40 35 mm culture dishes or five 96-well plates can be obtained from 20 postnatal rats.

2. *Preparation of neonatal rat cardiac myocyte cultures using collagenase and pancreatin dissociation with purification by elutriation*

This second method for preparation of neonatal rat cardiac myocytes uses a modified collagenase/pancreatin digestion procedure described by Harary and Farley,[8] and elutriation for purification of myocytes as described by Ulrich *et al.*[7] Rat pups are euthanized by decapitation. The hearts are removed and placed in 5 ml cold balanced salt solution (BSS: 0.81 mM $MgSO_4$, 117 mM NaCl, 5.3 mM KCl, 3.3 mM Na_2HPO_4, 5.6 mM glucose, 20 mM HEPES, 10 units ml^{-1} penicillin, and 10 μg ml^{-1} streptomycin at pH 7.5). The hearts are finely minced and rinsed twice with cold BSS. The minced hearts are transferred to a 125 ml Erlenmeyer flask containing a 1 inch sterilized stirring bar. An aliquot of digestion buffer (25 ml) consisting of 69 mg collagenase D (Boehringer Mannheim, Indianapolis, IN) plus

23 ml pancreatin NF (Gibco Laboratories, Grand Island, NY) per 200 ml BSS is added to the minced hearts.

The incubation flask is covered with sterile foil and placed in a 37°C water bath with gentle stirring. Three to four digestions are performed for 20 min each. After each digestion, the undigested heart tissue is allowed to settle. The supernatant, containing the isolated cells, is decanted into a sterile 50 ml centrifuge tube and kept on ice. Subsequent digestions of the remaining heart mince are accomplished by adding 25 ml digestion buffer per dissociation. The digestions are pooled, resuspended by inversion, and centrifuged at 400*g* for 5 min. The supernatant is discarded, and the pellet is resuspended in 20 ml Eagle's MEM. DNAse (20 units ml^{-1}) is added, and incubation is continued with gentle shaking at 37°C in a reciprocating water bath. A serum-free DNAse preparation should be used if the cells will be grown on laminin-coated glass coverslips. After 1 h, the cell suspension is filtered through a 60 μM nylon mesh into a sterile 50-ml polypropylene centrifuge tube. Filtration removes debris that may disrupt flow through the cell elutriator.

For purification by centrifugal elutriation, the cell suspension is transferred to a sterile 30 ml syringe and loaded into a centrifugal elutriator (Beckman Model J2-21M/E, Palo Alto, CA) at a rotor speed of 2000 rpm and a flow rate of 21 ml min^{-1}. BSS is the mobile phase. Rotor speed is maintained at 2000 rpm until turbidity has cleared the bubble trap (approximately 10 min). Speed is then decreased to 1850 rpm for 10 min to elute cellular debris. Subsequently, 10 min at 1580 rpm releases small cells like fibroblasts and endothelial cells. Myocytes are collected at 500 rpm for 10 min into four sterile 50 ml polypropylene centrifuge tubes. The collected myocytes are centrifuged at 400*g* for 5 min. The supernatant is discarded, and the cells resuspended in 5 ml culture medium (Eagle's MEM supplemented with 3% fetal calf serum, 6% horse serum, 10 units ml^{-1} penicillin, and 10 $\mu g\,ml^{-1}$ streptomycin).

Samples are pooled and an aliquot is taken to count the cells using a hemocytometer. We normally obtain $4\text{–}5 \times 10^7$ cells per 20 rat pups. Viability is 92–98% as determined by exclusion of 1% trypan blue. After diluting to 5×10^5 cells per ml, cells are plated on 35 mm culture dishes (10^6 cells per 35 mm), multiwell plates (75 000 cells per well), or glass coverslips (placed in a 35 mm dish). Glass coverslips must be coated with laminin because elutriated myocytes will not attach to untreated glass. To prepare coated coverslips, they are rinsed in 70% ethyl alcohol for 1 h and air-dried in a laminar flow hood for sterilization. Laminin (Collaborative Research, Bedford, MA) is diluted to 5 $\mu g\,ml^{-1}$ in culture media. Each coverslip is incubated for 1 hr at room temperature with 4–5 drops of diluted laminin. Myocytes are plated directly onto the residual laminin. Myocyte cultures are maintained in Eagle's MEM supplemented with 3% fetal calf serum, 6% horse serum, 10 units ml^{-1} penicillin, and 10 $\mu g\,ml^{-1}$ streptomycin. Culture medium is replaced every 48 h. Cells are grown in a humidified atmosphere (37°C) of 5% carbon dioxide and 95% air. Experiments can be conducted 4–6 days after initial plating of the myocytes.

B. Adult cardiac myocytes

The development of adult cardiac myocyte cultures stems from the idea that hearts from larger and older animals provide terminally differentiated myocyte that more closely resembles adult human myocytes.[9–11] Adult cell isolations frequently demonstrate a 'calcium intolerance' that causes isolated rod-shaped cells to hypercontract and lose viability when exposed to physiologic concentrations of calcium. Isolation of adult cardiac myocytes that retain an *in vivo* rod-shaped appearance is dependent on a number of variables. The quality of digestive enzyme seems particularly important. Other important variables include perfusion pressure, digestion time, temperature, electrolyte balance, and method of physical dispersion after perfusion. The difficulty of reliably obtaining large numbers of cardiac myocytes from adult sources has limited their use in cytotoxicity screening.

Overgrowth of fibroblasts and other non-muscle cells can occur within 3–5 days in culture. Cytosine arabinoside and other mitotic inhibitors are frequently used to restrict contamination by non-muscle cells. Cultured adult rat cardiac myocytes require several days in culture before spontaneous contractions are evident. Cultured adult rabbit cardiac myocytes require a couple of days in culture plus triiodothyronine-supplemented medium before spontaneous contractions are evident. A disadvantage of waiting several days before the cells begin spontaneous contractions is that the cells lose their *in vivo* rod-shaped morphology in culture. Adult rat cardiac myocyte rod-shaped morphology is essentially lost after 24 h in culture. Adult rabbit cardiac myocytes retain a rod-shaped morphology for up to 4 days in culture. Non-spontaneously contracting rod-shaped cells cells can be electrically stimulated to duplicate *in vivo* contractile activity. With the continued development of adult cardiac cell isolation techniques, investigators should be able to exploit the strengths of this model.

1. *Preparation of adult rabbit cardiac myocyte cultures*

Adult rabbit cardiac myocytes are isolated using a modified procedure described by Haddad *et al.*[9] White New Zealand rabbits weighing 3–4 kg are injected with heparin (250 units per kg body weight) via a 22 G butterfly catheter placed in the marginal ear vein. The animal is then anesthetized with 35 mg kg^{-1} Surital (Parke-Davis, Morris Plains, NJ) via the same route. The chest cavity is opened and immediately irrigated with ice-cold calcium-free buffer A (5 mM KCl, 110 mM NaCl, 1.2 mM NaH_2PO_4, 28 mM $NaHCO_3$, 25 mM HEPES, 30 mM glucose, 20 mM butanedione monoxime, 0.05 units ml^{-1} insulin, 250 mM adenosine, 1 mM creatine, 1 mM carnitine, 1 mM octanoic acid, 1 mM taurine, 2 units ml^{-1} heparin, 10 units ml^{-1} penicillin, and 10 mg ml^{-1} streptomycin at pH 7.3). The heart is removed and placed in 100 ml ice cold-buffer A where it is trimmed, cannulated, and flushed with 10 ml ice-cold buffer A.

The heart is then mounted on a modified Langendorf perfusion apparatus and retrogradely perfused for 5 min with buffer A saturated with 95% oxygen and 5% carbon dioxide at 37°C from a height of 100 cm at a rate of 25–35 ml min^{-1}. The perfusate is discarded. A digestion buffer (buffer B), consisting of buffer A without heparin and containing 25 mM $CaCl_2$, 68 units ml^{-1} collagenase type 2 (Worthington Biochemical, Freehold, NJ) and 70 units ml^{-1} hyaluronidase type 1-S (Sigma Chemicals, St Louis, MO) is perfused through the heart. The first 5 min of perfusate is discarded. After 5 min, buffer B is recirculated for 20 min. The ventricles are then separated with scissors below the atrioventricular junction. Four incisions towards the apex are made, and the tissue is gently agitated for 30 min in buffer C (buffer A without heparin and supplemented with 25 mM $CaCl_2$ and 0.5 mg ml^{-1} 1 : 250 trypsin) to release the rod-shaped myocytes.

The cell suspension is poured into 50 ml polypropylene tubes and centrifuged at 20*g* for 2 min. The supernatant is discarded and the cell pellets are pooled and resuspended in 50 ml buffer D (Joklik's medium and medium 199 (1 : 1 mixture) containing 20 mM butanedione monoxime, 1 mM creatine, 1 mM taurine, 1 mM octanoic acid, 1 mM carnitine, 0.05 units ml^{-1} insulin, 10 units ml^{-1} penicillin, and 10 mg ml^{-1} streptomycin). After 10 min, the cell suspension is centrifuged at 20*g* for 2 min and the resultant pellet is resuspended in buffer D supplemented with 0.5 mg ml^{-1} trypsin. The purpose of a second tyrpsin digestion is to digest hypercontracted cells that sediment with rod-shaped cells during centrifugation. After 30 min, the cell suspension is centrifuged at 20*g* for 2 min and the resultant pellet is resuspended in 15 ml nutrient medium (buffer D minus butanedione monoxime).

The cells are counted and diluted with nutrient medium to 50 000 cells ml^{-1}. Cells are plated at a density of 50 000 cells per cm^2 on laminin-coated glass coverslips. We typically preincubate culture surfaces for 1 h at room temperature with laminin (15 $\mu g\,ml^{-1}$) diluted in serum-free nutrient medium using 10 mg laminin per cm^2. The cell isolation procedure yields about 10^7 cells of which 70–80% are rod-shaped myocytes. Cell cultures are incubated in a humidified atmosphere of 5% carbon dioxide and 95% air at 37°C. Adult rabbit cardiac myocytes maintain a rod-shaped appearance for up to 6 days in culture, provided serum is excluded from the incubation medium. Adult rabbit myocytes begin to lose electrically stimulated contractile responses after their first day in culture. However, nutrient medium supplemented with 1 ng ml^{-1} triiodothyronine maintains stimulated contractile responses for up to 5 days in culture. For long-term culture (>4 days), proliferation of non-muscle cells must be inhibited with 10 μM cytosine arabinoside added during days 2–5 of the culture. We typically use 1- to 2-day cultured cells for cytotoxicity experiments.

III. END-POINT ASSAYS

A. Cell death assays

Cell death assays, often referred to as permeability assays, employ bulky charged molecules that normally cannot diffuse into and out of cells. These assays are based on dye exclusion (uptake of trypan blue or propidium iodide), dye inclusion (retention of calcein), and leakage of cytoplasmic enzymes (lactate dehydrogenase).

There are a number of dye exclusion assays that are used to assess plasma membrane integrity. The classical dye exclusion test utilizes trypan blue. Cells are incubated with trypan blue, and blue nuclear staining is assessed by conventional optical microscopy. The trypan blue assay is relatively easy and reliable, but is also time consuming and labor intensive. Thus, the trypan blue exclusion assay is not well suited for high sample screening. Fluorescent DNA-binding assays are attractive alternatives to the trypan blue assay. Propidium iodide and ethidium bromide homodimer are fluorescent charged compounds that are excluded from viable cells. Leaky plasma membranes allow these dyes to enter the cell, where they can then bind to double-stranded DNA. Once bound to DNA, they exhibit a red shift and an increase in fluorescence emission that can be used to quantify loss of viability in large populations.[12] Fluorescent DNA-binding assays can be conducted on cells cultured in 96-well microtiter plates using a multi-well fluorescence scanner.[13] These fluorescence-based dye exclusion assays provide a number of advantages. Plasma membrane integrity can be made monitored continuously over time from the same cells in a nondestructive manner. With a multi-well fluorescence scanner, the assays have a high degree of statistical accuracy, are easy to perform, and can be used to screen large numbers of samples. However, as in any fluorescence assay, appropriate controls must be performed to ensure that test agents are not themselves fluorescent or causing other interference with the fluorescent probe.

1. Propidium iodide dye exclusion assay

The propidium iodide dye exclusion assay is performed in a Krebs–Ringer–HEPES buffer (KRH: 115 mM NaCl, 5 mM KCl, 1 mM KH_2PO_4, 1.2 mM $MgSO_4$, 2 mM $CaCl_2$, and 25 mM HEPES at pH 7.4) containing 30 μM propidium iodide. In the absence of cells, propidium iodide exhibits an excitation maximum near 500 nm and an emission maximum near 625 nm. Binding of propidium iodide to DNA causes a red shift of the excitation maximum to 540 nm and the emission maximum to 640 nm, with a two- to threefold increase in fluorescence intensity. A multi-well fluorescence scanner equipped with appropriate excitation and emission filters can be used to record fluorescence from 24- or 96-well microtiter plates. For cytotoxicity screening, myocytes are cultured in 96-well microtiter plates (50 000 cells per well) and treated with varying concentrations of test agents. Typically, we scan plates every 15 or 30 min. Between measurements, plates are kept in a 37°C air incubator. Increasing fluorescence signifies loss of cell membrane integrity. Maximal change of fluorescence corresponds to 100% cell death. At the end of the experiment, 25 μM digitonin or 5 μM Triton X100 is added to each well to permeabilize all cells and label all nuclei with propidium iodide. Fluorescence is measured again to determine a value corresponding to 100% cell death. Percentage viability (V) is calculated as $V = 100\,(X-A)/(B-A)$ where A is initial fluorescence, B is fluorescence after addition of digitonin or Triton X100, and X is fluorescence at any given time. The propidium iodide asssay allows continuous measurements of cell viability over time. However, as in any fluorescence assay, appropriate controls must be performed to assure that test agents are not themselves fluorescent or cause any other fluorescence interference with the fluorescent marker.

2. Cytosolic enzyme release

Release of lactate dehydrogenase (LDH) is estimated from the conversion of NADH to NAD, after pyruvate addition, and is measured spectrophotometrically from the rate of decrease in 340 nm absorbance.[14] LDH release can also be measured in 96-well microtiter plates using an enzyme-linked immunosorbent assay (ELISA) reader. This is particularly helpful for high volume and high capacity cytotoxicity screening. We typically express cell damage as the percentage of total releasable enzyme. Permeabilization with 25 μM digitonin is a useful way to release total cellular content of LDH that is more reliable and reproducible than cell scraping and sonication. Since LDH is a sulfhydryl-dependent enzyme, appropriate control experiments should ascertain that the test agent does not directly inhibit LDH enzyme activity.

The reagents required for the LDH assay are a phosphate buffer, a solution of NADH, and a solution of pyruvic acid. A 0.1 M sodium phosphate buffer (pH 7.4) can be prepared from stock solutions of 0.2 M NaH_2PO_4 and 0.2 M Na_2HPO_4. Mix 190 ml of NaH_2PO_4 with 810 ml Na_2HPO_4 and dilute to a final volume of 2000 ml. A 25–50 ml sample of 3.5 mM NADH is prepared in 0.1 M sodium phosphate buffer. In addition, a 25–50 ml sample of 9 mM sodium pyruvate is prepared in 0.1 M sodium phosphate buffer. The NADH and sodium pyruvate solutions should be made fresh before each experiment. The NADH is light sensitive and should be kept on ice in an amber bottle or wrapped in aluminum foil.

To conduct the assay in a 3 ml cuvette, a 100 μl test sample aliquot is added to 2.5 ml 0.1 M phosphate buffer. Some 200 μl NADH solution is then added to the cuvette and the reaction is initiated by the addition of a 200 μl aliquot of sodium pyruvate solution. The absorbance is then monitored at 340 nm for about 5 min to determine the rate of oxidation of NADH.

The assay can also be performed in 96-well microtiter plates using an ELISA reader, especially if the instrument is interfaced with a computer and kinetic software. To each well, a 10 μl aliquot of test sample and a 15 μl aliquot of NADH solution is added to 200 μl phosphate buffer, the reaction is initiated by the addition of a 15 μl aliquot of sodium pyruvate solution, and the change in optical density is measured every 30 s. Since the data are commonly expressed as the percentage of the total, determination of the maximal releasable amounts of enzyme must be performed. We typically use 5 min exposure of 25 μM digitonin to permeabilize the sarcolemma and release total enzyme. Additional control experiments with LDH from permeabilized cells or pure enzyme should be performed to assure that the test agent does not inhibit the intrinsic activity of the enzyme.

B. Functional assays

1. *Contractile activity*

Measurement of spontaneous contractions in neonatal rat cardiac myocytes is a simple and effective functional test of contractile activity.[15] Beating rates are microscopically examined and are consistent, provided a constant temperature (37°C) is maintained on the microscope stage. Temperature control of the microscope stage can maintained by placing the microscope in a thermostatic Plexiglas chamber or by warming the microscope stage with an air heater. We typically culture cells on 35 mm culture dishes and dose with test agent(s) for a period of time followed by examination by phase contrast microscopy. Contractions are counted for a 10–15 s interval in four fields of view. Data are reported as beats per minute. Beating rates range between 150 and 200 beats per minute, with reproducibility from 3–4 day cultures being remarkably close.

2. *Intracellular reactive oxygen species*

Production of toxic oxygen radicals as potential mediators of cell injury has received considerable attention over the years. Here we describe a couple of methods that we have used to monitor the production of toxic oxygen radicals in cultured heart cells.[16] The basis of the assays are that reactive oxygen sensitive compounds are loaded into the cells which are converted to a product that can be measured using spectrophotometric or spectrofluorometric techniques. The first method uses nitroblue tetrazolium (NBT) as the oxidative marker, whereas the second method uses the fluorescent probe 2′,7′-dichlorofluorescin (DCF).

To monitor intracellular production of reactive oxygen species with NBT, myocytes are cultured in 35 mm plates and treated with test compound for a period of time followed by a 1.5 h incubation in 0.8 mM NBT. The cell monolayers are then rinsed with a physiological buffer and 0.5 ml water is added to the culture dish. The monolayer is scraped and collected into screw-top test tubes. The cells are sonicated and 0.5 ml pyridine is added to help solubilize the NBT–formazan product. The test tubes are vortexed and centrifuged. The supernatant is transferred to a quartz cuvette and the absorbance read at 550 nm to determine the concentration of NBT–formazan (molar absorptivity 30 000). Data are expressed as a percentage of the control or the amount of NBT-formazan per mg protein. The drawback of expressing the data per mg protein is that the colorimetric basis of the assay interferes with most protein assays. Thus, a second set of samples is required to conduct protein determinations.

To monitor intracellular production of reactive oxygen species with DCF, myocytes are cultured in 35 mm plates and treated with test compound for a period of time followed by a 30 min incubation in 15 μM 2′,7′-dichlorofluorescin diacetate (DCFDA). DCFDA is hydrolyzed by intracellular esterase to liberate the free acid (2′,7′-dichlorofluorescin: DCFH), which remains trapped in the cell. Reactive oxygen species then oxidize DCFH to the fluorescent tracer 2′,7′-dichlorofluorescein (DCF). The cell monolayers are then rinsed with a physiological buffer, and 1 ml 1% deoxycholate is added to lyse the cells. The lysates are transferred to a 3 ml disposable acrylate cuvette. Cuvettes containing the fluorescent tracer should be kept on ice and in the dark to minimize auto-oxidation of DCFH to DCF. The fluorescence of DCF is determined using 488 nm excitation and 525 nm emission. After an initial fluorescence reading, the lysates are incubated at 50°C for 1 h in the presence of 25 μl 1 N NaOH and 100 μl 30% hydrogen peroxide. The purpose of this second incubation is to ensure complete hydrolysis of DCFDA and to oxidize fully any remaining intermediate (DCFH) to the fluorescent product DCF. The fluorescent intensity of each sample is read again to determine the total amount of DCFDA loaded into the cells. Hence, data are expressed as the percentage of DCF formed from total DCFDA loaded.

3. *Cellular energy capacity*

The main energy supply of the heart is by mitochondrial β-oxidation of fatty acids. Since heart tissue quickly consumes ATP, toxicant-induced changes of ATP and other energy metabolism related enzymes are important to overall cell viability. Assays to estimate cellular energy capacity include measurements of glucose-6-phosphate dehydrogenase, mitochondrial integrity (MTT assay), oxygen consumption, mitochondrial membrane potential, and the proton motive force. Estimation of succinate dehydrogenase (MTT assay), mitochondrial membrane potential, and the proton motive force are discussed in the following sections.

4. *Succinate dehydrogenase activity (MTT assay)*

The MTT assay has been widely used to assess cell viability. However, one must consider that the enzymatic reduction of 3-[4,5-dimethylthiazole-2-yl]-2,5-diphenyltetrazolium bromide (MTT) to MTT-formazan is catalyzed by mitochondrial succinate dehydrogenase. Hence, the MTT assay is dependent on mitochondrial respiration and indirectly serves to assess the cellular energy capacity of a cell. The MTT assay is a colorimetric reaction that can easily be measured from cell monolayers that have been plated in 35 mm dishes or multi-well plates.

Cell cultures are incubated for 2 h in culture medium or in in a Krebs–Hensleit–HEPES buffer (115 mM NaCl, 5 mM KCl, 1 mM KH_2PO_4, 1.2 mM $MgSO_4$, 2 mM $CaCl_2$, and 25 mM HEPES at pH 7.4) containing 0.5 mg ml^{-1} MTT. After 2 h, the incubation buffer is removed and the blue MTT–formazan product is extracted with acidified isopropyl alcohol (0.04 N HCl). After 30 min extraction at room temperature, the absorbance of the formazan solution is read spectrophotometrically at 570 nm.

5. *Mitochondrial membrane potential*

Membrane potential fluorescent probes are positively charged compounds that distribute into negatively charged compartments in accordance with the Nernst equation:[17–19]

$$dy = -60 \log(F_{in}/F_{out})$$

where dy is membrane potential in millivolts and F_{in} and F_{out} are fluorophore concentrations inside and outside a specific cellular compartment. The validity of this method depends on ideal behavior of the fluorophore. Many fluorescent membrane potential dyes, such as rhodamine-123, quench when they accumulate in the mitochondria and show nonspecific binding independent of the electrical potential. Correction factors may be applied to correct for these effects. However, each correction factor introduces a new degree of uncertainty to the overall precision and accuracy. The newer-generation membrane potential fluorophores, such as tetramethylrhodamine methyl ester (TMRM), seem to lack these undesirable qualities and may be more suited for monitoring mitochondrial membrane potential.[20,21] Fluorescence measurements of TMRM by confocal microscopy (Fig. 9.2) has allowed us simultaneously to measure the mitochondrial membrane potential and the plasma membrane potential of living cells.[1]

Confocal microscopy can create images of a slice through a living cell that approach 0.5 μm in thickness. In conventional fluorescence microscopy, depth of field is much greater and light from out-of-focus planes degrades image resolution. The improved depth resolution of confocal microscopy results in rejection of out-of-focus light to produce images that are remarkably detailed. This improved resolving power permits measurement of the nernstian distribution of cationic fluorophores.

Under normal conditions, cardiac myocytes typically exhibit a plasma membrane potential of −90 mV and a mitochondrial membrane potential of up to −150 mV. The Nernst equation predicts that, at equilibrium, a 10 : 1 uptake ratio of the fluorophore corresponds to a −60 mV gradient, a 100 : 1 gradient to a −120 mV gradient, and so forth. These potentials are additive with respect to the cell exterior. Thus, at equilibrium,

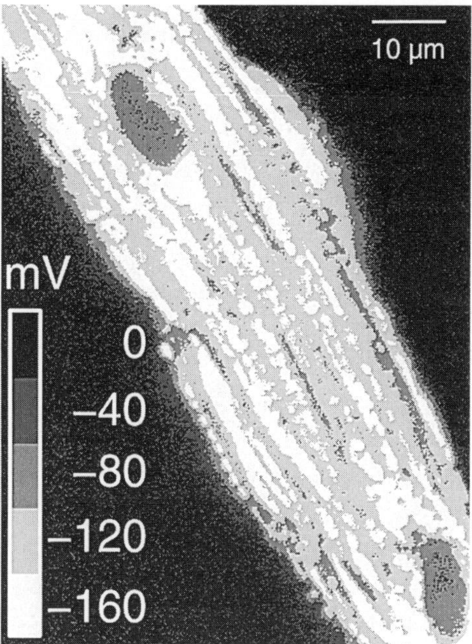

Fig. 9.2 Electrochemical potential determinations in cultured adult rabbit cardiac myocytes using TMRM and confocal microscopy. The image represents a non-drug-treated cell showing a plasma membrane potential of −80 mV and mitochondrial membrane potentials as great as −160 mV relative to the extracellular space.

mitochondria inside a living cardiac myocyte will be 240 mV more negative than the extracellular space. This −240 mV difference represents a 10 000 : 1 concentration gradient of the fluorophore. Typical 8-bit computer memories store up to 256 levels of light intensity per pixel, hence such large intensity gradients cannot be measured using a linear scale. This problem can be overcome by applying gamma circuits. Gamma circuits apply a logarithmic function to the output signal of the detector, thereby condensing a large signal range into the available 256 levels of video memory. Applying a gamma circuit, the broad-ranged fluoresence intensity of TMRM inside a cell can be converted to electrical potentials using the Nernst equation and displayed in pseudocolor.

To load TMRM into cultured cardiac myocytes, cells are incubated with 600 nm TMRM in culture medium for 20 min at 37°C. The cells are then placed on the microsope stage in Krebs–Ringer–HEPES buffer (KRH: 115 mM NaCl, 5 mM KCl, 1 mM KH_2PO_4, 1.2 mM $MgSO_4$, 2 mM $CaCl_2$, and 25 mM HEPES at pH 7.4) containing 150 nM TMRM to maintain equilibrium distribution of the membrane potential probe. Experiments are then initiated after an additional 15 min incubation. For membrane potential determinations, we use the Bio-Rad MRC-600 laser scanning confocal unit equipped with a Nikon Diaphot. TMRM is excited at 568 nm from an argon–krypton laser. To quantitate TMRM fluorescence using confocal microscopy, the reader is referred to Chacon *et. al.*,[1] for a detailed description of the method.

6. *Proton motive force*

The proton motive force ($d\mu H^+$) is comprised of two components, a mitochondrial membrane potential (dy) and a H^+ ion concentration gradient (dpH) across the mitochondrial membrane, where:

$$d\mu H^+ = dy + 60d\text{pH}$$

Confocal microscopy measurements of cells co-loaded with TMRM, to measure dy and SNARF®-1 to measure dpH, allows both components of $d\mu H^+$ to be evaluated within mitochondria of living cells.[1] SNARF-1 is a single excitation dual-ratio emission fluorescent probe used to measure intracellular pH. SNARF-1 is loaded into cells using its lipid-soluble acetoxymethyl ester derivative (SNARF-1-AM). Inside the cell, SNARF-1-AM is hydrolyzed by endogenous esterases to liberate free SNARF-1. Similar to other ion-sensitive fluorophores, SNARF-1 does not load exclusively into the cytosol. In particular, mitochondria, nucleus, lysosomes, and cytosol may load heavily with ion-reporting probes such as SNARF-1, thereby allowing measurements of pH within multiple compartments inside a living cell.

To load SNARF-1 into cultured cardiac myocytes, cells are incubated with 5 μM SNARF-1-AM for 45 min in culture medium at 37°C. The cells are washed twice and placed on the microsope stage in Krebs–Ringer–HEPES buffer (KRH: 115 mM NaCl, 5 mM KCl, 1 mM KH_2PO_4, 1.2 mM $MgSO_4$, 2 mM $CaCl_2$, and 25 mM HEPES at pH 7.4). Ratioed fluorescence emissions (584 nm: >620 nm), excited at 568 nm, are used to estimate pH against an *in situ* calibration. The reader is referred to Chacon *et al.*[1] for a more detailed description of intracellular pH measurements using SNARF-1 and confocal microsocpy.

To determine $d\mu H^+$ within in intact cell, measurements of dy and dpH across the mitochondria must be measured. For example, in the experiments of Figs 9.2 and 9.3, we can determine a mitochondrial $d\mu H^+$ of at least −140 mV in resting adult rabbit cardiac myocytes ($dy = -100$ mV and $d\text{pH} = 0.9$ units). Measurements of hydrogen ion gradients

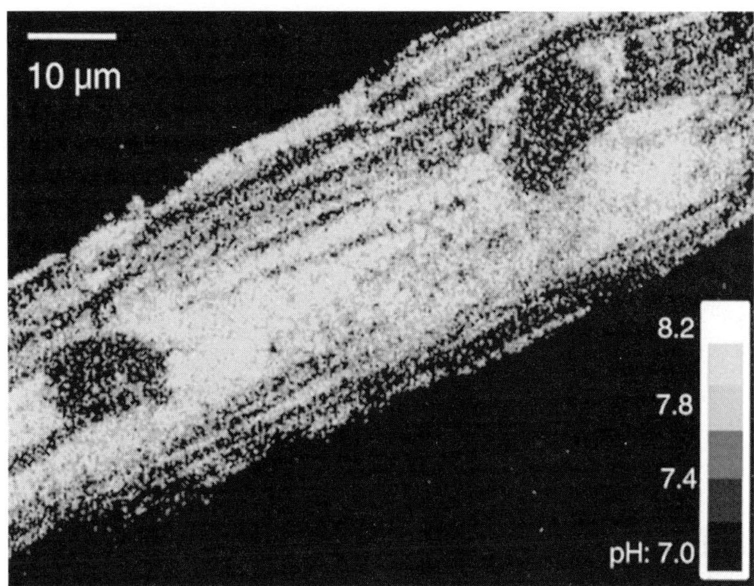

Fig. 9.3 Confocal imaging of cytosolic and mitochondrial pH in a cultured adult rabbit cardiac myocyte. Confocal images were collected to show the difference in pH between the mitochondrial and cytosolic compartments (ΔpH). The image shows a cytosolic pH of 7.0 with a mitochondrial pH between 7.8 and 8.1 (ΔpH = 0.8–1.1 units).

serve to define mechanisms of cytotoxicity. However, its practicality is limited in high-volume sample screening.

7. Calcium homeostasis

Calcium regulates various cell functions. Therefore, it is not surprising that a great deal of interest has been directed at studying alterations in intracellular calcium.[2,16,22]

The advent of calcium-selective fluorophores has facilitated quantitation of intracellular calcium levels using fluorescence microscopy. Interpretation of the fluorescence microscopy may be misleading since the dyes have been shown to sequester within intracellular organelles. In particular, mitochondria possess esterase and sequester the dyes when loaded as their ester derivatives. Should measurements of cytosolic calcium be conducted by conventional digitized fluorescence imaging, then efforts to minimize subcellular sequestration must be taken. On the other hand, one can take advantage of the subcellular localization of these dyes and the thin optical sectioning capabilities of confocal microscopy to image calcium levels within subcellular organelles of a living cell (Fig. 9.4). Fluorescence microscopy estimates of intracellular calcium levels are effective in mechanistic investigations but are limited in high-volume high capacity cytotoxicity screening.

IV. CONCLUSION

Primary cultures of cardiac myocytes are attractive models that can minimize the use of animals and reduce the cost of new product development. These models have a biological

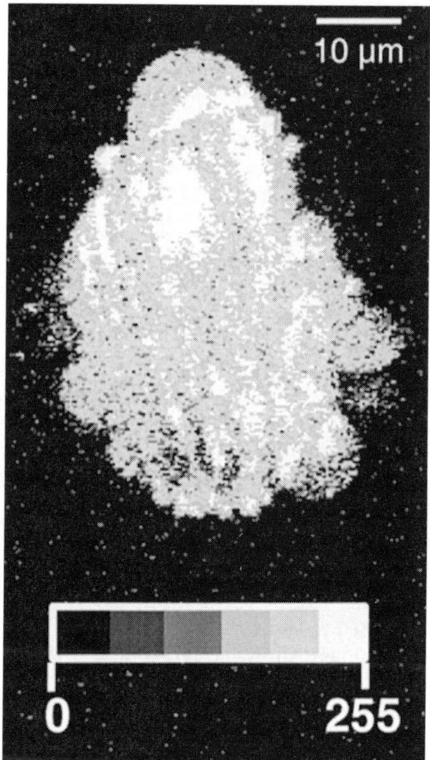

Fig. 9.4 Intracellular free calcium in a hypercontracted cardiac myocyte after 51 min chemical hypoxia. The gray scale represents fluorescence intensity. Mitochondrial calcium loading became prominent at the onset of hypercontraction. The white regions of the image showing the greatest fluorescence intensity were determined to be mitochondria by spatial localization of each image pixel with corresponding pixels from a TMRM image that was simultaneously acquired (not shown).

basis that links them to the *in vivo* biological response being modeled. We have reviewed different assays that could be used to assess pharmacological and toxicological responses of cardiac mycoytes in culture. These assays are essentially divided into two categories: those that measure alterations of physiological functions and those that measure cell death. Cell death is an abrupt all-or-nothing phenomenon that occurs as the consequence of abrupt breakdown of the plasma membrane. Once the dose and time dependency of cell death have been established, functional assays can proceed to identify the molecular and cellular mechanisms of action.

REFERENCES

1. Chacon, E., Reece, J. M., Nieminen, A.-L., Zahrebelski, G., Herman, B. and Lemasters, J. J. (1994) Distribution of electrical potential, pH, free Ca^{2+}, and volume inside cultured adult rabbit cardiac myocytes during chemical hypoxia: a multiparameter digitized confocal microscopic study. *Biophys. J.* **66:** 942–952.
2. Bond, J. M., Chacon, E., Herman, B. and Lemasters, J. J. (1993) Intracellular pH and Ca^{2+} homeostasis in the pH paradox of reperfusion injury to neonatal rat cardiac myocytes. *Am. J. Physiol.* **265:** C129–C137.

3. Acosta, D. and Ramos, K. (1984) Cardiotoxicity of tricyclic antidepressants in cultured rat myocardial cells. *J. Toxicol. Environ. Health* **14:** 137–143.
4. Spahr, R., Jacobson, S. L., Siegmund, B., Schwartz, P. and Piper, H. M. (1989) Substrate oxidation by adult cardiomyocytes in long-term primary culture. *J. Mol. Cell. Cardiol.* **21:** 175.
5. Probst, I., Spahr, R., Schweickhardt, C., Hunneman, D. H. and Piper, H. M. (1986) Carbohydrate and fatty acid metabolism of cultured adult cardiac myocytes. *Am. J. Physiol.* **250:** H853.
6. Wenzel, D. G., Wheatley, J. W. and Byrd, G. D. (1970) Effects of nicotine in cultured heart cells. *Toxicol. Appl. Pharmacol.* **17:** 774–785.
7. Ulrich, R. G., Elliget, K. A. and Rosnick, D. K. (1989) Purification of neonatal rat cardiac cells by centrifugal elutriation. *J. Tissue Culture Methods* **11:** 217–221.
8. Harary, I. and Farley, B. (1963) *In vitro* studies on single beating rat heart cells. I. Growth and organization. *Exp. Cell Res.* **29:** 451–465.
9. Haddad, J., Decker, M. L., Hsieh, L.-C., Lesch, M., Samarel, A. M. and Decker, R. S. (1988) Attachment and maintenance of adult rabbit cardiac myocytes in primary cell culture. *Am. J. Physiol.* **255:** C19–C27.
10. Welder, A. A., Grant, R., Bradlow, J. and Acosta, D. (1991) A primary culture system of adult rat heart cells for the study of toxicologic agents. *In Vitro Cell. Dev. Biol.* **27A:** 921–926.
11. Spieckermann, P. G. and Piper, H. M. (1978) *Isolated Adult Cardiac Myocytes.* Steinkopff Verlag Darmstadt, New York.
12. Gores, G. J., Nieminen, A.-L., Dawson, T. L., Herman, B. and Lemasters, J. J. (1988) Extracellular acidosis delays the onset of cell death in ATP-depleted hepatocytes. *Am. J. Physiol.* **255:** C315–C322.
13. Nieminen, A.-L., Gores, G. J., Bond, J. M., Imberti, R. I., Herman, B. and Lemasters, J. J. (1992) A novel cytotoxicity screening assay using a multi-well fluorescence scanner. *Toxicol. Appl. Pharmacol.* **115:** 147–155.
14. Mitchell, D. B., Santone, K.S. and Acosta, D. (1980) Evaluation of cytotoxicity in cultured cells by enzyme leakage. *J. Tissue Culture Methods* **6:** 113–116.
15. Acosta, D., Wenzel, D. G. and Wheatley, J. W. (1974) Beating duration of cultured rat heart cells as affected by drugs and other factors. *Phamacol. Res. Commun.* **6:** 263–271.
16. Chacon, E. and Acosta, D. (1991) Mitochondrial regulation of superoxide by calcium: an alternate mechanism for the cardiotoxicity of doxorubicin. *Toxicol. Appl. Pharmacol.* **107:** 117–128.
17. Emaus, R. K., Grunwald, R. and Lemasters, J. J. (1986) Rhodamine 123 as a probe of transmembrane potential in isolated rat-liver mitochondria: spectral and metabolic properties. *Biochim. Biophys. Acta* **880:** 436–448.
18. Lemasters, J. J., Nieminen, A.-L., Chacon, E., Imberti, R., Reece, J. M. and Herman, B. (1992) Use of fluorescent probes to monitor mitochondrial membrane potential in isolated mitochondria, cell suspensions, and cultured cells. In Lash, L. and Jones, D. P. (eds) *Mitochondrial Dysfunction*, Academic Press, San Diego, CA.
19. Chen, L. B. (1988) Mitochondrial membrane potential in living cells. *Ann. Rev. Cell Biol.* **4:** 155–181.
20. Ehrenberg, B., Montana, V., Wei, M.-D., Wuskell, J. P. and Loew, L. M. (1988) Membrane potentials can be determined from the Nernstian distribution of cationic dyes. *Biophys. J.* **53:** 785–794.
21. Lemasters, J. J., Chacon, E., Zahrebelski, G., Reece, J. M. and Nieminen, A.-L. (1992) Laser scanning confocal microscopy in living cells. In Herman, B. and Lemasters, J. J. (eds) *Optical Microscopy: New Technologies and Applications*, Ch. 12, pp. 339–354. Academic Press, San Diego, CA.
22. Chacon, E., Ulrich, R. and Acosta, D. (1992) A digitized-fluorescence-imaging study of mitochondrial Ca^{2+} increase by doxorubicin in cardiac myocytes. *Biochem. J.* **281:** 871–878.

10

Immunotoxicology Testing *In Vitro*

CLIVE MEREDITH AND KLARA MILLER

I.	Introduction	225
II.	Lymphocytes	226
III.	Antigen-presenting cells (accessory cells)	227
	A. Dendritic cells	227
	B. Monocytes and macrophages	228
IV.	Cytokines	229
V.	Immunotoxicology	231
VI.	Immunotoxicology *in vitro*	232
VII.	Conclusions	237
	Acknowledgement	239
	References	239

I. INTRODUCTION

The immune system has developed primarily as a defence against microbial invasion with a primary requirement to distinguish between 'self' and 'non-self'. It is this latter unique ability that has led to survival of the evolving species in a hostile environment and the capacity to develop specific responses to each intrinsic challenge at the same time as maintaining homoeostatic mechanisms.

The earliest manifestation of so-called innate immunity was phagocytosis, which is still the main defensive mode of action in primitive organisms. In higher vertebrates phagocytosis plays another important role, in the handling of senescent red blood cells and in the scavenger receptor function that is responsible for the uptake of apoptosed cells. Later in evolution innate immunity was amplified, first by the development of a vascular system that allowed phagocytosis and processing by both fixed and circulatory cells, and second by the development of a disseminated lymphoid system as well as of specialized primary and secondary lymphoid organs such as the thymus, spleen and lymph nodes. The lymphoid system also developed local lymphoid cell aggregates associated with the alimentary and respiratory tracts, commonly known as gut-associated lymphoid tissue (GALT) and bronchus-associated lymphoid tissue (BALT). The cells most commonly found in the lymphoid system are lymphocytes, consisting of two main populations, T and B, which develop along distinct differentiation pathways and are responsible for the remarkable

IN VITRO METHODS IN PHARMACEUTICAL RESEARCH
ISBN 0-12-163390-X

specificity of immune responses. They in turn do not function in isolation, and other cells known as accessory or antigen-presenting cells (APCs) are needed during initiation of the immune response.

To prevent inappropriate responses during such cell interactions, the immune system is controlled by a genetic region which codes for the major histocompatibility complex (MHC). The genes encoding MHC molecules are extremely polymorphic, there being at least 100 distinct alleles at some loci so that they distinguish one individual of a given species from another such individual. These 'antigenic' determinants are found on the membrane of lymphocytes and on most of the fixed tissue cells in the body, and regulate the ability to generate immune responses to both synthetic and naturally occurring antigens (host responsiveness) as well as ensuring histocompatibility restriction. Most importantly the MHC complex includes a set of polymorphic genes encoding class I and class II molecules (glycoproteins), whose essential function is to present antigenic peptides.

All cell populations that participate in immune reactions arise from stem cells in the bone marrow, as do other cell lines, such as polymorphonuclear leucocytes, which participate in immunological reactions through the release of chemical mediators and cytokines.

II. LYMPHOCYTES

Lymphocytes are functionally heterogeneous and consist of two main populations, T and B, concerned with cell-mediated or humoral immunity, respectively. T cells are generated in the thymus from precursors that have migrated from the bone marrow to the thymus.[1] Considerable mitotic activity occurs in the thymus, particularly in the cortex, and epithelial cells, fibroblasts, dendritic cells and macrophages of the thymus provide a microenvironment essential for differentiation to occur. Hormones secreted by thymus epithelial cells have been shown to have specific effects on the differentiation and functional activity of T cells. Cortical thymocytes have long been known to lack immunobiological activity, owing to lack of surface structures such as the T-cell receptor (TCR) complex found on mature cells. It is probable that part of the considerable death rate of cortical thymocytes is due to some cells failing to rearrange TCR genes effectively. The relatively small numbers of thymocytes present in the medullary region are phenotypically and functionally similar to peripheral T cells. It does not follow, however, that these cells are on the way out to the periphery, and some medullary thymocytes are known to remain resident in the thymus for long periods.[2]

About 80% of lymphocytes in human blood and 60% of those in peripheral lymphoid tissue are of T lineage, and most express either the T4 (CD4) or T8 (CD8) surface membrane antigen (cluster differentiation antigens). Cells bearing CD4 (helper cells) are concerned with activation of B cells and macrophages, and recognize antigen in association with MHC class II molecules. Cells within the CD4 population will provide 'help' for specific antibody production, whereas others are involved in cellular immunity. Their roles will be described in more detail later. The CD8 T-cell population is thought to have evolved principally to combat virus-infected cells by a direct cell–cell cytotoxic mechanism. They recognize peptides generated in the cell cytosol and displayed at the cell surface bound to MHC class I molecules to which the CD8 cells co-receptor binds. $CD8^+$ cells also have the capacity to act as 'suppressor' cells. Overactivity of suppressor T cells may result in an inability to respond to an antigenic challenge, while underactivity may allow the development of autoimmune manifestations.

B cells originate from pluripotent haematopoietic stem cells and differentiate into immunoglobulin-secreting plasma cells through a complex multistep ligand-driven process. The generation of B cells takes place in the bone marrow in mammals, and in the bursa of chickens (in which they were first identified). Immunoglobulin gene diversity in humans and rodents is created mainly by ongoing gene rearrangement in the bone marrow, followed by somatic hypermutation. In the chicken, immunoglobulin gene rearrangement is less complex and diversity is generated by somatic gene modifications. There is an extremely high rate of B-cell division in the bursa of birds and in the bone marrow of mammals but, as in the thymus, the newly generated cells undergo programmed cell death *in situ*.[3] It has been suggested that apoptosis is a consequence of non-functional immunoglobulin gene rearrangement and lack of surface immunoglobulin (sIg) expression. When newly formed B cells reach the peripheral tissues, their survival depends on activation by encounter with antigen, and the somatic rearrangement of receptor genes, which allows the generation of antigen receptors with diverse recognition capacities, ensures the specificity of the response. The mitotically activated B cells typically generate subclones, each making antibody of one of the immunoglobulin classes: IgM, IgG, IgA, IgD and IgE. Both newly formed and established B cells have the opportunity of responding to the antigen concerned, giving rise to antibody-secreting cells (plasma cells) and memory B cells.

In the generation of a T cell-dependent antibody response, T and B cells are engaged in an active reciprocal interchange between MHC class II and the TCR. Additional molecules, both on the cell membrane and in the cytosol, are needed to ensure efficient signal transduction, and an array of cell-surface differentiation antigens (CD) and accessory molecules has been identified on the surface of T and B cells.[4] Interestingly, the receptor-like glycoprotein CD45, expressed on both T and B cells, is involved in the antigen-driven activation of B cells as well as T-cell activation, and appears to play a role in the regulation of postactivation events associated with B-cell differentiation.[5] The relative contributions of primary and memory B cells in an immune response to a T-dependent antigen have been studied in rats.[6] Primary B cells are recruited only in the first few days after immunization, after which the response is sustained by long-lived cells belonging to memory clones.

Under some circumstances, and dependent on the state of differentiation, B cells may also, through the B-cell receptor (BCR) for antigens, process and present antigen to T cells. Recognition by the TCR would then lead to the binding of accessory molecules such as CD23 (FcεRII), CD28 and CD40 to their respective ligands.

III. ANTIGEN-PRESENTING CELLS (ACCESSORY CELLS)

A. Dendritic cells

Dendritic cells lack most conventional surface membrane markers associated with the macrophage lineage, but expression of MHC class II is very strong and hence they are often called 'professional' antigen-presenting cells (APCs). They are found in lymphoid tissues and in the interstitial epithelium of the lung and other non-lymphoid organs. Langerhans' cells, which also belong to the dendritic family,[7] are found in the epidermis of the skin. Activated dendritic cells are thought to be the most effective APCs because they are able to present the appropriate antigenic peptides in the context of constitutively expressed co-stimulatory signals,[8] migrating to lymph nodes after taking up antigen in the periphery. In the lung the

APC must be capable of efficiently sampling extracellular fluids within the airway and of directed migration to paracortical zones in the regional lymph nodes, and it must be highly efficient in activating naive T cells. As yet, it is not clear which cytokine plays the more important role in activation, maturation and/or migration of dendritic cells; granulocyte–macrophage colony-stimulating factor (GM-CSF), tumour necrosis factor (TNF) α and interleukin (IL) 1 have been implicated, and a recent report has suggested that IL-4 may play an important role.[9] Analogous to epidermal Langerhans' cells, airway and lung dendritic cells are restricted to antigen acquisition and processing *in situ* and only develop the capacity to present antigen to T cells after maturation and migration to the paracortical area of secondary lymphoid organs.[10]

B. Monocytes and macrophages

Monocytes and macrophages are defined as phagocytic mononuclear cells and are grouped together on the basis of having a common origin and similar cytochemistry. They are a very heterogeneous group of cells and macrophages from different sites display differences in secretion patterns and antigen presentation. For example, studies on fresh human alveolar macrophages and blood monocytes demonstrate differences in the release of cytokines.[11] Alveolar macrophages release low amounts of IL-1β in response to lipopolysaccharide (LPS) and high amounts of TNF-α, whereas blood monocytes release abundant amounts of IL-1β but low amounts of TNF. Another important difference between alveolar and serosal (pleural and peritoneal) macrophages is in the expression of MHC class II on the surface membrane: this is tenfold higher in peritoneal and pleural cell populations compared with that found on free-lying pulmonary cells.

Free-lying alveolar macrophages function well as phagocytic cells, and act primarily to regulate potentially damaging inflammatory responses in the lung. It has recently been postulated that the alveolar macrophage plays two important immunoregulatory roles.[12] During the afferent limb of the immune response they release cytokines critical for the production of functionally active dendritic cells and may also pass on the processed antigen to the dendritic cell, whereas during the efferent limb of the immune reaction they respond to products of sensitized T cells such as interferon (IFN) α to interact with T-helper cells in an antigen-specific, MHC-restricted manner or develop cytotoxic activity.

When activated, cells of the monocyte–macrophage lineage can kill neoplastic cells and/or elicit tumour-destructive reactions centred on the tumour vasculature. Activated cells spread more extensively on glass or plastic culture dishes and have a higher density of surface membrane receptors such as the IgG Fc receptor. Agents such as LPS have been shown to induce increased production and secretion of IL-1 and other cytokines, and macrophages that have been 'activated' by the products of antigen-specific lymphocyte activation are non-specifically more effective in ingesting and killing a wide range of bacteria.

Cells of monocyte–macrophages lineage recognize a great range of antigens, not only those of external origin, and have also been shown to be capable of oxidizing small molecules to immunogenic metabolites via the lipo-oxygenase pathway.[13] A protein antigen is usually broken down to a peptide fragment produced by ingestion and partial digestion with subsequent presentation of the processed antigen on the surface in conjunction with MHC class II. After processing there is synthesis of IFN-α, which induces increased expression of MHC class II, and IFN-α together with antigen provides a signal for the synthesis of low amounts of IL-1.

IV. CYTOKINES

Research over the last decades has shown conclusively that the immune network is regulated by cytokines, which may act as both messenger and effector molecules. Unlike more familiar soluble mediators such as hormones, which are mainly produced by one type of cell and act on another specific cell, cytokines can be produced by several different cell populations and are able to affect the proliferation and differentiation of diverse cell populations of other systems as well as the lymphoreticular one. Such processes inevitably involve complementary cell membrane recognition molecules, thus initiating receptor–ligand interactions with subsequent local release of mediators.

At least 13 major interleukins have now been identified as cytokines, as well as a number of growth factors affecting haematopoietic tissues, and three major types of interferons (Tables 10.1 and 10.2). Several other cytokines involved in inflammatory responses, such as TNF, have also been described. Research into the role of cytokines in immune regulation was greatly stimulated by the classification of T-helper cells into two groups, Th1 and Th2.[14] Th1 cells are now defined by their production of cytokines IL-2, IFN-γ and TNF-β, and Th2 cells are defined by their production of IL-4, IL-5, IL-6, IL-10 and IL-13; both cell types produce IL-3, TNF-α and GM-CSF. Th1 cells promote cell-mediated immune (CMI) reactions whereas TH2 cells are involved in the development of humoral immunity.

Because phagocytic cells precede the appearance of specific lymphocytes in the evolution of the immune response, it was recently been postulated[15] that the early T-cell response depends on the production of cytokines by macrophage-like phagocytic cells at an early stage of infection or antigen presentation.[16] Indeed, co-culture of T-helper cells with activated macrophages has been shown to result in the production of IFN-γ induced by macrophage-derived IL-12.[17] Furthermore, IL-2 has also been shown to be a potent stimulator of IFN-γ production by natural killer (NK) cells, suggesting that NK cells could play an intermediary role in polarizing the T-helper cell response. It may be that the earliest form of a cellular immune system comprised macrophage-like cells producing IL-12, together with IFN-γ producing NK cells, so as to protect the host against viral and other intracellular infection, whereas cells of the mast cell–basophil lineage (known to synthesize IL-4 and IL-5) evolved to counteract metazoan parasites such as helminths. By exploiting such divergent non-specific responses, the subsequent evolving adaptive T-cell responses would then give rise to the Th1-dependent CMI responses and TH2-dependent antibody–allergenic responses, respectively, that we know today.

To ensure a proper balance and flexibility of immune responsiveness each subset is able to inhibit its counterpart, i.e. IFN-γ directly inhibits proliferation of Th2 but not Th1 cells,[18] whereas IL-4 and IL-10 downregulate MHC class II expression by monocytes, reducing their antigen-presenting capacity and inhibiting cytokine production by Th1 cells. The establishment of Th2 dominance is dependent on early secretion of IL-4 by Th2 cells and by the secretion of IL-10, which also downregulates Th1 responses by suppressing the production of macrophage-derived IL-12.[19] IL-13 also downregulates the production of IL-12 and IFN-α by monocytes (which induce development of Th1 responses) and, like IL-4, it may therefore skew the development in favour of a TH2 response.[20] It must be emphasized that Th2 cells play a prominent role in immediate-type hypersensitivity as IL-4 is the critical stimulus inducing IgE production, and that polarization of Th1 responses is a major factor in the development of contact sensitization. A key switch that induces T cells to become Th1 cell is IL-12, which primes cells for IFN-γ production even in the presence of IL-4. The role and functions of different integrins and adhesion molecules will not be described in this chapter, but it is obvious that cytokines produced *in vivo* would be rapidly washed away

Table 10.1 Interleukins.

Name	Source	Main functions
IL-1α (membrane bound) IL-1β	Monocytes/macrophages, endothelial cells, fibroblasts, neuronal cells, glial cells, keratinocytes, epithelial cells	Activation, differentiation of cells involved in inflammation and immune responses; affects CNS and endocrine systems
IL-2	T cells	Stimulates T-cell proliferation and differentiation; enhances activity of NK and LAK cells; promotes proliferation and IgG secretion of activated B cells
IL-3	T cells, keratinocytes, mast cells, neuronal cells	Stimulates production and differentiation of macrophages, neutrophils, basophils, eosinophils and mast cells; supports proliferation of multipotential progenitor cells
IL-4	T cells, mast cells, basophils, macrophages	Induces differentiation of CD4 T cells to TH2 cells; induces proliferation and IgE, IgA secretion of B cells
IL-5	T cells, mast cells	Stimulates growth and differentiation of eosinophils
IL-6	Monocytes/macrophages, T-cells, hepatocytes, fibroblasts, endothelial cells, neuronal cells	Activates haematopoietic progenitor cells; induces increase in platelet numbers; stimulates production of acute-phase proteins
IL-7	Bone marrow cells, fetal liver cells	Supports growth of pre-B cells; stimulates proliferation and generation of cytotoxic T cells and LAK cells
IL-8	Monocytes, T cells, fibroblasts, endothelial cells, keratinocytes, neutrophils	Chemotaxin *in vitro* for neutrophils, T cells and basophils; activates neutrophils to release lysosomal enzymes
IL-9	T cells	Enhances *in vitro* survival of T-cell lines; enhances activity of mast cells
IL-10	T cells, macrophages, keratinocytes, B cells	Potent immunosuppressant of macrophage functions; enhances B-cell proliferation and immunoglobulin secretion
IL-11	Stromal fibroblasts	Synergizes with IL-3 and IL-4; stimulates synthesis of hepatic acute-phase protein
IL-12	B cells, macrophages	Induces differentiation of TH1 cells; stimulates growth of NK cells
IL-13	T cells	Inhibits inflammatory cytokine production by monocytes/ macrophages; induces B-cell growth and differentiation
IL-14	T cells	Inhibits proliferation of activated B cells; inhibits immunoglobulin secretion of mitogen-stimulated B cells

IL, interleukin; Ig, immunoglobulin; LAK, lymphokine-activated killer; NK, natural killer.

Table 10.2 Other individual cytokines.

Name	Source	Main functions
TGF-α	Macrophages, keratinocytes	Mitogenic for fibroblasts; angiogenic activity *in vivo*
TGF-β	Chondrocytes, platelets, fibroblasts, monocytes	Inhibits growth of many cell types; inhibits NK cell activity
TNF-α	Monocytes/macrophages, neutrophils, NK cells, LAK cells	Immunostimulant; mediates expression of genes for growth factors and cytokines
TNF-β	Lymphocytes	Similar to TNF-α
RANTES	T cells, platelets, renal epithelium	Chemoattracts monocytes, T cells and eosinophils; induces histamine release from basophils
GM-CSF	T cells, endothelial cells, fibroblasts, monocytes/ macrophages	Enhances proliferation of multipotential stem cells, monocytes, neutrophils and eosinophils
M-CSF	Monocytes/macrophages, fibroblasts, endothelial cells	Enhances proliferation of multipotential stem cells and monocytes
G-CSF	Monocytes/macrophages, fibroblasts, endothelial cells	Enhances proliferation of multipotential stem cells and neutrophils

TGF, transforming growth factor; TNF, tumour necrosis factor; GM-CSF, granulocyte–macrophage colony-stimulating factor.

without mechanisms to capture and immobilize certain cytokines on the endothelium, where they mediate activation and induction of other chemokines.[21] Cytokines produced within the tissues are also important inducers of leucocyte subset-specific adhesion.

V. IMMUNOTOXICOLOGY

If immunotoxicology is to play a significant role in the risk assessment of pharmaceutical and industrial chemicals, it is important that it can offer tests that are sensitive, specific and reproducible. At present there is a lack of agreement between toxicologists and scientists involved in immunotoxicology as to which tests are most appropriate in assessing and predicting the immunotoxicity of any given group of compounds. This is mainly due to the difficulties in applying conventional dose–response relationships to an integrated, interdependent system capable of reacting to changing circumstances. Furthermore, the effects of an agent on and within the immune system must be considered in relation to the effects and constraints imposed by antigen. Indeed, antigenic challenge is inseparable from immune reactivity; without antigen there is no immune response and the concept of immunotoxicology becomes meaningless. Thus, antigen not only adds another dimension to the dose effect of dose–response relationship: the requirement of antigen actually separates conventional toxicity from immunotoxicity. Whereas it is perfectly possible to examine the effect of an agent on lymphoid organ weight, for example, some form of antigen challenge must be considered if one wishes to address the effect of the agent on immune reactivity.

Recent advances in molecular biology have provided new *in vitro* and *in vivo* techniques for the detection and precise evaluation of immunotoxic events and processes that could offer significant advantages over existing procedures for determining immune reactivity. Indeed, assays can now be performed that eliminate the need for *in vivo* antigen challenge. As suggested above, they are based on the finding that the development of immune responses depends on precise cellular communication involving a series of soluble polypeptide mediators (cytokines), which include interleukins, lymphokines, growth factors and their receptors on the cell surface.

The necessity for developing such *in vitro* systems is particularly relevant for biotechnology-derived drugs. Monoclonal antibodies and proteins produced by recombinant DNA technology are not only powerful tools for biomedical research but many of them have human clinical applications. Assessment of the immunotoxicity of these biotechnology-derived molecules raises a series of new problems clearly distinct from those encountered with other chemicals. For instance, human IL-2 can bind to murine IL-2 receptors and support the proliferation of mouse T cells, but human IFN-γ and IFN-α are totally inactive in mouse or rats because of species differences in the structure of interferon receptors. Clinical experience, however, has shown that some of the recombinants may induce an acute inflammatory reaction, probably by triggering the synthesis of a series of cytokines. An important question, therefore, is whether it would be possible to design *in vitro* toxicity assays that could pinpoint some key cytokines and which might be developed as screening assays at an early stage of the preclinical development of such substances.

A large body of clinical and experimental data has already shown that induction of TNF-α is the pivotal event in the inflammatory syndrome induced by anti-CD3 monoclonal antibodies, and in the septic shock and several acute adverse reactions induced by other biotechnology products. TNF-α is the first cytokine to be released by LPS-activated monocytes, albeit in low amounts, and it upregulates subsequent production of IL-1, IL-6 and IL-8. Furthermore, IFN-γ produced by activated T cells synergizes with TNF-α in the activation of monocytes and endothelial cells and probably enhances the toxicity of TNF-α. A most encouraging development is recent evidence that blood mononuclear cell suspensions represent a highly sensitive system for the detection of TNF-α secretion as induced by monoclonal antibodies, although the kinetics of *in vitro* production is slower than expected from *in vivo* administration.[22]

VI. IMMUNOTOXICOLOGY *IN VITRO*

As can be seen from the preceding sections, the immune system is a highly complex entity involving a large number of cell types from varying lineages and is dependent for its normal function on subtle interactions between these cell types requiring both cell–cell contact and communication via soluble mediators and their receptors. Thus the whole immune system does not readily lend itself to modelling with *in vitro* techniques. Even though there have been great advances in cell culture technologies in recent years, with better understanding of the demands of cells for essential cytokines or growth factors for normal functioning, it is difficult to envisage any *in vitro* system that could mimic several of the properties of the whole immune system *in vivo*. Therefore, to make any progress in this field, it is necessary to break down immune function into a series of compartments, often related to known pharmacotoxicological effects of drugs and chemicals on specialized immune responses, from which can be developed appropriate *in vitro* systems to model specific facets of the immune system.

A second problem facing those who attempt to develop *in vitro* models of the immune system is that most immune manifestations require more than one exposure, with a defined time lag between the original exposure of the immune system and the clinical effect. Sometimes this is due to a two-stage process, e.g. hypersensitivity responses where the initial exposure to an allergen primes the system such that a magnified response, with clinical symptoms, occurs after a subsequent exposure. Clearly it is difficult to model such a response using *in vitro* systems that are essentially short-term experimental procedures. It is possible, however, to perform *ex vivo* procedures to model this process, e.g. the local lymph node assay (LLNA) where the complex priming stage is performed *in vivo* but where a correlate of the elicitation of contact allergy is performed *in vitro*.

In terms of immune suppression, the effect of an agent that induces a downregulation in response cannot be manifest until the immune system is subsequently challenged to perform a normal response. In humans this would occur when the immune system is called on to fight off an adventitious infection; this is normally modelled in experimental animals using a host resistance assay. It is difficult to envisage appropriate *in vitro* systems to model this procedure directly.

Instead we must further break down these compartments of the immune system so that we fundamentally understand the mechanisms by which normal functioning and responsiveness of that compartment is maintained. We must understand the role of cell–cell contact, the interactions between adhesion molecules, and the role of cytokines and their receptors. Then, even if it is not possible to model the precise interactions between immune cell types *in vitro* (due to limitations in available skills in cell culture technology), it is possible to identify the important pathways in selected immune responses and important markers of the process which can be used as surrogates for the whole complex response.

At present, there are a number of ongoing debates as to the role of *in vivo* immunotoxicology within the drug development process and within the regulatory testing process. As a relatively new discipline, immunotoxicology has found it hard to establish itself as a stand-alone requirement; rather it is seen by many as an adjunct to existing testing strategies. Regulatory authorities can request evidence of potential immunotoxicity but this is generally conducted in the course of repeat-dose studies and focuses on haematological parameters, organ weights and histopathological analysis of lymphoid tissue. There is no requirement for immune function testing unless there are certain indications in the conventional repeat-dose studies. There are various proposals for tiered testing strategies, e.g. the National Toxicology Program (NTP) Tier I/Tier II model, but these would be effected some way into the regulatory testing process. To be of real benefit to the pharmaceutical and chemical industry, there has to be development in the area of immune function tests which can aid in defining immunopharmacological efficacy as well as immunotoxicological potential, in tests that can aid in screening candidate molecules and ranking their immunopharmacotoxicological potential, and in tests that can be incorporated into in-house testing protocols to aid in the hazard identification and hazard assessment processes. There would be major economic advantages to the pharmaceutical and chemical industry, in terms of experimental costs as well as time, in the development and validation of appropriate *in vitro* systems to model the responsive components of the immune system.

It is important at this stage to distinguish between the two potential uses of *in vitro* test systems; this is particularly important for *in vitro* immunotoxicology. First, any appropriate *in vitro* screen (usually a mechanistic-based test) can be employed in the process of drug development to assist in screening candidate molecules for efficacy or for potential undesirable side-effects. In terms of immunotoxicology *in vitro*, there are many systems employed using isolated lymphocytes or monocytes which can be used in this type of procedure. It is not necessary that these tests be validated by rigorous interlaboratory trial, for they may be used by only a small number of organizations and are there to expedite the internal decision-making process about the development of potential new medicines or useful chemicals. At present, this is the area of highest opportunity for *in vitro* immunotoxicological test systems. Second, there is the use of *in vitro* techniques to assist in regulatory submission; here it is an absolute requirement that the test be relevant and well validated if it is to have any utility and is to make any worthwhile contribution to the reduction in animal experimentation. *In vitro* immunotoxicological tests have less immediate contribution to make here; indeed it is unlikely that they will contribute significantly to the regulatory process before there is a full-scale introduction of *in vivo* immunotoxicological testing as a required adjunct to repeat-dose studies. Because the validation process itself is extremely protracted and subject to multiple interpretation, we are not likely to see a true *in vitro* immunotoxicological test within the regulatory arena in the foreseeable future.

This is not to say that there is a lack of opportunity for *in vitro* immunotoxicology within the regulatory sector. As stated above, the local lymph node assay (LLNA) has been developed to perform the lymphocyte proliferation stage of contact sensitization *in vitro* and has been shown to be an effective test for identifying contact allergens.[23] In this type of *ex vivo* test, mice are exposed dermally in a sensitization phase and subsequently killed in order to isolate the lymphocytes from the draining lymph nodes. The proliferative capacity of the stimulated lymphocytes is shown to correlate well with the known sensitization potential of reference compounds. This assay has been subject to significant intra- and inter-laboratory validation exercises[24] and currently has an impact on regulatory toxicology in that positive responses can be accepted as diagnostic of sensitizing hazard. Is there any potential for further refining this assay such that it can be done entirely *in vitro*? Sadly, the answer must be no, at least in the short term, for in considering alternatives to the sensitizing phase of the LLNA, we confront one of the major challenges facing those who develop alternatives in immunotoxicology research – the problems of allergen processing and presentation *in vitro*. For sensitization to occur, it is necessary for the allergen to penetrate the skin, interact with APCs, undergo 'processing', and be presented in a suitable form to T lymphocytes. *En route*, the allergen induces the release of accessory factors which influence the magnitude of this response. Whilst there have been advances in understanding this process, certainly in terms of the requirement for epidermal cytokines,[25] the capacity to model the process *in vitro* is at present lacking.

Most of the work performed so far to characterize antigen-specific T cells has utilized lymphocytes from sensitized animals (or humans) and is designed either to study the role of Th1/Th2 clones[18] or to develop diagnostic tests for chemical allergy.[26] There have been some attempts to use exclusively *in vitro* systems, for example using naive T lymphocytes cultured in the presence of hapten-modified epidermal Langerhans' cells,[27] and such systems, based on an end-point of thymidine incorporation, offer some potential. The challenge is to culture potential APCs with allergen and necessary co-factors in order to achieve processing and presentation *in vitro*.

In terms of more general immunomodulatory properties, there have been many strategies to develop *in vitro* screening systems. One of the more promising was proposed by Steer *et al.*[28] using IL-2-containing medium from EL-4 thymoma cells to stimulate the IL-2-dependent T-cell line, CTLL-2, and to test the effects of 14 different chemicals on proliferation. By comparison with basal cytotoxicity in an unrelated cell line, clear distinctions could be made between the effects of chemicals known to be immunomodulatory and non-immunomodulatory agents. However, there were certain compounds, e.g. colchicine, which tested positive in this assay, yet have no known immunomodulatory activity *in vivo*, so it seems that a more specific end-point might be desirable for further development of this *in vitro* test. Some examples of *in vitro* assays used in immunotoxicology testing are given in Table 10.3.

Table 10.3 Examples of *in vitro* assays.

Assay	Objective	References
[^{3}H]thymidine uptake	Measure of lymphocyte proliferation	29, 30
Multiple end-point test battery	Screen for chemically induced dysfunction	31, 32
cDNA probes	Measure changes in expression of genes coding for immunoregulatory cytokines	33–35
Globulin-free human serum albumins	Evaluation of low-molecular-weight chemicals as potential respiratory allergens	36
Co-culture (mouse thymocytes on thymic epithelial monolayers)	Investigate cellular and molecular mechanisms of thymic atrophy	37, 38
Cell culture (mouse splenocytes and human peripheral blood mononuclear cells)	Evaluation of effects on lymphoproliferative and cytotoxic functions	39

The question of which species to use when considering the development of *in vitro* systems for immunotoxicology research and testing has always been a taxing one, particularly in view of the fact that most immunotoxicologists cannot agree on whether the mouse or the rat is the best *in vivo* model. There have been some attempts to establish multiple end-point approaches for *in vitro* immunotoxicity, based on the use of immunocompetent cells from C57Bl mice.[31] In this battery of tests, assays such as antibody-dependent phagocytosis of sheep red blood cells, macrophage TNF activity, NK cell activity, blastogenesis and IgM assays can be performed and have been shown to correlate with literature *in vivo* results for a class of compounds known as organophosphates.[32] This clearly represents a useful advance in the development of alternatives, although certain aspects such as metabolism (important for many organophosphates) are not considered in this system. The situation with regard to the testing of monoclonal antibodies (usually of murine origin) or recombinant cytokines is particularly complex because certain compounds have distinct species specificity and toxicity cannot be modelled in a test animal. Here mechanistic understanding and the development of validated *in vitro* approaches are prerequisite. Strategies for the design of appropriate predictive tests for monoclonal antibody toxicity have been presented recently.[40]

For *in vitro* toxicology, the possibility exists to use cells of human origin, e.g. peripheral blood mononuclear cells or appropriate cell lines, e.g. monocytic U937, HL60. There have been a number of considerations of the role of human cells within immunotoxicity testing[41] and recently a study has compared the effects of pharmaceutical agents on rodent splenocytes and human peripheral blood lymphocytes *in vitro*.[39] Both lymphoproliferative and cytotoxic functions were studied in response to the immunomodulatory drugs, azathioprine, cyclosporin A and dexamethasone, as well as the non-immunomodulators, cimetidine and furosemide. In general, *in vitro* assays performed within this study were representative of the *in vivo* situation, with the exception of NK cell activity in the rat for cyclosporin A.

In our own laboratory we have developed an approach to *in vitro* immunotoxicology which has some similarities to the aforementioned test systems but which is unique in that it relies on molecular end-points rather than functional assays. Our approach has been to focus on the expression of key immunoregulatory genes, mainly the cytokines and their specific receptors, in various compartmentalized models of immune cell systems. The advantage of this approach is that the end-points, i.e. cytokine expression analysis, are directly relevant to the functioning and responding immune system *in vivo* and thus permit direct correlations to be drawn between the behaviour of immune cells *in vivo*, *ex vivo* and *in vitro*. Our initial observations were based on the behaviour of rodent macrophage and splenic lymphocyte cultures in the presence of the immunomodulators, Biostim and cyclosporin A,[33] and we further showed that both kinetic and dose–response studies could be performed on these cells with a high sensitivity.[34] The principles of this type of analysis (molecular immunotoxicology) have been stated previously[42] and are based on: (a) the relevance of this type of analysis to the *in vivo* situation; (b) applicability to *in vivo*, *ex vivo* and *in vitro* cell populations from rodent or from human; and (c) the use of cDNA hybridization analysis to identify specific cytokine mRNAs and thus measure a cellular response within a narrow time window (due to the intrinsically short half-life of the mRNA species). A schematic of the techniques used is shown in Fig. 10.1.

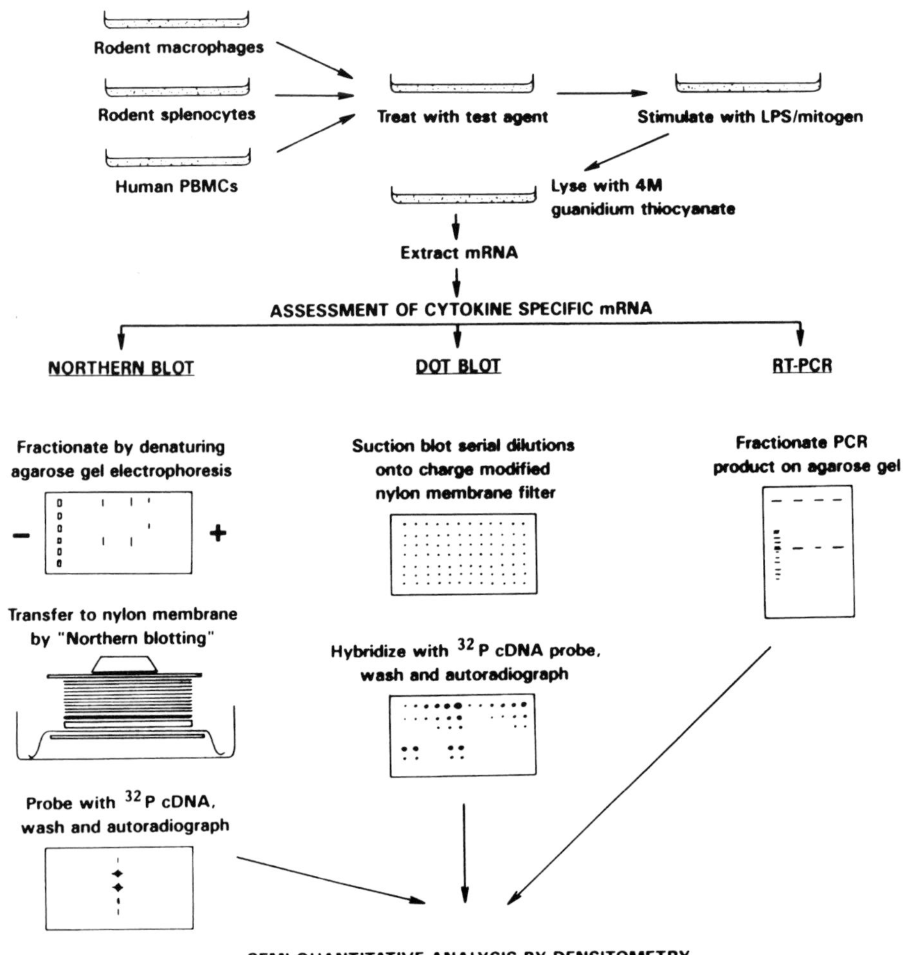

Fig. 10.1 Schematic diagram of the techniques used for *in vitro* molecular immunotoxicology in the authors' laboratory.

Using this type of analysis we have been able to show that, for the immunomodulators, azathioprine, cyclosporin A and Biostim, there are good correlations between the modulation of cytokine mRNA seen in isolated *in vitro* systems and modulation of cytokines seen when these compounds are administered *in vivo*.[43] As can be seen from Table 10.1, there is a whole range of cytokines currently identified, most of which can be incorporated as potential end-points into the expression analysis. However, it is clear that some cytokines have pivotal roles in the immune response, e.g. IL-2, whereas others have much more specific roles, e.g. IL-5 in the development of eosinophilia. Therefore it seems pertinent to include certain types of analysis, e.g. IL-2, IL-4, IFN-γ, IL-13 mRNA expression analysis into cell culture systems that are primarily lymphocytic, and IL-1α, IL-1β, IL-6 and TNF-α mRNA expression analysis into cell culture systems that are primarily monocytic. The expression of the relevant receptors cannot be ignored; although we have not yet identified a compound that directly upregulates or downregulates the expression of a cytokine receptor *in vitro*, we do see modulation of receptor expression within *in vitro* models of immune activation and it can act as a marker of immunomodulation, e.g. for the immunosuppressive organotin compound tributyl tin oxide.[44]

This type of molecular immunotoxicology analysis has found a number of applications within the development of *in vitro* tests for immunotoxicity,[35] particularly within research and development programmes funded by the European Union. There are a number of ongoing programmes that fully exploit this type of analysis, although certain drawbacks should be mentioned. Our knowledge of the whole complexity of the way in which cytokines regulate the immune system and the immune response is incomplete, particularly with respect to synergistic interactions, and it is not always possible to ascribe the expression of an individual cytokine to a specific immune function. No doubt our knowledge and understanding in this area will improve with the passing of time. At a technical level, there are some difficulties in achieving absolute quantitation of cytokine gene expression, particularly when performing multiple screening analyses, and therefore it is difficult to make interexperiment comparisons. Again, there are a number of developments underway, particularly with respect to the quantitation of reverse transcription–polymerase chain reaction (RT–PCR) products, and it is likely that these problems will be overcome in the near future.

VII. CONCLUSIONS

Immunotoxic reactions induced by xenobiotics usually involve several pathogenic mechanisms as xenobiotics can influence virtually every step of the immune response. In some situations, the manifestations of dysfunction may be primary, such as in allergic reactions or in autoimmune disease where the immune response is directed against one or more of the body's own constituents. In other cases, the consequences are likely to be secondary in that perturbation or impairment of immune function leads to inflammatory reactions or increased susceptibility to infection and perhaps to cancer. The various categories of immunotoxicity display different characteristics with regard to dependence on genetic variation in susceptibility, mode of antigen presentation and biochemical mechanisms.

These multiple levels of complexity explain why the development of *in vitro* tests in immunotoxicology are considered a real challenge. *In vitro* tests present a number of obvious advantages over *in vivo* tests on laboratory animals as they would contribute to spare animal lives in the toxicology field and, when using materials of human origin, avoid the problems related to interspecies variability in terms of susceptibility to immunotoxic compounds. Two major limitations often quoted when considering the development of *in vitro* tests are the impossibility of reproducing *in vitro* the complex microenvironment in which immune responses are initiated *in vivo*, and the non-specific toxic or stimulatory effects xenobiotics may have on immune cells. Nevertheless, evidence that the immune system is tightly regulated by cytokines and related molecular targets offers important new avenues for *in vitro* screening and for monitoring the potential immunotoxic effects of drugs and medicinal products. Development of new biotechnological tools such as cDNA probes, oligonucleotides and RT–PCR methodology also represent an innovation in respect to current methodology and will greatly contribute to developing *in vitro* model systems. Furthermore, the recent introduction of biotechnology-derived products as therapeutic agents underlines the importance of developing new methods to predict potentially damaging immune reactions.

As far as drug-induced immunosuppression is concerned, possible mechanisms to be considered include the interference of TCR-mediated transduction signalling, modulation of cytokine transcription, and mRNA degradation and the induction of apoptosis. For classical drugs, the major adverse effects on the immune system to be considered are autoimmunity and Type I hypersensitivity. Experimental autoimmune manifestations induced by mercurials, gold salts and D-penicillamine in rodents have been extensively characterized, especially in terms of genetic factors and T-cell involvement. Interestingly, the autoimmune abnormalities observed in these models are quite similar to those caused by the same agents in humans.[45] These animal models could therefore form the basis for developing predictive *in vitro* assays using lymphoid cells from animals that are genetically susceptible to or resistant to drug-induced autoimmunity *in vivo*.

There are no validated animal models for preclinical assessment of the potential of a drug to give rise to adverse reactions, and studies have therefore been limited to diagnosis of allergy in individuals who are already sensitized. Some *in vitro* tests such as measurement of proliferative responses of human lymphocytes in response to drugs are used, but they are rather insensitive and their reliability is doubtful. There is evidence that determination of cytokines (i.e. IL-2, IFN-γ, IL-10, IL-4, IL-5 and IL-6) is much more reliable when analysing drug-specific human T-cell responses in allergic drug reactions. Test systems are being developed (at least in one laboratory) to use a primary autologous mixture lymphocyte reaction in which responder peripheral blood mononuclear cells (PBMCs) from normal individuals are cultured with autologous drug-treated stimulator PBMCs. This test has potential for screening any compound for its capacity to generate T-cell determinants – although for some drugs a metabolic generating system will need to be incorporated.

The recent introduction of biotechnology-derived products as therapeutic agents raises new and difficult issues in this area and stresses the importance of developing new methods to predict immunotoxic reactions. In the case of OKT 3, for example, the antibody triggers a massive polyclonal activation of $CD3^+$ cells and monocytes, resulting in the systemic release of cytokines such as TNF, which has been shown to be responsible for severe first-dose reactions. This activating effect can be reproduced in *in vitro* in isolated PBMCs.

There are tremendous economic benefits in identifying proper *in vitro* models for the assessment of all categories of immunotoxicity, which in time would lead to the establishment of test procedures compatible with regulatory requirements. Indeed, should legislation ever become retrospective, there might be little alternative given the escalating costs of conventional animal experiments. The benefits of *in vitro* testing, however, lie not only in facilitating screening of potential immunotoxic effects but in improved risk assessment based on a true understanding of the mechanisms involved in the dysregulating of immune responses.

ACKNOWLEDGEMENT

Work in the authors' laboratory is supported by BIOTECHNOLOGY programme of the European Commission (contract no. BIO2-CT92-0316).

REFERENCES

1. Boyd, R. L. and Hugo, P. (1991) Towards an integrated view of thymopoiesis. *Immunol. Today* **12:** 71–79.
2. Nikolic-Jugic, J. (1991) Phenotypic and functional stages in the intrathymic development of alpha–beta T cells. *Immunol. Today* **12:** 65–70.
3. Vainio, O. and Imhof, B. A. (1995) The immunology and developmental biology of the chicken. *Immunol. Today* **16:** 365–369.
4. Robey, E. and Allison, J. P. (1995) T cell activation: integration of signals from the antigen receptor and co-stimulatory molecules. *Immunol. Today* **16:** 307–313.
5. Justement, L. B., Brown, U. K. and Lin, J. (1994) Regulation of B-cell activation by CD45 – a question of mechanism. *Immunol. Today* **15:** 399–406.
6. MacLennon, I. C. and Gray, D. (1986) Antigen-driven selection of virgin and memory B cells. *Immunol. Rev.* **91:** 61–85.
7. Austyn, J. M. (1987) Lymphoid dendritic cells. *Immunology* **62:** 161–170.
8. Janeway, C. A. Jr. (1992) The immune system evolved to discrimate infectious nonself from noninfectious self. *Immunol. Today* **13:** 11–16.
9. Sallusto, F. and Lanzavecchia, A. (1994) Efficient presentation of soluble antigen by cultured human dendritic cells is maintained by granulocyte/macrophage colony-stimulatory factor plus interleukin 4 and downregulated by tumor necrosis factor alpha. *J. Exp. Med.* **179:** 1109–1118.
10. McWilliam, A. S., Nelson, D. J. and Holt, P. G. (1995) The biology of airway dendritic cells. *Immunol. Cell Biol.* **73:** 405–413.
11. Wewers, M. D. and Herzyk, D. J. (1989) Alveolar macrophages differ from blood monocytes in human IL-1 beta release. Quantitation by enzyme-linked immunoassay. *J. Immunol.* **143:** 1635–1641.
12. Miller, K., Hudspith, B. N. and Meredith, C. (1992) Secretory and accessory cell functions of the alveolar macrophage. *Environ. Health Perspect.* **97:** 85–89.
13. Tonn, T., Goebel, C., Wilhelm, H. and Gleichmann, E. (1994) Gold kinetics under long-term treatment with gold (I) disodium thiomalate: a comparison in three different mouse strains. *Br. J. Rheumatol.* **33:** 724–730.
14. Mossman, T. R. and Coffman, R. L. (1989) TH1 and TH2 cells: different patterns of lymphokine secretion lead to different functional properties. *Ann. Rev. Immunol.* **7:** 145–173.
15. Garside, P. and Mowat, A. M. (1995) Polarization of Th-cell responses: a phylogenetic consequence of nonspecific immune defence? *Immunol. Today* **16:** 220–223.
16. Manetti, R., Barak, V., Piccinii, M.-P. *et al.* (1994) Interleukin-1 favours the *in vitro* development of type 2 T helper (Th2) human T-cell clones. *Res. Immunol.* **145:** 93–100.
17. de Magistris, M. T., Alexander, J., Coggeshall, M. *et al.* (1992) Antigen analog–major histocompatibility complexes act as antagonists of the T cell receptor. *Cell* **68:** 625–634.
18. Romagnani, S. (1992) Induction of TH1 and TH2 responses: a key role for the 'natural' immune response? *Immunol. Today* **13:** 379–380.
19. Evavold, B. D. and Allen, P. M. (1991) Separation of IL-4 production from Th cell proliferation by an altered T cell receptor ligand. *Science* **68:** 625–634.
20. Punnonen, J., Aversa, Y., Cocks, B. G. *et al.* (1993) Interleukin 13 induces interleukin 4-independent IgG_4 and IgE synthesis and CD23 expression by human B cells. *Proc. Natl Acad. Sci. U.S.A.* **90:** 3730–3734.

21. Butcher, E. C. (1991) Leukocyte–endothelial cell recognition: three (or more) steps to specificity and diversity. *Cell* **67:** 1033–1036.
22. Goldman, Y., Miller, K. and Bazin, H. (1995) How to predict adverse immune reaction induced by pharmaceutical compounds. *Trends Biotech.* **13:** 283–285.
23. Kimber, I., Mitchell, J. A. and Griffin, A. C. (1986) Development of a murine local lymph node assay for the determination of sensitising potential. *Fd. Chem. Toxicol.* **24:** 585–586.
24. Kimber, I., Hilton, J., Botham, P. A. *et al.* (1991) The murine local lymph node assay: results of an interlaboratory trial. *Toxicol. Lett.* **55:** 203–213.
25. Kimber, I. (1994) Chemical allergy: cellular and molecular mechanisms and novel approaches to predictive testing. *Toxicol. In Vitro* **8:** 987–990.
26. Stejskal, V. D. M., Cederbrant, K., Lindvall, A. and Forsbeck, M. (1994) MELISA – an *in vitro* tool for the study of metal allergy. *Toxicol. In Vitro* **8:** 991–1000.
27. Hauser, C. and Katz, S. I. (1988) Activation and expansion of hapten- and protein-specific T helper cells from non-sensitised mice. *Proc. Natl Acad. Sci. U.S.A.* **85:** 5625–5628.
28. Steer, S., Lasek, W., Clothier, R. H. and Balls, M. (1990) An *in vitro* test for immunomodulators. *Toxicol. In Vitro* **4:** 360–362.
29. Miller, K. and Atkinson, H. A. C. (1986) The *in vitro* effects of trichothecenes on the immune system. *Fd. Chem. Toxicol.* **24:** 545–549.
30. van Blamberg-van der Flier, B. M. E. and Scheper, R. J. (1990) *In vitro* tests with sensitised lymphocytes – relevance for predictive allergenicity testing. *Toxicol. In Vitro* **4:** 246–251.
31. Fautz, R. and Miltenburger, H. G. (1993) Immunotoxicity screening *in vitro* using an economical multiple endpoint approach. *Toxicol. In Vitro* **7:** 305–310.
32. Fautz, R. and Miltenburger, H. G. (1994) Influence of organophosphorus compounds on different cellular immune functions *in vitro*. *Toxicol. In Vitro* **8:** 1027–1031.
33. Meredith, C., Scott, M. P. and Miller, K. (1989) Immunotoxicology screening *in vitro*; modulation of expression of immunoregulatory genes. *Hum. Toxicol.* **8:** 411–412.
34. Meredith, C., Scott, M. P., Pekelharing, H. and Miller, K. (1990) The effect of Biostim (RU 41740) on the expression of cytokine mRNAs in murine peritoneal macrophages *in vitro*. *Toxicol. Lett.* **53:** 327–337.
35. Meredith, C. and Miller, K. (1994) Molecular immunotoxicology testing *in vitro*. *Toxicol. In Vitro* **8:** 1001–1005.
36. Gauggel, D. L., Sarlo, K. and Asquith, T. N. (1993) A proposed screen for evaluating low-molecular weight chemicals as potential respiratory allergens. *J. Appl. Toxicol.* **13:** 307–313.
37. Greenlee, W. F., Dold, K. H., Irons, R. D. and Osborne, R. (1985) Evidence for direct action of 2,3,7,8-tetracholoridebenzo-*p*-dioxin (TCDD) on thymic epithelium. *Toxicol. Appl. Pharmacol.* **79:** 112–120.
38. Cook, J. C., Dold, K. M. and Greenlee, W. F. (1987) An *in vitro* model for studying the toxicity of 2,3,7,8-tetracholoridebenzo-*p*-dioxin to human thymus. *J. Appl. Toxicol.* **13:** 307–313.
39. Lebrec, H., Roger, R., Blot, C., Burleson, G. R., Bohuon, C. and Pallardy, M. (1995) Immunotoxicological investigation using pharmaceutical drugs. *In vitro* evaluation of immune effects using rodent or human immune cells. *Toxicology* **96:** 147–156.
40. Revillard, J. P., Robinet, E., Goldman, M., Bazin, H., Latinne, D. and Chatenoud, L. (1995) *In vitro* correlates of the acute toxic syndrome induced by some monoclonal antibodies: a rationale for the design of predictive tests. *Toxicology* **96:** 51–58.
41. Kimber, I. and Cumberbatch, M. (1993) Human immune cells and *in vitro* immunotoxicity testing. In Rogiers, V., Sonck, W., Shepherd, E. and Vercruysse, A. (eds) *Human Cells and* In Vitro *Pharmacotoxicology*, pp. 185–195. Vubpress, Brussels.
42. Meredith, C. (1992) Molecular immunotoxicology. In Miller, K., Turk, J. and Nicklin, S. (eds) *Principles and Practice of Immunotoxicology*, pp. 344–356. Blackwell, Oxford.
43. Meredith, C. and Scott, M. P. (1994) Altered gene expression in immunotoxicology screening *in vitro*: comparison with *ex vivo* analysis. *Toxicol. In Vitro* **8:** 751–753.
44. Meredith, C., Bahra, P. S., Gorey, J. L., Scott, M. P. and Miller, K. (1991) The effect of tributyltin oxide (TBTO) on the expression of rat and murine cytokine mRNA *in vitro* and *in vivo*. *Human Exp. Toxicol.* **10:** 469.
45. Goldman, M., Druet, Ph. and Gleichmann, E. (1991) Th2 cells in systemic autoimmunity – insights from allergenic diseases and chronically-induced autoimmunity. *Immunol. Today* **12:** 223–227.

11

Cutaneous Pharmacotoxicology *In Vitro*

ROLAND ROGUET

I. Introduction 242
II. Biological models 242
  A. The dermis 242
    1. Isolation of dermal fibroblasts 242
    2. Fibroblast monolayer cultures 244
    3. Formation of the lattice or 'dermal equivalent' 244
    4. Commercial 'dermal equivalent' models 244
  B. The epidermis 244
    1. Isolation of interfollicular keratinocytes 245
    2. Conventional keratinocyte cultures 245
    3. Keratinocyte culture in three-dimensional systems 247
    4. Commercial models of reconstructed epidermis 248
  C. Epidermis and dermis: 'reconstructed skin' 249
  D. Excised skin 250
    1. Preparation of excised human skin 250
III. General phenomena involved in cutaneous pharmacotoxicology 250
  A. Percutaneous absorption 251
    1. Determination of the kinetics of transcutaneous permeation 252
    2. Determination of concentrations in skin structures 252
    3. Calculations and interpretation of results 253
  B. Cutaneous metabolism 254
    1. Measurement and effect of xenobiotics on cytochrome P450-dependent enzyme in cultured human keratinocytes 254
  C. Assessment of cutaneous toxicology 255
    1. 'Basal' cytotoxicity tests 256
    2. Tests based on cell's differentiated functions 257
    3. Tests based on the inflammatory process 258
IV. Conclusions and future perspectives 260
  Acknowledgements 261
  Appendix 261
  References 261

IN VITRO METHODS IN PHARMACEUTICAL RESEARCH
ISBN 0-12-163390-X

I. INTRODUCTION

The need to replace animals in cutaneous pharmacotoxicology, together with the desire to develop biological systems to understand the underlying mechanisms, has led to the emergence of methods based mostly on cell culture or excised skin models. Thus, in future, some of the beneficial or detrimental properties of dermatological products would be deduced from their mechanisms of action and not from clinical effects observed in animals (or occasionally humans).

Relative to many organs, such as the liver and kidneys, the skin is highly complex and heterogeneous in both histological and cellular terms. It also has the property of being directly in contact with the external environment, while at the same time being irrigated by the systemic circulation. The pharmacotoxicology of products administered by the systemic route and, above all, the transcutaneous route must therefore be taken into account. In the assessment of a given compound, not only its intrinsic activity but also its percutaneous absorption and possible metabolism by enzymes present in the viable skin layers must be considered. The activity of a compound is the sum of these different aspects, some being accessible *in vitro*.

When studying absorption, the stratum corneum is of crucial importance as it forms a barrier to exogenous substances, while the viable parts of the epidermis are essential for the metabolism of xenobiotics. All the different skin structures can be targeted by active substances, so most of the systems used in cutaneous pharmacotoxicology will mimic dermal and/or epidermal structures.

II. BIOLOGICAL MODELS

Two types of skin cell culture are currently feasible: classical systems using conventional culture dishes as a support, and systems reconstructing the three-dimensional structure of the different skin compartments. In the case of the reconstructed epidermis (composed of keratinocytes and eventually melanocytes) or reconstructed skin (composed of keratinocytes and fibroblasts), an immersion step is required for epidermal differentiation (Figs 11.1 and 11.2).

A. The dermis

Excluding the cells of the vascular endothelium, the dermis is composed mainly of fibroblasts. Fibroblasts from the papillary or reticular dermis have been used in pharmacotoxicity testing, the end-points being viability,[1] proliferation[2] or more specific functions such as collagen synthesis. Fibroblasts are simple to isolate from skin biopsy material, and their culture conditions[3] and use for *in vitro* toxicology studies are both well characterized.[4,5] They can be cultured in conventional two-dimensional (monolayer) or three-dimensional (lattice) systems.

1. *Isolation of dermal fibroblasts*

From explants Human skin is defatted using a scalpel. Then, with an electric dermatome, slices of 0.2 mm in thickness (epidermis) are eliminated. The underlying dermis is cut into

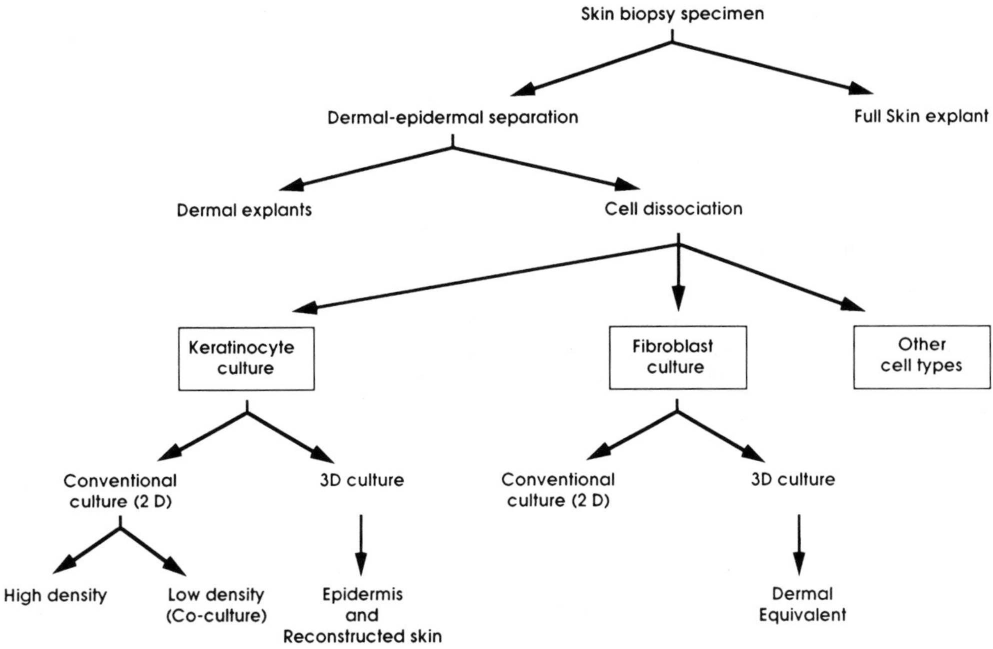

Fig. 11.1 Various types of skin cell culture.

pieces of about 1 mm^3. The explants (about six per 10 cm^2) are placed in the bottom of a Petri dish. After 30 min (attachment period) they are covered with culture medium (medium I: see appendix).

Enzymatic dissociation The fragments of dermis are digested with collagenase (2 mg ml^{-1}, 150 units mg^{-1}) for 3 h at 37°C with circular agitation in minimum essential medium (MEM) (20 mM HEPES) containing penicillin (75 units ml^{-1}) and fungizone (3.5 μg ml^{-1}).

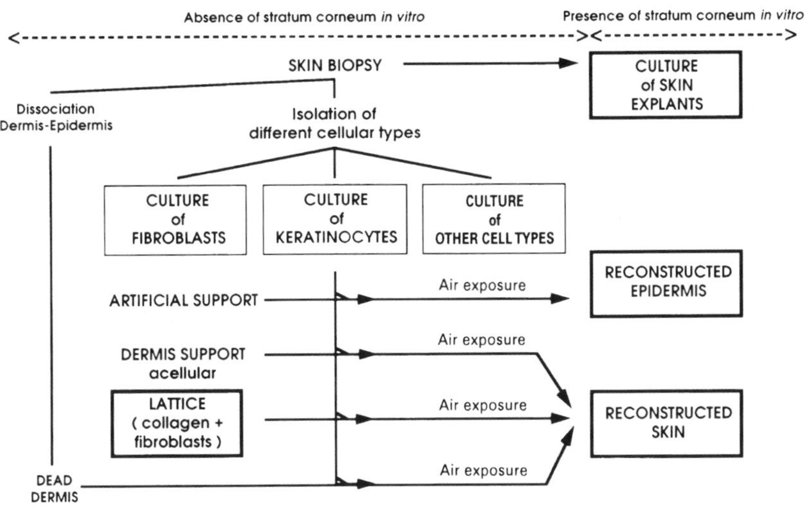

Fig. 11.2 Different types of skin cell system.

The cell suspension is then filtered through cheesecloth and the filtrate is centrifuged at 800*g* for 10 min. The pellet is resuspended in culture medium (see above) and viable cells are counted.

2. *Fibroblast monolayer cultures*

From explants Concentric proliferation is observed 6 days after seeding. The explant can be removed about 2–3 days later. A confluent monolayer is obtained 10 days after seeding.

Enzymatic dissociation The fibroblast suspension is seeded at a density of 2×10^4 cells per cm^2 in medium I (see appendix).

3. *Formation of the lattice or 'dermal equivalent'*

The lattice is obtained by contraction, in the presence of human fibroblasts, of a collagen solution in culture medium.[6] The initial collagen concentration varies in the literature from 0.4 mg ml^{-1} (reference 7) to 2.5 mg ml^{-1} (reference 8), while the initial fibroblast density varies from 1.25×10^4 to 4.5×10^5 cells ml^{-1}. A methodological study has shown that the optimum values of these two parameters are 2.9 mg ml^{-1} and 5×10^2 fibroblasts per ml, respectively.[9]

Preparation of the cell suspension See above.

Preparation of the collagen solution Collagen is obtained from rat tail tendons solubilized in 0.5 M acetic acid and dialysed for 3 days against Dulbecco's Modified Eagle's Medium (DMEM) (diluted 10 times), then centrifuged at 11 000*g* for 24 h at 4°C to eliminate microorganisms. The collagen solution is adjusted to 5.4 mg ml^{-1} in culture medium.

Formation of the lattice The fibroblast suspension (10^3 cells per ml) and collagen solution are mixed and gently vortexed, then placed in an untreated Petri cell culture dish. After 2 days the diameter of the lattice is about 40% of the initial diameter.

4. *Commercial 'dermal equivalent' models* (Fig. 11.3)

Bell's model This model[10] is marketed by Organogenesis (Living Dermal Equivalent – LDE) and consists of a lattice supported by a semipermeable membrane (e.g. Transwell).

The Naughton model This model[11] is marketed by Advanced Tissue Sciences (La Jolla, USA) (ATS) Skin^2 – ZK 1100). It is composed of human fibroblasts seeded on a nylon mesh. *In situ* secretion of collagen (and other macromolecules, including growth factors) by fibroblasts gives rise to the 'dermal equivalent'.

B. The epidermis

The normal epidermis is composed of keratinocytes, melanocytes, Langerhans' cells and Merkel cells. Most existing studies of cutaneous pharmacotoxicology have involved the first two cell types, especially keratinocytes.

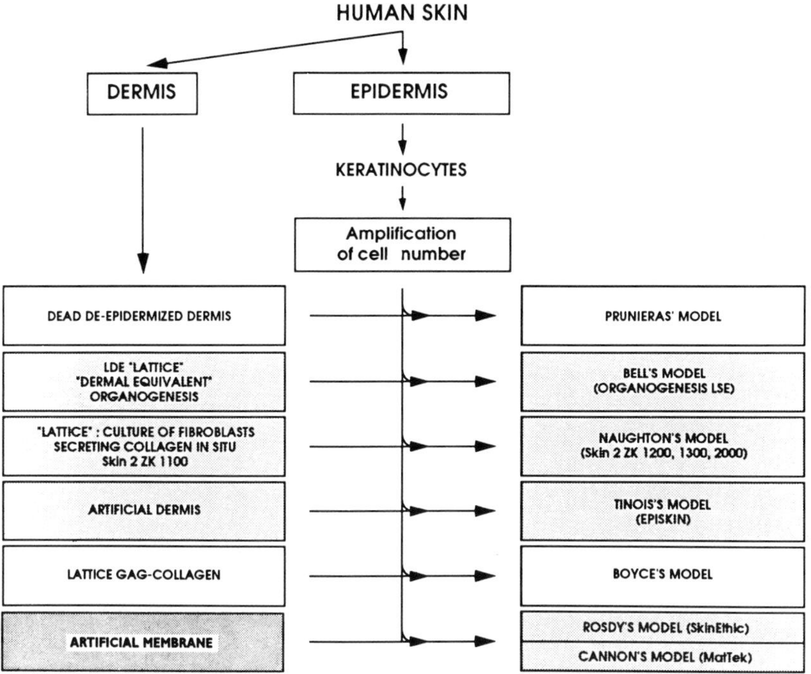

Fig. 11.3 Various *in vitro* models of reconstructed dermis, epidermis or skin equivalents. Shaded boxes show models that are currently or previously marketed.

1. *Isolation of interfollicular keratinocytes*[12]

Sterile skin is defatted with a scalpel. Slices of 0.4 mm are then cut with an electric dermatome and rinsed in DMEM containing HEPES and three successive concentrations of antibacterial/antifungal drugs, as follows: four times (30 min), twice (15 min) and once (10 min) the standard concentrations (penicillin 50 units ml^{-1}, streptomycin 50 $\mu g\,ml^{-1}$ and amphotericin B 2.5 $\mu g\,ml^{-1}$). The slices are then laid flat, epidermis uppermost, in a Petri dish containing a solution of 0.2% trypsin in phosphate-buffered saline (PBS) free of calcium and magnesium, and left overnight at 4°C. The following day the epidermis is peeled from the upper dermis and vortexed for 1 min. The cell suspension thus obtained is filtered through sterile cheesecloth, resuspended in 5 volumes of culture medium (see below) and centrifuged at 800*g* for 10 min. The pellet is resuspended in culture medium and viable cells are counted by the trypan blue method.

2. *Conventional keratinocyte cultures*

The culture conditions have been described in detail elsewhere.[13] In brief, two types of conventional keratinocyte culture can be envisaged: high- and low-density cultures.

High-density cultures These are pure keratinocyte cultures, as the other cell types of the epidermis (particularly melanocytes) disappear during the first few days.

After isolation, keratinocytes are seeded on a plastic support at a density of 2×10^5 viable cells per cm^2 in medium II (see appendix). The medium is renewed 5 h after seeding, then every 2 days.

(A defined medium is increasingly used for keratinocyte culture; it consists of MCDB 153 medium supplemented with epidermal growth factor (EGF) and pituitary extract (medium III: see appendix).[14] This medium (keratinocyte growth medium: KGM) is produced by Clonetics Laboratories, San Diego, USA.)

Under these conditions, confluence is obtained 2–4 days after seeding. After 1 week of culture, the presence of a multilayer structure (five or six cell layers) can be observed by means of electron microscopy, and corresponds to the beginning of cell differentiation (Fig. 11.4).

Low-density cultures[15,16] These are co-cultures of keratinocytes with 3T3 fibroblasts (Flow 03-405-F-CCL92) irradiated or treated with mitomycin to inhibit their proliferation. The 3T3 fibroblasts acts as a feeder layer for the keratinocytes. Under these conditions, keratinocytes maintain a strong growth capacity and can be cloned.

Use of 3T3 fibroblasts: 3T3 fibroblasts are seeded on to a plastic support at a density of 10^3 cells per cm^2 in medium IV (see appendix). When confluence is reached, they are rinsed in PBS and left in contact with mitomycin (10 $\mu g\,ml^{-1}$ DMEM). The cells are then rinsed free of calcium and magnesium in PBS, detached using a solution of trypsin and ethylene diamine tetra-acetic acid (EDTA), and resuspended in keratinocyte co-culture medium. They are then seeded at a density of 3×10^4 cells per cm^2 in co-culture medium (see appendix).

Isolated keratinocytes are seeded directly on to a layer of 3T3 fibroblasts treated with mitomycin, at a minimal density of 10^4 cells per cm^2 in co-culture medium (see appendix).

Pure keratinocyte cultures must be used for toxicological studies. They are obtained spontaneously in the case of high-density cultures and by selective removal of fibroblasts (in

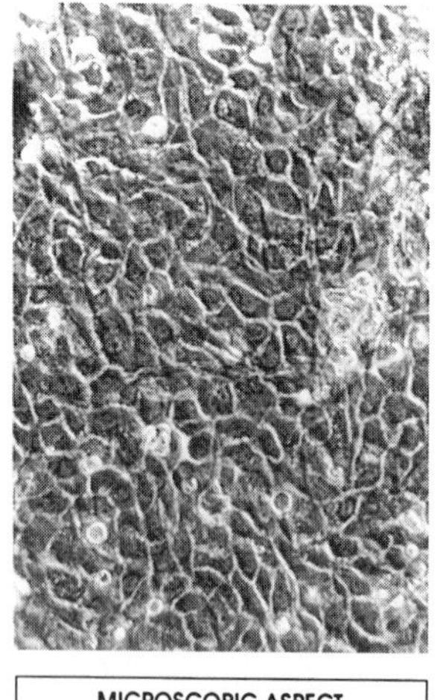

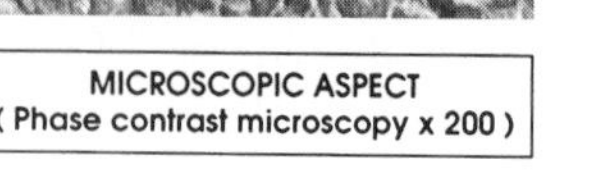

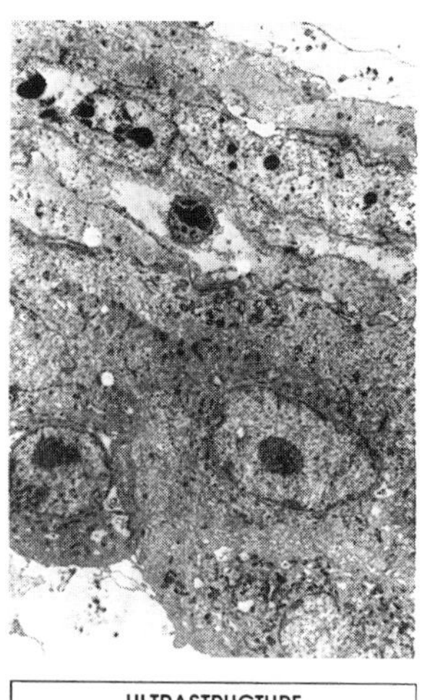

Fig. 11.4 Light microscopy and ultrastructure of normal human keratinocytes in culture. Human keratinocytes are cultivated as described in the text and examined after 2 weeks of culture. A mutilayered sheet with basal, spinous and granular cells can be observed. The final differentiation (stratum corneum) is not obtained in this condition.

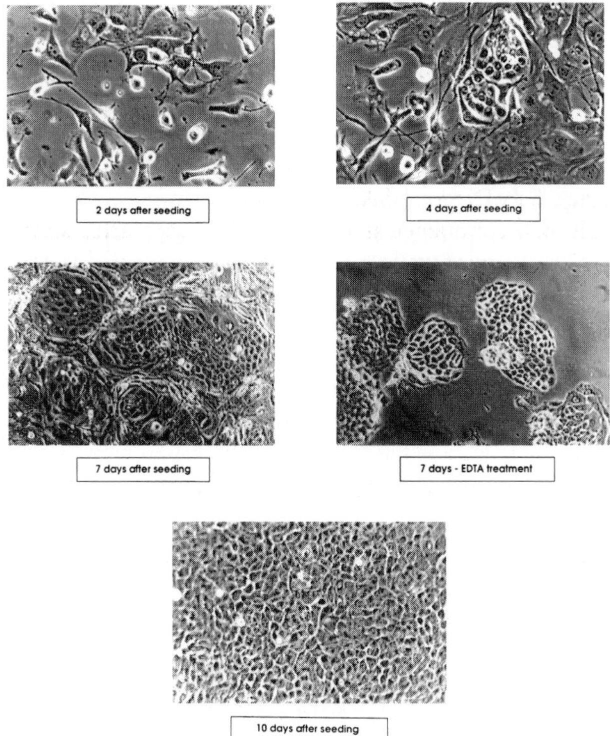

Fig. 11.5 Evolution of co-culture of normal human keratinocytes and mitomycin-treated 3T3 cells. EDTA (0.2%) treatment of subconfluence culture eliminated 3T3 cells after 7 days of culture. Three days later a completely confluent culture of pure keratinocytes can be observed.

the presence of EDTA) in the case of co-culture (Fig. 11.5). Both systems involve immersed cultures; thus the final keratinocyte differentiation stages are never reached. The advantages and limitations of these two types of culture for cutaneous toxicology studies are summarized in Table 11.1.

Table 11.1 Advantages and limitations of high- and low-density cultures of normal human keratinocytes.

Culture type	Advantages	Limitations
High initial density	Simple Differentiation characteristics maintained Inter-individual differences maintained	Need for abundant biopsies Number of assays limited Difficult to standardize
Low initial density	Large number of cells Possible to clone Possible to cryopreserve	Differentiation characteristics maintained? Xenobiotic metabolism maintained?

3. *Keratinocyte culture in three-dimensional systems*

The reconstructed epidermis is prepared according to the dead de-epidermized dermis (DDED) model.[17,18]

Preparation of the DDED Human skin is dermatomed and immersed in PBS free of calcium and magnesium for 7 days at 37°C. The epidermis is eliminated by peeling. The underlying dermis is killed by ten freeze–thaw cycles and stored at −70°C.

Keratinocyte seeding A stainless steel ring (1 cm in diameter) is placed on the dermis. Freshly isolated or subcultured keratinocytes are then seeded inside the ring at a density of 5×10^5 in medium V (see appendix). After 24 h the ring is removed and the cultures are kept immersed for 4 days. The culture is then placed on a metallic grid and exposed to air throughout the culture period. A differentiated, multilayered epidermis is obtained after 10 days of culture (Fig. 11.6).

4. *Commercial models of reconstructed epidermis* (Figs 11.3 and 11.6)

Rosdy's model[19] The keratinocyte support is a cellulose acetate (PIHA, Millipore). After 14 days of culture in chemically defined medium, a multilayer epithelium is obtained (20–25 cell layers). This model is currently sold by SkinEthic (Nice, France). Some of the classical markers of epidermal differentiation (keratin lipids) are present.

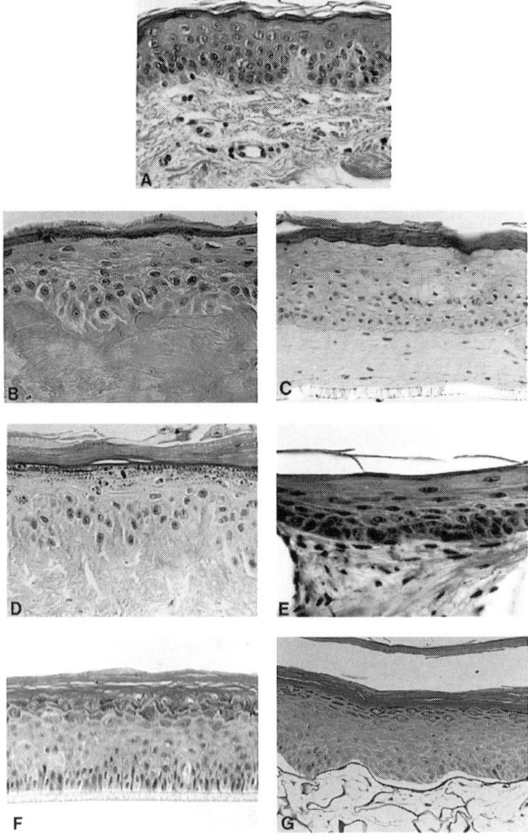

Fig. 11.6 Histology of normal and *in vitro* reconstituted human skin. A, normal human skin; B, Tinois's model (Episkin); C, Bell's model (Testskin LSE); D, Pruniéras's model (DDED); E, Naughton's model (ZK 1300); F, Rosdy's model (SkinEthic); G, Boyce's model. (Haematoxylin and eosin staining, original magnification ×60.)

Cannon's model[20] MatTek Corporation (Ashland, USA) produce an 'EpiDerm human skin model system' composed of normal human keratinocytes cultured on permeable Millipore membranes. In this model, some of the classical markers of epidermal differentiation (cytokeratins, pro-filagrin, keratohyaline granules) are present.

Tinois's model[21] In this model (Episkin; produced by Imedex, Chaponost, France), the dermal support is composed of human collagens I and III covered with a fine layer of collagen IV. The morphology of the reconstructed epidermis is similar to that of normal epidermis. Morphological studies have shown a multilayered epithelium composed of a well-organized basal cell layer, a spinous layer, a granular layer and stratum corneum. Characteristic epidermal ultrastructures have also been observed, including keratin filaments, tonofilaments, desmosomes, keratohyalin granules and membrane-coating granules. Markers of epidermal differentiation such as involucrin, filagrin, transglutaminase I and lipids characteristic of the stratum corneum (ceramides) have been detected.[22]

C. Epidermis and dermis: 'reconstructed skin'

These models are generally derived from dermal equivalent models (collagen plus fibroblasts); a reconstructed epidermis is formed by seeding keratinocytes on the surface (Figs 11.3 and 11.6).

Naughton's model[11] Models ZK 1200 and ZK 1300 (ATS; La Jolla, USA) were derived from Naughton's model ZK 1100.

Bell's model[10,23,24] The 'Living Skin Equivalent' (LSE; Organogenesis, Cambridge, USA) was derived from Bell's LDE model.

Boyce's model[25] This reconstructed skin model uses a collagen and chondroitine-6-sulfate support. Keratinocytes are seeded after treatment of the surface with collagen. Fibroblasts can later be seeded on the other side of the support.

As with the reconstructed epidermis, epidermal differentiation is obtained by an immersion step. These cultures possess dermal structures and viable cells and can thus be used for pharmacological studies of interactions between dermal and epidermal cells.

The advantages and limitations of three-dimensional cultures of human epidermis and reconstructed skin for pharmacotoxicological applications are summarized in Table 11.2.

Table 11.2 Advantages and limitations of three-dimensional cultures of human epidermis and reconstructed skin.

Advantages	Limitations
Involvement of stratum corneum barrier function in skin toxicity	Complexity of setting up cultures
Possibility of studying and/or modulating barrier function	High cost (commercial models)
Existence of an intraepidermal concentration gradient after topical application	
Long-term culture (10–30 days)	
Possibility of applying water-insoluble compounds, formulations or UV light	

D. Excised skin

These models are based on skin specimens maintained in culture. Skin is used whole or dermatomized to reduce the thickness of the dermis.[26,27] The main value of these models is that they facilitate studies of substances (or formulations) on biological materials in conditions simulating normal use (presence of the two or three skin compartments: epidermis, dermis and hypodermis). Above all, they take into account the presence of an intact stratum corneum. Although the size of the explants necessary for toxicity studies can be considerably reduced relative to the original technique,[28] these methods use a large surface of skin. In addition, the samples cannot be kept viable for more than a few hours.

In recent years Dannenberg and co-workers[29,30] have described a method by which human skin explants can be maintained in culture and used for several days. The main value of this technique is that it uses human skin. It has been used to assess a toxic agent (mustard gas) on the basis of morphological cell integrity (presence of perinuclear vacuoles), cell anabolism (leucine incorporation) and also inflammatory phenomena (release of inflammatory mediators, histamine and proteases).[31]

1. *Preparation of excised human skin*

For studies of percutaneous absorption, abdominal or breast skin specimens are stored at 4°C in sterile conditions in the absence of culture medium, between two sheets of aluminium foil, for no more than 12 h. The skin is defatted with a scalpel and its surface is delicately cleaned with soft cotton soaked in PBS.

For studies involving long-term survival in cell culture conditions (cytotoxicity, mediator release, etc.), biopsy specimens are stored in Hanks salt solution containing penicillin 1000 units ml^{-1} and streptomycin 1000 $\mu g\, ml^{-1}$. They are then cut into pieces of about 1 cm^2 and washed three times with the same solution. The explants are cultured for 24 h in Petri dishes containing culture medium VI (see appendix). The level of the medium is adjusted so that the surface of the explant is exposed to air.

Under the culture conditions described by Dannenberg *et al.*[30] the epidermis survives for 24 h at 36°C, while basal cells and hair follicles are viable for 3–4 days.

III. GENERAL PHENOMENA INVOLVED IN CUTANEOUS PHARMACOTOXICOLOGY

After topical application or accidental contact of a xenobiotic with the skin, activity (or toxicity) is conditioned by two, or eventually three, steps:

1. Percutaneous absorption by passage across the superficial layers of the epidermis (stratum corneum) towards the viable epidermal structures, dermis, hypodermis and, in some cases, systemic circulation.
2. Eventual metabolism by phase I and II enzymes present in the epidermis.
3. Interaction with epidermal and dermal structures, which can give rise to pharmacotoxic phenomena.

Each of these steps can be studied *in vitro* using the biological models described above. It must, however, be stressed that these models can provide information only on the potential action of the test product.

A. Percutaneous absorption

Cutaneous absorption is often measured with *in vitro* techniques, given the simplicity of the experimental conditions. However, the relevance of the results thus obtained to *in vivo* absorption depends strongly on the experimental conditions.

Biological models Although it is theoretically possible to use reconstructed human epidermis or reconstructed skin to measure percutaneous absorption, the relatively high permeability of the reconstructed stratum corneum in the different models tends to lead to an overestimation.[32] Pending the availability of reconstructed models with a barrier function corresponding to that observed *in situ*, determination of percutaneous absorption *in vitro* is based mainly on excised human skin. The latter can be used whole (epidermis plus dermis) or dermatomized. In the latter case, the epidermis and upper dermis are isolated by cutting the specimen parallel to the surface (350 μm thickness, corresponding to the distance between the skin surface and vessels).[33] In this way penetration can be determined down to the cutaneous vessels.

Measurement cells (Fig. 11.7) Several types of measurement cell are in routine use. They are composed of either one or two compartments. The one-compartment Franz cell[35] is increasingly used to study the penetration of substances with relatively poor absorption. The skin surface is exposed to the environment, so that products and formulations can be applied under conditions simulating real use. In addition, and contrary to two-compartment cells, the skin surface is not hydrated by the medium contained in the upper cell. A flow-through cell system[33] may be introduced to automate sample collection from a one-chamber cell (dynamic cell). This also promotes viability. The receptor fluid is manually or continuously pumped beneath the skin through a receptor of the skin compartment.

Choice of receptor fluid This is a crucial point when determining the cutaneous absorption of compounds *in vitro*. *In vivo*, hydrophobic compounds are taken up by the blood flow

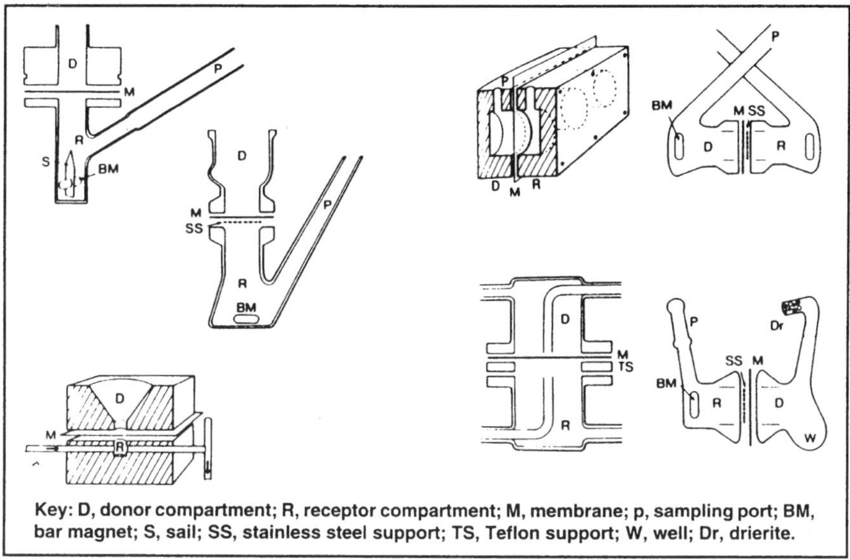

Fig. 11.7 Typical skin diffusion cells. From Cleary.[34]

perfusing the skin directly below the epidermis. When this type of compound is applied *in vitro* it may be absorbed by the skin but not evacuated *in vitro* by the underlying aqueous buffer solution. Analysis of the receptor fluid thus suggests that little or no penetration is taking place. In fact, for this type of compound, skin permeation rates seem to be measured more accurately when the receptor fluid contains 4% bovine serum albumin or a non-toxic concentration of surfactant.

Determining the quantity of compound in skin structures at the end of the penetration phase
After a fixed penetration phase and measurement of the amounts present in the receptor fluid, the quantity present in the skin can be determined (usually with radiolabelled compounds).

1. Determination of the kinetics of transcutaneous permeation

After homogeneous topical application of a known quantity of product or volume of solution, aliquots are taken at fixed times from the receptor volume and replaced with equal volumes of medium. The quantity of product that has passed through the skin is determined by counting in scintillation fluid (when a radiolabelled compound is used) or with a sensitive analytical method.

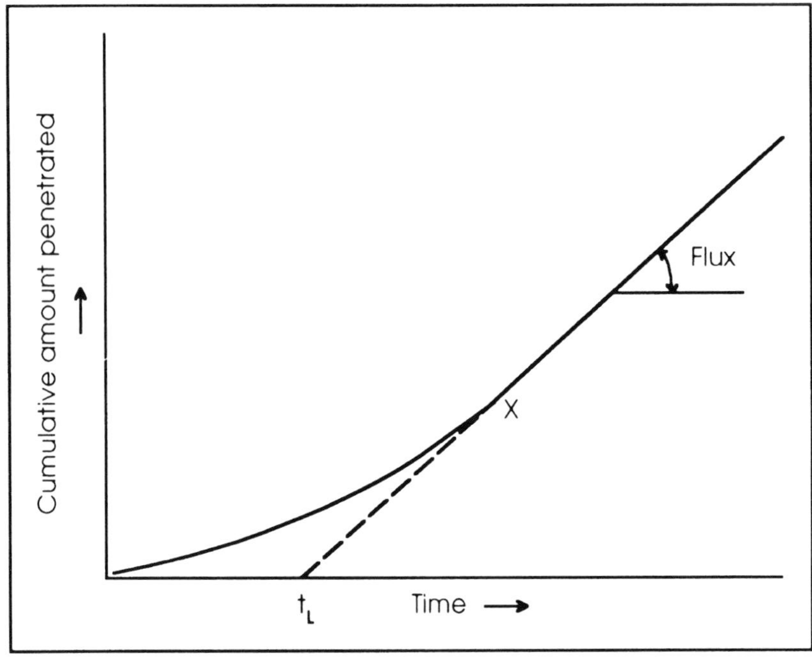

Fig. 11.8 Kinetics of *in vitro* skin penetration: time *versus* permeation, showing the approach to steady state and the lag time (t_L). Flux, flux of penetration at the steady state.

2. Determination of concentrations in skin structures[36]

After a defined period, excess compound remaining on the skin surface is removed by gentle wiping with dry cotton swabs. The skin specimen is then fixed on to a rubber stopper of suitable size and the horny layer is removed by about 20 strippings with adhesive tape.[37] (The concentration in the stratum corneum can be assessed by analysing the strips.[38]) The remaining skin specimen is frozen and one or more punch biopsies are taken and refrozen on a freeze microtome. Sixteen slices of 10 μm thickness are cut: these are regarded as epidermis. The rest of the specimen (the dermis) is cut into 40 μm slices; the thickness of the skin is determined from the number of slices. If a radiolabelled compound is used, each slice is placed in a counter vial and solubilized with Soluene 300. The radioactivity of each slice is then measured in a liquid scintillation counter. In the case of non-labelled compounds, the quantity in each slice can be determined by an analytical method.

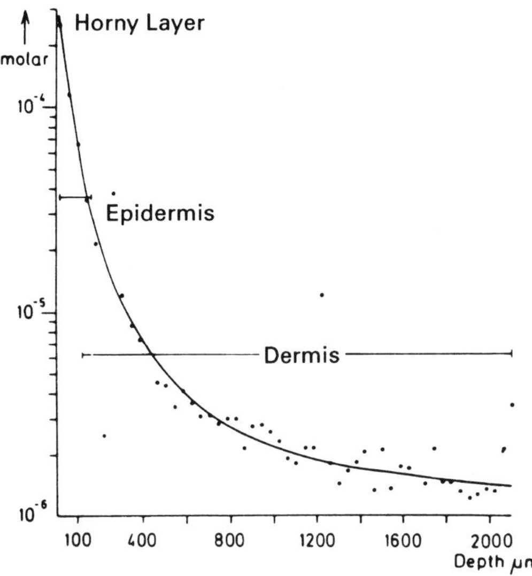

Fig. 11.9 Distribution of desoximetasone in human skin after topical application for 1000 min *in vitro*. From Schaefer and Schalla.[36]

3. *Calculations and interpretation of results*

Various parameters can be deduced from the penetration kinetics: indeed, the permeation rate J (amount of substance penetrating in a given time) can be calculated from the difference in the concentration (ΔC) between the surface (generally considered infinite) and the receptor medium. Passive diffusion of the compound across skin structures obeys Fick's law:

$$J = K_p \, (\Delta C)$$

where K_p is the permeability constant. In the case of small, at least slightly hydrophilic, molecules K_p depends on: (1) the partition coefficient (K) of the molecule between the stratum corneum and the vehicle in which it is solubilized; (2) the diffusion constant (D) in the stratum corneum; and (3) the thickness (e) of the stratum corneum:

$$K_p = \frac{K \times D}{e}$$

Thus, such techniques can be used to determine important constants of transcutaneous penetration (penetration rate, lag time period) (Fig. 11.8).

At diffusion steady state, the distribution of the substance in the epidermis and upper dermis is represented by a steep diffusion gradient with a semilogarithmic plot appearing no more linear (Fig. 11.9). Analysis of the different parts of the curve (stratum corneum, epidermis and dermis) is used to calculate the amounts in each of these compartments. Thus, in studies of distribution kinetics, compounds with strong affinity for the stratum corneum will have similar values in this compartment, whereas those with strong affinity for the dermis (steroids, etc.) will accumulate in it. Thus, *in vitro* studies of transcutaneous penetration can provide information on some of the essential characteristics of xenobiotic absorption through excised skin and, in the near future, reconstructed skin.

B. Cutaneous metabolism

During transepidermal passage, some xenobiotics undergo enzymatic transformation which may influence their kinetics of penetration and can lead to activation or detoxification. Most of this biotransformating activity is located in the living cells of the epidermis, which are capable of hydrolysis (esterase activity), reduction, oxidation (hydroxylation) and conjugation.[39,40] The two latter functions are particularly involved in the metabolism of xenobiotics and endogenous molecules, and have been detected in the epidermis and in isolated and cultured keratinocytes.[41,42]

The presence of different forms of cytochrome P450[43–45] and phase II-related enzyme activities[44,46] have been demonstrated both in keratinocytes and in conventional and three-dimensional culture.

After characterization of the metabolic capacities of *in vitro* epidermal culture systems (two- or three-dimensional), two important applications can be envisaged:

1. The *in vitro* metabolization of foreign or endogenous compounds by cultivated human keratinocytes or excised skin.[47–49]
2. Investigation of the effect of topically applied drugs on the metabolic activity of enzymes (induction or inhibition). With regard to imidazole derivatives, for example, induction of ethoxycoumarin-O-de-ethylase (ECOD) activity at low doses has been shown in human cultivated keratinocytes[44] in agreement with *in vivo* data[50] (Fig. 11.10).

1. *Measurement and effect of xenobiotics on cytochrome P450-dependent enzyme in cultured human keratinocytes*

Conventional (two-dimensional) culture Human keratinocytes were cultivated as previously described. Cells were treated with tested agents dissolved in a culture medium containing dimethylsulfoxide (DMSO) (maximum final concentration 0.5%) for different times before determination of enzyme activity. Then, cultures of human keratinocytes were washed in keratinocyte growth medium (KGM) to remove the culture medium and loose cells, and the compound being tested and the substrates 7-ethoxycoumarin and 7-ethoxyresorufin dissolved in ethanol were added to KGM (maximum final concentration of ethanol 1%). After incubation, the reaction was terminated by removing the reaction mixture. The fluorescence of the different substrates was measured by fluorescence spectrophotometry, a standard curve being established for each.

Three-dimensional model cultures Different concentrations of agents solubilized in KGM were applied to the surface of the epidermis for the chosen length of time, and were then

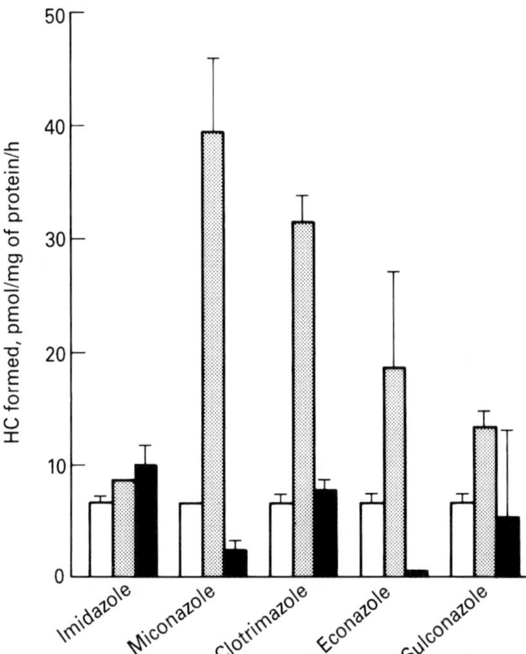

Fig. 11.10 Effect of imidazole derivatives on ethoxycoumarin-O-de-ethylase (ECOD) activity in cultured human keratinocytes. Imidazole compounds dissolved in ethanol (final concentration 1%) were added to the culture medium for 24 h and ECOD activity was then measured. Values are mean ± s.d. of three experiments. □, Control; ▒, 1 μM; ■, 10 μM.

eliminated by rinsing before determination of enzyme activity. In the case of pharmaceutical emulsion (non-water soluble), 20 mg was applied per square centimetre of epidermis for the selected time and then eliminated by rinsing with PBS. 7-Ethoxycoumarin-O-de-ethylase activity was measured by applying 220 nmol of substrate in 150 μl of culture medium (containing 1% ethanol) to the surface of reconstructed epidermis. The amount of 7-hydroxycoumarin produced was measured in the underlying culture medium (KGM) by spectrofluorometric detection.

C. Assessment of cutaneous toxicology

The main reactions involved in cutaneous toxicology are: non-immunological contact dermatitis (due to irritation) and immunological contact dermatitis (due to sensitization); pigment alteration; comedogenesis; and carcinogenesis.

Carcinogenesis is still studied mostly in animal models. The possibility of transfecting human epidermal cells with genes that increase their sensitivity to malignant transformation does, however, hold promise for the development of *in vitro* systems.

Comedogenesis is assessed *in vivo* by the formation of a stopper in the hair follicle ostium of the mouse external ear canal. No *in vitro* culture models are yet capable of replacing this test, as the formation of hair follicles in culture is at a very early stage of development.

In the field of pigment changes, i.e. hypopigmentation or hyperpigmentation, recent experiments with cultured human melanocytes, and studies of pigmentation using co-cultures of functional keratinocytes and melanocytes, suggest that a screening model should soon become available (R. Schmitt and M. Regnier, personal communication).

Immunological contact dermatitis *in vitro* involves two essential phases: (1) presentation of the antigen to T lymphocytes during the sensitization phase; and (2) migration of activated cells towards the lymph nodes in response to signals emitted during subsequent topical applications of the sensitizing antigen. To reproduce these reactions, it would be necessary to 'educate' *in vitro* naive lymphocytes, induce them to proliferate and then to recognize the specific antigen. Antigen presentation in the epidermis is ensured by Langerhans' cells, which can select and position the antigenic motif, leading to T-lymphocyte activation. We now know how to extract and purify Langerhans' cells, but are as yet unable to maintain their functional properties in culture. This problem depends mainly on a number of sequential factors brought into play in an order that remains to be determined. The difficulty of reproducing these complex phenomena *in vitro* is clear, and the development of an alternative method in this area will be a lengthy process.

Non-immunological contact dermatitis (irritant dermatitis) is the field in which most progress has been made. The methods used for its evaluation *in vitro* are based on the models described above (conventional two- and three-dimensional cultures of fibroblasts and/or keratinocytes). They are used to assess the two main parameters of skin reaction: acute primary irritation linked to reversible inflammatory phenomena, and necrosis leading to irreversible tissue changes.

Until recently, only cell viability could be studied in cell culture. As a result, the irritancy of a test substance was assessed in terms of its necrotic potential (tested at a high concentration). The recent elucidation of the mechanisms underlying skin inflammation, especially pro-inflammatory mediators and their production by epidermal cells, has led to mechanistic tests reflecting phenomena demonstrated *in vivo* during non-immunological irritation.

There are two types of test for cell viability or dysfunction as applied to fibroblasts or keratinocytes in classical or three-dimensional culture: (1) tests of basal cytotoxicity, which are common to all animal cells; and (2) tests related to specific dysfunction of epidermal cells.

1. *'Basal' cytotoxicity tests*

These tests are more or less specific for different types of cell damage and are widely used to assess cytotoxicity for a large range of cell types. They are based on undifferentiated cell functions and can be applied to skin cells, especially fibroblasts and keratinocytes. The methodology and interpretation of the results (dose–effect curves) are similar to those used for other cell types described in this book.

Tests based on cell membrane integrity

Plasma membrane: The release of cytosolic enzymes such as lactate dehydrogenase (LDH) is commonly used as an index of plasma membrane damage. This method is simple, rapid and easy to automate.[51] Artefacts due to interactions between the test product and enzyme activity (denaturation of LDH by surfactants, for example) can be detected by measuring intracellular and extracellular activity or by measuring the activity of a known amount of LDH after incubation with the test product.

Lysosomes and the plasma membrane: The technique most commonly used is that described by Borenfreund and Puerner,[52] based on the uptake of a cationic dye (neutral red) by lysosomes. Xenobiotics that alter cell or lysosome membranes produce a fall in neutral red uptake and binding. This highly reproducible and sensitive test can be automated and combined with other cytotoxicity tests.

The metabolic activity of cells can be assessed at various levels. The action of xenobiotics can be measured by means of techniques based on cell physiology or the synthesis of specific macromolecules.

Tests based on cell's intermediary metabolism These include cell respiration tests using a Clark electrode, and measurement of pH variations in the medium due to metabolic activity. This latter method has been automated in the form of a microphysiometer, a device capable of detecting very small pH variations. In addition, it appears suited for determining the reversibility of cell damage.[53]

Tests based on mitochondrial activity This technique is based on the reduction of a tetrazolium salt catalysed by mitochondrial enzyme systems and has been reported to reflect cell growth and xenobiotic cytotoxicity.[54] Although simple, reproducible and readily automated, this method is subject to certain artefacts.[55]

Tests based on cell proliferation These tests include cell counting methods (or assays reflecting the number of cells present in the culture) and the assessment of DNA synthesis with radionucleotide probes. Cell counting can be difficult with keratinocytes, given the problems of isolating them after culture. Determination of biochemical markers (protein assay by Bradford's method[56]) or of DNA synthesis by the L 4′,6-diamidino-2-phenylindole (DAPI) method[57] reflects cell numbers more accurately. DNA synthesis is measured by estimating labelled thymidine incorporation in the acid-insoluble fraction of cell material[12] or by immunohistological methods with monoclonal antibodies directed against bromo-deoxyuridine (BrdU), a pyrimidine analogue of thymine incorporated in DNA.[58]

An important parameter of cell proliferation is growth capacity, defined as the ratio between thymidine incorporation and the amount of DNA present in the culture.[12]

2. *Tests based on cell's differentiated functions*

Tests based on the differentiated functions of keratinocytes are mainly used to assess the pharmacological properties of compounds (retinoic acid and its derivatives, for example). Duffy and Flint[59] have proposed a simple test for determining the effect of compounds on the differentiation of XB-2 cells, an epithelial cell line derived from a mouse teratoma. This method simultaneously provides information on the degree of cell keratinization (specific keratin staining with rhodamine B), cell proliferation (Nile blue staining), cell toxicity (MTT test, neutral red uptake and LDH release) and cell stratification (ultrastructural studies). By comparing given criteria in XB-2 and 3T3 cells, it appears that keratinization, LDH release and stratification are the parameters most closely reflecting skin irritation. The choice of irritant (retinol), although effectively an irritant *in vivo*, makes it difficult to extrapolate these observations because of their inherent pharmacological properties. However, in another study of 19 compounds, nine of which were irritant *in vivo*, the same authors obtained only one false-positive and one false-negative result by combining these different parameters.[60]

3. Tests based on the inflammatory process signaling

In addition to the assessment of neutrophil granule release and histamine release by mast cells, other *in vitro* tests based on one or several phases of the inflammatory process involved in skin irritation are now under development.

When activated by various irritants, keratinocytes are capable of expressing or overexpressing the production and release of some inflammatory mediators.[61] Thus, changes in the plasma membrane can lead to the release of arachidonic acid metabolites after lipo-oxygenase activation (12-1,2 hydroxyeicosatetraenoic acid (HETE), 15-HETE, leukotriene B_4, prostaglandin (PG) E_2 and PGD_2).[62,63] The production of cytokines – tumour necrosis factor (TNF)α and β,[64,65] interleukin (IL) 1 and IL-6,[66,67] and granulocyte–macrophage colony-stimulating factor (GM-CSF)[68] – by keratinocytes exposed to an irritant has been demonstrated *in vivo* and *in vitro*. Most of these factors have an exocrine action on dermal or epidermal cells (Langerhans' cells), modifying their growth, differentiation or expression of surface antigens. They can also have endocrine activity by stimulating the secretion of other factors, modulating the expression of their own receptors or stimulating the growth of keratinocytes themselves (for a review see Luger *et al.*).[66]

The importance of these reactions in the onset of skin irritation has led researchers in this field to envisage the assay of certain inflammatory mediators produced *in vitro* by keratinocytes: '. . . the first of a second generation of *in vitro* irritancy tests'.[69]

Various methods have been described to assess inflammatory mediator production by keratinocytes.

Production of arachidonic acid metabolites This can be determined by the radioactivity of culture supernatants after incorporation of radiolabelled arachidonic acid. This simple method was developed by DeLeo *et al.*[70] and accurately predicts the irritant potential of surfactants.[71] Coupled with high-performance liquid chromatography methods, it can be used to identify arachidonic acid metabolites formed after application of irritant agents (benzoyl peroxide) on skin equivalents.[72]

Biological assays of inflammatory mediators Some such assays have mainly been applied to interleukins; for example, concentration-dependent stimulation of certain thymocyte lines by interleukins (mouse thymocyte amplification assay; MTA), first shown by Gery *et al.*,[73] can be used to assay IL-1 and anti-IL-1 activity or TNF-α. This method has been widely used to assay the IL-1 produced by keratinocyte or organ cultures after the action of an irritant.[31,74]

Other biological methods can be used to appreciate the overall physiological effect of the mediators thus released, in terms of their chemotactic potency. The chemotactism of arachidonic acid derivatives (12-HETE, PGE_2 and PGD_2) and interleukins for polymorphonuclear leucocytes has formed the basis for a detection test. Using a two-compartment chamber (Boyden chamber), the presence of these agents is quantified by counting peritoneal neutrophils fixed to or contained in the membrane separating the neutrophils from the chemotactic stimulus. Although only semiquantitative, this method has the advantage of reflecting the biological effect of mediators in inflammatory processes *in vivo*.

Specific assays of certain inflammatory mediators in culture supernatants or in the intracellular compartment can be performed by means of radioimmunological or immunoenzymological methods. For example, after treatment of human keratinocytes with irritative agent, an increase in the intracellular IL-1 concentration has been shown[67] (Fig. 11.11). This increase in intracellular mediator concentrations is an early and sensitive event that occurs at subcytotoxic irritant concentrations. In three-dimensional keratinocyte culture

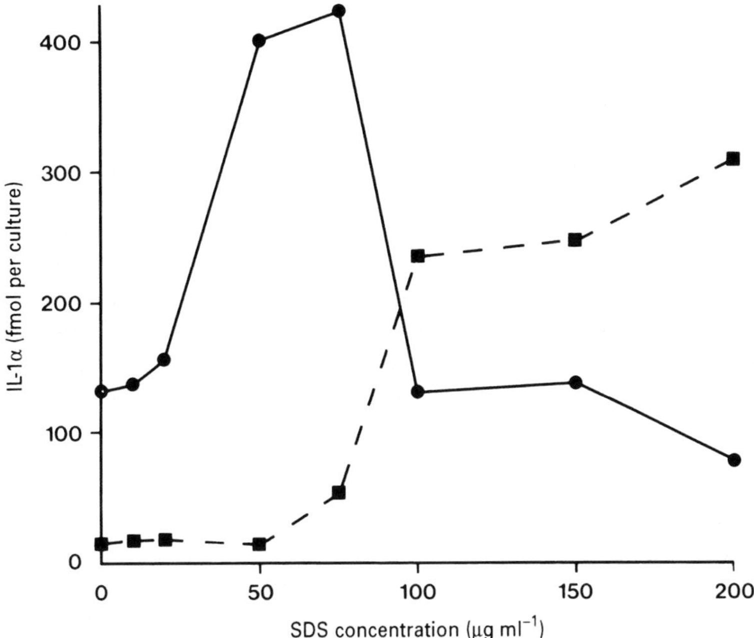

Fig. 11.11 Production of interleukin (IL) 1α according to the dose of sodium dodecyl sulfate (SDS) administered. ●, Intracellular IL-1α; ■, extracellular IL-1α.

systems (reconstructed epidermis), a release of IL-1α after administration of surfactants or UVB has been shown.[75–77] Moreover, a relationship has been found between the release of IL-1α by reconstructed epidermis and the *in vivo* irritative potential of surfactants[78] (Fig. 11.12).

Although highly specific, these methods simply detect the presence of a given mediator, not its physiological activity.

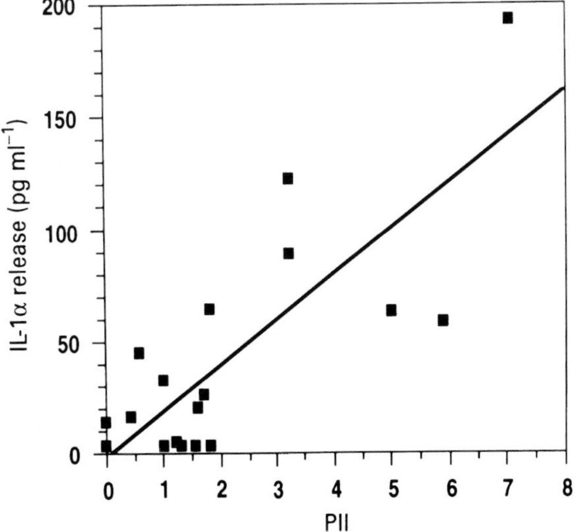

Fig. 11.12 Correlation between the production of interleukin (IL) 1α by a human reconstituted epidermis and *in vivo* cutaneous irritative potential of surfactants. PII, primary irritative index.

Determination of intracellular mediator content (or the cell-associated fraction) Culture media were collected, centrifuged to eliminate detached cells, and the supernatants were stored at −80°C for determination of inflammatory mediators in the extracellular compartment. Some 2 ml of fresh medium was added on the cellular sheet and immediately frozen in liquid nitrogen. Frozen cells were mechanically harvested and sonicated with a cell disrupter (Sonifier B-20). Cell lysates were centrifuged (5000*g* for 30 min) and the amount of mediator (IL-1α or/and PGE_2) in the supernatant was evaluated by means of radio-immunoassay or enzymoimmunoassay.

Determination of mediators released into the culture medium
Inflammatory mediators can be determined in the culture medium of conventional keratinocyte cultures, as well as in the underlying culture [medium of three-dimensional keratinocyte cultures as described before (page 258)].

IV. CONCLUSIONS AND FUTURE PERSPECTIVES

As with other organs, *in vitro* methods for studying cutaneous pharmacotoxicology require reliable models closely resembling human structures and/or functions. The choice of end-points relevant to the *in vivo* situation is also a crucial factor. These two elements are the cornerstones of successful 'alternative' methods.

With regard to cutaneous pharmacotoxicology, the use of excised human skin remains a necessity for certain applications, but will be increasingly limited by ethical considerations. The development of three-dimensional culture systems reproducing normal skin structure and suited to the topical application of cosmetic or dermatological preparations in conditions simulating their routine use is a considerable step forward. These experimental models or commercially available, have the advantage of using human starting materials, but require some improvement. Most are limited to a reconstructed epidermis as a basis for keratinocyte culture, and the barrier function of the stratum corneum to xenobiotics is less efficient than *in vivo* situation. In addition, the introduction of melanocytes as the incorporation of Langerhans' cells will extend the possible ties of these models.

While the end-points for percutaneous absorption and metabolism are well defined, those of irritancy are still at the experimental stage. The assessment of percutaneous absorption *in vitro* with the different models (excised and reconstructed skin) is subject to fundamental pharmacodynamic rules. The study of skin metabolism *in vitro* (after validation of the models relative to normal skin) is limited only by the analytical methods currently used to identify the different metabolites. Concerning skin irritancy (contact dermatitis), where *in vivo* phenomena are more complex and involve a large number of cell types, the mechanistic approach adopted in recent years is no doubt the most promising, even though the choice of specific markers of irritation remains controversial.

Few validation studies of the systems available for the predictive assessment of the different aspects of cutaneous toxicity have been undertaken. Concerted evaluation of protocols for percutaneous absorption were started in November 1994 under the auspices of the European Centre for the Validation of Alternative Methods (ECVAM). In contrast, international validation of methods for predicting skin irritancy and cutaneous metabolism has not yet begun.

In conclusion, we are now in possession of elaborate, reproducible, reconstructed epidermis and skin culture systems. Some improvement is required for these models for specific purposes, and this will require a thorough evaluation of their existing capabilities.

ACKNOWLEDGEMENTS

The author thanks Ms Grandidier for reviewing technical procedures included in the manuscript. The secretarial assistance of Ms Boissier is greatly appreciated.

APPENDIX

Culture media

Medium I: DMEM containing penicillin 75 units ml^{-1}, streptomycin 75 $\mu g\,ml^{-1}$, fungizone 3.7 $\mu g\,ml^{-1}$ and 10% fetal calf serum (FCS).
Medium II: MEM with Earle's salts, 10% FCS, 0.1% penicillin 50 U/nl, streptomycin, 1%, 50 μg/nl sodium pyruvate and 1% glutamine.
Medium III: MCDB 153 plus (for 1 litre of medium) bovine pituitary extract (4 ml, 7.5 mg protein per ml), human epidermal growth factor 1 μg, insulin 5 mg, hydrocortisone 1 mg, gentamicin 25 mg and amphotericin 25 μg.
Medium IV: DMEM containing 10% FCS, 0.1% penicillin, streptomycin, 1% 50 μg/ml sodium pyruvate and 1% glutamine.
Medium V: MEM with Earle's salts, sodium pyruvate 1 mM, L-glutamine 200 mM, penicillin 100 units ml^{-1}, streptomycin 100 $\mu g\,ml^{-1}$ and 10% FCS.
Medium VI: RPMI 1640 containing glutamine 300 $mg\,l^{-1}$ and supplemented with penicillin 100 units ml^{-1}, streptomycin 100 $\mu g\,ml^{-1}$ and glutamine 2 mM.

REFERENCES

1. Cornelius, M., Dupont, C. and Wepierre, J. (1991) *In vitro* cytotoxicity tests on cultured human skin fibroblasts to predict the irritation potential of surfactants. *ATLA* **19:** 324–336.
2. Boullard, A., Roguet, R., Kermici, M. and Giacomoni, P. U. (1990) Effet des irradiations UV-A et UV-B sur la croissance et la synthèse de l'ADN de fibroblastes humains en culture. *J. Med. Nucl. Biophys.* **14:** 169–171.
3. Ham, R. G. (1980) Dermal fibroblasts. *Methods Cell Biol.* **21A:** 255–275.
4. Lamont, G. S., Bagley, D. M., Kong, B. M. and De Salva, S. (1989) Developing an alternative to the Draize skin test – comparison of human skin cell responses to irritants *in vitro*. In Goldberg, A. (ed.) *Alternative Methods in Toxicology*, Vol. 7, pp. 175–181. Mary Ann Liebert, New York.
5. Ponec, M., Haverkart, M. and Soei, Y. L. (1990) Use of keratinocyte and fibroblast culture for toxicity studies of topically applied compounds. *J. Pharm. Sci.* **79:** 312–316.
6. Hull, B. E., Sher, S. E., Rosen, S. *et al.* (1983) Structural integration of skin equivalents grafted to Lewis and Sprague-Dawley rats. *J. Invest. Dermatol.* **81:** 429–436.
7. Grinnel, F. and Lamke, C. R. (1984) Reorganization of hydrated collagen lattices by human skin fibroblasts. *J. Cell Sci.* **66:** 51–63.
8. Schor, S. L. (1980) Cell proliferation and migration on collagen substrats *in vitro*. *J. Cell Sci.* **41:** 159–175.
9. Rompré, P., Auger, F. A., Germain, L. *et al.* (1990) Influence of initial collagen and cellular concentrations on the final surface area of dermal and skin equivalents. A Box-Behnken analysis. *In Vitro Cell. Dev. Biol.* **26:** 983–990.
10. Bell, E., Ivarsson, B. and Merrill, C. (1979) Production of tissue-like structure by contraction of collagen lattices by human fibroblasts of different proliferative potential *in vitro*. *Proc. Natl Acad. Sci. U.S.A.* **76:** 1274–1278.
11. Naughton, G. K., Jacob, L. and Naughton, B. A. (1989) A physiological skin model for *in vitro* toxicity studies. In Goldberg, A. (ed.) *Alternative Methods in Toxicology*, Vol. 7, pp. 183–189. Mary Ann Liebert, New York.

12. Pruniéras, M., Delescluse, C. and Régnier, M. (1976) Growth and differentiation of postembryonic mammalian epidermal keratinocytes in culture. In Robert, L. (ed.) *Frontiers of Matrix Biology*, pp. 52–73. S. Karger, Basel.
13. Régnier, M., Pruniéras, M. (1988) Culture de cellules épidermiques. In Adolphe, M. and Barlovatz-Meimon, G. (eds) *Culture de cellules animales. Méthodologie, Applications*, pp. 181–193. Inserm Ed, Paris, France.
14. Boyce, S. T. and Ham, R. G. (1985) Cultivation, frozen storage and clonal growth of normal human epidermal keratinocytes in serum-free media. *J. Tissue Culture Methods* **9**: 83–93.
15. Rheinwald, J. G. and Green, H. (1975) Serial cultivation of strains of human epidermal keratinocytes. The formation of keratinizing colonies from single cells. *Cell* **6**: 331–344.
16. Rheinwald, J. G. and Green, H. (1977) Epidermal growth factor and the multiplication of cultured human epidermal keratinocytes. *Nature* **265**: 421–424.
17. Pruniéras, M., Régnier, M. and Schlotterer, M. (1979) Nouveau procédé de culture de cellules épidermiques humaines sur derma homologue ou hétérologue – préparation de greffons recombinés. *Ann. Chir. Plast.* **24**: 357–362.
18. Pruniéras, M., Régnier, M. and Woodley, D. (1983) Methods for cultivation of keratinocytes with an air–liquid interface. *J. Invest. Dermatol.* **81**: 28S–33S.
19. Rosdy, M. and Clauss, L. C. (1990) Complete human epidermal cell differentiation in chemically defined medium at the air–liquid interface on inert filter substrates. *J. Invest. Dermatol.* **95**: 409–414.
20. Cannon, C. L., Neal, P. J., Southee, J. A., Kubilus, J. and Klausnez, M. (1994) New epidermal model for dermal irritancy testing. *Toxicol. In Vitro* **8**: 889–891.
21. Tinois, E., Tillier, J., Gaucherand, M., Dumas, H., Tardy, M. and Thivolet, J. (1991) *In vitro* and post-transplantation differentiation of human keratinocyte growth on the human type IV collagen film of a bilayed dermal substitute. *Exp. Cell Res.* **193**: 310–319.
22. Tinois, E., Gaetani, Q., Gayraud, B., Dupont, D., Rougier, A. and Pouradier Duteil, X. (1994) The Episkin model: successful reconstitution of human epidermis *in vitro*. In Rougier, A., Goldberg, A. M. and Maibach, H. I. (eds) In Vitro *Skin Toxicology – Irritation, Phototoxicity, Sensitization*, pp. 133–141. Mary Ann Liebert, New York.
23. Bell, E. (1984) *Tissue-equivalent and Method for Preparation Thereof*. US Patent no. 4 485 096 27.
24. Bell, E., Gay, R., Swiderek, M., Class, T. *et al.* (1989) Use of fabricated living tissue and organ equivalents as defined higher order systems for the study of pharmacologic responses to test substances. In Wilson, G. and Davis, S. (eds) *Pharmaceutical Applications of Cell and Tissue Culture*, pp. 131–137. Plenum Press, New York.
25. Boyce, S. T., Christianson, D. and Hansbrough, J. F. (1988) Structure of a collagen-GAG skin substitute optimized for cultured human epidermal keratinocytes. *J. Biomater. Res.* **22**: 939–957.
26. Kao, J., Hall, J. and Holland, J. M. (1983) Quantitation of cutaneous toxicity – an *in vitro* approach using skin organ culture. *Toxicol. Appl. Pharmacol.* **68**: 45–56.
27. Helman, R. G., Hall, J. W. and Kao, J. K. (1986) Acute dermal toxicity – *in vivo* and *in vitro*: Comparisons in mice. *Fund. Appl. Toxicol.* **7**: 94–100.
28. Bartnik, F. G., Pitterman, W. F., Mendorf, N., Tillman, U. and Künstler, K. (1990) Skin organ culture for the study of skin irritancy. *Toxicol. In Vitro* **4**: 293–301.
29. Nakamura, M., Rikimaru, T., Yano, T. *et al.* (1990) Full-thickness human skin explants for the toxicity of topically applied chemicals. *J. Invest. Dermatol.* **95**: 325–332.
30. Dannenberg, A. M., Jr. and Moore, K. G. (1994) Toxic and allergic skin reactions, evaluated in organ-cultured full-thickness human and animal skin explant. In Rougier, A., Goldberg, A. M. and Maibach, H. I. (eds) In vitro *Skin Toxicology – Irritation, Phototoxicity, Sensitization*, pp. 351–366. Mary Ann Liebert, New York.
31. Rikimaru, T., Nakamura, M., Yano, T. *et al.* (1991) Mediators, initiating the inflammatory response, released in organ culture by full-thickness human skin explants exposed to the irritant sulfur mustard. *J. Invest. Dermatol.* **96**: 888–897.
32. Roguet, R., Régnier, M., Cohen, C., Dossou, K. G. and Rougier, A. (1994) The use of *in vitro* reconstituted human skin in dermatoxicity testing. *Toxicol. In Vitro* **8**: 635–639.
33. Bronaugh, R. and Collier, S. (1993) *In vitro* methods for measuring skin permeation. In Zatz, J. L. (ed.) *Skin Permeation: Fundamentals and Applications*, pp. 93–113. Allured Publishing, Wheaton, USA.
34. Cleary, G. W. (1993) Transdermal drug delivery. In Zatz, J. L. (ed.) *Skin Permeation*, pp. 207–237. Allured Publishing, Wheaton, USA.
35. Franz, T. J. (1975) On the relevance of *in vitro* data. *J. Invest. Dermatol.* **64**: 190–200.

36. Schaefer, H. and Schalla, W. (1980) Kinetics of percutaneous absorption of steroids. In Mauvais-Jarvis, P., Vickers, C. F. H. and Wepierre, J. (eds) *Percutaneous Absorption of Steroids*, pp. 53–66. Academic Press, New York.
37. Zesch, A., Nordhaus, R. and Schaefer, H. (1972) Zur Krontrolle des Hornschitabrisses durch Widerstandsmessungen. *Archiv für Dermatologische Forschung* **242:** 398–402.
38. Rougier, A., Dupuis, D., Lotte, C., Roguet, R. and Schaefer, H. (1983) *In vivo* correlation between stratum corneum reservoir function and percutaneous absorption. *J. Invest. Dermatol.* **81:** 275–278.
39. Bickers, D. R., Dutta-Chouckry, T. and Mukhtar, H. (1982) Epidermis: a site of drug metabolism in neonatal rat skin. *Mol. Pharmacol.* **29:** 234–247.
40. Mukhtar, H. and Bickers, D. M. (1981) Drug metabolism in skin: Comparative activities of the mixed-function oxidases, ethoxide hydratone and glutathion S-transferase in liver and skin of neonatal rat. *Drug Metab. Dispos.* **9:** 311–314.
41. Coomes, M. W., Norling, A. M., Pohl, R. J., Muller, D. I. and Fouts, J. R. (1983) Foreign compound metabolism by isolated skin cell from the hairless mouse. *J. Pharmacol. Exp. Ther.* **225:** 770–777.
42. Raffali, F., Rougier, A. and Roguet, R. (1994) Measurement and modulation of cytochrome P-450 dependent enzyme activity in cultured human keratinocytes. *Skin Pharmacol.* **7:** 345–354.
43. DiGiovanni, J., Miller, D. R., Singer, J. M., Viaje, A. and Slaga, T. J. (1982) Benzo(a)pyrene metabolism in primary cultures of mouse epidermal cells and untransformed and transformed epidermal cell lines. *Cancer Res.* **42:** 2579–2586.
44. Pham, M. A., Magdalou, J., Totis, M., Fournel-Gigleux, S., Siest, G. and Hammock, B. D. (1989) Characterization of distinct forms of cytochromes P-450, epoxide metabolizing enzymes and UDP-glucuronosyltransferases in rat skin. *Biochem. Pharmacol.* **38:** 2187–2194.
45. Roguet, R., Cotovio, J., Kremers, P., Rougier, A., Pouradier Duteil, X. and Leclaire, J. (1995) Cytochrome P-450 enzyme activities and testosterone metabolism in a reconstituted human epidermis. *Toxicol. In Vitro* **8:** 95–102.
46. Pham, M. A., Magdalou, J., Siest, G. *et al.* (1990) Reconstituted epidermis: a novel model for the study of drug metabolism in human epidermis. *J. Invest. Dermatol.* **94:** 749–752.
47. Kao, J., Patterson, K. and Hall, J. (1985) Skin penetration and metabolism of topically applied chemicals in six mammalian species, including man: an *in vitro* study with benzo(a)pyrene and testosterone. *Toxicol. Appl. Pharmacol.* **81:** 502–516.
48. Ademola, J. I., Chow, C. A., Wester, R. C. and Maibach, H. I. (1993) Metabolism of propanolol during percutaneous absorption in human skin. *J. Pharm. Sci.* **82:** 767.
49. Cormier, M., Ledger, P. W., Marty, J. P. and Amkraut, A. (1991) *In vitro* cutaneous biotransformation of propanolol. *J. Invest. Dermatol.* **97:** 447–453.
50. Merk, H. F., Kaufmann, I., Vögel, F., Röwert, J. and Jungiger, H. (1987) Influences of imidazoles on cutaneous cytochrome P-450 activity after topical and systemic application. *Skin Pharmacol.* **1:** 184–189.
51. Ponsoda, X., Jover, R., Castell, J. V. and Gomez-Lechon, M. J. (1991) Measurement of intracellular LHD activity in 96-well cultures: a rapid and automated assay for cytotoxicity studies. *J. Tissue Culture Methods* **13:** 21–24.
52. Borenfreund, E. and Puerner, J. A. (1984) A simple quantitative procedure using monolayer cultures for cytotoxicity assays (HTD/RN-90). *J. Tissue Culture Methods* **9:** 7–9.
53. Catroux, P., Rougier, A., Dossou, K. G. and Cottin, M. (1993) The silicon microphysiometer for testing ocular irritancy *in vitro*. *Toxicol. In Vitro* **7:** 465–473.
54. Mossman, T. (1983) Rapid colorimetric assay for cell growth and survival – application to proliferation and cytotoxicity assays. *J. Immunol. Methods* **65:** 55–63.
55. Vistica, D. T., Skehan, P., Scudiero, D., Monks, A., Pittman, A. and Boyd, M. R. (1991) Tetrazolium-based assays for cellular viability. A critical examination of selected parameters affecting formazan production. *Cancer Res.* **51:** 2515–2520.
56. Bradford, M. (1976) A rapid and sensitive method for the quantification of microgram quantities of protein utilising the principle of protein dye binding. *Anal. Biochem.* **72:** 248–255.
57. Meyer, J. C. and Grundmann, H. (1984) Fluorimetric determination of DNA in epidermis and cultures fibroblasts, using 4′-6-diamidino-2-phenylindole (DAPI). *Arch. Dermatol. Res.* **276:** 52–56.
58. Oku, T., Takigawa, M. and Yamada, M. (1987) Cell proliferation kinetics of cultured human keratinocytes and fibroblasts measured using a monoclonal antibody. *Br. J. Dermatol.* **116:** 673–679.

59. Duffy, P. A. and Flint, O. P. (1987) *In vitro* dermal irritancy test. In Atterwill, C. K. and Steele, C. E. (eds): In vitro *Methods in Toxicology*, pp. 279–297. Cambridge University Press, Cambridge.
60. Duffy, P. A., Flint, O. P., Orton, T. C. and Fursey, M. J. (1986) Initial validation of an *in vitro* test for predicting skin irritancy. *Fd. Chem. Toxicol.* **24:** 517–518.
61. Parish, W. E. (1990) Inflammatory mediators applied to *in vitro* toxicity – studies on mediator release and two-cell system. *Toxicol. In Vitro* **4:** 231–241.
62. Galey, C. I., Ziboh, V. A., Marcello, C. L. and Voorhees, J. J. (1985) Modulation of phospholipid metabolism in murine keratinocytes by tumour promoter, 12-O-tetradecanoyl-phorbol-13-acetate. *J. Invest. Dermatol.* **85:** 319–323.
63. Stanley, P. L., Steiner, S., Havens, M. and Tramposch, K. M. (1991) Mouse skin inflammation induced by multiple topical applications of 12-O-tetradecanoylphorbol-13-acetate. *Skin Pharmacol.* **4:** 262–271.
64. Higley, H., Ellingsworth, L. and Voorhees, J. J. (1992) Differential modulation of transforming growth factor $\beta 1$ expression and mucin deposition by retinoic acid and sodium lauryl sulfate in human skin. *J. Invest. Dermatol.* **98:** 102–108.
65. James, L. C., Moore, A. M., Wheeler, L. A., Murphy, G. M., Dowd, P. M. and Greaves, M. W. (1991) Transforming growth-factor α – *in vivo* release by normal human skin following UV irradiation and abrasion. *Skin Pharmacol.* **4:** 61–64.
66. Luger, T. A., Köck, A., Danner, M., Colot, M. and Micksche, M. (1985) Production of distinct cytokines by epidermal keratinocytes. *Br. J. Dermatol.* **113:** 145–156.
67. Cohen, C., Dossou, K. G., Rougier, A. and Roguet, R. (1991) Measurement of inflammatory mediators produced by human keratinocytes *in vitro*: a predictive assessment of cutaneous irritation. *Toxicol. In Vitro* **5:** 407–410.
68. Gallo, R. L., Staszewski, R., Sauder, D. N., Knisely, T. L. and Granstein, R. D. (1991) Regulation of GM-CSF and IL-3 production from murine keratinocyte cell line PAM 212 following exposure to ultraviolet radiation. *J. Invest. Dermatol.* **97:** 203–209.
69. Duffy, P. A. (1989) Irritancy testing: a cultured approach. *Toxicol. In Vitro* **3:** 157–158.
70. DeLeo, V. A., Harber, L. C., Kong, B. M. and De Salva, S. J. (1987) Surfactant induced alteration of arachidonic acid metabolism of mammalian cells in culture. *Proc. Soc. Exp. Biol. Med.* **184:** 477–482.
71. DeLeo, V. A., Honson, D., Scheide, S., Kong, B. J. and De Salva, S. J. (1989) The effect of surfactants on the metabolism of choline phospholipids in human epidermal keratinocytes in culture. *J. Toxicol. Cut. Ocular Toxicol.* **8:** 227–240.
72. Dykes, P. J., Edwards, M. J., O'Donovan, M. R., Merret, V., Morgan, H. E. and Marks, R. (1991) *In vitro* reconstruction of human skin – the use of skin equivalents as potential indicators of cutaneous toxicity. *Toxicol. In Vitro* **5:** 1–8.
73. Gery, I., Gershon, R. K. and Waxman, B. H. (1972) Neutralization of the lymphocyte response to mitogens – the responding process. *J. Exp. Med.* **136:** 128–135.
74. Gueniche, A. and Ponec, M. (1993) Use of human skin cell cultures for the estimation of potential skin irritants. *Toxicol. In Vitro* **7:** 15–27.
75. Cohen, C., Dossou, K. G., Rougier, A. and Roguet, R. (1994) Episkin: an *in vitro* model for the evaluation of the phototoxicity and the sunscreen photoprotective properties. *Toxicol. In Vitro* **8:** 669–671.
76. Nelson, D. and Gay, R. J. (1993) Effects of UV irradiation on a living skin equivalent. *Photochem. Photobiol.* **57:** 830–837.
77. Roguet, R., Cohen, C. and Rougier, A. (1994) A reconstituted human epidermis to assess cutaneous irritation, phototoxicity and photoprotection *in vitro*. In Rougier, A., Goldberg, A. M. and Maibach, H. I. (eds) In Vitro *Skin Toxicology – Irritation, Phototoxicity, Sensitization*, pp. 83–97. Mary Ann Liebert, New York.
78. Roguet, R., Cohen, C., Dossou, K. G. and Rougier, A. (1993) Episkin, a reconstituted human epidermis for assessing *in vitro* the irritancy of topically applied compounds. *Toxicol. In Vitro* **8:** 283–291.

12

Ocular Irritation

HORST SPIELMANN

I. Introduction 265
II. Use and limitations of the Draize rabbit's eye test 266
III. Refinement of the Draize rabbit's eye test 268
  A. The low-volume eye test 268
  B. Changes of OECD guideline no. 405 268
  C. Integrated eye irritancy testing strategy for new chemicals within the framework of the European notification procedure 269
IV. *In vitro* alternatives for assessing ocular irritation 271
  A. Organotypical models 272
    1. The HET-CAM test 272
    2. The CAMVA 274
    3. The BCOP test 274
    4. The isolated rabbit eye (IRE) test 275
    5. The chicken enucleated eye test (CEET) 276
  B. Cell and tissue testing methods 277
    1. The neutral red uptake test 277
    2. The red blood cell (RBC) haemolysis test 278
    3. The fluorescein leakage test 279
    4. The silicon microphysiometer (SM) test 280
    5. The tissue equivalent test 280
  C. Physicochemical tests 281
    1. The EYTEX test 281
V. Validation of *in vitro* alternatives to the Draize eye test 282
VI. Conclusions and future perspectives 284
References 285

I. INTRODUCTION

For more than 50 years the Draize rabbit's eye test has been used as the standardized animal assay for ocular safety assessment. In 1944 Draize and co-workers[1] at the US National Institutes of Health developed the assay in which a systemic numerical scoring system is used to quantify ocular irritation. The scoring system of the Draize eye test allows assessment of

IN VITRO METHODS IN PHARMACEUTICAL RESEARCH
ISBN 0-12-163390-X

the full spectrum of eye irritation properties of test materials, ranging from non-irritating to severely irritating and corrosive properties. Today, the Draize eye test is still the world-wide standard for assessing the ocular irritation of new chemicals. The test has been standardized at the international level, e.g. by the Organization for Economic Cooperation and Development as OECD guideline no. 405[2] 'Acute eye irritation/corrosion', and it is the most widely used test for classification and labelling of chemicals according to their ocular safety. This is essential information on toxicology which has to be determined with all new chemicals, as accidental ocular exposure may occur in the workplace and wherever the product is being used by the consumer. Without this information, new chemicals and products can be neither produced nor introduced on to the market.

The eye is a very sensitive organ, not only in humans but also in laboratory animals. For the past 20 years the Draize rabbit's eye test has, therefore, been criticized more than any other toxicological test in animals by the animal welfare movement. Moreover, the Draize eye test has also been criticized for two scientific reasons: on the one hand for the subjectivity of the method and on the other for overpredicting the response in humans. Thus, over the past 20 years toxicologists in industry and academia have attempted to develop non-animal methods that can be used for ocular safety assessment. It has been a great challenge so far to develop *in vitro* methods that are simple to perform and provide reproducible results which are sufficient for ocular risk assessment in humans.

In this chapter the use and limits of the Draize eye test are described briefly, as this information has to be taken into account when developing *in vitro* alternatives that are acceptable for regulatory purposes. The major part of the chapter gives an outline of the most promising non-animal methods which are currently undergoing validation. Finally, the current use of *in vitro* alternatives for in-house safety testing and for regulatory purposes is discussed.

II. USE AND LIMITATIONS OF THE DRAIZE RABBIT'S EYE TEST

The spectrum of irritancy covered by the Draize rabbit's eye test ranges from assessment of corrosivity and/or severe damage to the eye, to mild and moderate irritation to the eye, to non-irritant chemicals that do not require any labelling. Thus it has to be taken into consideration that the Draize eye test is used in toxicology for a variety of purposes. It is, on the one hand, used to identify chemicals that may cause damage to the eye and have to be labelled for regulatory purposes to avoid accidental ocular damage. On the other end of the scale this animal test is carried out to assess ocular safety of cosmetics and of drugs to be used in the treatment of ocular diseases.

Due to the world-wide use of the Draize eye test for assessing a wide range of toxicological end-points, a considerable number of scoring systems has been developed to evaluate reactions of the rabbit's eye in the Draize eye test. For example, data obtained in one country in the Draize eye test for a given purpose may have to be repeated to meet the requirements of a regulatory agency in another country for classification and labelling. Moreover, the Draize eye test may have to be carried out in different ways depending on the use of the product, for example according to guidelines for safety assessment of industrial chemicals, cosmetics or drugs. Thus the ocular irritancy of a given chemical determined in the Draize eye test may be assigned to different categories of classification and labelling. To give a few examples, in the USA the maximum average score (MAS) scoring system with a scale ranging from 0 to 110 is used for regulatory purposes (Federal Hazardous Substance Act 1974)[3] and in Europe the EU classification scheme,[4] while an additional scoring system was developed for cosmetics testing in the Draize eye test by Kay and Calendra.[5]

Due to low reproducibility the Draize eye test has been criticized heavily from the scientific point of view. The criticism is based on a blind validation trial which was carried out more than 20 years ago with a standardized set of test chemicals in 24 experienced laboratories in the USA.[6] Fig. 12.1 gives an example for three chemicals tested in this validation trial on intralaboratory and interlaboratory variability in the results of the Draize eye irritation test in rabbits. It is important to note in Fig. 12.1 not only the high variability of the data but also that each of the three test chemicals was assigned at least by one of the laboratories to be either severely irritant or non-irritant, with the majority of laboratories providing results between the two extremes.

Recently, a similar variation of Draize eye test data to be used as reference was observed within the world-wide EC/Home Office validation study on alternatives to the Draize eye test.[7] Even the best available Draize eye test data showed a high variability in the medium range of irritation, while good reproducibility was observed both at the upper end for severely irritating chemicals and at the lower end of the Draize scale for non-irritating ones.

Taking these results into account one may wonder why the Draize eye test is still popular and has not been replaced by more reproducible methods. The most important reason for staying with the system is the test object, which is the living eye. According to the Draize scale of evaluation, all adverse reactions are recorded in every tissue of the eye, including long-term effects up to 21 days after exposure. The results obtained in the Draize eye test can, therefore, easily be compared to the situation in the human eye. The higher sensitivity of the rabbit eye in comparison with the human eye adds to the safety of the test, which is an

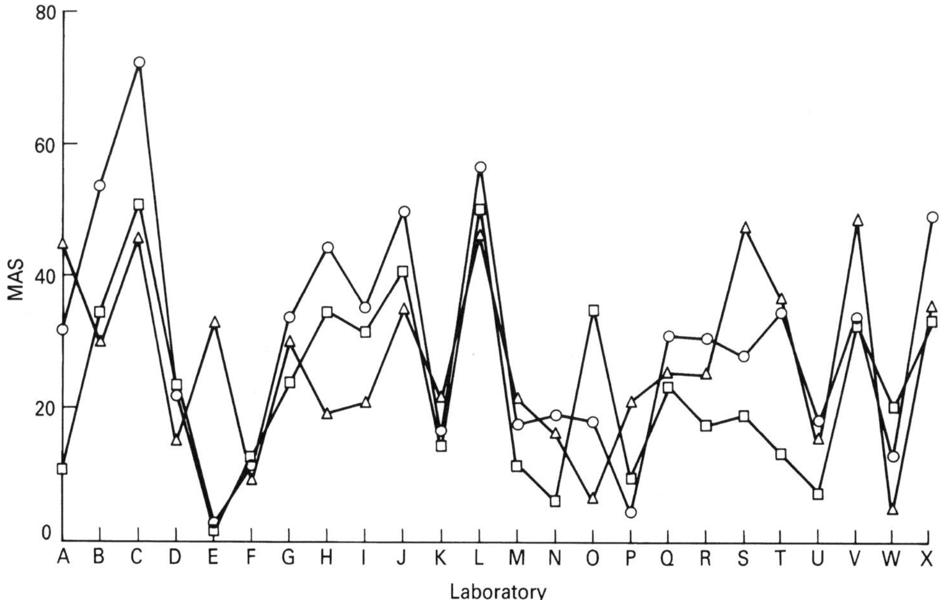

Fig. 12.1 Validation of the Draize eye test in 24 laboratories in the USA. Draize eye test data in rabbits were evaluated according to the maximum average score (MAS) scale (0–110) with a cut-off value of 20 to discriminate between non and mild irritants, and values greater than 60 indicating severe ocular irritants, while irritant chemicals are located between 40 and 60, i.e. >40 and <60. To show the variability of the Draize eye test, results are given for three chemicals (△, chemical 1; ○, chemical 2; □, chemical 3) all of which are exceeding both the limits of MAS >40 and <20, one of them is even exceeding the limits of MAS >60 and <20. From Weil and Scala.[6]

advantage when judging from the viewpoint of both the liability of the producer and also of safety assessment of the regulator.

III. REFINEMENT OF THE DRAIZE RABBIT'S EYE TEST

In toxicology the current scientific concept for developing alternatives to testing in animals is the '3Rs' concept of Russel and Burch,[8] who suggested in their book on principles of humane testing a sequence of refining, reducing and replacing a given animal test. In the field of ocular irritation testing, the first step would be the refinement of the Draize eye test and the final goal is the replacement of this test by one or more non-animal tests. To reduce suffering of rabbits in the Draize eye test, and also the numbers of animals used, the procedure was modified to give information that is more predictive of the response in humans and less stressful for the test animals.

A. The low-volume eye test

As indicated above, the results of the Draize eye test are biased towards overpredicting human risk. From the technical viewpoint this may be due to the amount of material and the site to which it is applied. In the standard Draize eye test 100 μl or 100 mg of test material is applied to the conjunctival sac of the rabbit eye. In a study on the influence of the volume of test material, Griffith *et al.*[9] demonstrated that 0.01 ml of test substance applied directly to the cornea produce an irritation response similar in magnitude and duration to the response in humans. From this study the authors working at Procter and Gamble (USA) developed the low-volume eye test (LVET), which is different from the classical Draize eye test in three aspects: 0.01 ml is applied instead of 0.1 ml; the test chemical is applied directly to the cornea and not into the conjunctival sac; and the eyelids are not held shut right after treatment.

Results obtained in the LVET were compared with literature data from human exposure, and by comparing the response in human volunteers and rabbits.[10] The data showed clearly that human ocular response was more accurately predicted from the LVET than from the standard Draize test protocol. The same study also proved that the LVET is, of course, less stressful for the rabbits because it produces less irritation and allows shorter recovery times.

The LVET has not reached wide acceptance outside the USA, probably because the OECD changed guideline no. 405 'Acute eye irritation/corrosion' in 1987[2] as far as severely eye irritating chemicals are concerned at the time when the LVET was still being developed and validated.

B. Changes of OECD guideline no. 405

In 1987 the OECD has updated OECD guideline no. 405 ('Acute eye irritation/corrosion')[2] to reduce suffering of rabbits in the Draize eye test. According to the new version, careful consideration needs to be given to all available information on a substance to minimize testing of substances under conditions that are likely to produce severe reactions. The following information should be evaluated:

1. Physicochemical properties and chemical reactivity, resulting in strongly acidic (< 2) or alkaline (> 11.5) pH in the eye.
2. Results from skin irritation studies indicating definite corrosive or severe skin irritancy in a dermal study.
3. Results from well-validated alternatives studies indicating potential corrosive or severe irritating properties.

Test materials indicating a high irritation potential need not be tested in the Draize eye test and can be classified and labelled for regulatory purposes without performing the test. Regulatory agencies within EU countries are routinely accepting the escape clause defined in OECD guideline no. 405 under nos 1 and 2. However, because no well-validated alternative method has so far been accepted by regulatory agencies at the international level, a series of validation studies on Draize alternatives has been initiated in many member countries of the EU and the OECD to identify severely eye-irritating materials.

The approaches developed are driven by both scientific and ethical considerations. To give an example, the isolated rabbit eye (IRE) test,[7] which is well established in the UK as an alternative to the Draize eye test, has not been taken up by the other EU member states because the procedure for killing rabbits in a humane way to obtain their eyes for testing purposes seems unacceptable from an ethical point of view outside the UK. In Germany, even the use of eyes obtained from the slaughterhouse is not an accepted alternative, in contrast to the use of bovine eyes in the BCOP (bovine cornea opacity and permeability) test in France[11] and of chicken eyes in the CEET (chicken enucleated eye) test in the Netherlands.[12]

For the reasons described, some well-established and nationally validated *in vitro* assays are accepted by regulatory authorities of a few EU member states according to recommendation no. 3 of the updated version of OECD guideline no. 405.[2] Regulatory authorities in the UK are accepting the isolated rabbit eye test as a well-validated alternative method; the BCOP test is accepted in France and Belgium, and the HET-CAM (hens egg test at the chorion allantoic membrane) assay in Germany.

C. Integrated eye irritancy testing strategy for new chemicals within the framework of the European notification procedure

To reduce testing of severely eye-irritating materials in the Draize eye test, regulatory authorities in Germany have developed a stepwise strategy for eye irritation testing within the EU according to recommendation no. 3 of the updated version of OECD guideline no. 405.[13] In the stepwise procedure, a sequence of physicochemical as well as *in vivo* and *in vitro* toxicological data is being taken into account for evaluation of the eye irritation potential of new chemicals. Within this procedure chemicals that give a positive result in one of the steps of the procedure are classified and labelled according the EU classification scheme ‘R 41: Risk of severe damage to eyes’.[4] On the other hand, all chemicals that give negative results in each of the steps will have to undergo *in vivo* testing in the Draize rabbit's eye test.

The following stepwise strategy has proven useful (Fig. 12.2).

Step 1: Measurement of pH Eye irritation properties of strongly acidic (pH < 2) or alkaline (pH > 11.5) chemicals can be labelled ‘R 41’ without any testing *in vivo*.

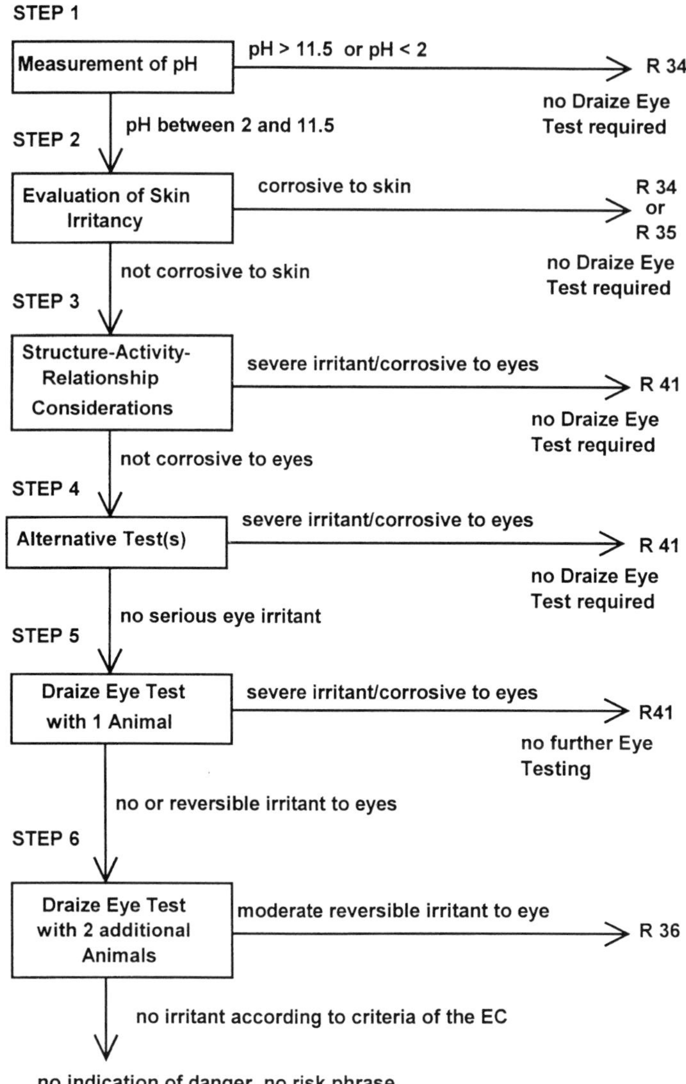

Fig. 12.2 Eye irritancy testing strategy for new chemicals within the notification procedure of the European Union. From Schlede and Gerner.[13]

Step 2: Evaluation of skin irritancy Eye irritiation properties of substances corrosive to skin need not be tested for eye irritation and can be labelled 'R 41' without testing in the Draize eye test.

Step 3: Structure–activity relationship considerations Theoretical considerations on qualitative structure–property relationships and structural activity relationship (SAR) modelling are taken into consideration, usually in combination with Step 4.

Step 4: In vitro *methods and alternative tests* Results of validated alternative methods for predicting severe eye irritation and corrosion effects to eyes can be sufficient for labelling chemicals 'R 41' without any testing in animals.

Step 5: Draize eye test with one animal If the result shows severe irritation or corrosion to the eye, no further testing is required within the EU and the chemical can be labelled 'R 41' without any further testing.

Step 6: Draize eye test with two additional animals This step has to be performed when less severe effects are seen in step 4 on the eyes of the single animal used in Step 5.

The stepwise procedure described is used for regulatory purposes in a few EU member states. There are, however, differences as far as *in vitro* assays are accepted by the national competent authorities. This is due to differences in experience with specific *in vitro* assays at the national level. Taking into account experience from a national validation trial in Germany, the HET-CAM assay is accepted as a well-validated *in vitro* alternative to the Draize eye test by German regulators for predicting serious damage to the eye and labelling with the risk-phrase 'R 41: Risk of serious damage to eyes'.[13] For similar reasons, in France and Belgium the national competent authorities are accepting *in vitro* data obtained with the BCOP assay, and regulatory authorities in the UK accept data obtained with the isolated rabbit eye assay.

IV. *IN VITRO* ALTERNATIVES FOR ASSESSING OCULAR IRRITATION

During the past decade many *in vitro* models have been developed to replace the Draize eye test. As outlined above, the eye is a very complex organ capable of a wide range of responses to injury. It seems, therefore, unlikely that a single *in vitro* assay will be able to cover all toxic responses of an organ as complex as the eye. It seems most likely that replacement of the Draize eye test can be achieved only by a battery consisting of multiple *in vitro* tests with a wide spectrum of end-points. The end-points will have to cover the major responses of the eye to chemical damage and the tests will have to be reproducible and easy to conduct.

Development of such a complete battery of *in vitro* assays will not be easy, because our understanding of the basic cellular and molecular mechanisms of eye irritation is limited. Therefore, it is still difficult to develop mechanistically based assays. Moreover, some of the essential components charcteristic of eye irritation cannot yet be modelled *in vitro*, for example inflammation, repair, scarification and even pain. However, promising *in vitro* tests have been developed which cover essential parts of the reaction spectrum of the eye, either at the upper end to identify severely irritating chemicals or at the lower end for non-irritant materials. Such assays are used within laboratories of the industry as screens within a tiered testing approach. The use of these *in vitro* systems, more complex tissue culture systems, improved bioanalytical systems and a better understanding of the toxicological reactions at the molecular level will lead to more sophisticated *in vitro* systems for assessing ocular irritation. At the same time, use of the Draize eye test will decrease and in years to come the *in vivo* test may not have to be performed at all.

Although the range of tests proposed for replacing the Draize eye test is wide, they can easily be categorized into organotypical models, cell and tissue assays, and physicochemical tests. The organotypic models usually provide complex information comparable to the situation in the eye. However, they are often performed as *ex vivo* tests where the organs are obtained from animals that were bred and killed specifically for the *in vitro* test. In contrast, in cell and tissue assays, and also in physicochemical tests, usually only a single end-point is measured but no animal has to be killed for testing.

A. Organotypical models

1. *The HET-CAM test*

Principles of the method and basic testing procedure The HET-CAM test is an organotypical test in which test materials are applied to the sensitive chorion allantoic membrane (CAM) of chicken eggs on day 9 of embryonation. It is assumed that acute irritating effects on the small vessels and protein membranes of this soft tissue membrane are similar to effects induced by the same chemicals in the eye. The HET-CAM test, which was originally developed by Luepke,[14] is well established in the cosmetics industry in Europe, and several variations of the original HET-CAM assay have been developed (e.g. for classification of severely eye irritating chemicals according to EU regulations).

In most HET-CAM protocols, three end-points are determined to assess the ocular irritating properties of test materials on the CAM: *haemorrhage*, *lysis* and *coagulation*. Several variants of the HET-CAM assay protocols have been developed to allow testing of materials with different physicochemical properties. Of the three most widely used protocols, two have been developed for transparent materials (the reaction time method and determination of the irritation threshold) and one for non-transparent materials and solids (the end-point measurement method). As initially suggested by Luepke,[14] all HET-CAM protocols utilise an observation period of 5 min (300 s) and the three end-points of haemorrhage, lysis and coagulation for assessing the reaction at the CAM.

The most widely used method is the *reaction time method*, in which the time of appearance of each of the three end-points is determined up to 5 min after application of undiluted or 10% diluted test material.[14,15] The second method is the *threshold method*, in which the concentration at appearance of the three end-points is assessed,[15,16] and the third is the *end-point measurement* method for insoluble materials, in which the CAM is exposed to test materials for 5 min and, after they have been carefully rinsed off, the CAM is examined for severity of haemorrhage, lysis and coagulation.[14,15]

Different scoring systems have been developed for the different HET-CAM test protocols. Luepke's original HET-CAM scale,[14] ranging from 0 to 21, is still most widely used. It is a weighted scale in which coagulation is given a higher weight than haemorrhage and lysis, and in which reaction values greater than 10 are classified as severe eye irritation.

Application of the method

Non-irritant and mildly irritant materials (e.g. cosmetics): The HET-CAM test is an established method in many cosmetics companies in Europe, particularly in France and Germany, for in-house safety assessment of raw materials and formulations. The *in vitro–in vivo* correlation is very good in the area of mild to non-irritating test materials. According to in-house experience reported by leading companies of the European cosmetics industry (e.g. Beiersdorf, Henkel and L'Oreal), the HET-CAM test shows a better *in vitro–in vivo* correlation than any other *in vitro* alternative to the Draize eye irritation test.[17]

Fig. 12.3 gives an example obtained with 42 surfactant-based chemicals and formulations from one of the leading cosmetic manufacturers.[18] In this plot Pearson's linear correlation coefficient for *in vitro* HET-CAM results versus *in vivo* Draize eye test data is almost perfect ($r = 0.86$; highly significant) up to a value of 45 in the MAS–Draize eye test scale, which is

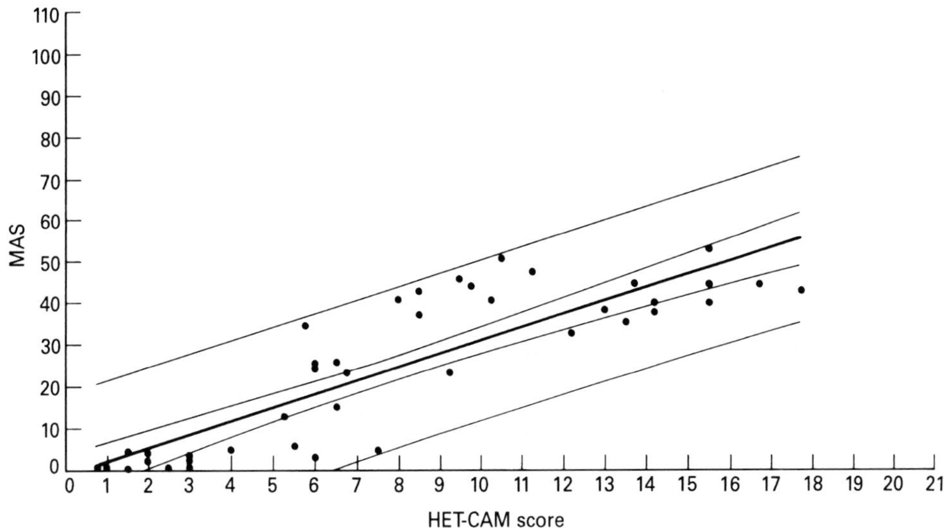

Fig. 12.3 *In vitro–in vivo* correlation between the HET-CAM test according to Luepke[14] and the maximum average score (MAS) of the Draize eye test for 42 water-soluble surfactants and surfactant-based formulations. Data were produced in-house in a laboratory of the European cosmetics industry (Pearson's linear correlation analysis 0.86, $P < 0.001$). The linear regression line of the regression and of the prediction of a single MAS value are shown. The *in vivo* data set covers only the lower spectrum of irritation in the Draize eye test (MAS 0–45).

graded 0–110. The data in Fig. 12.3 indicate that, at the lower end of the MAS scale in the range of non-irritating to mildly irritating substances, the HET-CAM test be used to predict the Draize eye scores for surfactants. Therefore, the HET-CAM test is the most important *in vitro* test within various batteries used to assess eye irritation potential in many cosmetics companies in Europe.[17]

Classification of severely eye-irritating materials: To assess severely irritating materials at the upper end of the MAS scale (MAS > 60) and for classification according to EU regulations as 'R 41: Risk of severe damage to eyes',[4] other HET-CAM protocols have been developed and validated. In a national validation study in Germany of alternatives to the Draize eye test, a HET-CAM protocol for classifying and labelling chemicals as 'severely irritating to the eye' according to EU regulations (i.e. as R 41) was developed and validated successfully.[15,16]

Discriminant analysis revealed that, among the end-points routinely determined in the HET-CAM test, coagulation of a 10% solution was the best discriminating factor for identifying severely eye-irritating chemicals, and coagulation of undiluted chemicals for the less water-soluble ones.[19] Stepwise discriminant analysis allowed the development of an *in vitro* testing strategy for identifying severely eye-irritating chemicals from coagulation data of the HET-CAM test. Results obtained with 200 chemicals under blind conditions suggest that this approach will provide an acceptable predictivity for regulatory purposes. Regulatory authorities in Germany have agreed to accept classification of severely eye-irritating chemicals with this HET-CAM protocol.[13]

Limitations of the method It has to be stressed that there is no standard HET-CAM test protocol that can be used for replacing the Draize eye test but that specific HET-CAM protocols have been developed to cover the many applications of the Draize eye test. Each of the HET-CAM protocols has its limitations. A HET-CAM protocol that can successfully be used for safety testing of cosmetics may not be appropriate for classifying severely eye-irritating materials, and vice versa. It is, therefore, important to identify specifically the area in which the HET-CAM assay will be used to replace the Draize eye test. If this is taken into consideration, the HET-CAM assay can be used to replace the Draize eye test for in-house testing and for regulatory purposes.

Although it has been claimed that solid and insoluble material can be handled in the HET-CAM assay, these materials generated problems in validation trials as the results were not sufficiently reproducible. This is particularly the case for sticky test materials.

2. The CAMVA

Principles of the method and basic testing procedure The chorion allantoic membrane vascular assay (CAMVA) is the second CAM-based assay. It was developed in 1985 by Leighton *et al.*[20] and refined according to the requirements of an industrial laboratory by Bagley *et al.*,[21] and to the use of eggs on day 10 of embryonation rather than day 14.

In contrast to the HET-CAM assay, in the CAMVA only vascular effects on the CAM are recorded; 30 min after dosing the CAM is examined for hypoaemia (ghost vessels), hyperaemia (capillary injection) and haemorrhage. If a vascular effect of any degree is observed, the egg is considered positive. The concentration of test material inducing a positive response in 50% of eggs (RC_{50}) is calculated by probit analysis.

Regression analysis of the *in vitro–in vivo* correlation of the same test materials tested in the CAMVA on days 14 and 10 of embryonation revealed that the 14-day CAMVA predicts higher *in vivo* scores than the 10-day CAMVA within the entire range of ocular irritancy.[19]

Application of the method In the cosmetics industry in the USA, the CAMVA has been used successfully to predict the eye irritation potential of alcohol-containing formulations; it is less accurate for predicting the eye irritation potential of oil or water emulsions. In a few companies, the CAMVA serves as a screen for eye irritation potential. To assess the ocular irritation potential of a new product within a company, historical data of similar products are first evaluated and the eye irritation potential of the product ingredients are assessed; thereafter the CAMVA serves as a screen.[21]

Limitations of the method Materials containing polyethylene glycol typically result in false-positive results. Insoluble material can be tested only by experienced laboratories. The CAMVA has not undergone systematic validation; therefore, objective information on the limits of the method is not yet available. Although the CAMVA has been used successfully for safety assessment of cosmetics, there is no information on the application of the CAMVA in other areas of eye irritation testing, e.g. for the classification of severely eye-irritating materials.

3. The BCOP test

Principles of the method and basic testing procedure In the BCOP test, which was developed recently by Gautheron *et al.*,[11] bovine corneas from eyes freshly collected from a local abattoir are used to assess the eye-irritating properties of test materials. Two end-points are determined in the BCOP assay: opacity and permeability of isolated corneas. The corneas are freshly prepared and mounted in special holders, which consist of an anterior and a posterior chamber. Both chambers are filled with simple culture medium and test material is applied to the anterior chamber of the holder. Corneas are exposed for 1 h.

Change in opacity was the only end-point determined when the BCOP assay was originally developed. Later, measurement of permeability was added, as visualized by the application of a fluorescent dye.[11]

In the *opacity measurement*, change in light transmission passing through the cornea is determined with an opacitometer and expressed as a numerical opacity value. In the *permeability measurement*, which is performed immediately after the opacity measurement, the permeability of the cornea is determined by exposure to fluorescein for 90 min. Special protocols for solids and surfactants have been developed, in addition to the standard protocol for liquids.

Application of the method The BCOP test score was derived empirically by Gautheron and modified during a validation trial.[22] It is based on the Kay and Calendra classification scheme[5] for data obtained *in vivo* in the Draize eye irritation test in rabbits, and the following classification has been derived from testing cosmetics as well as industrial chemicals:[22]

0–25	mildly irritant
25.1–55	moderately irritant
55.1–80	severely irritant
$\geq$ 80.1	very severely irritant

In a validation study funded by the EU in 12 laboratories with 52 test chemicals, an *in vitro–in vivo* correlation of 0.73 was obtained between the BCOP and MAS test scores of the Draize eye test.[22]

The BCOP assay is used routinely for in-house safety assessment in laboratories of the cosmetics and drug industry in France and Belgium and it has become popular in the USA. It is also used for regulatory purposes in a few of these companies, to classify and label chemicals as 'severely irritating to the eye' according to EU regulations (R 41).[4] The BCOP assay is easy to learn and to establish; it is also cheap to conduct, and validation trials have shown that the data are reproducible among laboratories.[22]

Limitations of the method In the EU validation study, all four false-negative results were on solids and three of four false-positive findings were from liquids.[22] Thus, the methodology may have to be modified to cover all the physical forms of test substances. Neutralization and buffering of solids by the culture medium, which is used to solubilize solids, may also have to be taken into account. There seems to be a tendency to overestimate the irritating properties of alcohols in the BCOP assay.

4. *The isolated rabbit eye (IRE) test*

Principles of the method and basic testing procedure The isolated rabbit eye (IRE) assay is specific for corneal effects. Damage to the cornea is assessed by measuring corneal thickness as an index of swelling. The IRE test was initially developed in 1981 by Burton *et al.*[23] and the recently standardized protocol of the IRE test[24] is well established in toxicology laboratories in the UK.

Rabbits are humanely killed and the eyes are removed immediately after death and mounted in moist, temperature-controlled chambers. After a period of stabilization, the eyes are exposed to the undiluted test material for 10 s, after which they are thoroughly rinsed with saline. The mean opacity scores and the percentage corneal swelling are determined at 1 h and 4 h after treatment with a slit-lamp biomicroscope fitted with a depth-measuring attachment, or an ultrasonic pachymeter. In addition, the penetration of fluorescein dye into the cornea can be measured by applying fluorescein solution to the cornea for 10 s, after which excess dye is rinsed away.

High numerical values should correlate with high *in vivo* irritancy. The degree of swelling is used to grade the severity of response, in that any chemical causing more than 15% corneal swelling at any time after treatment is considered to have the potential to cause severe ocular irritation *in vivo*.

Application of the method The test is ideally suited to investigations on undiluted test materials (solids, liquids and insoluble materials). The IRE test is currently used in the UK as the second step of a tiered approach in which cytotoxicity is determined first. Chemicals that are predicted to be severe irritants proceed for confirmation to the second tier of testing, the IRE assay.[24] For assessment of chemicals hazardous to the eye, the *in vitro* identification of potentially severe effects in this tiered approach is accepted by regulatory agencies in the UK without the need to conduct Draize eye tests in rabbits. In an evaluation of IRE test data by a review panel of the IRAG (US Inter Regulatory Agency Group) Working Group on organotypic models for the assessment of ocular irritation,[25] it was confirmed that the IRE assay is a good screen for severely irritating materials but is poor at discriminating between such materials and those of low irritation potential. However, it was concluded that the IRE test seems to have practical application in screening for severely irritating materials.[25]

Limitations of the method No technical difficulties are usually experienced in the performance of the test. As a predictive tool across the whole range of eye irritation, the IRE test alone is of no practical value for predicting irritation potential. As described above, it can be used successfully as an in-house screen for severely eye-irritating materials within a battery of *in vitro* assays.

5. The chicken enucleated eye test (CEET)

Principles of the method and basic testing procedure The chicken is a suitable species of abattoir animal to act as an eye donor for the assessment of eye irritation potential of test materials. Since 1992, the CEET has been incorporated in standard toxicity testing at a contract laboratory as a prescreen for the Draize eye test.[12] The effects of test materials are assessed following application to the corneas of enucleated chicken eyes.

Heads of spring chickens are collected at a local abattoir. Within 2 h of killing, enucleated eyes are placed in a superfusion apparatus, which keep the eyes in good condition for at least 6 h. Test compound is applied to the cornea of at least three eyes in a single dose of either 30 μl (liquids, gels and pastes) or 30 mg (solids) for 10 s. Eyes are examined for corneal thickness and swelling at 0, 30, 75, 120, 180 and 240 min after treatment, using a fixed scoring system. Fluorescein retention by damaged epithelial cells is scored at 30 min post-treatment only. All examinations are carried out with a slit-lamp microscope, such as is normally used in human ophthalmoscopy.

The mean percentage of corneal swelling and the mean corneal opacity value for all test eyes are calculated for the observation time points at 30, 75, 120, 180 and 240 min. The mean fluorescein retention value for all test eyes is calculated for the observation time point at 30 min only. Morphological effects on the cornea are also recorded.

Based on the maximum mean scores defined for corneal swelling, corneal opacity and fluorescein retention by damaged epithelial cells, the irritation potential of the compound (ranging from not irritating to severely irritating), is assessed using the CEET classification system.

Application of the method With the results of the CEET, an irritation index can be calculated which takes into account the maximum mean scores of the three parameters measured, i.e. corneal swelling, corneal opacity and fluorescein retention. The CEET irritation index can range from 0 to 200.

At present, the CEET is routinely used in-house in a contract laboratory as a screen for eye irritation before the standard Draize eye test. Depending on the results in the CEET, which are available within 6 h, a decision can be made to conduct an *in vivo* assay. In the Netherlands the competent regulatory authorities accept classification of severely eye-irritating test materials as 'R 41' according to EU regulations in the CEET test without performing the Draize eye test in rabbits.

Limitations of the method With hydrophobic compounds, a special protocol has been successfully explored, consisting of multiple exposures or removing the aqueous liquid from the cornea as much as possible, just before application, ensuring a more intense contact with the compound.

There may not be a chicken abattoir in close proximity to the laboratory. Several options are available to overcome this problem: moving experimental set-up (which is small and does not require much space) to the slaughterhouse, using end-of-lay birds instead of spring chickens, and using other kinds of birds (e.g. turkeys).

B. Cell and tissue testing methods

1. *The neutral red uptake test*

Principles of the method and basic testing procedure The neutral red uptake (NRU) cytotoxicity test is based on the observation that some materials which are damaging to the eye appear to be cytotoxic to a number of cell types *in vitro*. Surface-active agents are expected to be cytolytic at different concentrations, depending on their irritancy potential. The NRU cytotoxicity testing procedure is based on the work of Borenfreund and Puerner[26] and permanent cell line mouse 3T3 cells are selected because of their ease of maintenance.

The concentration of test material resulting in a 50% inhibition of neutral red uptake (NRU_{50}) is determined by extrapolation from the dose-response curve. The NRU_{50} values are given in micrograms per millilitre of test material.

Application of the method The exact use of the assay to predict ocular irritation depends on the purpose of testing and the experience of the user. For personal care products, the assay has been used to select formulations for development and to qualify final products for use on human panelists.

Like other cytotoxicity assays, the NRU assay is reproducible with water-soluble materials. Therefore, many laboratories perform the NRU cytotoxicity assay as an essential part of a battery of *in vitro* tests or in a tiered approach of *in vitro* screening for ocular irritation. The NRU assay is well established in batteries of *in vitro* assays to identify non-irritiant materials in the cosmetics industry and it is also used as the first step of tiered *in vitro* testing strategies to identify severely eye-irritating materials, for example in combination with the IRE assay[24] or the HET-CAM assay.[19]

To predict ocular irritation from cytotoxicity data, a graph is usually constructed of historical animal eye irritation data versus 3T3 *in vitro* cytotoxicity data. Materials whose *in vivo* ocular irritation potential is unknown are tested *in vitro*, and the projected *in vivo* score is extrapolated from the graph. It is important to have a sufficient database for various chemical classifications, because the relationship between cytotoxicity in 3T3 cells and the *in vivo* response appears to vary with chemical class.

Limitations of the method False-negative results are obtained if test materials are not water soluble or at least water miscible. In addition, materials with high or low pH values are likely to be less toxic in the NRU cytotoxicity assay owing to the buffering capacity of the culture medium. Moreover, test materials with high acid or alkaline reserve, and also reactive species such as hypochloride, may react with the culture medium and therefore, be underpredicted.

2. *The red blood cell (RBC) haemolysis test*

Principles of the method and basic testing procedure In the RBC assay, which was developed in 1987 by Pape *et al.*[27] for *in vitro* ocular irritancy testing of surfactants, membrane damage is assessed by measuring the leakage of haemoglobin from red blood cells incubated with test material under standard conditions. In the original protocol of the RBC assay, human erythrocytes were used; it was shown by Lewis *et al.*[28] that the assay can also be carried out with red blood cells from rabbits.

In the RBC assay, protein denaturation is measured by determining the reduction in absorbance at 541 nm (oxyhaemoglobin absorption maximum) with increasing concentration of test substance. The degree of denaturation can be determined in a range-finding study, and lysis of the erythrocyte membrane is subsequently assessed at concentration intervals selected from the results of the range-finding study.

In the RBC, membrane damage (lysis) is expressed as the H_{50} value (the concentration causing 50% haemolysis relative to the totally lysed sample). Denaturation is expressed as D_{low} (the lowest concentration causing denaturation – a 10% decrease in absorbance at 541 nm) and D_{max} (the maximum percentage denaturation seen at any concentration tested).

Application of the method The end-points determined in the RBC, H_{50} and D_{low} are inversely correlated with maximum average score (MAS), and D_{max} is positively correlated with MAS. Most of the materials used to evaluate the RBC assay have been surfactants. The end-points determined in the RBC assay are, therefore, specific to this class of chemicals. In a few companies of the cosmetics industry in Europe, the RBC assay is used in conjunction with other non-animal approaches and structure–activity information in the assessment of ocular safety of surfactants and surfactant-based finished products before they are tested on human volunteers without previous testing in animals.

Limitations of the method As with all cell-based assay systems, protocols are not yet available to handle both water-soluble and water-insoluble test materials. Limited evaluations have been carried out on vehicles suitable within the RBC assay.

3. *The fluorescein leakage test*

Principles of the method and basic testing procedure In the fluorescein leakage assay, which was developed in 1988 by Tchao,[29] the loss of transepithelial impermeability of a confluent monolayer of Madin-Darby canine kidney (MDCK) cells following exposure to irritant materials is measured by determining the degree of leakage of fluorescein across the cell monolayer. In the fluorescein leakage test, MDCK cells are grown to confluence on microporous filters in commercial cell culture inserts with an apical and basal culture chamber. The cells are exposed to high concentrations of test material for 1 min and 'leakage' of fluorescein into basal culture can be measured spectrophotometrically. Thus, the fluorescein leakage test is thought to model disruption of the integrity of the corneal epithelium by chemicals that may be potentially irritant to the eye.

The damage caused is determined by the amount of fluorescein that leaks through the confluent layer over a set period of time. The percentage of leakage is expressed relative to controls and fluorescence intensity is determined in a fluorescence measurement system, using excitation and emission wavelengths of 485 and 530 nm, respectively.

Sodium fluorescein leakage across the treated cell layer into the basal chamber is assessed either spectrophotometrically[29,30] at 492 nm or spectrofluorometrically (excitation 485 nm, emission 530 nm;).[31] Results are expressed either as FL_{20} or FL_{50} values,[30,31] reflecting the dose of test agent causing either 20% or 50% leakage, respectively, of sodium fluorescein through the monolayer.

Application of the method The FL_{20} and FL_{50} values are used to rank the toxicities of test chemicals. The lower the FL_{20} or FL_{50} value, the more toxic the material is to the eye. Although several protocols of the method have been evaluated, there are not sufficient data to make a proper judgement of the potential use of the fluorescein leakage assay as a screen or replacement, although there is an indication that the assay may develop into a suitable screen for surveying surfactants, alcohols and severe irritants. The strengths of the assay are that it is based on epithelial function, modelling responses of corneal epithelium with epithelial cell layers grown on cell inserts to enhance differentiation. Moreover, it is rapid, simple and without the need for specialized equipment. It seems suitable for inclusion into a battery of assays to assess ocular effects.

Limitations of the method A standard procedure for the fluorescein leakage assay is not yet available because the method has not been validated sufficiently. Mild materials are most suitable for testing with this assay. The method is limited to epithelial or endothelial cells. An artificial break of the monolayer can yield false-positive results, and delayed effects may be underestimated with the usual procedure.

One of the greatest difficulties is the handling of viscous, non-toxic materials, because they are almost impossible to remove after the initial 1 min exposure. Strong acids or alkalies may also cause damage owing to pH effects alone rather than specific chemical toxicity. Only materials that are either in solution or in suspension can be tested with the fluorescein leakage test. Solids cannot sufficiently be tested, as they cannot be easily removed from the cell surface after the exposure period. Non-aqueous materials or materials insoluble in mineral oil cannot be tested and corrosive materials at the normal set dose ranges are likely to kill the cell monolayer.

4. *The silicon microphysiometer (SM) test*

Principles of the method and basic testing procedure The silicon microphysiometer (Molecular Devices Corporation, Menio Park, CA) is based on a light-addressable potentiometric sensor that allows indirect measurement of real-time changes in cellular metabolism. The instrument provides continuous monitoring of the rate at which living cells inside a flow-through chamber excrete acidic metabolites as a normal part of energy metabolism. In contrast to other *in vitro* tests, the SM test assesses functional cell changes occurring at sublytic concentrations of test compounds.

In the SM test, the rate of cellular metabolism (acid metabolite production) is measured in murine L929 fibroblasts in a flow-through chamber within the microphysiometer instrument.[32,33] Cells grown on culture inserts are exposed to increasing concentrations of test substances, diluted in culture medium, for approximately 810 s per dose. The acidification rate is measured immediately after washout of each dilution of test sample from the chamber. The end-point of the test, the MRD_{50} value, is determined from dose–response curves relating test substance concentration. MRD_{50} values are expressed in units of $\log_{10}$ $\mu g\ ml^{-1}$, where MRD_{50} is defined as the dose of test substance required to produce a reduction in metabolic (acidification) rate to 50% of baseline control levels.[32]

Application of the method The SM test appears suitable for ocular irritancy screening of liquid, water-soluble surfactants and surfactant-based products.[33–35] It has been proposed as a screening method in the cosmetics industry for liquid, water-soluble, surfactant-containing materials, such as personal care and household cleaning products, to be used as part of a tiered testing process. From a practical standpoint, the primary use of the data is comparative as *in vitro* responses of a new product and the benchmark are compared, to predict whether the new product has the same, more or less irritancy potential.

Limitations of the method The test is limited in its ability to handle aqueous-insoluble substances. An important aspect of this is that the new product and the benchmark need to have a similar chemical composition. Wide use of the method is limited because of the need for expensive instrumentation. The MS test has so far not been used to identify severely eye-irritating materials, nor to distinguish severely irritating from moderately irritating materials.

5. *The tissue equivalent test*

Principles of the method and basic testing procedure The assay is based on the use of a human dermal fibroblast/epidermal keratinocyte co-culture grown on a nylon mesh which is commercially available as the skin[2] model ZK 1200 (Advanced Tissue Sciences, La Jolla, CA). Because this model shows characteristics of mucosal epithelium, it is considered to be closer to *in vivo* tissue than monolayer cultures.

The end-points assessed in the system are cytotoxicity determinations, either in the methyl-thiazol-diphenyl-tetrazolium bromide (MTT) assay or as leakage of lactate dehydrogenase (LDH) and prostaglandin (PG) E_2 release as an indication of inflammatory response.[36] To determine the three biochemical end-points, test kits are available from the manufacturer of the tissue equivalent assay. MTT assay proved to be the most appropriate end-point for ocular irritancy testing in the tissue equivalent assay.[36]

Application of the method The skin^2 ZK 1200 tissue equivalent assay has the advantage of being able to handle a wide range of physical types of materials, such as granules, powders, solids and liquids, including water-soluble and -insoluble materials at extremes of pH. It has been useful as a screen for household cleaning and personal care products when MTT is used as end-point. In addition, the method seems to be able to distinguish severely irritating from mildly irritating chemicals.[36]

The assay is used in-house in the cosmetics industry as a prescreen in a tiered system for identifying severe irritants or for the prediction of broad irritancy classes from non-irritating to mildly, moderately and severely irritating.[36]

Limitations of the method Some types of materials may interfere with the LDH assay and measurement of PGE_2 release; more work is required to substantiate or refute the utility of these end-points. The skin^2 ZK 1200 tissue equivalent assay is fairly expensive because it is patented and only available commercially. However, the system can be shipped world-wide by express air freight and provides reproducible results. The high price has restricted its use to laboratories of the industry which are also using the system for the whole spectrum of local toxicity testing.

C. Physicochemical tests

1. *The EYTEX test*

Principles of the method and basic testing procedure The EYTEX system (In Vitro International, Irvine, USA) is a commercially available *in vitro* alternative test to replace the Draize eye test for evaluation of ocular irritation.[37] It is a patented biochemical assay in which changes of relevant macromolecules upon exposure to chemicals and fomulations are used to predict *in vivo* eye irritancy. The mechanism of the EYTEX assay is supposed to be based on alterations in the conformation and hydration of an ordered protein-based macromolecular matrix.[37]

Small quantities of test sample, when presented to EYTEX reagent, produce a turbidity which mimics the response of the protein in the cornea during corneal injury or ocular irritation. The turbidity, measured in a spectrophotometer, is compared with that produced by eye irritant standards of known Draize score. The EYTEX Draize equivalent (EDE) score is determined from a calibration curve.

Several protocols have been developed to allow testing of a broad spectrum of materials. The three most widely used protocols are the upright membrane assay (UMA), the rapid membrane assay (RMA) and the alkaline membrane assay (AMA). The UMA protocol is a broad-range screening protocol for samples with a 10% dilution and $pH < 8.0$. The AMA protocol is used for samples with 10% dilution and $pH > 8.0$. The RMA protocol is used for surfactants and when a sample does not qualify in the UMA protocol.

Qualification of sample data is most important when the EYTEX system is used. Qualification is the processs whereby an assay is considered technically valid if it adheres to specified performance standards. The EYTEX system requires qualification of both the assay protocols and the sample. Sample qualification problems are normally overcome by repeating the assay at a lower concentration, selected from a prior concentration screen.

Application of the method The result of an EYTEX assay is the EYTEX Draize equivalent (EDE), read directly from a calibration curve of Draize 24 h maximum score versus optical density, plotted from the known calibration standard run at the same time as the sample. The EDE may then be used to predict the irritancy potential of the sample by comparison with *in vivo* data and classifications.

The major advantage of the EYTEX assay is its ability to test materials of various physicochemical states (e.g. solids). It is also fairly rapid and is reasonably inexpensive. Because the EYTEX assay has been used for in-house testing world-wide in laboratories of the chemical, cosmetics and drug industry, a huge database of EYTEX data has been developed.

Limitations of the method Although good correlation between *in vitro* and *in vivo* data has been reported by the manufacturer, Bruner *et al.*[32] found no significant correlation between the *in vivo* irritancy potential of 17 commercial products and chemicals and the EYTEX system. Moreover, under blind testing conditions in a formal validation study with 60 chemicals, the EYTEX assay did not provide data corresponding sufficiently with *in vivo* Draize eye test data.[7]

Validation studies revealed that, among surfactants, magnesium-neutralized surfactants are greatly overestimated in the EYTEX test, particularly when tested on their own.[7,32] This problem is not as great as with other surfactants or materials. Carbohydrate materials, particularly multicarboxylated ones, are also overestimated by the EYTEX system.

V. VALIDATION OF *IN VITRO* ALTERNATIVES TO THE DRAIZE EYE TEST

To achieve regulatory acceptance by national and international regulatory authorities, toxicity test procedures have to undergo formal validation in a ring trial under blind conditions. The scientific basis of the validation procedure was defined in 1990 by American and European experts in the field at the CAAT/ERGATT workshop on the validation of toxicity testing procedures.[38] Although most of the validation studies on *in vitro* alternatives to the Draize eye test have followed the recommendations of the CAAT/ERGATT workshop, so far none of these methods has been accepted for regulatory purposes at international level (e.g. the OECD has not incorporated them into the OECD Guidelines for Testing of Chemicals[2]). Results of the major validation trials of *in vitro* alternatives to the Draize eye test will briefly be summarized.

Validation of the HET-CAM and NRU cytotoxicity test in Germany From 1988 to 1992 a formal validation study was carried out in Germany on two *in vitro* methods for ocular irritancy testing established in laboratories of the chemical industry, the HET-CAM assay and the NRU cytotoxicity test. The goal of the study was to prove that severely eye-irritating chemicals can successfully be classified 'R 41' according to EU Directive 61/458/EEC on the classification, packaging and labelling of dangerous substances.[4] The study, which was carried out in ten laboratories and on a broad spectrum of chemicals, showed that the two assays provided reproducible data.[16] Modern biostatistical methods, such as stepwise discriminant analysis, allowed an *in vitro* testing strategy to be developed to identify R 41 chemicals by combining coagulation data of the HET-CAM assay with cytotoxicity data.[18] The results obtained with 200 chemicals under blind conditions suggest that this approach will provide an acceptable sensitivity, predictivity and percentage of false data for severely eye-irritating chemicals.

European validation trial of the BCOP test In 1991–3 the BCOP test was validated in a formal validation trial under blind conditions at the European level to determine the capability and possible limitations of the method for predicting ocular irritancy of a large set of chemicals.[22] The study was sponsored by DG XI of the EU, with 12 laboratories participating and 52 test chemicals of a wide range of structure, and both physicochemical and irritation properties. The prediction rate was high at 84%, and sensitivity and specificity of the assay were also greater than 84%. All the 'false negatives' were solids and all the 'false positives' were liquids, indicating that the protocol may have to be adjusted to the physicochemical nature of test materials. Given the number of products evaluated and the reproducibility within and among laboratories, the results of the validation trial confirm that the BCOP assay is very useful for screening chemicals for ocular irritation.[22]

Validation studies of in vitro *procedures for ocular irritancy testing established in the cosmetics industry in Europe and the USA* Five laboratories of the cosmetics industry in Europe and the USA evaluated five potential alternatives (silicon microphysiometer, Microtox test, NRU cytotoxicty test, CAMVA and HET-CAM assay) to the Draize eye test established as in-house tests with 32 materials for household cleaning, personal care and cosmetics.[34] The object of the evaluation, which was not carried out under blind conditions, was to establish the usefulness of the five methods as *in vitro* procedures for ocular irritation testing. Reproducibility of the five tests could not be assessed because most of the tests were carried out only in a single laboratory. The results demonstrated that, for the materials tested, all the assays showed some promise in the prediction of eye irritation as an alternative to the Draize eye test.[34] A similar result was obtained in a validation study of the US SDA (Soap and Detergent Manufacturers' Association), which involved nine in-house tests and 22 test materials including solvents, surfactants, oxidizing agents and cleaning products.[39]

Validation study of in vitro *procedures for ocular irritancy testing established in the Japanese cosmetics industry* In the first phase of a validation trial of the Japanese Cosmetic Industry Association, 12 alternative methods to the Draize eye test underwent preliminary validation with nine coded cosmetic ingredients (Draize MAS score 0–78) in 20 laboratories.[40] Intralaboratory and interlaboratory variances were small and correlation coefficients between *in vitro* methods and the Draize MAS scores were high (Pearson's rank correlation coefficient > 0.9) indicating that all of the organotypic and cell culture assays described can handle surfactants sufficiently well.[40] This result is not surprising because *in vitro* alternatives to the Draize eye test have predominantly been developed in laboratories of the cosmetics industry.

In-house validation of in vitro *testing strategies for ocular irritancy testing in the cosmetics industry* In a study on the relevance and reliability of ten *in vitro* methods for ocular safety assessment established in-house at a leading cosmetics company (L'Oreal, France), it was reported that ocular irritation seems to be best predicted by the HET-CAM test, especially haemorrhage, followed by cell culture-based methods (e.g. protein content and cytotoxicity measurement and the silicon microphysiometer test, the latter methods being related[41]). For assessment of recovery the BCOP test provided the most relevant information. Biostatistical analysis of *in vitro–in vivo* correlations, including partial least squares (PLS) regression analysis, showed that, when combined, the HET-CAM test and the BCOP test explained 93% of the variance in the MAS score of the Draize eye test.

In the biggest cosmetics company in the USA (Procter and Gamble), a tiered testing approach has been established for in-house testing, starting with historical data analysis and physicochemical characterization of a new formulation, and followed by an *in vitro* test battery to assess ocular irritation potential.[42] Depending on information from the non-animal data set, a safety assessment is performed which may require limited *in vivo* conformation by using the Draize eye test in one to three rabbits.

According to the Animal Protection Act in Germany, since 1987 animal tests for the safety assessment of decorative cosmetics are not to be conducted. Therefore, ocular safety assessment of cosmetics ingredients and formulations can take into account only historical and physicochemical data, and results from *in vitro* tests for eye iritation. The spectrum of *in vitro* assays established in laboratories of the cosmetics industry in Germany usually consists of the NRU cytotoxicity test, the HET-CAM test and the RBC assay.

World-wide EU/Home Office validation study of nine in vitro *alternatives to the Draize eye test* From 1992 to 1994 a world-wide international validation study on nine alternatives to the Draize eye test was conducted in 37 laboratories on 60 coded chemicals, sponsored by the EU and the British Home Office.[7] The principal goal of the study was to establish whether or not one or more of the nine non-animal tests (Table 12.1) could be used to replace the Draize eye test for all severely irritating materials or for severely irritating materials belonging to specific classes, to replace the animal test completely for chemicals with or without regard to chemical class. Preliminary analysis of the data suggests that, with the possible exception of predicting the irritancy of surfactants, none of the nine tests met any of the four performance goals. Although the Draize eye test data of the 60 test chemicals selected for the study had to meet the highest quality criteria, they showed significant interanimal variability, particularly in the mid-range of the MAS Draize score. Not unexpectedly, evaluation of the results revealed that the *in vivo* Draize eye test data used in the analysis of *in vitro–in vivo* correlations were too variable to be relied on.

Table 12.1 *In vitro* methods evaluated in the EU/Home Office international validation study on alternatives to the Draize eye test for classification and labelling of chemicals.[7]

Organotypical tests
HET-CAM test
Bovine corneal opacity and permeability test
Isolated rabbit eye test
Chicken enucleated eye test
Physicochemical and cellular tests
EYTEX test
Neutral red uptake cytotoxicity test
Red blood cell haemolysis test
Fluorescein leakage test
Silicon microphysiometer test

VI. CONCLUSIONS AND FUTURE PERSPECTIVES

Despite the discouraging result of the EU/Home Office validation trial,[7] industry uses many of the alternative methods quite successfully for in-house purposes, such as in product selection and in stepwise integrated procedures to identify severely eye-irritating materials. One reason why in-house testing is successful might be that testing is restricted to materials produced in the company with narrow ranges of chemistry. In addition, in-house testing is performed in the full knowledge of the physicochemical properties of the test materials, so that deficiencies in the alternative test can be avoided. In contrast, experience has shown that, in formal validation studies with coded chemicals, test materials are quite often handled most inappropriately owing to lack of information on physicochemical properties, which usually are not provided to keep the study unbiased.

No single test or test battery currently established can replace the use of animals in ocular safety. However, depending on the toxicological problem to be evaluated, several *in vitro* assays are appropriately established to make reliable safety assessments for ocular irritancy for a given group of chemicals and a specific purpose, for example to distinguish between severe and mild irritation or between non-irritating and mildly irritating materials.

Integrated tiered testing strategies for ocular irritancy testing are established in Europe to classify chemicals for regulatory purposes as severely irritating to the eye, which require testing in only a limited number of rabbits in the Draize eye test if the *in vitro* results are negative. Similar tiered testing strategies are estabished world-wide in laboratories of the cosmetics industry to identify non-irritating cosmetic ingredients and formulations. However, in some countries these *in vitro* procedures are used in parallel with *in vivo* testing, whereas in other countries confirmation by *in vivo* testing in the Draize eye test is exceptional.

In the USA, the LVET is well established for assessing the ocular safety of chemicals. Although the LVET is an *in vivo* test, in which the test material is applied to the rabbit's eye, the method allows a considerable reduction in suffering of the animals. Thus, in cases where the Draize eye test cannot yet be replaced by non-animal methods for scientific reasons, the LVET is the only acceptable, well-validated reduction alternative.

If complete elimination of animal use for ocular safety assessment is to be achieved, a better understanding of ocular tissue repair, inflammation and alterations at the cellular level is needed. Progress in tissue culture technique, cellular and molecular biology, and analytical techniques will lead us closer to the goal of completely replacing the Draize eye test by non-animal methods.

REFERENCES

1. Draize, J. H., Woodard, G. and Calvery, H. O. (1944) Methods for the study of irritation and toxicity of substances applied topically to the skin and mucous membranes. *J. Pharmacol. Exp. Ther.* **82:** 377–390.
2. OECD (1981, 1987, 1994) *Guidelines for Testing of Chemicals: Guideline No. 405 'Acute eye irritation/corrosion'*. OECD Publication Office, Paris.
3. Federal Hazardous Substances Act (1974) Test for eye irritants. In *Code of Federal Regulations*, Title 16, paragraph 1500,42,295. Code of Federal Regulations 295, Washington, DC.
4. European Economic Community (1983) Commission Directive 61/458/EEC on the Classification, Packaging and Labelling of Dangerous Substances.*Official Journal of the European Community* L 257/1.
5. Kay, J. H. and Calendra, J. C. (1962) Interpretation of eye irritation tests. *J. Soc. Cosmet. Chem.* **13:** 281–289.
6. Weil, C. S. and Scala, R. A. (1971) Study of intra- and interlaboratory variability in the results of rabbit eye and skin irritation tests. *Toxicol. Appl. Pharmacol.* **19:** 276–360.
7. Balls, M., Botham, P. A., Bruner, L. H. and Spielmann, H. (1995) The EC/Home Office validation study on alternatives to the Draize eye irritation test for the classification and labelling of chemicals. *Toxicol. In Vitro* **9:** 871–929.
8. Russel, W. M. S and Burch R. L. (1959) *The Principles of Humane Experimental Technique.* Methuen, London.

9. Griffith, J. F., Nixon, G. A., Bruce, R. D., Reer, P. J. and Bannan, E. A. (1980) Dose–response studies with chemical irritants in the albino rabbit eye as a basis for selecting optimum testing conditions for predicting hazards to the human eye. *Toxicol. Appl. Pharmacol.* **55:** 501–513.
10. Freeberg, F. E., Nixon, G. A., Reer, P. J. *et al.* (1986) Human and rabbit eye responses to chemical insult. *Fundam. Appl. Toxicol.* **7:** 626–634.
11. Gautheron, P., Dukic, M., Alix, D. and Sina, J. (1992) Bovine cornea opacity and permeability test: an *in vitro* assay of ocular irritancy. *Fundam. Appl. Toxicol.* **18:** 442–449.
12. Prinsen, M. K. and Koeter, H. B. W. M. (1993) Justification of the enucleated eye test with eyes of slaughter house animals as an alternative to the Draize eye irritation test with rabbits. *Food Chem. Toxicol.* **13:** 69–76.
13. Schlede, E. and Gerner, I. (1995) The Draize eye test and progress in development and acceptance of alternatives to this test in Europe. In Goldberg, A. M. and van Zutphen, L. F. M. (eds) *The World Congress on Alternatives and Animal Use in the Life Sciences: Education, Research, Testing*, pp. 333–336. Mary Ann Liebert, New York.
14. Luepke, N. P. (1985) Hen's egg chorioallantoic membrane test for irritation potential. *Food Chem. Toxicol.* **23:** 287–291.
15. Spielmann, H., Gerner, I., Kalweit, S. *et al.* (1991) Interlaboratory assessment of alternatives to the Draize eye irritation test in Germany. *Toxicol. In Vitro* **5:** 539–542.
16. Spielmann, H., Kalweit, S., Liebsch, M. *et al.* (1993) Validation study of alternatives to the Draize eye irritation test in Germany: cytotoxicity testing and HET-CAM test with 136 industrial chemicals. *Toxicol. In Vitro* **7:** 505–510.
17. Rougier, A., Cottin, M., de Silva, O., Catroux, P., Roguet, R. and Dossou, K. G. (1994) The use of *in vitro* methods in the ocular irritation assessment of cosmetic products. *Toxicol. in Vitro* **8:** 893–906.
18. Spielmann, H., Liebsch, M., Moldenhauer, F. *et al.* (1996) IRAG working group 2 report: CAM-based assays. *Food Chem. Toxicol.* (in press).
19. Spielmann, H., Liebsch, M., Moldenhauer, F. H. G., Holzhütter, H. G. and de Silva, O. (1995) Modern biostatistical methods for assessing *in vitro/in vivo* correlation in a validation trial on *in vitro* alternatives to the Draize eye test. *Toxicol. In Vitro* **9:** 549–556.
20. Leighton, J., Nassauer, J. and Tchao, R. (1985) The chick embryo in toxicology: an alternative to the rabbit eye. *Food Chem. Toxicol.* **23:** 293–298.
21. Bagley, D. M., Rizvi, P. Y., Kong, B. M. and Salva, S. J. (1991) Factors affecting use of the hen's egg chorionallantoic membrane as a model for predicting eye irritation potential. *J. Toxicol. Cutaneous and Ocular Toxicology* **10:** 95–104.
22. Gautheron, P., Giroux, J., Cottin, M. *et al.* (1994) Interlaboratory assessment of the bovine corneal opacity and permeability (BCOP) assay. *Toxicol. In Vitro* **8:** 381–392.
23. Burton, A. B. D., York, M. and Lawrence, R. S. (1981) The *in vitro* assessment of severe eye irritants *Food Chem. Toxicol.* **19:** 471–480.
24. Lewis, R. W., McCall, J. C. and Botham, P. A. (1994) Use of an *in vitro* test battery as a prescreen in the assessment of ocular irritancy. *Toxicol. In Vitro* **8:** 75–79.
25. Gad, S. C., Chamberlain, M., Gautheron, P., Prinsen, M. and Shadduck, J. (1996) Organotypic models for the assessment/prediction of ocular irritation. Report of IRAG Working Group 1. *Food Chem. Toxicol.* (in press).
26. Borenfreund, E. and Puerner, J. A. (1995) Toxicity determined *in vitro* by morphological alteration and neutral red absorption. *Toxicol. Letters* **24:** 119–224.
27. Pape, W. J. W., Pfannenbecker, U. and Hoppe, U. (1987) Validation of the red blood cell test system as an *in vitro* assay for the rapid screening of irritation potential of surfactants. *Mol. Toxicol.* **1:** 525–536.
28. Lewis, R. W., McCall, J. C. and Botham, P. A. (1993) A comparison of two cytotoxicity test for predicting the ocular irritancy of surfactants. *Toxicol. In Vitro* **7:** 155–158.
29. Tchao, R. (1988) Trans-epithelial permeability of fluorescein *in vitro* as an assay to determine eye irritants. In Goldberg, A. M. (ed.) *Alternative Methods in Toxicology. Vol. VI, Progress in* In Vitro *Toxicology*, pp. 271–283. Mary Ann Liebert, New York.
30. Shaw, A. J., Clothier, R. H. and Balls, M. (1990) Loss of transepithelial impermeability of Madin-Darby canine kidney (MDCK) cells as a determinant of ocular irritancy potential. *ATLA* **18:** 145–151.
31. Rhoads, L. S., Cook, J. R., Patrone, L. M. and Van Buskirk, R. G. (1993) A human epidermal model that can be assayed employing a multiple fluorescent assay and the CytoFluor 2300. *J. Toxicol. Cutaneous and Ocular Toxicology* **12:** 87–108.

32. Bruner, L. H., Miller, K. R., Owicki, J. C., Parce, J. W. and Muir, V. C. (1991) Testing ocular irritancy *in vitro* with the silicon microphysiometer. *Toxicol. In Vitro* **5:** 277–284.
33. Catroux, P., Rougier, A., Dossou, K. G. and Cottin, M. (1993) The silicon mycrophysiometer for testing ocular toxicity *in vitro*. *Toxicol. In Vitro* **7:** 465–469.
34. Bagley, D. M., Bruner, L. H., de Silva, O. *et al.* (1992) An evaluation of five potential alternatives *in vitro* to the rabbit eye irritation test *in vivo*. *Toxicol. In Vitro* **6:** 275–284.
35. Bruner, L. H., Kain, D. J., Roberts, D. A. and Parber, R. D (1991) Evaluation of seven *in vitro* alternatives for ocular safety testing. *Fundam. Appl. Toxicol.* **17:** 136–149.
36. Osborne, R., Perkins, M. M. and Roberts, D. A. (1995) Development and intralaboratory evaluation of an *in vitro* human cell-based test to aid ocular irritancy assessments. *Fundam. Appl. Toxicol.* **28:** 139–153.
37. Gordon, V. C. (1992) The scientific basis of the EYTEX system. *ATLA* **20:** 537–548.
38. Balls, M., Blaauboer, B., Brusick, D. *et al.* (1990) Report and recommendations of the CAAT/ ERGATT workshop on the validation of toxicity test procedures. *ATLA* **18:** 313–326.
39. Bagley, D. M., Booman, K. A., Bruner, L. H. *et al.* (1994) The SDA alternatives program phase III: comparison of *in vitro* data with animal eye irritation data on solvents, surfactants, oxidizing-agents, and prototype cleaning products. *J. Toxicol. Cutaneous and Ocular Toxicology* **13:** 127–155.
40. Ohno, Y., Kaneko, T., Kobayashi, T. *et al.* (1994) First-phase validation of the *in vitro* eye irritation tests for cosmetic ingredients. *In Vitro Toxicol.* **7:** 89–94.
41. Cottin, M., Dossou, K. G., de Silva, O. *et al.* (1995) Relevance and reliability of *in vitro* methods in ocular safety assessment. In Goldberg, A. M. and van Zutphen, L. F. M. (eds) *The World Congress on Alternatives and Animal Use in the Life Sciences: Education, Research, Testing*, pp. 323–332. Mary Ann Liebert, New York.
42. Bruner, L. H. (1992) Ocular irritation. In Frazier, J. M. (ed.) In Vitro *Toxicity Testing – Applications to Safety Evaluation*, pp. 149–190. Marcel Dekker, New York.

13

Phototoxicity of Drugs

MIGUEL A. MIRANDA

I. Sunlight and photobiological effects 290
II. Photosensitization in humans 290
III. Phototoxicity and photoallergy 291
IV. Drugs with phototoxic or photoallergic side-effects 291
V. Mechanisms of photosensitization reactions 293
VI. Photophysical studies of drugs 295
VII. Photochemistry of drugs 296
VIII. Animal models for testing photosensitizing drugs *in vivo* 299
IX. *In vitro* assays for potentially photosensitizing drugs 299
A. Spectrophotometric analysis 300
B. Photohaemolysis 300
C. *Candida albicans* phototoxicity test 301
D. Photodynamic lipid peroxidation 301
E. Histidine photo-oxidation 302
F. Photodamage to fibroblasts 304
G. Photocleavage to DNA 304
H. Photodegranulation of mast cells 305
I. Photo–basophil–histamine release test 305
J. Photoinhibition of thymidine incorporation into human lymphocytes . . . 305
K. Photo-enhanced generation of reactive oxygen species by human phagocytes 305
X. General strategy for *in vitro* phototoxicity testing 306
XI. Experimental procedures: how to do it 307
A. Photolytic degradation of drugs 307
B. Cytotoxicity of drug photoproducts 308
C. Drug-derived peroxides: fluorimetric determination and biological effects 308
D. Photoperoxidation of linoleic acid in the presence of drugs 309
E. Photohaemolysis test 309
F. *Candida albicans* phototoxicity test 310
G. Histidine photodegradation 310
H. Photodamage to fibroblasts 310
XII. Summary 311
Acknowledgement 312
References 312

IN VITRO METHODS IN PHARMACEUTICAL RESEARCH
ISBN 0-12-163390-X

I. SUNLIGHT AND PHOTOBIOLOGICAL EFFECTS

Solar energy has been essential to the development and evolution of life on earth. It can produce the so-called photobiological effects on microorganisms, plants, animals and humans. For such effects, the most relevant spectral regions are UVB (290–320 nm) and UVA (320–400 nm). Shorter wavelength radiation ($\lambda < 290$ nm) is efficiently filtered by the atmosphere (mainly by the ozone layer) and does not reach the earth's surface. Sunlight contains radiation of wavelength longer than 400 nm, but its biological effectiveness is much lower.[1,2]

Upon exposure of the skin to natural solar radiation, most of the incident UVB rays are absorbed in the stratum corneum. In contrast, a considerable part of the UVA rays can reach the dermis, where the presence of capillary blood vessels allows interaction with the whole body.[1,3,4] There, an essential requirement for the occurrence of photobiological effects is absorption of the radiation. This is based on the first law of photochemistry (Grotthus' law), which states that only absorbed light can initiate a photochemical reaction. Valuable information on the ability of a given substrate to absorb light is provided by its absorption spectrum. In this context, UVB radiation is very injurious to biological systems, owing to the strong absorbance of proteins and nucleic acids close to this region. Conversely, UVA and visible radiation are weakly absorbed by the biomolecules and, accordingly, these wavelengths are less damaging.[5] Such a situation can be altered by the incorporation of photosensitizers, which are substances capable of mediating photobiological effects after exposure to normally ineffective radiation. The photosensitizers become photochemically activated, and there is no direct absorption of light by the biomolecules.[4,6]

II. PHOTOSENSITIZATION IN HUMANS

Photosensitization can give rise to abnormal reactions of the skin, due to the exposure to UV or visible radiation and an exogenous chemical.[3,6,7] The incidence of this type of undesired effect is increasing every year[8–11] as a consequence of the considerable number of new chemicals entering the environment (drugs, cosmetics, industrial chemicals). Also, changes in living habits and the evolution of social and cultural standards have led to an unusual exposure to natural solar radiation and artificial sunlamps. Human data have been generated in three ways: (a) case reports; (b) photopatch tests; and (c) systemic provocative phototests.[12–15]

Isolated cases of photodermatitis induced by exogenous chemicals appear regularly in the scientific literature. Although they probably represent a very small fraction of the photosensitivity disorders that actually occur, their characterization provides high-quality primary data which have to be continuously collected and incorporated into databases.

More systematic information has been obtained by photopatch testing, which is usually performed in patients with suspected photosensitivity. It consists in the application of the test chemical to the skin of the back, followed by irradiation with predetermined light doses. The results are evaluated after different time intervals, according to an established score based on the skin reaction pattern. Systematic studies of this type have been conducted in large multicentre trials, using similar methodologies and a common list of potential photosensitizers.[13] The derived rank orders (based on the frequency of reactions) reflect to a certain extent the photosensitizing potential of the test substances.

A limitation of the above method is that false-negative results are frequently obtained with systemic photosensitizing drugs. In these cases, detection is achieved by means of the systemic provocative phototest.[16] This involves the medication of patients with controlled drug doses and subsequent irradiation of different skin sites with measured amounts of light within selected wavelength ranges. Readings are made for erythema and any abnormal morphological skin changes after periodical time intervals. This is a useful diagnostic tool, but is limited to a small number of patients and test substances.

III. PHOTOTOXICITY AND PHOTOALLERGY

Phototoxicity and photoallergy are the two major types of photosensitization reported by photodermatologists.[1,3,4,6,7,17–19] Phototoxic effects appear more frequently and do not involve an immunological mechanism. They should occur in all individuals provided their skin contains the photosensitizer at the appropriate concentration and is exposed to sufficient light. Usually, the clinical picture associated with phototoxicity includes burning, itching, erythema, oedema, hyperpigmentation and desquamation. These reactions are confined to the exposed areas of the skin and appear immediately after the first exposure. Cellular damage may occur either in the epidermis (if the photosensitizer is topically applied) or in the dermis (with a systemic photosensitizer). The term photoirritation is used to describe phototoxic reactions in the skin which are produced with topically applied substances following exposure to light.[17–19]

Photoallergy to chemicals is much less common than phototoxicity, although it is still important in interest and severity. The photoallergic response, which depends on individual immunological status, is developed in some patients as a modified ability of the skin to react to the combined effect of sunlight plus a photosensitizer. It is associated with a cell-mediated immune response.[11] Some clinical manifestations are erythema, eczema and/or vesiculo-bullous eruption. These cutaneous responses are usually restricted to the exposed parts of the skin, but can be extended to the unexposed areas, including previously sensitized distant sites. They do not occur after the first treatment with chemical and light; rather, there is an induction period of 1 or 2 weeks before skin reactivity can be demonstrated. Other specific features of photoallergy are the possibility of passive transfer and the requirement of lower doses of both photosensitizer and radiation energy to produce the photobiological effect.[17,18]

IV. DRUGS WITH PHOTOTOXIC OR PHOTOALLERGIC SIDE-EFFECTS

Many drugs are known to induce phototoxic and/or photoallergic responses after either systemic or topical application (see Table 13.1 for representative examples). As this property is shared by a wide variety of drugs with diverse pharmacological activities and different structural formulae, it has been difficult to establish satisfactory structure–activity relationships.[1,3,19] Thus, to advance satisfactory predictions a deeper understanding of the molecular mechanisms involved in these phenomena appears necessary. Such information is essential for the development of reliable assay methods to screen for the photosensitizing potential of new drug candidates. Until now, the pharmaceutical industry has not had to take this toxicological aspect into account; however, the increasing number of problems will probably prompt governments to include systematic phototoxicity testing in the guidelines for drug safety evaluation.

Table 13.1 Photosensitizing drugs.

Structural group	Paradigmatic compound	Pharmacological activity	Type of application	Type of side-effect
Arylacetic acids	Diclofenac	NSAID	Systemic Topical	Phototoxicity
Arylpropionic acids	Benoxaprofen	NSAID	Systemic Topical	Phototoxicity Photoallergy
Benzodiazepines	Chlordiazepoxide	Tranquillizer	Systemic	Phototoxicity Photoallergy
Dibenzoazepines	Protryptiline	Antidepressant	Systemic	Phototoxicity
Fibrates	Fenofibrate	Antilipidaemic	Systemic	Phototoxicity Photoallergy
Furocoumarins	Methoxypsoralen	PUVA therapy	Systemic Topical	Phototoxicity
Oxicams	Piroxicam	NSAID	Systemic Topical	Phototoxicity Photoallergy
PABA and derivatives	PABA	Sunscreen	Topical	Photoallergy
Phenothiazines	Chlorpromazine	Neuroleptic	Systemic	Phototoxicity Photoallergy
Quinolines	Chloroquine	Antimalarial	Systemic	Phototoxicity
Quinolones	Nalidixic acid	Antibacterial	Systemic	Phototoxicity
Sulphonamides	Sulfanilamide	Antibacterial	Systemic	Phototoxicity Photoallergy
Tetracyclines	Demethylchlorotetracycline	Antibiotic	Systemic	Phototoxicity
Thiazides	Hydrochlorothiazide	Diuretic	Systemic	Phototoxicity Photoallergy

Among the photosensitizing drugs listed in Table 13.1, the non-steroidal anti-inflammatory 2-arylpropionic acids (Fig. 13.1) deserve special mention. Because these agents have been designed to inhibit inflammation, the paradoxical fact that they can elicit inflammatory responses in conjunction with light is hardly acceptable.[1,20] In addition, the incidence of photosensitization disorders associated with 2-arylpropionic acids is higher than with other types of drug, which constitutes a matter for current concern.[20,21] The above

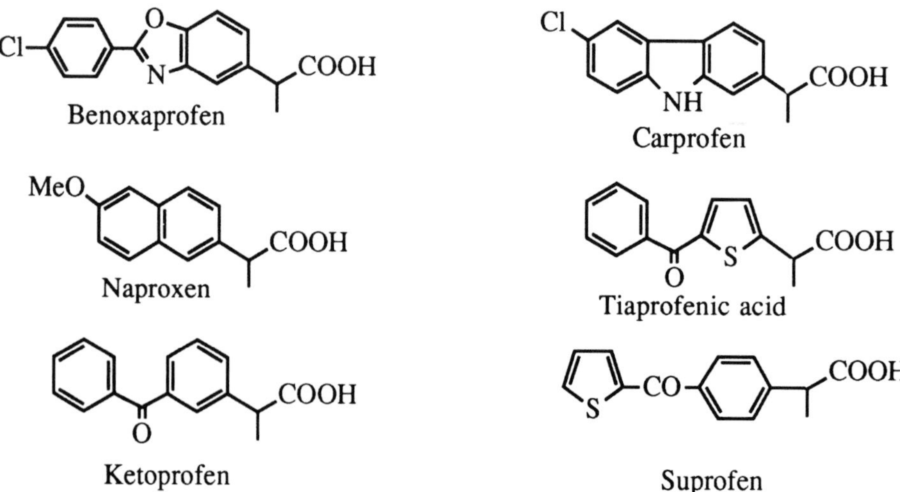

Fig. 13.1 Chemical structures of the non-steroidal anti-inflammatory 2-arylpropionic acids with *in vivo* photosensitizing properties.

reasons have led us to make preferential use of the information available on these drugs to illustrate the general aspects of the topic.

V. MECHANISMS OF PHOTOSENSITIZATION REACTIONS

The first event in photosensitization by drugs (D) is the absorption (A) of a photon, which promotes the drug to its excited singlet state ($^1D^*$). This is a high-energy species, which can undergo deactivation via different pathways[1,6,22–24] (Fig. 13.2):

(a) fluorescence emission (FL);
(b) internal conversion (IC) to the ground state;
(c) intersystem crossing (ISC) to an excited triplet state ($^3D^*$);
(d) ionization to give a radical cation plus an ejected electron ($D^{\cdot+} + e^-$);
(e) unimolecular reactions such as fragmentation to free radicals ($R^\cdot$) or transformation into photoproducts (P);
(f) intermolecular processes, such as energy transfer, electron transfer or chemical reactions (for instance cycloadditions). The partner reactants are usually a biomolecule (B) or oxygen present in the medium.

After intersystem crossing (path (c)), the resulting excited triplet ($^3D^*$) can undergo similar deactivation processes:

(g) phosphorescence emission (PH);
(h) ISC to the ground state;
(i) ionization (to give $D^{\cdot+} + e^-$). This is less favoured from the thermodynamic point of view than ionization from $^1D^*$, because of the lower energy of $^3D^*$;
(j) unimolecular photochemical reactions leading to free radicals ($R^\cdot$) or stable photoproducts (P);
(k) intermolecular processes (energy transfer, electron transfer or chemical reactions). Owing to the higher half-lives of triplet states, these processes are more likely to occur than those taking place from $^1D^*$.

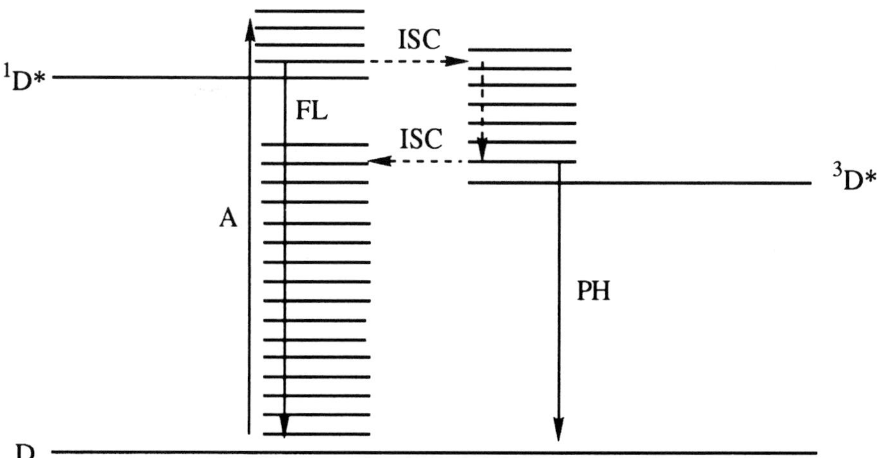

Fig. 13.2 Diagram showing generation of the excited states involved in photosensitization by drugs, as well as their main photophysical deactivation pathways. See text for explanation of abbreviations.

Processes (d), (e), (j) and (k) are more frequently involved in mechanisms of photosensitization by drugs (Figs 13.3 and 13.4). The so-called type I and II mechanisms are oxygen dependent. The former is based on initiation of a chain reaction by free radicals, whereas the latter is associated with singlet oxygen. By contrast, type III photosensitization

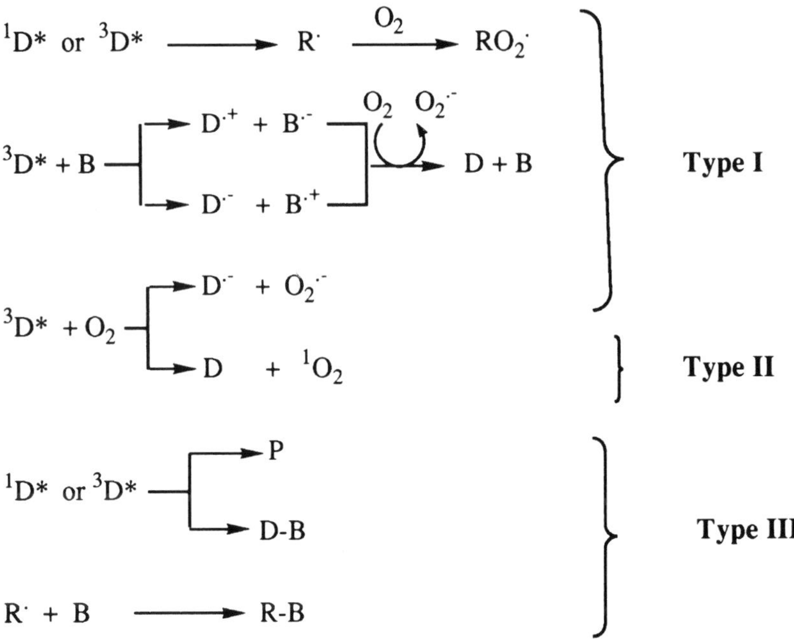

Fig. 13.3 Reaction mechanisms most frequently involved in photosensitization by drugs. Type I and II mechanisms are oxygen dependent. The former proceeds via radical chain, while the latter is associated with singlet oxygen. Type III mechanism does not require the presence of oxygen.

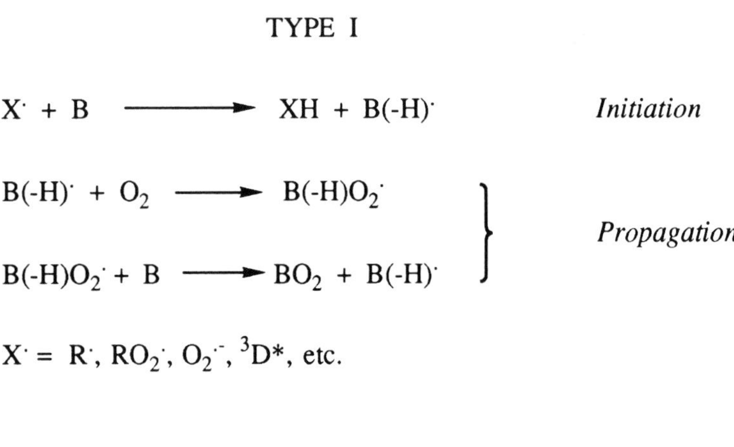

Fig. 13.4 Characteristic secondary reactions of type I and II mechanisms. They involve interaction of free radicals or singlet oxygen with the target biomolecules.

processes do not involve oxygen. Instead, stable photoproducts of the drug or covalent photoadducts of the drug to biomolecules are in the origin of the observed photobiological effects.

This is still a simplified picture of the molecular basis of photosensitization. Sometimes, complications arise from the fact that the photoactive compound may be a metabolite[7,25,26] rather than the parent drug. In rare cases, administration of a photochemically inactive drug can induce an abnormal accumulation of certain endogenous biomolecules (bilirubin, porphyrins, etc.), which at high concentrations are able to act as photosensitizers.

Because a detailed understanding of the molecular mechanisms of photosensitization by drugs is essential to anticipate and prevent the appearance of phototoxic or photoallergic side-effects, any systematic investigation in this field should start with a careful photochemical study of the drug of interest. This includes isolation of the photoproducts, identification of the intervening excited states and reactive intermediates, and photoreactions with biological targets.

VI. PHOTOPHYSICAL STUDIES OF DRUGS

A considerable amount of data on the mechanism of action of photosensitizing drugs can be obtained from the study of their radiative processes; in this way it is possible to know how excitation occurs and how the resulting excited states behave. Determination of the UV–visible absorption spectra is important, as only absorbed light can initiate a photochemical reaction. These spectra can be easily obtained in a few minutes, using low-cost instruments. Emission spectroscopy is also very informative, and the required technology has advanced enormously over the past decades through introduction of the time-resolved mode. It is possible to calculate the singlet and triplet excited state energies from the wavelengths of the fluorescence or phosphorescence maxima, respectively. Emission quantum yields, radiative lifetimes and quenching parameters provide valuable information on the excited states, such as generation efficiency, duration and reactivity.[23]

Complementary studies on the photophysical properties of a photosensitizing drug can be performed by means of flash photolysis.[27–30] With this technique, the drug is subjected to a very short pulse of intense radiation produced by a flashlamp or laser. This generates an instantaneous high concentration of excited molecules, which are directly observed by emission or absorption spectroscopy. As the pulse duration is much shorter than the decay processes, the fate of excited states can be followed in real time. Hence, flash photolysis allows determination not only of excited state energies and lifetimes or triplet quantum yields, but also of triplet–triplet absorption spectra. Moreover, it can be extended to the generation and detection of other transient species such as free radicals, which survive for a period much longer than the radiation pulse and possess characteristic absorption features. This is particularly useful to monitor a photochemical reaction in which both the formation and decay of short-lived intermediates are followed as a function of time.

An alternative method for detecting triplet excited molecules and measuring triplet quantum yields is electron spin resonance (ESR). With this technique, a magnetic field is applied to remove the degeneracy of spin sublevels of species with unpaired electrons. Then, excitation with microwave radiation promotes transitions between these sublevels, giving rise to spectroscopic signals.[27] Many of the intermediates involved in photosensitization reactions are chemical entities with one or more unpaired electrons (triplets, radicals, radical pairs, radical ions, etc.) and can be detected by ESR.[28] As a general limitation, such intermediates must be present in appreciable concentrations and persist for relatively long times in order to be detected by ESR. This can be achieved by the use of rigid media or matrix isolation instead of fluid solutions.

Chemically induced dynamic nuclear polarization (CIDNP) is a more sensitive technique for establishing the photolytic generation of radical pairs in solution.[27] Either enhanced absorption or emission are observed in the nuclear magnetic resonance (NMR) spectra of the irradiated samples, as a consequence of the non-equilibrium population of nuclear spin states associated with recombination of the radical pairs or scavenging of the free radicals after diffusional separation. An important advantage of CIDNP is that the structural information inherent to NMR is preserved, which provides valuable data on the chemical nature and origin of the photogenerated radicals.[31]

VII. PHOTOCHEMISTRY OF DRUGS

Most frequently, the photochemical reactivity of a drug is established by steady-state photolysis. The course of photoreactions can be followed by absorption spectroscopy and also by gas chromatography (GC) or high-performance liquid chromatography (HPLC). The resulting reaction mixtures are resolved by means of preparative chromatographic methods, to give the pure photoproducts. Their structures are assigned by NMR, infrared (IR) or mass spectrometry (MS). Isolation and identification of photoproducts is important because it allows proposals to be made regarding photochemical mechanisms and the short-lived reactive intermediates involved. In addition, the photoproducts may exhibit toxicity in the dark or act as photosensitizers in their own right.

The photochemical transformations of a wide number of drugs have been illustrated in a well-documented review.[32] Hence, our attention will be focused on the non-steroidal anti-inflammatory 2-arylpropionic acids, because of their interest as representative compounds in the field of photosensitization by drugs. It has been shown that these compounds undergo photodecarboxylation, to afford complex mixtures of photoproducts.[28,29,33–48] Their formation involves the intermediacy of free radicals and drug-derived peroxides. In addition, reactive oxygen species such as singlet oxygen and/or superoxide radical anion are produced. Depending on the structure of the aryl substituent, other photochemical reactions can also occur. The above results are summarized in Figs 13.5 and 13.6 for ketoprofen, a member of the group containing the benzophenone chromophore.

In certain cases, cellular damage by stable photoproducts has been proposed as a major mechanistic route in photosensitization by drugs. A clear example is the tranquillizer chlordiazepoxide, which photoisomerizes to an oxaziridine. This compound is moderately stable and its *in vitro* toxicity in the dark correlates very well with the phototoxicity of chlordiazepoxide.[3,25,32] Likewise, the formation of *p*-hydroxymethylaminobenzene sulfonamide upon irradiation has been found to be responsible (at least in part) for the photosensitization by sulfanilamide.[1,3] Formation of toxic photoproducts also plays a role in the adverse photobiological effects induced by chlorpromazine and the tetracyclines.[49]

This does not appear to be the case with 2-arylpropionic acids. Although, as a general rule, the most toxic photoproducts in different *in vitro* assays are the decarboxylated 1-hydroxyethyl derivatives,[37,39,42,45] the concentrations required to produce cellular damage are not likely to be reached in the tissues.[36] Therefore, the formation of toxic photoproducts probably constitutes a minor contribution to the well-established *in vivo* photosensitization by these drugs.

However, it is interesting to note that some members of the group (benoxaprofen, tiaprofenic acid, suprofen and ketoprofen) undergo decarboxylation upon light exposure,

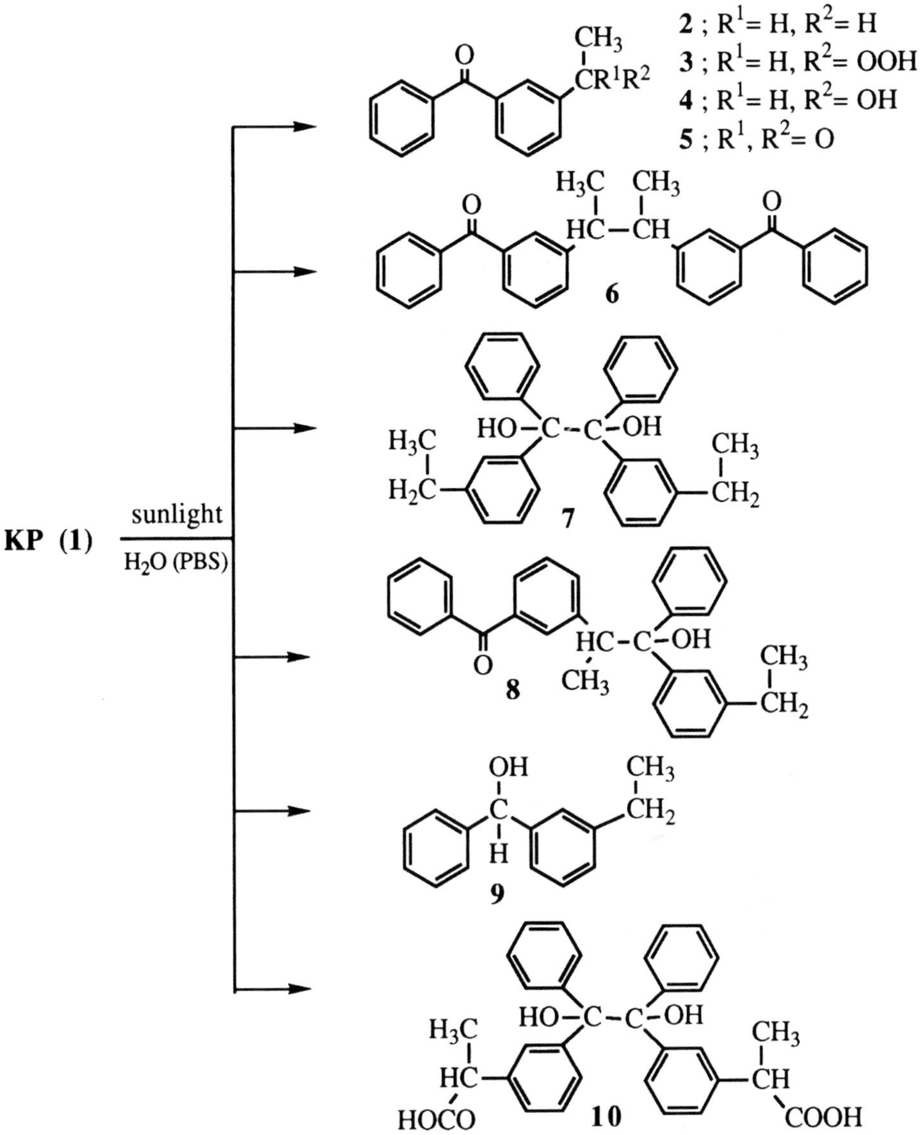

Fig. 13.5 Chemical structures of the photoproducts of ketoprofen, a representative 2-arylpropionic acid. Both photodecarboxylation products and dimers arising from initial hydrogen abstraction by the benzophenone chromophore are formed.

giving mainly photoproducts with an ethyl side-chain.[29,35,39,40,47,50] It has been convincingly demonstrated that these lipophylic photoproducts accumulate in cell membranes, where they produce cell lysis upon light exposure.[50–52] Thus, photobiological activity might be associated in these cases with the formation of photoproducts with high photosensitizing ability.

Both the parent drugs and the photoproducts are able to induce photosensitization via intermediate free radicals or active oxygen species involved in their photochemistry, by the well-known type I or type II mechanisms. The role of drug-derived peroxides has also been discussed.[39]

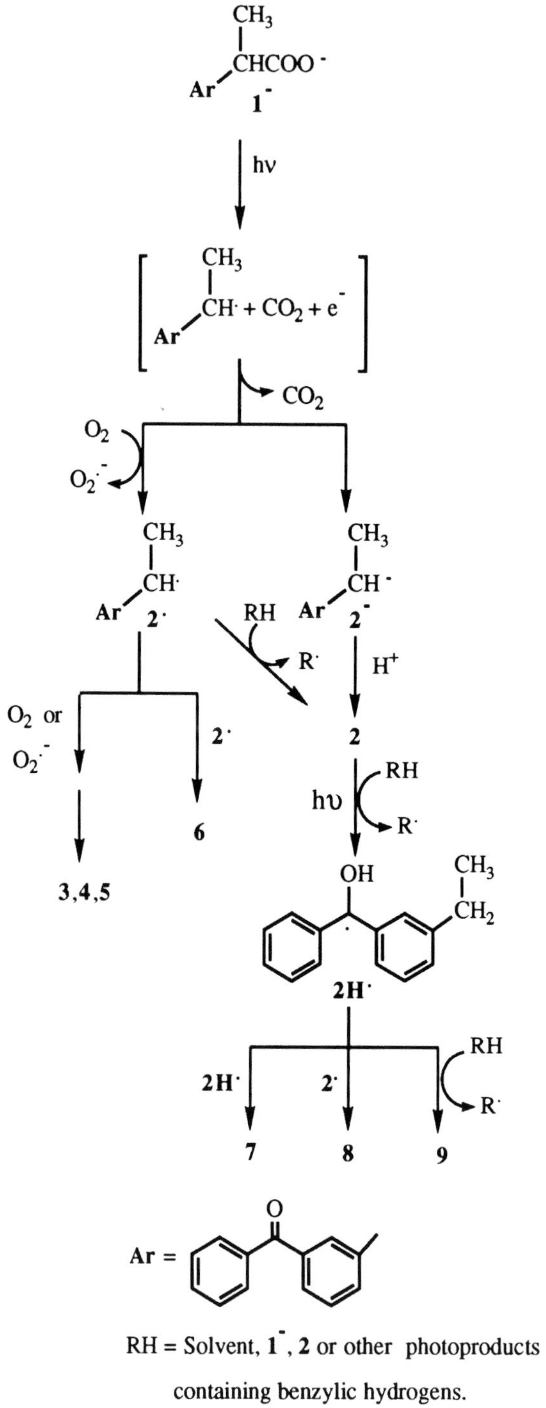

Fig. 13.6 Photochemical mechanism illustrating the different reaction pathways that ultimately lead to the isolated ketoprofen photoproducts.

VIII. ANIMAL MODELS FOR TESTING PHOTOSENSITIZING DRUGS *IN VIVO*

The possibility of using *in vivo* assays based on animal models in the prediction of a potential photobiological risk is higher for phototoxicity than for photoallergy. As the latter is idiosyncratic in nature, none of the existing *in vivo* methods is sufficiently reliable and reproducible to advance its development in humans. Usually, a drug is labelled as photoallergic on the basis of accumulated clinical evidence.[4,10,11,17,18] Although experimental studies performed with laboratory animals have led to some advancement in the understanding of the immunological mechanisms underlying photoallergy, animal models are not sufficiently predictive to detect photoallergic drugs with proven effectiveness.

In the case of phototoxicity, *in vivo* methods based on animal models have been employed for predictive purposes with an acceptable degree of success.[19,53–55] This is attributable to the fact that phototoxicity is dose dependent and hence it can appear in any living organism exposed to the combined effect of sunlight and a photosensitizer. Thus, phototoxic reactions have been induced in laboratory animals after epidermal, intraperitoneal or oral administration of phototoxic compounds followed by irradiation with different light sources (xenon or mercury arc lamps, fluorescent tubes, monochromatic light sources, etc.).

Most frequently used species are mice and guinea-pigs, although rabbits, hamsters and several other animals have been employed as well. Hairless rats, mice and guinea-pigs are now available; their use avoids problems of hair removal. Evaluation of the phototoxic reaction is dependent on the species used. In mice, it involves the quantitative assessment of oedema, by measuring either the weight increase of an exposed organ (tail, skin, etc.) or its increase in thickness (skin, ear). By contrast, in guinea-pigs erythematous reactions are more pronounced.

Although the above *in vivo* methodology has been found to be suitable for several phototoxic drug groups, the use of animals is expensive, time consuming and requires a considerable degree of technical ability. Moreover, testing in animals is difficult to standardize, owing to variability in a number of factors such as species, skin properties, hair characteristics and metabolic patterns. Moreover, there is an ethical barrier to the unjustified or excessive use of experimental studies with laboratory animals, which has become increasingly reduced and restricted by recent regulatory guidelines.[19]

IX. *IN VITRO* ASSAYS FOR POTENTIALLY PHOTOSENSITIZING DRUGS

The photosensitizing potential of new drugs should be detected at an early stage of their development by means of a simple, rapid, inexpensive and sensitive assay requiring readily available materials. Such an assay should be easily adaptable to a routine procedure, in order to screen a large number of molecules for photosensitizing ability. All these requirements can, in principle, be fulfilled by *in vitro* methods.[1,19,23]

In this context, it is again convenient to differentiate between phototoxicity and photoallergy. *In vitro* prediction of the latter entails more difficulties and hence it has been the subject of a rather limited number of studies, mainly dealing with photobinding of drugs to proteins.[56–60] Some good correlations between photoallergenicity and the formation of drug–protein photoadducts have been obtained, but the predictive value and general validity of these assays remain to be demonstrated, in view of the lack of an *in vitro* equivalent of the complex immunological responses of whole living organisms.

In vitro testing of phototoxicity has attracted much more attention. A considerable number of methods has been developed both for general screening purposes and for elucidation of specific mechanisms. Simple UV-spectrophotometric analysis provides useful preliminary information and allows non-absorbing compounds to be labelled as non-phototoxic. However, more reliable *in vitro* approaches typically consist of the exposure of a biological target to the photosensitizer plus UV radiation, followed by evaluation of the produced effects by measurement of an adequate end-point. Photohaemolysis and photo-induced yeast growth inhibition are old and well-established *in vitro* assays supported by large databases. Other tests systems involve co-irradiation of the photosensitizer either with cells (fibroblasts, keratinocytes, hepatocytes, lymphocytes, etc.) or with isolated biomolecules (polyunsaturated fatty acids, simple amino acids, proteins, DNA).

Recently, several *in vitro* phototoxicity assays have been included in a multicentre validation study conducted by COLIPA, the European cosmetics manufacturers' association, under the auspices of the EU.[19] After developing standard protocols, the responses obtained with 20 test chemicals were compared. The assays were evaluated according to a number of factors, such as predictive ability or reliability of the results, and classified into different priority categories. A few selected assays have been recommended for further validation (e.g. neutral red uptake using Balb/c 3T3 fibroblasts, photohaemolysis, histidine photo-oxidation or photobinding to proteins), whereas others have been dismissed.

As stated above, we shall focus our attention on 2-arylpropionic acids as representative photosensitizing agents, trying to describe the most interesting applications of *in vitro* methodologies to this family of non-steroidal anti-inflammatory drugs.

A. Spectrophotometric analysis

This preliminary method[61] is based on mathematical calculations which consider the mass of ingested drug (M), the extinction coefficient at the wavelength of interest (ε) and the radiation dose to which the patient may be exposed (H). The photosensitivity index (PI) is defined as $PI = M\varepsilon H$. At 320 nm, the calculated PI of 2-arylpropionic acids decreases in the order benoxaprofen > tiaprofenic acid > naproxen > ketoprofen > ibuprofen. Extension of this analysis to cover the whole solar spectrum can be done, but such refinement does not produce alterations in the above rank order. As the method is simple and expedient, it may be useful as a preliminary assay. However, it must be kept in mind that, although light absorption is a prerequisite for photosensitization, there are many possible energy-wasting channels to deactivate excited states. Hence, it is quite possible that a strongly absorbing substance is not able to act as a photosensitizer. This explains why the photoprotecting ability of sunscreens is not intrinsically bound to a high photosensitivity index.

B. Photohaemolysis

Photohaemolysis, which is probably the oldest *in vitro* phototoxicity test, reflects impairment of the function and integrity of cellular membranes after exposure to light plus a photosensitizing chemical.[62,63] Since the introduction of this assay, many variations have been devised and different end-points have been used to evaluate the results. With anti-inflammatory 2-arylpropionic acids, photohaemolysis has been quantified in two ways:

(1) as the release of haemoglobin, through the absorbance of the supernatants (after centrifugation) at 540 nm; and (2) by the decreasing number of intact red blood cells, which is proportional to the optical density at 650 nm. Application of this assay (method 1) to benoxaprofen, carprofen, ibuprofen, ketoprofen and naproxen produced different results depending on the irradiation wavelengths.[64] In the UVA range, ketoprofen was the most active drug; by contrast, benoxaprofen exhibited the highest activity upon irradiation with UVB light. Independent studies with method 2 have confirmed the phototoxicity of benoxaprofen, naproxen, ketoprofen and carprofen.[35,36,41–43,65,66] Using the same protocol, photohaemolysis has been observed to occur with suprofen and tiaprofenic acid.[44,67] The variations produced by withdrawal of oxygen or incorporation of different additives (radical scavengers, singlet oxygen quenchers, etc.) are related to the involved photosensitization pathways, which allows this model system to be employed for mechanistic investigations.

An intrinsic limitation of this test system is associated with the fact that it detects photosensitization only at the cell membrane level. Hence, false-negative predictions must be expected for compounds acting via photodamage to DNA or other biological targets different from the membrane components. However, the photohaemolysis assay is rapid and easy to perform, and its wide use has produced a large database.

C. *Candida albicans* phototoxicity test

Photosensitized *Candida albicans* growth inhibition[68,69] is evaluated as the diameter of the yeast-free zone. Such inhibition is assumed to indicate injury to DNA. Upon application of this assay to 2-arylpropionic acids at 0.1% concentration,[64] a higher activity was observed for naproxen, carprofen and benoxaprofen than for ketoprofen or ibuprofen. In a separate study, tiaprofenic acid was found to have a higher phototoxic index than naproxen.[70] As several modifications of this test have been developed, it is difficult to find standardized conditions.[71] Besides, the sensitivity may depend on the strain employed, and the predictive ability is not sufficiently satisfactory (many phototoxic compounds are not detected). From a technical point of view, the pathogenic nature of this yeast is a source of concern because of the risk for contamination in the laboratory. This is obviously a drawback for introduction of the technique in pharmaceutical companies.[19] In spite of the above limitations, the information generated with *C. albicans* phototoxicity testing can be useful, because it complements the data obtained by photohaemolysis.

D. Photodynamic lipid peroxidation

The photosensitizing potential of drugs is frequently related to their photodynamic properties, defined as the ability to mediate light-induced oxidation of biological substrates in the presence of oxygen. In this context, photoperoxidation is known to produce detrimental effects on cell membranes, so it must play an important role in skin phototoxicity.[72]

Lipids are good model systems to quantify photodynamic lipid peroxidation *in vitro*. On this basis, haemoglobin-free ghost membranes[73] and pure linoleic acid[35,36,40,67] have been employed to assess the phototoxicity of 2-arylpropionic acids. The linoleic acid method is particularly interesting because it is simple and expedient and involves the use of a well-defined reaction medium. Moreover, by the addition of radical scavengers, singlet oxygen quenchers or other mechanistic probes, it is possible to determine the photosensitization pathways involved.[35,36,40,74]

In aqueous solution, tiaprofenic acid and suprofen are able to photosensitize linoleic acid peroxidation (determined spectrophotometrically, through the appearance and subsequent increase of a band corresponding to the conjugated dienic hydroperoxides at 233 nm), whereas ibuprofen is not active in this model system (Fig. 13.7). This shows a good correlation with existing clinical data.[40,67] A similar effect has been observed for ketoprofen.[35,36] In this case, a type I mechanism appears to be responsible for the observed photoperoxidation, because it is inhibited dramatically by butylated hydroxyanisole (BHA) and reduced glutathione (GSH) (Fig. 13.8) but it is not affected by diazabicyclooctane (DABCO). The operating mechanism is depicted in Fig. 13.9.

The linoleic acid photoperoxidation assay is very simple and easy to perform. It appears suitable for mechanistic studies rather than for general screening of phototoxicity, owing to the fact that it is designed to detect photosensitization at the membrane level. Thus, damage to DNA or other cell constituents may pass unnoticed.

E. Histidine photo-oxidation

Histidine is a good probe for type II photodynamic effects, because it is a rather specific substrate for singlet oxygen. It is known that the photosensitized oxygenation of this amino acid produces cleavage of the imidazole ring, although the initial oxidation products have not been isolated. The histidine photo-oxidation assay involves determination of the amino acid remaining after irradiation in the presence of a potentially phototoxic compound.[75] This is achieved by means of the so-called Pauly reaction, which consists of the diazo coupling between histidine and the nitrosation product of sulphanilic acid. Formation of the

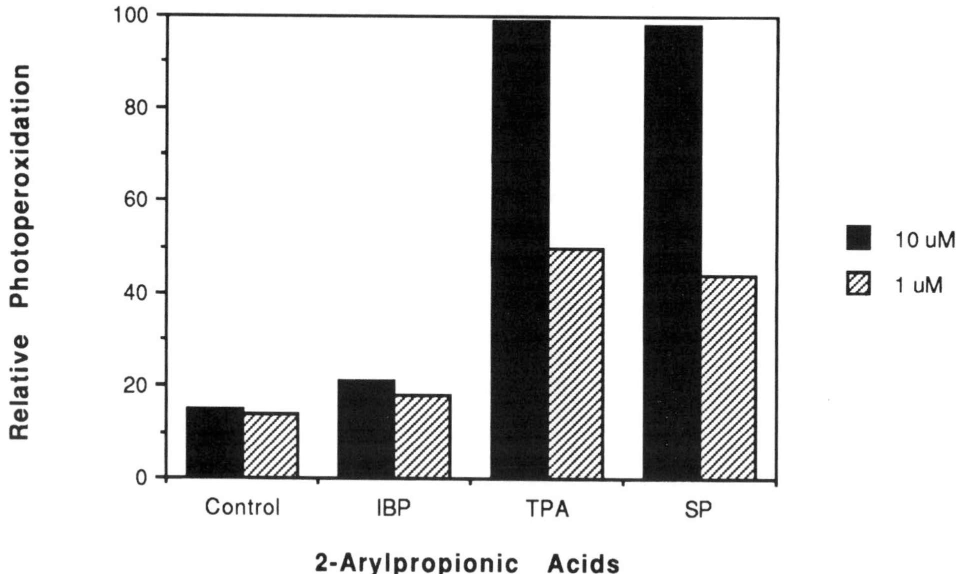

Fig. 13.7 Peroxidation of linoleic acid photosensitized by a series of 2-arylpropionic acids. Formation of conjugated diene hydroperoxides is monitored by the increasing absorbance at 233 nm. The control is linoleic acid irradiated in the absence of drugs, under the same conditions.

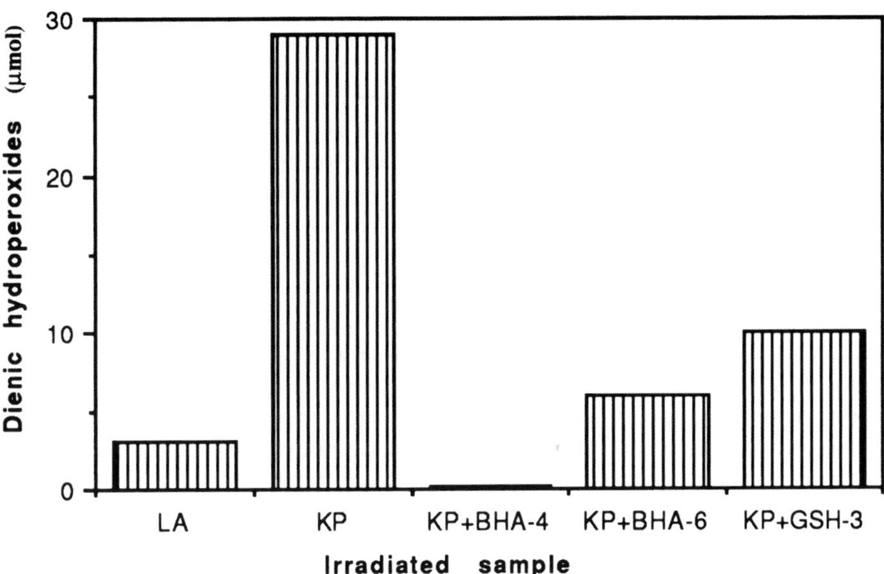

Fig. 13.8 Type I photosensitized peroxidation of linoleic acid (LA) mediated by ketoprofen (KP). A marked inhibition of the reaction is observed upon addition of free radical scavengers such as butylated hydroxyanisole (BHA) or reduced glutathione (GSH).

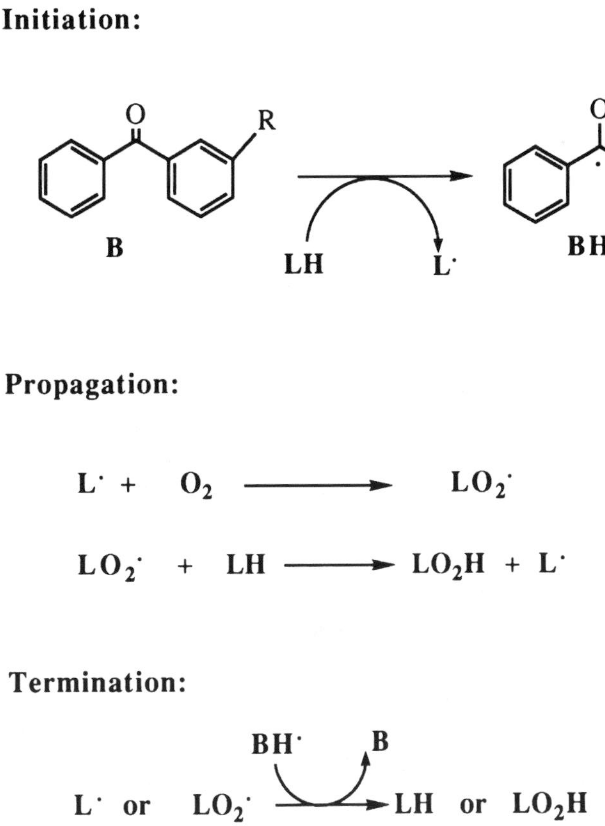

Initiation:

$$\mathbf{B} \xrightarrow[\ \mathrm{LH}\ \to\ \mathrm{L}^{\cdot}\ ]{} \mathbf{BH}^{\cdot}$$

O, R, B, LH, L·, OH, R, BH·

Propagation:

$$\mathrm{L}^{\cdot} + \mathrm{O_2} \longrightarrow \mathrm{LO_2}^{\cdot}$$

$$\mathrm{LO_2}^{\cdot} + \mathrm{LH} \longrightarrow \mathrm{LO_2H} + \mathrm{L}^{\cdot}$$

Termination:

$$\mathrm{L}^{\cdot} \text{ or } \mathrm{LO_2}^{\cdot} \xrightarrow{\ \mathrm{BH}^{\cdot}\ \to\ \mathrm{B}\ } \mathrm{LH} \text{ or } \mathrm{LO_2H}$$

Fig. 13.9 Radical chain mechanism justifying ketoprofen-photosensitized linoleic acid peroxidation. The benzophenone chromophore is thought to play a key role in this process.

corresponding azo compound is accompanied by development of a red colour, which is measured spectrophotometrically.

The histidine phototoxicity test allows the positive identification of many photosensitizers, including several 2-arylpropionic acids[76,77] such as tiaprofenic acid, suprofen and ketoprofen. However, it is more suitable as a mechanistic test than as a general screening test, because of its selectivity for type II photosensitizing substances.

F. Photodamage to fibroblasts

A different type of approach to phototoxicity testing involves exposure of selected target cells to the simultaneous effect of potential photosensitizers and UV radiation. This is followed by evaluation of the produced cellular damage by means of an adequate end-point. Several cell systems have been tried (fibroblasts, keratinocytes, lymphocytes, hepatocytes, etc.), but the most promising results have been obtained with fibroblasts, either as cultured cells or as continuous cell lines (3T3 or A431). Two types of toxicity end-points have been used: (a) cell viability, determined either through the mitochondrial dehydrogenase conversion of a tetrazolium salt (MTT) to a coloured formazan product or by means of the neutral red uptake;[19,78,79] and (b) membrane damage, by measuring the decrease of intracellular lactate dehydrogenase (LDH) activity as indicator of enzyme leakage.[36,50]

Concerning the application of these phototoxicity tests to 2-arylpropionic acids, it has been found that co-irradiation of tiaprofenic acid or ketoprofen with cultured human fibroblasts produces photodamage to the cell membranes, as indicated by the LDH method.[36,50] In an independent study conducted with 3T3 cell lines, a significant decrease in cell viability (MTT test) was observed upon irradiation in the presence of benoxaprofen.[78,79]

In summary, phototoxicity assays based on skin cells such as fibroblasts appear promising for screening purposes. Further validation is advisable to assess their validity with a wider range of phototoxins. An interesting research field may be the use of these systems to elucidate phototoxicity mechanisms and to detect cell perturbations or dysfunctions prior to cell death (level of cellular antioxidant defence systems, release of inflammatory mediators, etc.).

G. Photocleavage of DNA

UVB irradiation at 300 nm in the presence of non-steroidal anti-inflammatory drugs (NSAIDs) can produce enhanced strand breaks of bacteriophage ϕX174 supercoiled DNA.[80–82] As the efficiency of photocleavage decreases in oxygenated media, it appears that active oxygen species are not involved. According to the experimental data, either energy transfer or electron transfer mechanisms are involved. The activity rank order of 2-arylpropionic acids (ketoprofen > naproxen > benoxaprofen) is different from that obtained with other *in vitro* tests (for instance, in photohaemolysis with UVB the order is benoxaprofen > ketoprofen > naproxen).[64]

Although in principle this is not a specific assay for phototoxicity, it allows the detection of photochemical activity of the test compounds and thus can give rise to occasional correlations with *in vivo* phototoxicity data. Instead, the measurement of photodamage to DNA can be more suitable for predicting potential photomutagenicity; however, extrapolation to *in vivo* behaviour requires consideration of additional factors such as metabolism, cell penetration or membrane uptake.

H. Photodegranulation of mast cells

Because phototoxicity is frequently associated with urticaria, histamine release from skin mast cells may play an important role in the process. This has been the rationale for the design of some *in vitro* phototoxicity tests.[52,83] For instance, benoxaprofen photosensitizes concentration-dependent degranulation of rat peritoneal mast cells. The release of histamine can be measured by means of spectrofluorometric methods.[52] Likewise, when rat serosal mast cells (from the peritoneal and pleural cavities) are incubated with [^{3}H]serotonin, washed and UVA-irradiated in the presence of benoxaprofen, the radiactive mediator resulting from mast cell degranulation is detected in the supernatants.[83] The method has been tested with some other phototoxins; however, its general applicability remains to be explored in more systematic studies.

I. Photo–basophil–histamine release test

Suspensions of human leucocytes are used in this case as the model system, and photosensitized release of histamine from the cells to the supernatant (measured spectrofluorimetrically after derivatization) serves again as an end-point for identifying phototoxic drugs.[84] Within the series of 2-arylpropionic acids, activity has been found to decrease in the order ketoprofen > carprofen > tiaprofenic acid > benoxaprofen. No significant effect has been detected for indoprofen. This rank order is subjected to alteration, depending on the UVA exposure times and drug doses. As the method has been employed in a limited number of cases, further testing is required to evaluate its potential as a general assay for phototoxicity screening.

J. Photoinhibition of thymidine incorporation into human lymphocytes

Inhibition of [^{3}H]thymidine incorporation into mitogen-stimulated peripheral blood mononuclear cells (mostly lymphocytes) has been used as indicator of photobiological risk.[85] In this case, a chain process initiated by binding of the mitogen to cellular membranes results in DNA synthesis and blastogenesis. Cell dysfunctions affecting this process produce an inhibition of [^{3}H]thymidine incorporation. Such an effect has been demonstrated upon UVA irradiation of lymphocytes in the presence of a variety of test chemicals, including benoxaprofen. This assay uses readily available cells and relatively simple methodologies. In addition, it is able to detect both injury to the membranes and nuclear damage. However, there is considerable individual variation in the sensitivity of lymphocytes, which constitutes a major drawback.

K. Photo-enhanced generation of reactive oxygen species by human phagocytes

Benoxaprofen photosensitization of human polymorphonuclear leucocytes produces an increase in spontaneous membrane-associated oxidative metabolism. This has been demonstrated using end-points such as superoxide generation (reduction of ferricytochrome *c* in the presence of superoxide dismutase) or luminol-enhanced chemiluminescence.[86] It has been suggested that these pro-oxidative properties are directly related to the anti-inflammatory activity in the case of benoxaprofen and related NSAIDs. Hence, an adequate balance should be established to retain the desired pharmacological properties while minimizing the phototoxic side-effects. This confirms the convenience of evaluating the photosensitizing potential of new drugs, especially in the group of anti-inflammatory 2-arylpropionic acids.

X. GENERAL STRATEGY FOR *IN VITRO* PHOTOTOXICITY TESTING

The following aspects should be taken into account for the systematic *in vitro* evaluation of a potentially phototoxic drug (Fig. 13.10):

1. Sunlight absorption by the drug, as indicated by the overlap of its UV–visible light spectrum with the solar radiation at the earth's surface.

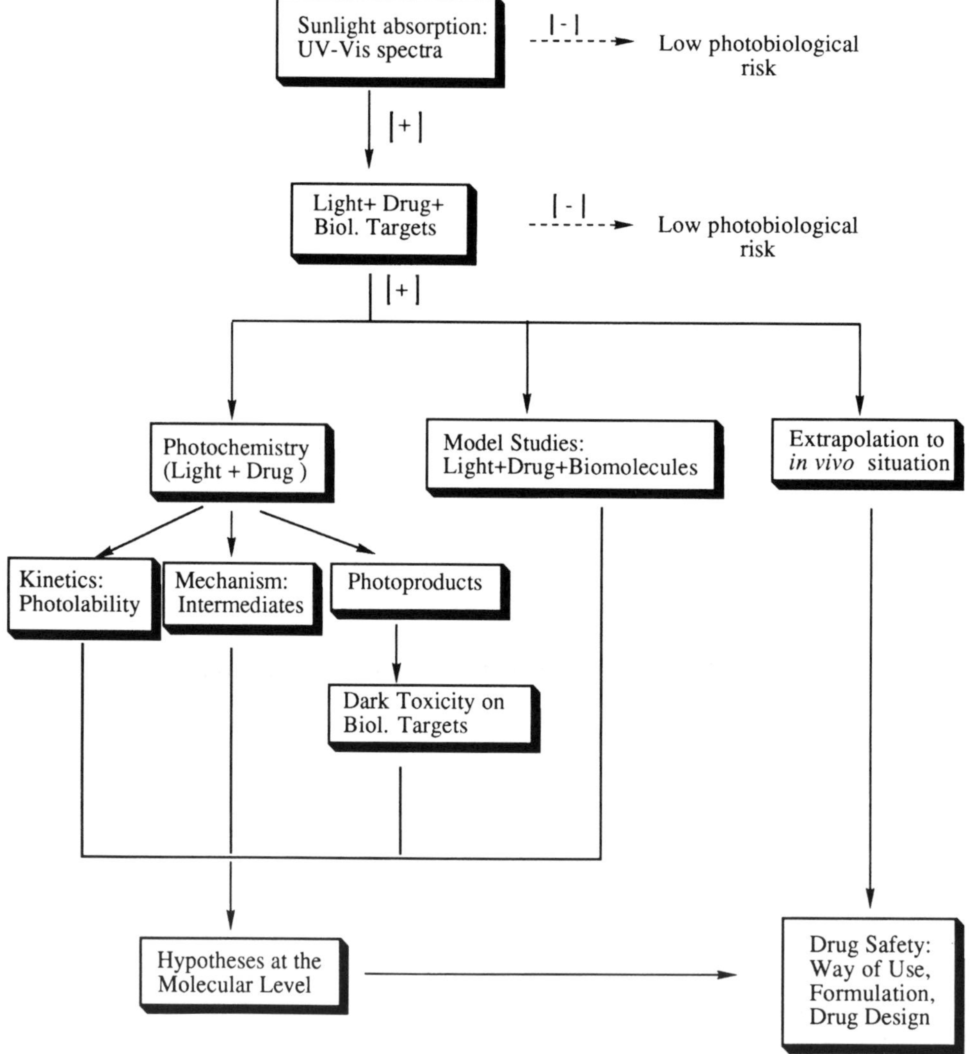

Fig. 13.10 General strategy for assessing the phototoxic risk of new drugs by means of *in vitro* methods.

2. Photochemistry of the drug (photodegradation in different media, identification of the photoproducts, chemical and spectroscopic evidence for the involvement of highly reactive intermediates, etc.).
3. Effects of the photoproducts on target cells (both as irradiation mixtures and as the isolated individual components).
4. Photochemical interaction of the drug with relevant biomolecules (lipids, proteins, DNA, or their simple building blocks).
5. Co-irradiation of the drug with cells or other biological test systems (photosensitized damage, alteration, dysfunction, etc.).
6. Extrapolation of *in vitro* data to the *in vivo* situation.
7. Structure–activity relationships (identification of the chromophores responsible for phototoxicity, quantitative correlations).
8. Recommendations for a possible decision (selection between several drug candidates, improvement of drug formulation by the addition of photostabilizers or radical scavengers, proposal of modified structures, etc.).

At first sight, such a study may appear very time consuming and difficult to perform, as it requires an interdisciplinary approach. However, when negative responses are obtained at the early phases of the study the problem can be simplified dramatically. Obviously, the lack of sunlight absorption by a drug (phase 1) allows the study to be stopped and is sufficient to label the drug as non-photosensitizing. In the case of light-absorbing drugs, it is still possible that negative results are obtained in the screening tests (phase 5: photohaemolysis, photodamage to fibroblasts, etc.), and then a detailed mechanistic investigation (phases 2–4) can be superfluous. Finally, the part of the work dealing with extrapolations, predictions and recommendations (phases 6–8) has to be limited to selected photoactive drugs, after obtaining detailed information on their photochemical and photobiological properties.

XI. EXPERIMENTAL PROCEDURES: HOW TO DO IT

To illustrate the development of the different study phases outlined above, some typical procedures are given below. Owing to space limitations, the information is restricted to essential aspects of the methods instead of providing detailed descriptions of the experiments. Additional data can be found in the cited literature. As usual, antiinflammatory 2-arylpropionic acids are taken as the representative group.

A. Photolytic degradation of drugs

Procedure A Tiaprofenic acid (1 mmol) was dissolved with an equimolar amount of NaOH, and the resulting solution was made up to 300 ml with phosphate-buffered saline (PBS) (50 mM, pH 7.2).[39] Irradiation was performed in an immersion well photoreactor for 1 h, through a Pyrex sleeve, using a 125 W medium-pressure mercury lamp as light source. The photoreactor was kept at 37°C during irradiation. The crude photomixture was extracted with methylene chloride. After evaporation of the organic phase, the photoproducts were isolated by column chromatography, using hexane and ethyl acetate as eluent. Three photoproducts were identified (compounds with ethyl, acetyl and 1-hydroxyethyl side-chains). Their structures were assigned on the basis of IR ^{1}H-NMR, ^{13}C-NMR and MS spectral data.

Procedure B Ketoprofen (5 mmol) was dissolved in 500 ml PBS, placed in an open Pyrex flask and exposed to natural sunlight. The progress of the reaction was monitored by taking aliquots after different irradiation times. These aliquots were acidified and extracted with methylene chloride. The resulting extracts were analysed by thin layer chromatography (TLC), HPLC and GC/MS.[35] An almost complete consumption of the drug was observed after 1 h. Owing to the lower solubility of the photoproducts, the solution became unclear and then an oily phase was formed. Column chromatography of the photomixture and subsequent repurification of the fractions by semipreparative HPLC, using hexane and ethyl acetate as eluent, allowed separation of nine different photoproducts. Their structures (see Fig. 13.5) were assigned on the basis of IR ^{1}H-NMR, ^{13}C-NMR, MS and UV–visible spectral data.

B. Cytotoxicity of drug photoproducts

The crude reaction mixture obtained upon irradiation of naproxen, as well as isolated individual components, was assayed for cytotoxic effects on cultured fibroblasts (Balb/3T3 C-31, ATCC: CCL163).[39,45] These cells were initially cultured until confluence on 3.5 cm plastic dishes in Dulbecco's modification of Eagle's culture medium (DMEM) supplemented with 10% fetal calf serum (FCS) and kept in a carbon dioxide/oxygen cell incubator at 37°C. The compounds were dissolved in acetone and added, in variable concentrations, to the cultures. The cytotoxic effects were evaluated by two criteria: cell viability (trypan blue exclusion test) and leakage to culture medium of LDH. The photoproducts with acetyl and 1-hydroxyethyl side-chains (1 mM) produced a marked release of intracellular LDH (35% and 50%, respectively). Under the same conditions, the parent drug was inactive.

C. Drug-derived peroxides: fluorimetric determination and biological effects

Peroxides were determined by a method based on the peroxidase-catalysed oxidation of the non-fluorescent dichlorodihydrofluorescein to the fluorescent dichlorofluorescein, and was performed directly with aliquots of the crude aqueous photomixtures obtained from naproxen and tiaprofenic acid (3 mM), degassed under vacuum, exhaustively purged with argon and kept at 0°C until use.[39] Samples of these photomixtures were diluted (1 : 10–1 : 100) in degassed distilled water and then aliquots of 20 μl were added in triplicate to 96-well plates. A measured amount of the assay solution (0.36 μmol dichlorodihydrofluorescein and 1 unit peroxidase in 180 μl of 50 mM phosphate buffer pH 7.2) was also added to each well with a multichannel pipette under argon atmosphere. The plate was sealed with black adhesive tape. After 30–120 min incubation in the dark, fluorescence was measured at room temperature with a microplate reader (Cytofluor 2300, Millipore), using 485 nm light for excitation and 530 nm for emission. Hydrogen peroxide was used as a reference compound and added to wells in increasing concentration up to 3000 pmol per well. The measured fluorescence was proportional to the amount of hydrogen peroxide present in the samples. Using this methodology, the crude photomixture of naproxen was shown to contain a higher concentration of peroxide than the photomixture of tiaprofenic acid.

The biological effects of naproxen peroxides were evaluated by the depletion of cellular glutathione concentration in rat hepatocytes. The cells were incubated for 20 h with the peroxides and then intracellular GSH was determined by the formation of fluorescent adducts with monochlorobimane, using a fluorescence microplate reader (excitation 390 nm, emission 460 nm). To investigate the ability of catalase and *N*-acetylcysteine to prevent cell death of hepatocytes treated with naproxen peroxides, cell viability was measured after 20 h incubation with the MTT test.

D. Photoperoxidation of linoleic acid in the presence of drugs

Duplicate solutions of linoleic acid (10^{-3} M) in PBS, containing variable amounts of tiaprofenic acid or suprofen (in the range 10^{-8} to 10^{-4} M) were irradiated through Pyrex with a 400 W mercury lamp, keeping the temperature at 37°C by means of a thermostated bath.[40] The reaction was monitored by UV spectrophotometry, following the appearance and subsequent increase of a new absorption maximum at a wavelength of 233 nm, due to the conjugated dienic hydroperoxides derived from linoleic acid. The controls were solutions (10^{-3} M) of linoleic acid alone and of drugs alone, at the corresponding concentrations, irradiated under the same conditions, as well as non-irradiated. The irradiated samples containing linoleic acid plus tiaprofenic acid or suprofen gave rise to significant formation of hydroperoxides (10^{-4} M). A clear relationship was found between this response and both the drug dose and irradiation times (10–120 min).

E. Photohaemolysis test

Procedure A Red blood cells (RBCs), obtained from human volunteers not taking any drug, were washed in physiological saline and centrifuged at 2000 rpm for 10 min.[64] This procedure was repeated three times. Then, buffered drug solutions (10 ml portions, 1–400 μg ml^{-1}) were transferred to plastic cups and 20 μl RBCs added. Duplicate samples of the resulting suspensions, as well as a sample containing only the drug solution, were exposed to UV radiation (UVA or UVB fluorescent lamps). A standard radiation dose not causing haemolysis in the absence of drug was used. After exposure was complete, the samples were incubated in the dark for 30 min. The suspensions were then centrifuged for 10 min at 2000 rpm and 4 ml of the supernatant was mixed with 1 ml Drabkin's solution ($Fe_3Fe(CN)_6$ 200 mg, KCN 50 mg, KH_2PO_4 140 mg, surfactant Triton X100 0.5 ml diluted with distilled water to 1000 ml, pH 7.2–7.4) in order to convert all types of haemoglobin to methaemoglobin, which is able to form the stable pigment cyanmethaemoglobin with a maximum absorbance at 540 nm. The samples were read at this wavelength with a conventional spectrophotometer. A control sample with 100% haemolysis consisted of 20 μl RBCs in 12.5 ml of Drabkin's solution.

Procedure B Solutions of ketoprofen (30 μM) in PBS were transferred to plastic cuvettes and human RBCs were added so that the resultant suspension had an optical density (OD) of about 0.5 at 650 nm (3.6×10^6 cells per ml). Duplicate samples were exposed to UV radiation through Pyrex glass using a 400 W mercury lamp as light source for periods ranging between 10 and 180 min. Cells received on average about 4 mW per cm^2 as determined by ferrioxalate actinometry. The haemolysis rate and percentage haemolysis were determined, after gentle turning of the cuvettes, with a conventional spectrophotometer by measuring the decreasing OD at 650 nm.[36] More than 90% photohaemolysis was observed after 1 h irradiation. Control experiments showed that no haemolysis occurred when RBCs were incubated for 4 h with ketoprofen in the dark or when they were irradiated for 4 h without drug.

F. *Candida albicans* phototoxicity test

Test drugs were dissolved in ethanol, dimethylsulfoxide or acetone.[64] A given volume of a 0.05–10% solution was applied to 7.5 mm filter paper discs. The latter were transferred to Sabouraud agar plates where a suspension of a fresh culture of *C. albicans* had been evenly spread. The plates (duplicate samples) were exposed to UVA radiation (1 mW per cm^2). The controls were samples kept in the dark and the vehicle alone. After exposure was complete, the diameter of the yeast-free zone was measured.

G. Histidine photodegradation

Solutions of tiaprofenic acid in 10% propylene glycol in PBS (0.01 M, pH 7.4) were mixed with the same amount of L-histidine monochloride solution (0.61 mM) in PBS. These mixtures were bubbled with oxygen and irradiated with the light of a psoralens and ultraviolet A radiation (PUVA) unit (365 nm, 16 mW per cm^2). When irradiation was complete, the samples were incubated in the dark at room temperature for 30 min. Histidine was determined by a modified Pauly reaction. For this, 200 μl of test solution was made up to 2 ml with PBS; 200 μl of 1% sulfanilic acid in 0.87 N HCl and 200 μl of 5% sodium nitrite were added and the mixture was left for 10 min; 0.6 ml of 20% sodium carbonate was then added and, after a further 2 min, 2 ml of ethyl alcohol. The OD of the final solution was read at 530 nm in a spectrophotometer against a control; the remaining histidine was determined from a standard curve.[76]

H. Photodamage to fibroblasts

Procedure A Balb/C 3T3 cells, clone 31 (ICN-Flow) were cultured in 96-well microtitre plates. After 24 h, the culture medium (DMEM) was removed, cells were washed twice in Earle's balanced salt solution (EBSS), and eight concentrations of the test drug (dissolved in EBSS) were added. Insoluble drugs can be dissolved in dimethylsulfoxide (DMSO) before use and added at a maximum concentration of 1% DMSO in EBSS. After pre-incubation with the test drug for 1 h, the cells were exposed to UVA (1.67 mW per cm^2) for 50 min (5 J cm^{-2}) using a SOL500 light source (H-1 filter). A second set of plates, in which the cells had been treated with the same drug, was kept in the dark for the same period. The EBSS was then replaced with DMEM (without drug) and neutral red uptake (NRU) was determined 24 h later. Cytotoxicity was derived from the concentration resulting in a 50% reduction in cell viability (IC_{50}).[19]

Procedure B Human fibroblasts (MRC-5) were initially cultured until confluence on a 96-well microplate using DMEM supplemented with 10% FCS and kept in a carbon dioxide/oxygen cell incubator at 37°C. Before the irradiation experiment the plate was carefully rinsed with fresh culture medium without serum. Ketoprofen was added in variable concentrations (0.01–1 mM) to 96 wells of cultured fibroblasts. Subsequently the latter were irradiated through Pyrex glass with a 125 W mercury lamp for 4 h at 37°C and the controls were kept in the dark. Cytotoxic effects were evaluated by measuring the intracellular enzymatic activity of LDH.[36] A marked difference in toxicity was observed between the irradiated cells and the respective non-irradiated controls. The decrease in LDH activity was significant at drug concentrations of 0.1 mM or higher.

Procedure C Cells (A431 epidermal cell line) were maintained in standard tissue culture flasks and subcultured into 96-well microtitre plates, at a density of 5×10^3 cells per well, for all assays.[78,79] Culture medium used was DMEM supplemented with L-glutathione 2 mM, penicillin 100 units ml^{-1}, streptomycin 100 $\mu g\, ml^{-1}$, and 10% (v/v) FCS. Cell cultures were incubated at 37°C in a carbon dioxide/oxygen (5 : 95) humidified atmosphere. After incubating overnight, medium was discarded and replaced with treatment medium (phenol red-free MEM with 10% FCS) containing the test drug at a previously determined highest no-effect concentration. Control wells received medium only. Plates were preincubated for 4 h to equilibrate and were then exposed to the UV radiation provided by an Oriel 1000 W solar simulator. The cells were then incubated for a further 20 h and cell viability was assayed by the MTT test. The ID_{50} values (UV dose reducing the viability to 50% of control level) were derived from the dose–response curves obtained for each test compound.

XII. SUMMARY

The incidence of undesired phototoxic side-effects associated with the use of drugs is clearly increasing. Patients, dermatologists, pharmaceutical companies and health authorities are rightly concerned by this problem and would like to be informed on the inherent risk of each specific drug. Although systematic phototoxicity testing is still not included in the guidelines for the safety evaluation of new drug candidates, this situation will probably change in the near future. Determination of the phototoxic potential is particularly important for topically applied drugs and also for certain drug families, such as non-steroidal anti-inflammatory agents.

Although *in vivo* methods can, in principle, be suitable for such a purpose, they are expensive, time consuming and difficult to standardize. Besides, there is a trend to restrict the use of animals for ethical reasons. By contrast, *in vitro* phototoxicity assays can be simple, inexpensive, sensitive and easily adaptable to a routine procedure. Among them, photohaemolysis and photodamage to fibroblasts (with NRU, MTT or LDH estimation as end-points) appear very promising for general screening. However, they have advantages and limitations, and still require further study. Both assays have been included in an ongoing EU/COLIPA validation trial.

A better understanding of the molecular basis of phototoxicity must be achieved in order to improve the predictive ability. Thus, the introduction of new phototoxicity end-points (for instance, release of inflammatory mediators) able to detect early cellular responses prior to irreversible damage might result in an increased sensitivity. On the other hand, the adequate use of chemical or biochemical assays specific for each possible mechanistic route might allow classification of phototoxic drugs according to their mode of action and allow correlations to be made between the involved photochemical mechanism and the observed biological effects. This information can be very useful in the improvement of drug formulation (for instance, adding a photostabilizer, a free radical scavenger or a singlet oxygen quencher). Finally, identification of the substructures (chromophores) responsible for phototoxicity and the establishment of quantitative structure–activity relationships would enable the introduction of modifications in drug design, leading to a more favourable benefit–risk ratio.

ACKNOWLEDGEMENT

Financial support from the Fondo de Investigaciones Sanitarias (grant FIS 95 1498) is gratefully acknowledged.

REFERENCES

1. Miranda, M. A. (1992) Phototoxicity of drugs. In Castell, J. V. and Gómez-Lechón, M. J. (eds) In Vitro *Alternatives to Animal Pharmaco-Toxicology*, pp 239–270. Farmaindustria, Madrid.
2. Robberecht, R. (1989) Environmental photobiology. In Smith, K. C. (ed.) *The Science of Photobiology*, 2nd edn, pp. 135–154. Plenum Press, New York.
3. Beijersbergen van Henegouwen, G. M. J. (1981) The interference of light in pharmacotherapy. *Pharm. Weekbl. [Sci.]* **3:** 85–95.
4. Epstein, J. H. (1989) Photomedicine. In Smith, K. C. (ed.) *The Science of Photobiology*, 2nd edn, pp. 155–192. Plenum Press, New York.
5. Grossweiner, L. I. and Smith, K. C. (1989) Photochemistry. In Smith, K. C. (ed.) *The Science of Photobiology*, 2nd edn, pp. 47–78. Plenum Press, New York.
6. Spikes, J. D. (1989) Photosensitization. In Smith, K. C. (ed.) *The Science of Photobiology*, 2nd edn, pp. 79–110. Plenum Press, New York.
7. Beijersbergen van Henegouwen, G. M. J. (1991) Systemic phototoxicity of drugs and other xenobiotics. *J. Photochem. Photobiol. B.* **10:** 183–210.
8. Harber, L. C. and Bickers, D. R. (1988) *Photosensitivity Diseases: Principles of Diagnosis and Treatment.* Saunders, Philadelphia, PA.
9. Johnson, B. E (1987) Light sensitivity associated with drugs and chemicals. In Jarrett, A. (ed.) *The Physiology and Pathophysiology of the Skin*, pp. 2541–2606. Academic Press, San Diego, CA.
10. Johnson, B. E. (1992) Drug and chemical photosensitization. In Marks, R. and Plewig, G. (eds) *Environmental Threat to the Skin*, pp. 57–66. Martin Dunitz, London.
11. Johnson, B. E. and Ferguson, J. (1990) Drug and chemical photosensitivity. *Semin. Dermatol.* **9:** 39–46.
12. Diffey, B. L., Daymond, T. J. and Fairgreaves, H. (1983) Phototoxic reactions to piroxicam, naproxen and tiaprofenic acid. *Br. J. Rheumatol.* **22:** 239–242.
13. Hölzle, E., Neumann, N., Hausen, B. *et al.* (1991) Photopatch testing: the five-year experience of the German, Austrian and Swiss photopatch test group. *J. Am. Acad. Dermatol.* **25:** 59–68.
14. Przybilla, B., Ring, J., Schwab, U., Galosi, A., Dorn, M. and Braun-Falco, O. (1987) Photosensibilisierende Eigenschaften nichtsteroidaler Antirheumatica im Photopatch-Test. *Hautarzt* **38:** 18–25.
15. Serrano, G., Fortea, J. M., Latasa, J. M., Sanmartín, O., Bonillo, J. and Miranda, M. A. (1992) Oxicam-induced photosensitivity. Patch and photopatch testing studies with tenoxicam and piroxicam photoproducts in normal patients and in piroxicam–droxicam photosensitive patients. *J. Am. Acad. Dermatol.* **26:** 545–548.
16. Hölzle, E., Plewig, G. and Lehman, P. (1986) Photodermatoses: diagnostic procedures and their interpretation. *Photodermatology* **4:** 109–114.
17. Epstein, J. H. (1983) Phototoxicity and photoallergy in man. *J. Am. Acad. Dermatol.* **8:** 141–147.
18. Epstein, J. H. and Wintroub, B. U. (1985) Photosensitization due to drugs. *Drugs* **30:** 42–57.
19. Spielmann, H., Lovell, W. W., Hölzle, E. *et al.* (1994) *In vitro* phototoxicity testing. The report and recommendations of the ECVAM Workshop 2. *ATLA* **22:** 314–348.
20. Kochevar, I. E. (1989) Phototoxicity of nonsteroidal antiinflammatory drugs: coincidence or specific mechanism? *Arch. Dermatol.* **125:** 824–826.

21. Kaidbey, K. H. and Mitchell, F. N. (1989) Photosensitizing potential of nonsteroidal anti-inflammatory agents. *Arch. Dermatol.* **125:** 783–786.
22. Laustriat, G. (1986) Molecular mechanisms of photosensitization. *Biochimie* **68:** 771–778.
23. Moysan, A., Miranda, M. A., Morliere, P. *et al.* (1994) Evaluation of phototoxicity: from *in vitro* to *in vivo*. In Rougier, A., Goldberg, A. M. and Maibach, H. I. (eds) In Vitro *Skin Toxicology (Methods in Irritation, Phototoxicity and Sensitization)*, pp. 185–194. M. A. Liebert, New York.
24. Paillous, N. and Comtat, M. (1988) Electron transfer in drug-induced photosensitization processes. In Fox, M. A. and Chanon, M. (eds) *Photoinduced Electron Transfer*, Vol. D, pp. 578–607. Elsevier, Amsterdam.
25. Bakri, A., Beijersbergen van Henegouwen, G. M. J. and Chanal, J. L. (1983) Photopharmacology of the tranquilizer chlordiazepoxide in relation to its phototoxicity. *Photochem. Photobiol.* **38:** 177–183.
26. Miranda, M. A., Boscá, F., Vargas, F. and Canudas, N. (1994) Photosensitization by Fenofibrate. II. *In vitro* phototoxicity of the major metabolite. *Photochem. Photobiol.* **59:** 171–174.
27. Gilbert, A. and Baggott, J. (1991) *Essentials of Molecular Photochemistry*. Blackwell, Oxford.
28. Moore, D. E. and Chappuis, P. P. (1988) A comparative study on the non-steroidal anti-inflammatory drugs, naproxen, benoxaprofen and indomethacin. *Photochem. Photobiol.* **47:** 173–180.
29. Navaratnam, S., Hughes, J. L., Parsons, B. J. and Phillips, G. O. (1985) Laser flash and steady state photolysis of benoxaprofen in aqueous solution. *Photochem. Photobiol.* **41:** 375–380.
30. Navaratnam, S., Parsons, B. J. and Hughes, J. L. (1993) Laser flash photolysis of benoxaprofen and its analogues 1. Yields of triplet states and singlet oxygen in acetonitrile solutions. *J. Photochem. Photobiol. A.* **73:** 97–103.
31. Marko, J., Vermeersch, G., Febvay-Garot, N., Caplain, S. and Lablache-Combier, A. (1983) ^{1}H and ^{13}C photo-CIDNP study of aqueous chloropromazine and analogs. *Photochem. Photobiol.* **38:** 169–175.
32. Greenhill, J. V. and McLelland, M. A. (1990) Photodecomposition of drugs. *Prog. Med. Chem.* **27:** 51–121.
33. Boscá, F., Miranda, M. A., Vañó, L. and Vargas, F. (1990) New photodegradation pathways for naproxen, a phototoxic nonsteroidal anti-inflammatory drug. *J. Photochem. Photobiol. A.* **54:** 131–134.
34. Boscá, F., Miranda, M. A. and Vargas, F. (1992) Photochemistry of tiaprofenic acid, a nonsteroidal anti-inflammatory drug with phototoxic side effects. *J. Pharm. Sci.* **81:** 181–182.
35. Boscá, F., Miranda, M. A., Carganico, G. and Mauleon, D. (1994) Photochemical and photobiological properties of ketoprofen associated with the benzophenone chromophore. *Photochem. Photobiol.* **60:** 96–101.
36. Boscá, F., Garganico, G., Castell, J. V. *et al.* (1995) Evaluation of ketoprofen (R, S and R/S) phototoxicity by a battery of *in vitro* assays. *J. Photochem. Photobiol. B.* **99:** 1–6.
37. Castell, J. V., Gómez-Lechón, M. J., Miranda, M. A. and Morera, I. M. (1987) Photolytic degradation of ibuprofen. Toxicity of the isolated photoproducts on fibroblasts and erythrocytes. *Photochem. Photobiol.* **46:** 991–996.
38. Castell, J. V., Gómez-Lechón, M. J. Miranda, M. A. and Morera, I. M. (1992) Phototoxicity of non-steroidal anti-inflammatory drugs: *in vitro* testing of the photoproducts of butibufen and flurbiprofen. *J. Photochem. Photobiol. B.* **13:** 71–81.
39. Castell, J. V., Gómez-Lechón, M. J., Grassa, C., Martínez, L. A., Miranda, M. A. and Tárrega, P. (1993) Involvement of drug-derived peroxides in the phototoxicity of naproxen and tiaprofenic acid. *Photochem. Photobiol.* **57:** 486–490.
40. Castell, J. V., Gómez-Lechón, M. J., Grassa, C., Martínez, L. A., Miranda, M. A. and Tárrega, P. (1994) Photodynamic lipid peroxidation by suprofen and tiaprofenic acid. *Photochem. Photobiol.* **59:** 35–39.
41. Costanzo, L. L., De Guidi, G., Condorelli, G., Cambria, A. and Famà, M. (1989) Molecular mechanism of naproxen photosensitization in red blood cells. *J. Photochem. Photobiol. B.* **3:** 223–235.
42. Costanzo, L. L., De Guidi, G., Condorelli, G., Cambria, A. and Famà, M. (1989) Molecular mechanism of drug photosensitization – II. Photohemolysis sensitized by ketoprofen. *Photochem. Photobiol.* **50:** 359–365.
43. De Guidi, G., Chillemi, R., Costanzo, L. L., Giuffrida, S. and Condorelli, G. (1993) Molecular mechanisms of drug photosensitization. 4. Photohemolysis sensitized by carprofen. *J. Photochem. Photobiol. B.* **17:** 239–246.

44. De Guidi, G., Chillemi, R., Costanzo, L. L., Giuffrida, S., Sortino, S. and Condorelli, G. (1994) Molecular mechanism of drug photosensitization. 5. Photohemolysis sensitized by suprofen. *J. Photochem. Photobiol. B.* **23:** 125–133.
45. Miranda, M. A., Morera, I., Vargas, F., Gómez-Lechón, M. J. and Castell, J. V. (1991) *In vitro* assessment of the phototoxicity of anti-inflammatory 2-arylpropionic acids. *Toxicol. In Vitro* **5:** 451–455.
46. Pietta, P., Manera, E. and Ceva, P. (1987) High-performance liquid chromatographic determination of ketoprofen degradation products. *J. Chromatogr.* **390:** 454–457.
47. Reszka, K. and Chignell, C. F. (1983) Spectroscopic studies of cutaneous photosensitizing agents – IV. The photolysis of benoxaprofen, an anti-inflammatory drug with phototoxic properties. *Photochem. Photobiol.* **38:** 281–291.
48. Vargas, F., Rivas, C., Miranda, M. A. and Boscá, F. (1991) Photochemistry of the non-steroidal anti-inflammatory drugs, propionic acid derived. *Pharmazie* **46:** 767–771.
49. Kochevar, I. E. (1981) Phototoxicity mechanisms. *J. Invest. Dermatol.* **76:** 59–64.
50. Castell, J. V., Gómez-Lechón, M. J., Hernández, D., Martínez, L. A. and Miranda M. A. (1994) Molecular bases of drug phototoxicity: photosensitized cell membrane damage by the major photoproduct of tiaprofenic acid. *Photochem. Photobiol.* **60:** 586–590.
51. Kochevar, I. E., Hoover, K. W. and Gawienowski, M. (1984) Benoxaprofen photosensitization of cell membrane disruption. *J. Invest. Dermatol.* **82:** 214–218.
52. Sik, R. H., Paschall, C. S. and Chignell, C. F. (1983) The phototoxic effect of benoxaprofen and its analogs on human erythrocytes and rat peritoneal mast cells. *Photochem. Photobiol.* **38:** 411–415.
53. Ljunggren, B. and Lundberg, K. (1985) *In vivo* phototoxicity of non-steroidal antiinflammatory drugs evaluated by the mouse tail technique. *Photodermatology.* **2:** 377–382.
54. Maurer, Th. (1987) Phototoxicity testing – *in vivo* and *in vitro*. *Fd. Chem. Toxicol.* **25:** 407–414.
55. Nilsson, R., Maurer, T. and Redmond, N. (1993) A standard protocol for phototoxicity testing. Results from an interlaboratory study. *Contact Dermatitis* **28:** 285–290.
56. Barratt, M. D. and Brown, K. R. (1985) Photochemical binding of photoallergens to human serum albumin: a simple *in vitro* method for screening potential photoallergens. *Toxicol. Lett.* **24:** 1–6.
57. Lovell, W. W. (1993) A scheme for *in vitro* screening of substances for photoallergic potential. *Toxicol. In Vitro* **7:** 95–102.
58. Miranda, M. A., Castell, J. V., Gómez-Lechón, M. J., Hernández, D. and Martínez, L. A. (1995) Photobinding of drugs to cells as an indicator of potential photoallergy. *Toxicol. In Vitro* **9:** 499–503.
59. Schoonderwoerd, S. A. and Beijersbergen van Henegouwen, G. M. J. (1987) Irreversible photobinding to skin constituents after systemic administration of chlorpromazine to Wistar rats. *Photochem. Photobiol.* **46:** 501–505.
60. Schoonderwoerd, S. A., Beijersbergen van Henegouwen, G. M. J., Persons, C. C. M., Caffieri, S. and Dall'Acqua, F. (1991) Photobinding of 8-methoxypsoralen, 4,6,4′-trimethylangelicin and chlorpromazine to Wistar rat epidermal biomacromolecules *in vivo*. *J. Photochem. Photobiol. B.* **10:** 257–268.
61. Diffey, B. L. and Brown, S. (1983) A method for predicting the phototoxicity of non-steroidal anti-inflammatory drugs. *Br. J. Clin. Pharmacol.* **16:** 633–638.
62. Barth, J., Hofmann, C. and Fickweiler, E. (1977) Untersuchungen zur fotohämolytischen Potenz von Pharmaka und Industriesubstanzen. *Dermatol. Monatsschr.* **163:** 613–618.
63. Kahn, G. and Fleischaker, B. (1971) Red blood cell hemolysis by photosensitizing compounds. *J. Invest. Dermatol.* **56:** 85–90.
64. Ljunggren, B. (1985) Propionic acid-derived non-steroidal antiinflammatory drugs are phototoxic *in vitro*. *Photodermatology* **2:** 3–9.
65. Condorelli, G., De Guidi, G., Giuffrida, S. and Costanzo, L. L. (1993) Photosensitizing action of nonsteroidal antiinflammatory drugs on cell membranes and design of protective agents. *Coord. Chem. Rev.* **125:** 115–127.
66. Condorelli, G., Costanzo, L. L., De Guidi, G., Giuffrida, S., Rizzarelli, E. and Vecchio, G. (1994) Inhibition of photohemolysis by copper(II) complexes with SOD-like activity. *J. Inorg. Biochem.* **54:** 257–265.
67. Miranda, M. A., Castell, J. V., Gómez-Lechón, M. J. and Martínez, L. A. (1993) *In vitro* photoperoxidation as an indicator of the potential phototoxicity of non-steroidal anti-inflammatory 2-arylpropionic acids. *Toxicol. In Vitro* **7:** 523–526.
68. Daniels, F. (1965) A simple microbiological method for demonstrating phototoxic compounds. *J. Invest. Dermatol.* **44:** 259–263.

69. Kavli, G. and Volden, G. (1984) The *Candida* test for phototoxicity. *Photodermatology* **1:** 204–207.
70. Horikawa, E. and Miura, T. (1988) Phototoxic index of drugs determined by *Candida* growth inhibition. *J. Dermatol.* **15:** 523–526.
71. Knudsen, E. A. (1985) The *Candida* phototoxicity test. The sensitivity of different strains and species of *Candida*, standardization attempts and analysis of the dose–response curves for 5- and 8-methoxypsoralen. *Photodermatology* **2:** 80–85.
72. Girotti, A. W. (1990) Photodynamic lipid peroxidation in biological systems. *Photochem. Photobiol.* **51:** 497–509.
73. Hoshino, T., Ishida, K., Irie, T., Hirayama, F. and Uekama, K. (1988) Reduction of photohemolytic activity of benoxaprofen by *β*-cyclodextrin complexations. *Journal of Inclusion Phenomena* **6:** 415–423.
74. Vargas, F., Canudas, N., Miranda, M. A. and Boscá, F. (1993) Photodegradation and *in vitro* phototoxicity of fenofibrate, a photosensitizing anti-hyperproteinemic drug. *Photochem. Photobiol* **5:**, 471–476.
75. Johnson, B. E., Walker, E. M. and Hetherington, A. M. (1986) *In vitro* models for cutaneous phototoxicity. In Marks, R. and Plewig, G. (eds) *Skin Models, Models to Study Function and Disease of Skin*, pp. 264–281. Springer, Berlin.
76. Figueiredo, A., Fontes Ribeiro, C. A., Gonçalo, M., Poiares Baptista, A. and Teixeira, F. (1993) Experimental studies on the mechanisms of tiaprofenic acid photosensitization. *J. Photochem. Photobiol. B.* **18:** 161–168.
77. Martínez, L. A. (1995) Desarrollo de un modelo *in vitro* para el estudio del potencial fotosensibilizador de nuevos fármacos en humanos. Los ácidos 2-arilpropiónicos como grupo modelo. *Ph D Thesis, Universitat de Valencia.*
78. Duffy, P. A., Bennett, A., Roberts, M. and Flint, O. P. (1987) Prediction of phototoxic potential using human A431 cells and mouse 3T3 cells. *Mol. Toxicol.* **1:** 579–587.
79. Duffy, P. A., Bennett, A., Roberts, M. and Flint, O. P. (1989) The prediction of phototoxic potential using human A431 cells and mouse 3T3 cells. *Altern. Methods Toxicol.* **7:** 327–335.
80. Artuso, T., Bernadou, J., Meunier, B. and Paillous, N. (1990) DNA strand breaks photosensitized by benoxaprofen and other non-steroidal antiinflammatory agents. *Biochem. Pharmacol.* **39:** 407–413.
81. Artuso, T., Bernadou, J., Meunier, B., Piette, J. and Paillous, N. (1991) Mechanism of DNA cleavage mediated by photoexcited non-steroidal antiinflammatory drugs. *Photochem. Photobiol.* **54:** 205–213.
82. Paillous, N. and Vicendo, P. (1993) Mechanisms of photosensitized DNA cleavage. *J. Photochem. Photobiol. B.* **20:** 203–209.
83. Gendimenico, G. J. and Kochevar, I. E. (1984) Degranulation of mast cells and inhibition of the response to secretory agents by phototoxic agents and ultraviolet radiation. *Toxicol. Appl. Pharmacol.* **76:** 374–382.
84. Przybilla, B., Schwab-Przybilla, U., Ruzicka, T. and Ring, J. (1987) Phototoxicity of non-steroidal anti-inflammatory drugs demonstrated *in vitro* by a photo–basophil–histamine-release test. *Photodermatology* **4:** 73–78.
85. McAuliffe, D. J., Morison, W. L. and Parrish, J. A. (1983) An *in vitro* test for predicting the photosensitizing potential (PSP) of various chemicals. *Altern. Methods Toxicol.* **1:** 287–307.
86. Anderson, R. and Eftychis, H. A. (1986) Potentiation of the generation of reactive oxidants by human phagocytes during exposure to benoxaprofen and ultraviolet radiation *in vitro*. *Br. J. Dermatol.* **115:** 285–295.

14

In Vitro Genotoxicity and Cell Transformation Assessment

IAN DE G. MITCHELL AND
ROBERT D. COMBES

I. Introduction 318
A. Objectives and scope 318
B. Genotoxicity 318
C. Genotoxicity testing rationale 320
D. History 320
E. Test battery concept 321
F. Guidelines, tests and regulatory requirements 321
G. Harmonization of guidelines 322
II. Test methodology 322
A. Generalizations 322
B. Current core tests 324
1. Bacterial tests for gene mutation 324
2. Mammalian cell tests for gene mutation 326
3. Mammalian cell tests for cytogenetic damage 328
4. New techniques for scoring chromosome aberrations 331
C. Supplementary genotoxicity tests 331
1. Structure–activity analysis 331
2. Tests for DNA damage 332
3. *In vitro* micronucleus test 335
4. Yeast tests for gene mutation, mitochondrial mutation, recombination and aneuploidy 335
5. Cell transformation 336
6. Human data (biomonitoring) 338
III. Potential new *in vitro* assays 338
A. Use of improved cell lines 338
1. New cell lines with targets 339
2. Cell lines with altered metabolizing potential 339
IV. Data analysis 339
A. Introduction 339
B. Assay validity 340
C. Do control and treated groups differ? 340
D. Is a response biologically important? 341
E. Data interpretation 342
V. Conclusions 344
References 345

IN VITRO METHODS IN PHARMACEUTICAL RESEARCH
ISBN 0-12-163390-X

I. INTRODUCTION

A. Objectives and scope

The main purpose of this chapter is to examine the role of *in vitro* methods in genotoxicity testing and to determine the relevance of the results obtained to the overall toxicological evaluation of pharmaceutical compounds. This objective will be achieved by indicating the principles underlying the core battery of *in vitro* genotoxicity assays used for regulatory purposes. Also information on several supplementary assays is described and advice given as to how these are utilized as adjuncts to the main tests, either for regulatory or in-house requirements. In addition, the relationship between genetic effects and cell transformation will be considered in terms of the end-points measured and inferences that may be drawn. Detailed protocols are not given here, but references are provided to where these have been described extensively in the published literature. However, principles of design, data collection and analysis are discussed in more detail.

B. Genotoxicity

Genotoxicity can be defined as toxic changes originating from effects on DNA. Such changes can arise via covalent binding of a chemical to DNA, leading to specific DNA base adducts, or by a physical alteration in DNA, for example nucleotide strand breakage. Intrinsic genotoxic chemicals, therefore, share the common property of being electrophilic, either directly or after some form of activation, thereby having the capacity to react with DNA, which is an intracellular nucleophile. Mutations can arise either directly from these lesions or may originate from errors in their repair. However, not all chemicals reacting with DNA prove eventually to be genotoxic. Some damage may be repaired in an error-free way. Other changes may be neutral in their effects or lethal (and hence unimportant to the organism at the frequency with which they usually occur). Furthermore, genotoxic changes can also arise indirectly, via interference with molecules or enzymes which are involved in DNA synthesis or chromosomal segregation (and these may not be electrophilic). The various possibilities are shown in Fig. 14.1. Genotoxins, therefore, are compounds that react either directly or indirectly with DNA to cause non-lethal, deleterious heritable changes in the structure, number or arrangement of genes. The specific types of lesion arising from these changes are shown in Fig. 14.2; gene mutations arising from changes in gene structure and chromosomal effects are indicative of changes in the arrangement or number of genes. When genotoxins react with DNA directly, the process is often, but not always, a single 'hit' stochastic process, whereby there is a finite chance of any interaction with DNA causing an effect. Alternatively, more than one 'hit' may be needed to produce an effect, either because of DNA error-free repair or because the effect on DNA is indirect via a target molecule with a high degree of redundancy. In such cases there will be a threshold response, below which there is no effect.

The potential ability of an agent to cause genotoxic changes should be testable in any organism or cell where DNA forms the basis of its inheritance. Unfortunately, this assumption ignores differences in the way organisms take up and metabolize (detoxify or activate) xenobiotics such as drugs. Many compounds are insufficiently reactive to be genotoxic without being first metabolized, especially by the cytochrome P450 mixed function oxidase (MFO) enzyme family present in many tissues, particularly the liver. Most

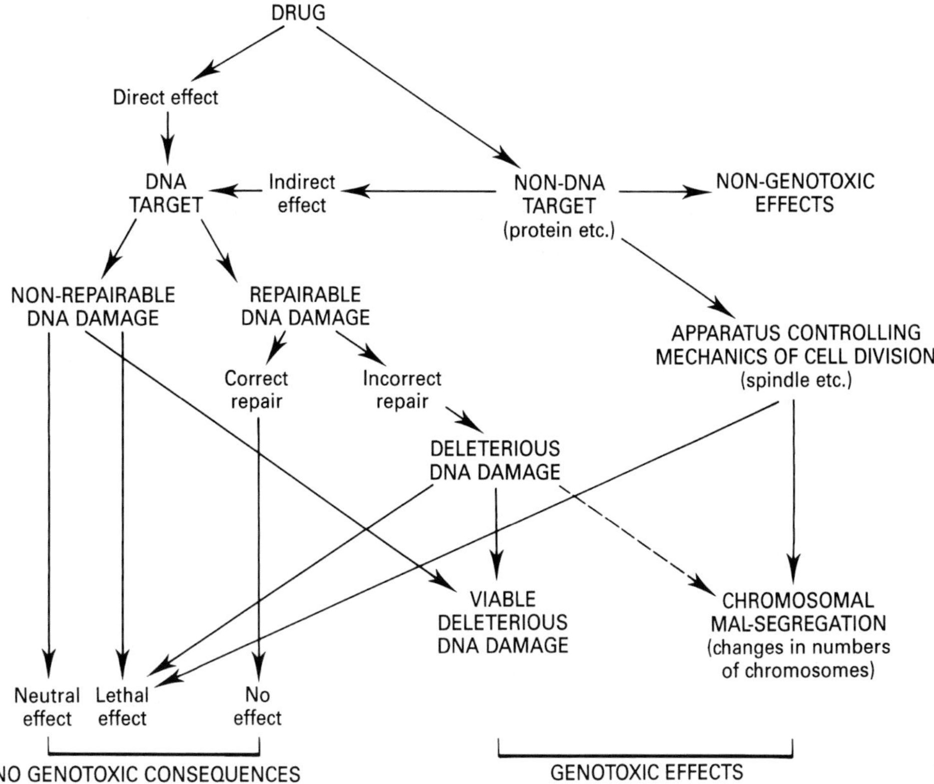

Fig. 14.1 Events leading to genotoxic responses.

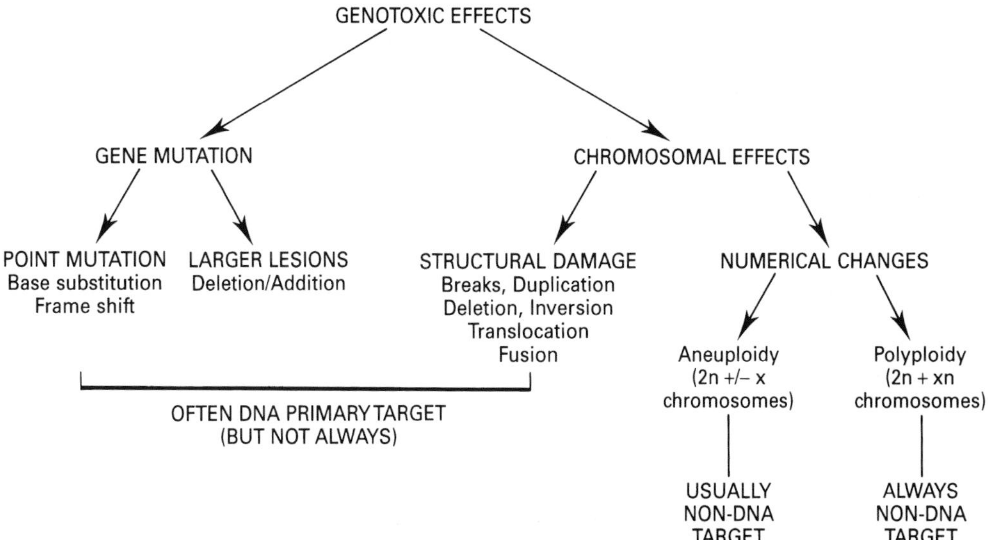

Fig. 14.2 Sub-divisions of genotoxic effects.

indicator cell lines used for *in vitro* genotoxicity assays lack much or all of this metabolizing capacity and it is necessary to use exogenous sources, the most common of which is a post-mitochondrial supernatant from enzyme-induced rat liver. It has become routine, therefore, to add mammalian liver homogenates and various co-factors to *in vitro* systems[1–6] to mimic mammalian phase I metabolism. However, interspecies differences in metabolism, the lack of phase II metabolism (usually detoxification) and the absence of the intracellular integration of these processes can all reduce the predictive value of *in vitro* assays.

The mechanistic relationship between mutation and carcinogenic processes has led to the universal adoption of mutagenicity assays to predict carcinogenicity, as mutations of oncogenes and tumour suppressor genes are involved in carcinogenesis.[7–9] As a result, genetic toxicology is now a major scientific discipline and has become an integral component of regulatory requirements, providing a rapid and relatively cheap way of screening large numbers of putative mutagens and carcinogens. Genotoxicity tests are the only *in vitro* assays that are currently part of routine regulatory packages. This is because the target molecule is known, unlike the situation in most other areas of toxicity testing.

C. Genotoxicity testing rationale

The importance of assays for genotoxicity goes well beyond its involvement in cancer. In almost any disease, where a single aberrant cell can lead eventually to a cascade of events and overt disease, there is the possibility of involvement of genotoxic changes. Furthermore, many of these diseases exhibit late onset, with the initiating insult separated from the appearance of the disease by many years. Activity in genotoxicity tests may, therefore, be the only warning of possible long-term toxic effects of a pharmaceutical compound. For example, genotoxic events seem likely to be involved in the aetiology of several somatic conditions including a component in the formation of cardiovascular disease via atherosclerotic plaques,[10,11] in autoimmune diseases,[12,13] in some slow neurodegenerative diseases[14–16] and in some diseases associated with mitochondrial defects.[17] In addition there is the possibility of inducing heritable disease. The original impetus for conducting genetic toxicology tests for regulatory purposes was the fear that genetic defects induced in germline cells of exposed parents would be inherited, causing a large increase in genetically defective individuals,[18] particularly from recessive genes. There has, however, been no evidence of an increase in heritable disease arising from exposure to any known environmental factor, so this aspect has declined in importance.

Thus, initially, most focus was directed at detecting germ cell mutagens. However, with the increasing realization of a mechanistic relationship between mutagenesis and somatic disease (particularly carcinogenesis), more attention has been paid to detecting somatic cell mutagens. There are, in fact, examples of chemicals whose tumorigenicity in rodents was demonstrated eventually, after being predicted by earlier positive genotoxicity assays.[19]

D. History

The discipline of genetic toxicology was developed in the late 1960s, even though demonstrations of the genetic effects of ionizing radiation and chemicals by Muller and Auerbach, respectively, had been made earlier.[20,21] Twenty-five years ago, extensive data on the histidine operon in the bacterium *Salmonella typhimurium* were obtained, and tester strains using this reversion system coupled with an exogenous mammallian oxidative metabolizing system[2] were developed for mutagenesis and carcinogenesis studies.[22,23] In the 1980s the basis of the science and its regulatory role received a setback when the correlation between genotoxicity and carcinogenicity was found to be considerably worse than initially supposed as a result of the National Cancer Institute/National Toxicology Program (NCI/NTP) and other trials.[24–26] However, this situation was restored by the realization of the existence of genotoxic and non-genotoxic carcinogens.[27,28] This restored faith in genotoxicity testing as surrogate assays for the 'important' (genotoxic) carcinogens, when coupled with an appreciation of the limitations of the rodent carcinogenicity bioassays.[29,30] With a more realistic appreciation of its advantages and limitations,[31] genotoxicity testing has now become a major scientific discipline.

E. Test battery concept

No test system can detect all genotoxins; all assays have significant blind spots. *In vitro* assays are also oversensitive and can generate positive results of no, or limited, relevance to the intact animal. This is probably because penetration to the target molecule is easier *in vitro* and exogenous mammalian oxidative metabolism is highly biased to activation (phase I metabolism[5]), and lacks the detoxification phases. Also, such assays are prone to oversensitivity as they: (a) lack mechanisms for transport of compounds and metabolites from the target site; (b) are not subject to immune responses; and (c) suffer from the possibility of spurious data due to the use of high test compound concentrations and other artefactual situations such as excessive toxicity and osmotic effects (see below). As a result there are very few *in vivo*-positive–*in vitro*-negative compounds.

The consequence of these observations is the tiered battery approach to testing. *In vitro* assays are used early on as they are quick and cheap, and negative data give a high degree of confidence in the safety from a genotoxic aspect. Less sensitive (insensitive) and more expensive animal assays are used later in testing, sometimes to confirm the *in vitro* negatives and sometimes to put in perspective *in vitro* positive data. Thus, *in vitro* assays are used for screening so that fewer compounds will need to be tested by the more time-consuming and costly *in vivo* methods.

F. Guidelines, tests and regulatory requirements

For the above reasons, guidelines for mutagenicity testing generally entail an initial *in vitro* screen comprising bacterial gene mutation and a test for chromosomal damage, in cultured mammalian cells.[32] The results from these *in vitro* assays are confirmed by further testing, using short-term, animal, *in vivo* protocols, usually in rodents,[33] and evolved from suggestions first proposed by Bridges.[34] The scheme described above covers the broad outline for regulatory testing for most countries. However, there are more than 100 potential genotoxicity tests[35] and regional differences exist in the exact nature of testing strategies and their deployment (see Aardema[36] for updated world-wide regulatory guidelines for all types of compounds). Importantly, requirements will vary almost on a case-by-case basis and will depend on the substance being tested, its intended usage and likely human exposure levels. For example, with new pharmaceuticals up to three or four tests can be required, comprising one for gene mutation in bacteria, one for gene mutation in mammalian cells *in vitro* and one for chromosomal effects in cultured mammalian cells, followed by cytogenetic analysis in rodent bone marrow.

G. Harmonization of guidelines

There has been considerable recent interest in harmonizing regulatory guidelines for genotoxicity testing.[37] Aspects of harmonization of genotoxicity test guidelines have been the subject of two recent reports: the International Workshop on Standardization of Genotoxicity Test Procedures (Melbourne, Australia, February 1993),[38] and the International Conference on Harmonization (ICH) of Technical Requirements for Registration of Pharmaceuticals for Human Use – Notes for Guidance on Specific Aspects of Regulatory Genotoxicity Tests.[39,40] These efforts follow earlier initiatives for pharmaceuticals.[41] Increased harmonization will reduce the numbers of animals used by lowering the need for repeat testing to satisfy more than one regulatory agency.

Although universal agreement on strategy and protocol design was rarely attained, there has been an increasing measure of consensus on these issues. The content of the core battery for pharmaceuticals and the timing of the tests plus their general principles are currently being defined by the ICH. They are recommendations, currently at the draft stage, and are intended to supersede all national guidelines. At the time of writing, it is uncertain whether two or three *in vitro* assays will be required before first human dosing. These are Ames (bacterial) tests plus *in vitro* cytogenetic and (probably) gene mutation assays in mammalian cells. If these tests are negative, an *in vivo* assay is needed before phase I (volunteers) or phase II (early clinical) trials can be conducted. With any *in vitro*-positive data, at least one more *in vivo* assay is needed, possibly with some extra *in vitro* supplementary tests to investigate the positive data. With any positive results it is prudent to ensure that the genotoxicity battery is complete before dosing to volunteers (see section on biomonitoring).

Recommended test methodologies are given in a whole series of national guidelines which define minimal criteria for the design, execution and interpretation of individual assays. These are written by professional bodies, such as the American Society for Testing of Materials[42] and the various environmental mutagen societies, for example the UK Environmental Mutagen Society.[43–46] Detailed background information and advice on protocols can be found in other diverse publications, especially Kilbey *et al.*[47] and Venitt and Parry.[48] Generally, methodologies given by the Organisation of Economic Cooperation and Development (OECD),[49] which are currently being updated (in draft at the time of writing) and the EEC[50] are based on expert recommendations of the professional bodies mentioned above. Also, it is useful to be aware of the Japanese requirements.[51,52] The most detailed sources are to be found in standard operating procedures (SOPs); a set of SOPs covering some commonly used mutagenicity tests has been published.[53] As stated above, only the outline methodology of tests will be given, with notes of useful modifications and critical factors for the proper conduct of a study, many of which are not published. Recently, a set of protocols has been published for some of the more commonly used genotoxicity assays.[54–57]

II. TEST METHODOLOGY

A. Generalizations

In vitro assays follow a straightforward general format (Fig. 14.3). Despite differing in detail, the outline and key points are similar throughout:

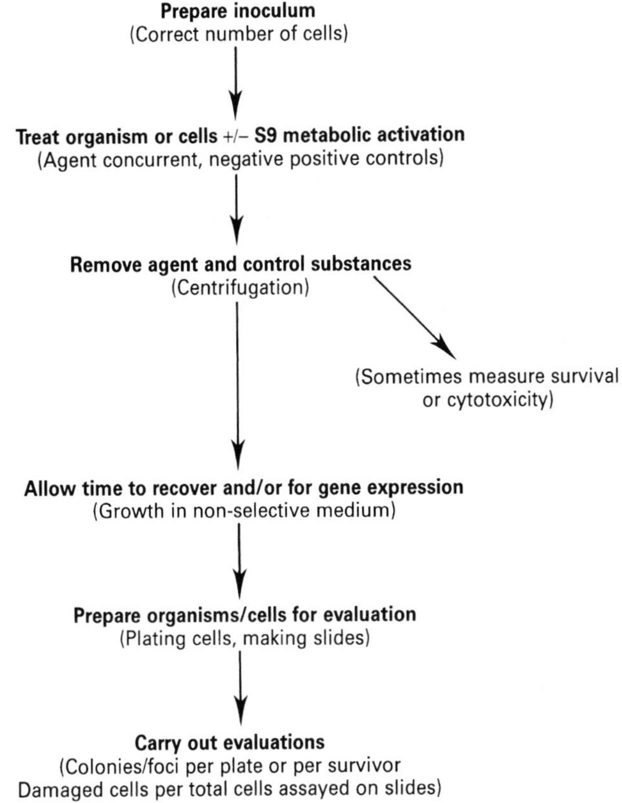

Fig. 14.3 Generalized methodology.

1. There must be the right number of cells or organisms in the inoculum: too few and the assay becomes variable; too many and the assay may become insensitive and difficult to score.
2. Treatments should be in low protein medium or suspension (to avoid binding and possible inactivation of the compound under test).
3. Extreme conditions of cytotoxicity, osmolality, pH and temperature, for example, must be avoided as such testing environments can often lead to artefactual positive results, particularly in mammalian cell cultures.[58–61]
4. Tests should have sufficient numbers of experimental units (e.g. plates, flasks or tubes) in each group, to allow assessment of within-test variability; absolute minimum two, ideally at least four.
5. At least three, and preferably five, concentrations spaced at about two- to threefold concentration intervals should be analysed. The highest concentration assayed should be limited by toxicity, solubility or the highest (limit) concentration recommended in guidelines, usually 5000 μg per ml or per plate.
6. Sufficient numbers of the measured end-point(s) (e.g. cells, colonies, foci, chromosomes) must be assessed, so that zero values are very rare for each experimental unit. Too few mutants per experimental unit will result in variable data. Ideally, values should exceed about 16 per group of (two or more) experimental units. However, once the number exceeds about 100, there is little increase in accuracy in scoring more cells.

7. Tester cells nearly always lack mammalian oxidative (phase 1) metabolic competence. Assays, therefore, usually must be conducted in the presence of an exogenous metabolizing system, normally S9 (as well as in its absence), to remedy this deficiency. However, S9 is toxic to cultured cells and treatments including it should not exceed 4–6 h.
8. Tests must include negative and positive controls, both with and without metabolic activation (S9) if used.
9. Assays should be repeated at least once (each on a separate occasion).
10. Literature references given in this chapter should be consulted for the experimental details of media, cell numbers, treatment time, recovery and expression time, as well as general incubation times.

It should be noted that there are some exceptions to the generalized methodology. In Ames (bacterial) agar plate methodology,[3] the treatment, recovery and selection phases are all combined on the agar plate, whereas in the rarely used bacterial fluctuation test[62] the underlying methodology differs markedly in concept.

B. Current core tests

1. *Bacterial tests for gene mutation*

Reverse mutation assay in Salmonella typhimurium *and* Escherichia coli The most commonly used strains are histidine-requiring auxotrophs of *S. typhimurium* and tryptophan-requiring auxotrophs of *E. coli*.

The principles of the test are as follows.[63] A high titre of exponentially growing auxotrophic cells of different tester strains, sensitive to reversion by induction of base-pair, frame shift and suppressor mutations (particularly for *E. coli*) are each exposed to test compound with and without an exogenous metabolizing system (usually S9), and incubated on agar medium which permits only prototrophic revertants to form colonies on a background lawn of non-revertants. The numbers of prototrophic revertant colonies are counted as a measure of mutation (and also general toxicity as evidenced by a decline below control numbers). The extent of the background lawn of residual growth of non-revered bacterial cells is noted (checked microscopically if necessary), as a measure of general toxicity. Induced mutation by the test compound is assumed if there is a biologically significant increase in the number of colonies present on treated compared with concurrent controls. There should be a definite background lawn of growth present; evident reduction in extent of the lawn indicates a bactericidal effect, and may lead to spurious results. A flow diagram for typical test methodology is shown in Fig. 14.4.

The main experiment should be preceded by an initial toxicity test to define a range of test compound concentrations for use in the main test. It is important for the top dose level to be the highest one that is possible, limited by toxicity, solubility or is the limit concentration recommended in regulatory guidelines (5000 μg per plate). Other important points are the general ones cited under the Data Analysis section and:

1. All testing procedures should be conducted in controlled lighting as certain compounds can be photoactivated and also certain light sources are themselves mutagenic.

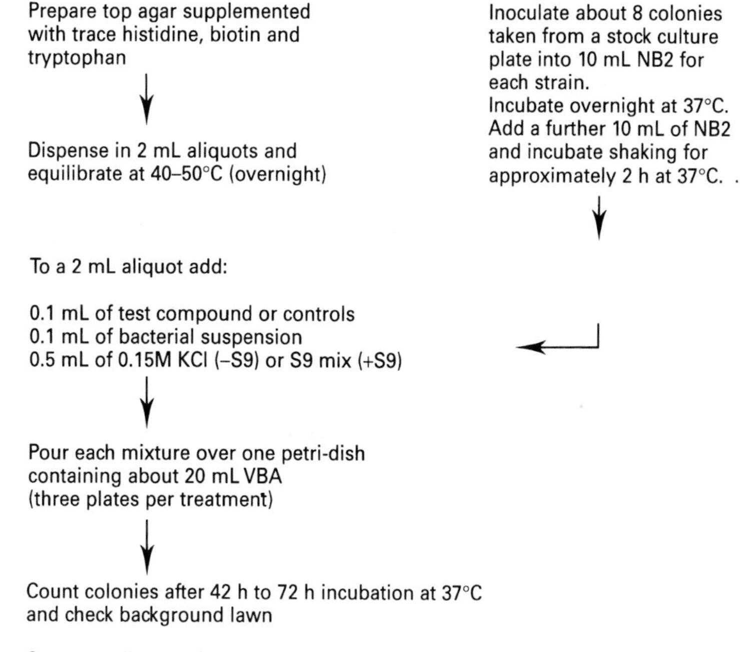

Fig. 14.4 Agar plate assay with *Salmonella typhimurium* (histidine reversion) and *Escherichia coli* (tryptophan reversion).

2. Extremely toxic levels giving no or very thin lawns can result in an increase in auxotrophic (non-mutant) macrocolonies. These toxic levels should be avoided. When in doubt the macrocolonies can be tested for growth (prototrophic mutant) or lack of growth (auxotrophic non-mutant) on histidine-deficient medium.
3. A quick assessment of data can be made using the fold-increase approach in which a dose level is considered to be mutagenic if it results in a two- to threefold, or greater, increase in the revertant count, compared with the negative control. Where high numbers of spontaneous colonies are recovered (e.g. with tester strains TA100, 102 and 104) the necessary fold increase for a positive effect can be lower.
4. Protocols appropriate for the physicochemical properties of the test material should be employed. For example, protocols for testing vapours and gases are given in the published recommendations cited above.

In summary, interpretation of Ames plates should be undertaken according to the general strategy as follows:

(a) For acceptance of data, spontaneous counts could fall within recommended and laboratory historical ranges.
(b) Positive control counts must be at least three times the vehicle control counts.
(c) There must be four or more dose levels with no significant toxicity and two or more plates uncontaminated for each dose level.
(d) For a clear negative result, mean plate counts must be less than 1.5-fold those for the concurrent vehicle control (some prefer not to use a lower limit and apply statistical analysis to any value over control) and for a clear positive result the mean plate counts should be at least threefold the concurrent vehicle counts.

(e) For equivocal results (e.g. increases over control between 1.5- and threefold) the strategy in the Data Analysis section should be followed.

Critical protocol factors for the *Salmonella* assay are discussed by Gatehouse[64] and Gatehouse *et al.*[63] Some of these affect the results obtained only quantitatively, while others change the outcome of a test in a qualitative way.

Protocol and genetic system variations The standard test can be conducted using several modifications to the protocol to increase the sensitivity of the assay to certain mutagens. Such variations include liquid preincubation, and treat-and-plate protocols, the fluctuation and host-mediated assays, as well as the use of different S9/co-factors, strains and genetic systems, such as forward mutation systems to avoid feeding effects.[32,63,65–67]

Prescreening for Salmonella *mutagenicity* During early stages of pharmaceutical development, it is likely that only very small quantities of several candidate compounds will be available. It may be advantageous to have mutagenicity date to aid compound selection and to identify any potentially active impurities. Such data must, however, be used with extreme caution; compounds should almost never be rejected simply on the basis of bacterial mutagenicity data. For prescreening in-house, the emphasis is on identifying activity using rapid, sensitive protocols, reduced in size (from those needed for regulatory purposes) to take account of the small amounts of material that may be available. It is also important to have details of test material chemical structure and sample characteristics, such as likely contaminants, to facilitate the design of the reduced protocol and choice of tester strains. A typical reduced Ames test might consist of the two strains with the broadest specificity, e.g. TA100 and TA98 (with and without S9), with assays done only once using two plates per concentration. Assuming a top dose level of 5 mg per plate, three dose levels (+/− S9), two plates per dose, a preliminary toxicity assay (one strain and one plate per dose) test, the minimum total quantities of test material required would be only 100 mg compared with about 1.5 g for a regulatory test. Published methods for industrial prescreening include the use of the gradient plate assay.[68]

2. *Mammalian cell tests for gene mutation*

Gene mutations can be assayed in cultured mammalian cells, and several genetic systems and cell assays are available; the principal ones[69] are outlined below.

Forward mutation in mouse lymphoma L5178Y cultures at the thymidine kinase locus (clone 3.7.2.C $TK^{+/-}$ cells) In this assay,[70,71] exponentially growing $TK^{+/-}$ cells (heterozygous at the thymidine kinase (tk) locus) are used. These are sensitive to the toxic nucleoside base analogue, trifluorothymidine (TFT), as a result of its cellular uptake followed by conversion to the toxic monophosphate by thymidine kinase. Cells are exposed to test compound with or without an exogenous metabolizing system, followed by an incubation period to allow expression of any forward mutations to give homozygous $TK^{-/-}$ cells which can divide to form TFT-resistant colonies, $TK^{-/-}$ cells remain viable by synthesizing thymidine phosphates de novo (by an alternative pathway). Colonies resistant to TFT are counted to evaluate mutation. Colonies arising in the absence of TFT are also counted to determine survival. These data are used to calculate mutant frequency (MF: number of mutant colonies per 10^x survivors, where $x = 5$–7). In the standard suspension assay method, cell treatment and expression of mutations occurs in liquid culture before plating into soft agar, and toxicity is determined by measuring cloning efficiency and suspension growth (expressed as relative total growth (RTG)). A significant increase in MF over vehicle control, in the absence of excessive lowering of RTG (to below about 10%) is taken as evidence of mutagenesis. A standard protocol is shown in Fig. 14.5. Note the flask, not the dish, is the experimental unit for statistical analysis. (This methodology can also be used for assessing HGPRT mutation (see next section) by increasing cell numbers about fivefold and selecting on 6-TG agar.)

Various modified protocols have been produced, including the microwell or fluctuation assay[69] and the *in situ* method[72] in which cells are plated into soft agar immediately after treatment and centrifugation, so that mutants are immobilized, and are not diluted out during gene expression. Small and large colony variants arise, due to differing growth rates of various mutants. There is evidence at the molecular level that small colonies result from

Mammalian Cell Mutation Assay at the Thymidine Kinase Gene Locus of L5178Y TK +/– Mouse Lymphoma Cells

Day 0 Centrifuge, at 280 g for 5 min, exponentially growing cells and resuspend, at a concentration of 1×10^6 cells per mL, in medium consisting of 50% conditioned medium and 50%* ROP.

↓

Distribute 6 mL of cell suspension to each treatment tube and 4 mL of S9 mix or ROP to the appropriate cultures. This gives a cell concentration of 6×10^5 per mL.

↓

Add 100 μL solvent control, treatment solution or positive control to the appropriate cultures from 100-fold concentrated stock solutions.

↓

Incubate for 4 hours at 37°C in a shaking water bath/roller incubator.

↓

Centrifuge cells from each culture, wash twice in R10P and resuspend in 20 mL of R10P+ to give a cell concentration of 3×10^5 per mL. Incubate at 37°C.

↓

Day 1 Adjust cells to 3×10^5 per mL by taking cell counts and replacing appropriate volume of cell culture with fresh medium. Incubate at 37°C for approximately 24 hours.

↓

Day 2 Count cells and adjust to 5×10^5 per mL in preparation for cloning.

Dilute cells 0.1 mL into 10 mL R10P# Add 40 μL (200 cells) to each of three 100 mm Petri dishes. Add 25 mL of cloning medium containing molten 0.25% BBL agar to each Petri dish. Cool at room temperature for 30 minutes then place dishes into a 5% CO_2 incubator at 37°C.

In subdued lighting. Add 1 mL of cells to each of three 100 mm Petri dishes. Add 24 mL of cloning medium containing molten 0.25% BBL agar and 4 μg/mL TFT to each Petri dish. Cool at room temperature for 30 minutes then place dishes in a 5% CO_2 incubator at 37°C.

Colonies are counted when they have reached sufficient size.

Cells may be left for 20–30 minutes at this stage to acclimatise.
* ROP = RPMI 1640 medium without horse serum
+ RIOP = as ROP plus 10% horse serum

Fig. 14.5 Mammalian cell mutation assay at the thymidine kinase gene locus of L5178Y TK +/– mouse lymphoma cells.

chromosomal damage, and that gene mutations give large colonies[73] but this distinction is not absolute.[74] Nevertheless, as some compounds induce predominantly one type of colony, it is important to use conditions optimal for the recovery and enumeration of all colonies.[75] The assay has been criticized for generating positive results for compounds negative for rodent carcinogenicity. However, in terms of genotoxicity, it is sensitive to agents inducing a wide spectrum of genetic damage and, when conducted well, does not give rise to many unique (false) positives.

Other mammalian gene mutation systems One of the other, most widely used, tests is the sex-linked HGPRT mutation assay in the male Chinese hamster ovary (CHO) or fibroblasts (V79) cell lines.[69] These cells are hemizygous (single gene copy) for the hypoxanthine–guanine–phosphoribosyl–transferase locus ($HGPRT^{+}$), and therefore are sensitive to the toxic effects of the base analogue, 6-thioguanine (6-TG), owing to its cellular uptake and conversion to the toxic monophosphate. After treatment, with and without a metabolizing system, any cells undergoing forward mutation to $HGPRT^{-}$ (recessive mutant) remain viable, because guanine phosphates are synthesized by an alternative pathway *de novo*. After incubation, such mutated cells give rise to 6-TG-resistant colonies to provide a measure of mutation, while colonies arising in the absence of 6-TG give an indication of overall survival. Surviving cells and 6-TG^{r} colonies are counted to give the proportion of mutants (MF), as in the mouse lymphoma TK+/− assay. Both treatment and expression phases of the assay can be performed with cells in suspension, or as monolayers. Metabolic cooperation between cells can arise using the monolayer assay, via the passage through intercellular gap junctions from 6-TG sensitive into 6-TG^{r} cells, thereby reducing the numbers of mutant cells arising and complicating data interpretation.[76] The key disadvantage of this assay is the low spontaneous frequency of mutation at the HGPRT locus, so that it is almost impossible to start with enough cells in the inoculum. As a consequence the assay is very variable and insensitive.

A further mammalian cell gene mutation assay, the AS52/XPRT system, is undergoing evaluation as an alternative to both of the above assays; it has the increased sensitivity of the L5178Y assay, apparently without some of its complications.[77]

3. *Mammalian cell tests for cytogenetic damage*

In vitro cytogenetic regulatory assays involve analysing cells at metaphase, and can be subdivided into tests using permanent cell lines, usually derived from Chinese hamsters e.g. ovary CHO and lung (CHL) cell lines, and those using primary cells usually of human origin (e.g. lymphocytes). It is uncertain which cell type is best.[78] Treatment can be either in suspension culture (using tubes or flasks) or on slides or coverslips in dishes. It should be noted that the culture vessel or dish is the experimental unit for statistical purposes, and not the individual slides prepared for microscopy.

The use of Chinese hamster cell lines makes culturing easier and quicker, and scoring only 22 chromosomes per cell is much simpler than dealing with 46 (as in the case of human lymphocytes). However, Chinese hamster cell lines are usually karyotypically unstable, having a modal chromosome content, whereas human cells are stable and likely to be more relevant when extrapolating to humans, e.g. for thresholds or no-effect levels. Such considerations do not matter so much for assessing chromosomal structure damage, but are crucial in assessing the relevance of polyploidy to safety.

Detailed methodologies for Chinese hamster cell lines and human lymphocytes are given in several publications[59,79–81] and are outlined in Figs 14.6 and 14.7. It is important to

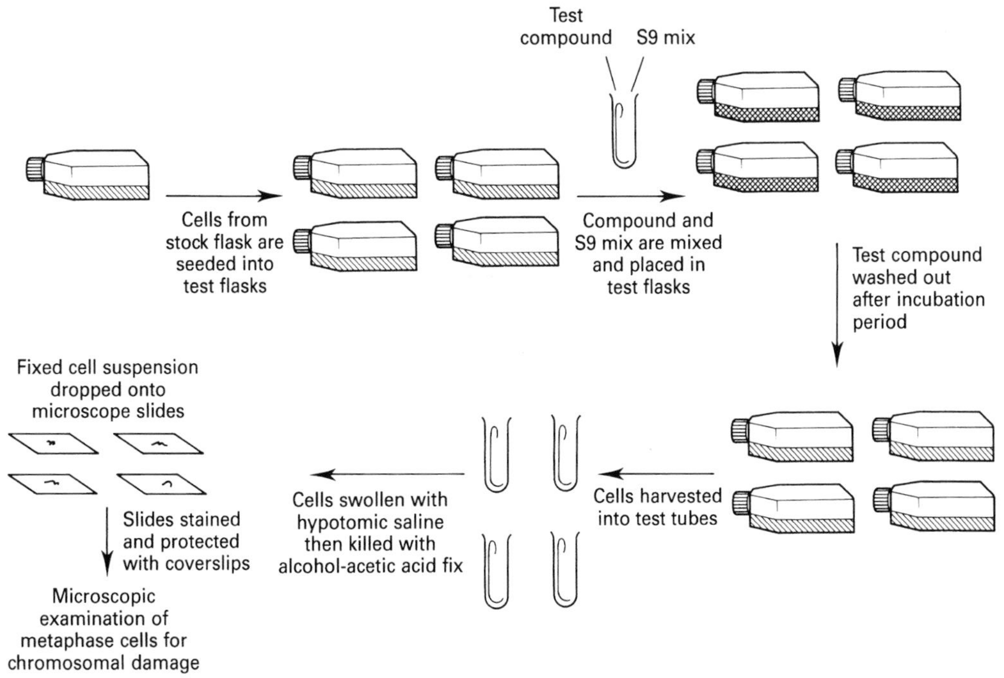

Fig. 14.6 Chromosomal aberration assay with Chinese hamster ovary cells in vitro.

understand that cells have to undergo DNA replication in order for chemically induced DNA lesions to be manifested as chromosome damage leading to aberrations, micronuclei or sister chromatid exchanges. Methods are based on exposing dividing cells to test agent (with or without S9), culturing for about 1.5 cell cycles, and then treating with a spindle inhibitor (colcemid or colchicine) to accumulate cells in metaphase. Cells are harvested (by trypsinization to detach and separate them into suspension for slide or coverslip methodology), swelled in hypotonic saline, fixed in alcohol–acetic acid, concentration by centrifugation, stained and scored under the light microscope for both structural and numerical aberrations[59] (Fig. 14.6). Important features of these assays are detailed in the Generalizations section of Test methodology. In addition:

(a) Normally three (or more) concentrations are tested; the highest should give more than 50% inhibition of the mitotic index (MI; proportion of cells in division), and/or decrease of some other measure of inhibition of cell growth, or increased mortality. (Alternatively, solubility may limit the top concentration, or a limit concentration set by guidelines may be used.)

(b) Cells should be sampled about 1.5 cell cycles after the start of treatment; ideally the cell cycle time should be checked in each experiment, but in practice a value determined at 'some time' in the testing laboratory will do. Calculation of cell cycle is usually by bromodeoxyuridine (BUdR) incorporation,[82] but this is more complex than might be expected.[83]

The following end-points are scored: (a) the total aberrations per cell; and (b) the frequency of aberrant cells (excluding accessory data). A statistically significant increase in (b) over concurrent vehicle control values is assumed to indicate **cytogenetic activity of the**

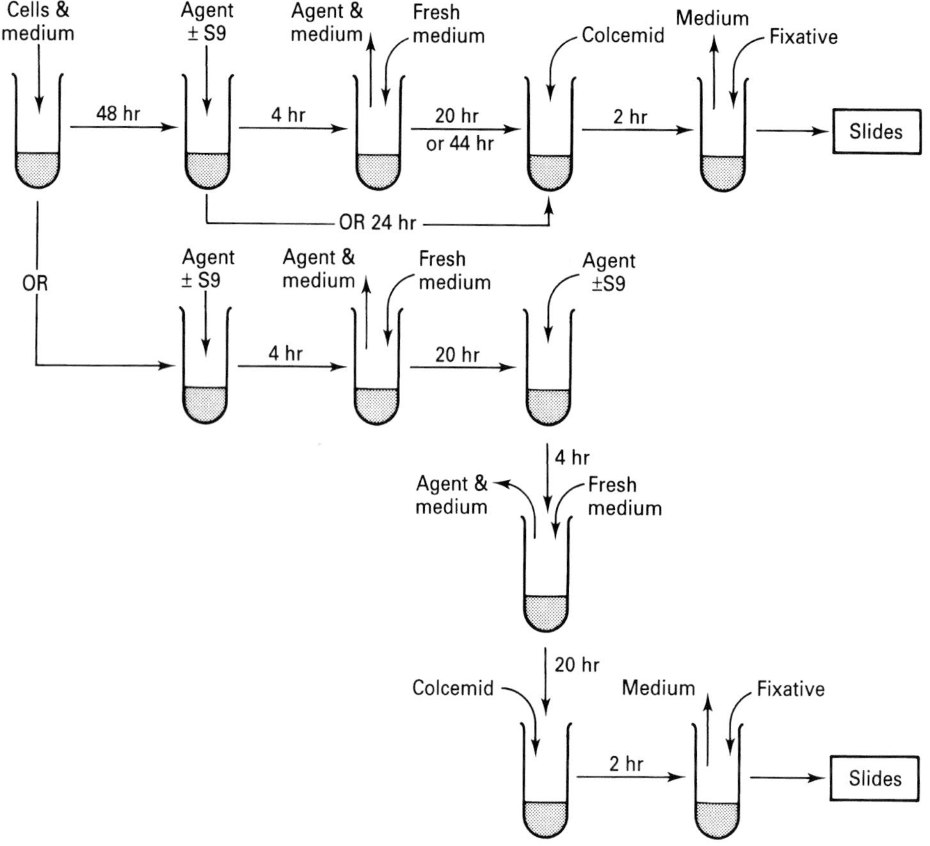

Fig. 14.7 Variations in lymphocyte metaphase analysis.

test compound, unless effects are found only at highly toxic concentrations. The following extra points should be noted:

1. It is debatable whether a late sampling after three or four cell cycles is needed. Evidence is sparse and may well depend on what cell type and agents are being used.[84] Current opinion (International Conference of Harmonisation) seems to be inclined towards using only the earlier (1.5) cell cycle time (usually about 20–24 h after treatment initiation).
2. It should be noted that most of the recommended methods for scoring aberrations are similar, a key difference being the differentiation of gaps and breaks. All recommended methods suggest that a discontinuity in a chromosome of more than one chromatid width is needed to upgrade a gap to a break. Most recommendations[59] require evidence of displacement as well. We think this is an added, unnecessary complication and favour basing the difference simply on size of discontinuity.[85] The reason for the concern about gaps is that they can be due merely to reversals in the coiling arrangement of chromatin, rather than to a discrete discontinuity in the chromosome with potential genetic consequences.
3. Ideally at least 200 metaphases per treatment or control should be analysed for structural damage to chromosomes (breaks in chromosomes and chromatids, interchanges, dicentrics, ring chromosomes and fragments), scored and recorded. It is also useful to score as accessory data, gaps and, where possible (primary cells only),

polyploidy should be assessed by scanning 2000 metaphases. Hyperdiploidy (cells with a chromosome number exceeding the normal diploid complement) and hypodiploidy (cells with a chromosome number less than the normal diploid complement) can be scored as markers of aneuploidy (loss or gain of chromosomes). However, hypodiploidy, in particular, can be caused by technical artefacts, so the results should be used as accessory data only.

4. During statistical analysis, to avoid the serious problem of an excessive number of comparisons (see Data analysis section), it is preferable to combine all structural damage (excluding accessory data), and to express the results as numbers of cells with or without structural damage. Although some guidelines suggest that analysis should be performed both including and excluding accessory data, we recommend that accessory data should normally be excluded to avoid confusion. Polyploidy (whole number multiples of the basic, normal chromosome complement) occurring at or near therapeutic levels should be analysed as a separate end-point, and treated as an important (not accessory) lesion.[86]
5. To increase the power of the analysis, it is useful to perform duplicate negative controls.

4. *New techniques for scoring chromosome aberrations*

In recent years, substantial improvements have been made to facilitate traditional light microscope methods for scoring chromosomal damage. These include application of fluorescence *in situ* hybridization (FISH) and image analysis[87,88] to permit automation and increased speed of scoring. FISH[89,90] involves preparing single-stranded nucleic acid sequences of interest which are labelled with fluorochrome conjugated 'reporter' molecules and then used as probes by reannealing them with denatured regions of the chromosome with complementary base sequences immobilized on a microscope slide. After incubation, fluorescent signals are visible as fluorescing dots at any sites of probe hybridization against a total DNA background. The process of localizing and highlighting specifically any region of the chromosome or the entire genome in this way is known as 'chromosome painting'. Also, centromeric probes can be used for rapid detection of chromosomes lacking centromeres, and whole chromosome paints can be prepared to facilitate detection of numerical aberrations.

C. Supplementary genotoxicity tests

1. *Structure–activity analysis*

There are several ways of looking at the structure of a molecule to assess whether it is likely to be genotoxic and/or carcinogenic. Strictly these are not *in vitro* methods but are included as non-animal techniques. Methods include pattern recognition, where certain aspects of chemical structure are known to be indicative of genotoxicity or carcinogenicity,[91] and this principle has been used to construct a rule-based computer program, DEREK.[92] DEREK is a knowledge-based expert system, and several mutagenicity rules have been written.[93] Automated rule-induction systems also exist, where molecules are dismantled into fragments and the frequency with which such fragments occur in genotoxic and inactive molecules is determined. An example is the computer-aided structural evaluation program, CASE.[94,95] Alternative systems based on the use of physicochemical parameters (e.g. octanol–water partition coefficient) and molecular orbital considerations[96–98] have been used, as well as systems based on likely metabolism due to interaction with specific isozymes of cytochrome P450.[99,100]

When used on their own these systems have limited prospective predictivity for genotoxicity, although there are signs that using them in combination with other approaches and tests may prove useful.[101,102] In particular, a CASE structural analysis system combined with computerized assessment of physicochemical and molecular orbital parameters, and with a metabolic assessment program built in, should be a significant advance. Such a system is being developed in Klopman's laboratory (personal communication). These systems are discussed in detail by Combes and Judson.[103]

2. *Tests for DNA damage*

Interaction with DNA (adduction), can be measured directly using several molecular techniques, while indirect methods are available for detecting the consequences of such interaction in terms of stimulation of DNA strand breakage or DNA repair synthesis.

Direct tests for DNA damage

Molecular techniques DNA damage, in the form of covalently bound adducts, can be measured in any cell capable of division. Moreover, the repair of such adducts can be monitored by analysing cellular DNA at different post-exposure times. Procedures for monitoring DNA adduction are divisible into those suitable for quantification of adducts and those designed to permit adduct characterization.[104] DNA binding requires the use of radioactive test compound,[105] which is often available during the early stages of pharmaceutical testing. However, association of radiolabel with extracted DNA can be due to metabolic recycling and incorporation via the nucleotide pool. Thus, it is necessary to demonstrate the presence of adducts with chromatography – a time-consuming process. DNA adduction can be demonstrated without radiolabelled test material by using the technique of ^{32}P post-labelling, summarized below.

After exposure, DNA is isolated, purified and enzymatically digested into its constituent nucleoside 3′-monophosphates. These are converted into 5′ ^{32}P-labelled biphosphates (phosphorylation) by reaction with gamma [^{32}P]ATP and T4 polynucleotide kinase. The normal and adducted nucleosides are separated by multidirectional anion exchange thin layer chromatography (TLC) on polyethyleneimine cellulose plates. Modified adducted bases are detected as extra spots on autoradiograms of the TLC plates, and are quantified by Czerenkov counting using scintillation or densitometry. Adduct levels are related to the total number of nucleotides. Various methods have been tried to enhance assay sensitivity, after enrichment of adducts by butanol extraction or nuclease P1 treatment, and by separating adducts using high-performance liquid chromatography. Background levels of endogenous adducts (I compounds) present in DNA from untreated cells must be defined and taken into account when interpreting data. Some modifications to the methodology have extended the range of bulky and non-bulky adducts detectable. Nevertheless, because the assay is sensitive, problems in interpreting autoradiograms can arise. Another disadvantage of the assay is that it is necessary to use relatively high levels of β-emitting ^{32}P. The post-labelling technique can be useful for establishing mechanisms of weak and unexpected genotoxicity, seen with conventional assays, for example induction of DNA adducts in cultured mammalian cell to facilitate interpretation of mutagenicity data.[106] However, it should be noted that the method is not suitable for the detection of all adducts, particularly small ones e.g. crucially, methyl adducts from alkylation.

Limited identification of adducts can be achieved with the above approach. However, they also can be characterized by means of analytical chemistry and immunoassay with polyclonal and monoclonal antibodies.[107,108] These molecular techniques are extremely sensitive, with detection levels varying from 1 in 10^6 to 1 in 10^{10} nucleosides. Only very small amounts of DNA are required and adduction can be determined in any tissue.

DNA strand breaks can be measured in individual mammalian cells using microgel electrophoresis single cell gel electrophoresis (SCGE),[109] by embedding them in agarose gel on a microscope slide and subjecting them to detergent and high salt concentration lysis under alkaline conditions, causing nucleotide strand unwinding for single-strand breaks, or neutral conditions, for double-strand breaks. The DNA is electrophoresed and damage is scored by measuring the distance of migration from the cell nucleus to the anode after ethidium bromide staining and fluorescence determination. Distinct tails are seen and the technique is referred to as the 'comet assay'. This sensitive technique is being evaluated for its use in genotoxicity testing, and has the potential of a highly sensitive, cheap and rapid way of directly detecting DNA damage. The problem is that cytotoxicity and cell death can cause the production of 'comets' via indirect damage of DNA, thereby confounding interpretation of positive data.

Indirect tests for DNA damage Stimulation of DNA repair can be measured, either by the increased susceptibility to toxicity of repair-deficient strains compared with their otherwise isogenic repair-proficient parent cells, or by detecting and quantifying some stage of repair, such as unscheduled DNA synthesis (UDS) or the presumed intermediate consequences of DNA strand breakage – sister chromatid exchange (SCE).

Microbial tests for DNA repair: In these tests, DNA damage is detected by measuring differential growth inhibition of repair-proficient and -deficient strains in the presence of a putative genotoxin. This method has been used in microorganisms, especially bacteria[110] with strains of *E. coli* and *Bacillus subtilis* (e.g. rec^- or pol^- assays), and less frequently in fungi, such as yeast. The principle of the test is as follows. Concentrations of test compound causing DNA damage, which is reparable in a repair-proficient strain surviving the exposure, will be lethal to cells of a repair-deficient strain, which is unable to repair the damage. This assumes the latter strain is otherwise genetically identical (isogenic). Differential toxicity, manifested as either zones of inhibition on agar or growth in liquid culture, is expressed as the relative survival of the respective strains. Significantly greater toxicity to a repair-deficient strain, under the same exposure conditions and number of DNA replications, is taken as evidence of induction of DNA repair.

The major protocols used for the assay involve either agar diffusion (with zones of inhibition measured) or liquid suspension (with growth measured either with a vital dye or by colony counting). Careful use of positive and negative controls is required. Negative results may be due to lack of agar diffusion of test compound, and therefore absence of toxicity to either strain should be scored as 'no test'. Some promutagens have been found to be positive without the need for S9, particularly in the *B. subtilis* assay, although better results have been obtained with a modified spore assay.[111] This approach is particularly suitable for testing toxic compounds, because it relies on differential toxicity as an end-point and allows a distinction to be made between toxicity due to both genotoxic and other mechanisms. The main difficulty is ensuring that strains are isogenic and that the repair deficiency does not make the bacteria more susceptible to cytotoxic as well as genotoxic effects.

Unscheduled DNA synthesis: UDS occurs when DNA damage results in repair DNA synthesis. This usually involves excision of a small portion of a nucleotide strand bearing the lesion followed by filling of the gap (by DNA polymerase) and ligation. UDS can be measured in a variety of mammalian cell types, such as rodent hepatocytes, HeLa cells and lymphocytes.[112] The principle of the assay is as follows.

DNA repair synthesis, occurring in non-replicating cells as a result of induction of DNA damage, is measured by autoradiography or scintillation counting of incorporated tritiated thymidine. Silver grains over the cytoplasm are subtracted from those over the nucleus in the former method, giving numbers of net nuclear grains (NNGs). The mean NNG count, and the proportion of cells in repair ($NNG > 5$) in treated cells, is compared with that in cells from concurrent negative control cultures. With the exception of metabolically competent primary hepatocytes, it is necessary to add an exogenous metabolizing system to cultures of cells, but promutagens should always be included as positive controls. UDS should be distinguished from scheduled DNA, or S phase, synthesis (SDS) resulting from bulk replication, which occurs at cell division. Therefore, where possible, autoradiography is preferable to scintillation counting (unless it is possible totally to eliminate SDS). However, with autoradiography it is important not to score disrupted cells, where cytoplasmic loss can give spuriously low grain counts.

Sister chromatid exchange: DNA repair also can lead to strand breaks which result in cytogenetic effects such as SCEs. These arise as a result of intrachromosomal events involving symmetrical exchanges occurring along the chromosome by some, as yet obscure, mechanism. SCEs can be detected in mammalian cells, for example lymphocytes, CHO cells, or any dividing cells. The principles of the test are as follows. Treated cells undergo two divisions with the thymidine analogue bromodeoxyuridine (BUdR). During the first division, one of the two DNA chains of each chromatid becomes labelled, and after the second division two chains of one chromatid are labelled, while only one chain of its sister chromatid is labelled. Chromosome preparations are then stained, most commonly with the fluorescent stain Hoechst 33258 and Giemsa. DNA which is substituted with BUdR in both strands is poorly stained by Giemsa and appears light under the microscope, whereas DNA substituted in one strand is darker. During the repair of lesions at replication it is thought that chromatids exchange fragments of duplex DNA, thereby giving alternate switches of light and dark staining along the chromatids (SCE). Various parameters that can be measured include the numbers of SCEs per chromosome and per cell. The former measure is considered to be a more accurate indication of the amount of DNA damage. For a positive result there should be a statistical increase in SCEs relative to vehicle controls observed in 30–50 cells per culture. BUdR concentration and the treatment time can be varied to improve detection of SCEs. Although it is thought that the formation of SCEs is unlikely to have any direct genetic consequence, they are considered indicative of cytogenetic damage due to strand breakage and DNA repair, and the assay has proved useful for biomonitoring human exposure. SCEs are easier to identify than aberrations, although their visualization requires a more complicated procedure than that necessary to detect structural aberrations. SCEs occur more frequently than structural aberrations after treatment with low concentrations of a wide range of chemicals, especially those causing DNA adducts. However, certain clastogens are unable to induce SCEs. Although the formation of exchanges relies on the presence of a lesion at replication, and this mitigates against their formation in G0 (resting lymphocytes), SCE analysis of peripheral lymphocytes is likely to continue to be a widely used method of biomonitoring.[113]

3. In vitro *micronucleus test*

The rodent *in vivo* bone marrow micronucleus assay forms a major component of regulatory genotoxicity testing schemes. In recent years, there has been interest in developing *in vitro* micronucleus assays to supersede the more technically demanding metaphase analysis methods. An appropriate protocol has yet to be developed,[114] although the assay works well in certain laboratories using human lymphocytes and should prove useful under certain circumstances, particularly for identifying aneugens for which there is no currently acceptable assay.[115]

A micronucleus comprises a portion of chromatin surrounded by a separate nuclear membrane which arises either by condensation of acentric chromosomes that remain separate at anaphase due to their inability to attach to the spindle at cell division, or by exclusion of intact centric chromosomes from anaphase segregation, for example as a consequence of centromere malfunction or spindle disruption. Therefore, micronuclei represent the disruption of small amounts of decondensed chromatin, each micronucleus surrounded by its own nuclear membrane and maintained separately from the nucleus. Thus, the existence of raised numbers of micronuclei is evidence of prior induction of structural chromosome damage or of changes in chromosome number.

Numbers of micronucleated cells are scored, using a variety of staining methods (e.g. May–Grünwald). Cytochalasin B has been used to accumulate binucleate cells, thereby helping to ensure that micronuclei are scored in cells that have divided just once after exposure.[116] The two types of micronuclei that are produced (those containing whole chromosomes and those with chromosomal fragments) can be distinguished cytologically by means of centromeric antibody markers.[117] If the centromeric kinetochore is undamaged, centromeres stain positively with fluorescently labelled anti-kinetochore antibodies, whereas chromosomal fragments lacking a kinetochore are not stained. If necessary, anti-kinetochore antibody staining data can be confirmed by using other techniques such as *in situ* hybridization with centromeric DNA probes. Thus, by distinguishing kinetochore-positive and -negative micronuclei, it is possible to score chemically induced clastogenic and aneugenic events separately. This is because chromosomal breakage often produces micronuclei lacking centromeres and associated kinetochores, whereas aneugenesis always results in centromere and kinetochore-positive micronuclei.

Although human lymphocyes are the commonest cells to which the *in vitro* micronucleus assay is applied, other cells have been used. Fritzenschaf *et al.*[118] observed that an assay involving the induction of micronuclei in cultured Syrian hamster embryo (SHE) cells using 75 chemicals gave 89% concordance with *in vivo* micronucleus data, when the same chemicals were used. Some investigators have used cultured L5178Y mouse lymphoma cells to assess genotoxicity by the induction of micronuclei.[119]

4. *Yeast tests for gene mutation, mitochondrial mutation, recombination and aneuploidy*

The unicellular microbe yeast provides several advantages for studying genetic toxicology compared with bacteria. First, several different genetic end-points can be measured, and it is easy to culture with a short generation time, as well as having stable haploid and diploid phases. Furthermore, the results obtained are likely to be more relevant to human hazard, than using bacteria, because yeasts have a eukaryotic cellular organization, including chromosomal organization of DNA as well as cytochrome P450-mediated metabolism. Although yeast cells have endogenous activation capacity, this is relatively low and varies with cell cycle, so that addition of S9 to tests may be necessary. Yeast assays are not widely used despite these advantages, and the main use has been as an alternative to bacterial assays for antibiotics.

The most useful tests in yeast have been described in detail by Zimmermann *et al*[120] and Brooks *et al.*[121] Therefore, the methods will not be described in detail but certain key factors will be highlighted. Most assays are in *Saccharomyces cerevisiae*, with *Schizosaccharomyces pombe* as a rare alternative. Treat-and-plate methodology (as described in the General section and see Fig. 14.3), is nearly always used, with end-points being enumeration of protrophic revertant colonies or toxin-resistant colonies. Occasionally non-selected (recombinant) colonies are assessed. Gene mutation can be assayed in *S. cerevisiae* using either reverse or forward mutation systems. In general, the forward mutation assays are of more use than reverse mutation. Workable methodology and expected spontaneous frequency data are given by Mehta and Von Borstel[122] for reverse mutation in a multiply marked strain, and by Mitchell and Gilbert[123] for forward mutation at three loci (*can, ada* and *cyh*).

S. cerevisiae is the only organism in which mitochondrial mutation or deletion can be measured easily, because it can survive without mitochondria. As a consequence, mitochondrial mutation (rho^-) or deletion (rho^0) can be detected as small (petite) colony phenotype, although doubts have been expressed about the relevance of such mutations to genotoxicity. Some protagonists[124] claim that the induction of petite mutants is relevant for predicting carcinogenicity. However, it seems that the relevance of mitochondrial mutation in yeast is more likely to be associated with some of the known human diseases caused by mitochondrial defects[17] and possibly associated with ageing.

Recombination (exchange of genetic material) could be an important genotoxic lesion in terms of cancer and autoimmune disease (see Introduction and Sengstag[125]). This phenomenon occurs normally during meiosis, but also can occur during mitosis as mitotic crossing over (MCO). MCO occurs either between two different genes (reciprocal recombination) or between two mutant sites within the same gene (gene conversion, or non-reciprocal recombination, due to the unequal ratios of progeny phenotypes arising). These forms of recombination are not detected as overt chromosomal exchanges at metaphase in mammalian cells. Yeast, together with the fruit fly *Drosophila melanogaster*,[126–128] provide the only practical means for measuring this type of lesion. The commonest assays in yeast for its detection are mitotic recombination and mitotic gene conversion in yeast.[129–131] The usual end-points scored are growth of prototrophic colonies on selective medium and the presence of coloured mutant colonies, or colony sectors. Although the exact mechanism whereby MCO occurs is unknown, its frequency is increased by genotoxins stimulating genetic exchanges, presumably via induction of DNA strand breaks.

Aneuploidy also can be detected in yeast.[130,132] However, the toxicological relevance of aneuploidy induction in fungi is dubious, first because the nuclear membrane is involved in the fungal mitotic apparatus, and some membrane-active agents act as fungal aneugens, and second because fungal tubulin differs from that in mammals thereby possibly altering the sensitivity of the system to mammalian aneugens.

5. *Cell transformation*

Cell transformation assays are difficult to define in terms of target molecules, or of the sequential processes related to cancer aetiology (initiation, promotion and progression),[133] and even the latter concept is likely to be an oversimplification.[29,134,135] Certainly the escape from mitotic control is a key characteristic of *in vivo* initiation and *in vitro* primary cell immortalization, and both these phenomena are likely to involve genotoxic events,[136,137] probably related to overcoming the barriers of replicative senescence and cell (apoptotic) senescence.[138–141] Investigations on immortalized cell lines probably cover only the reversible (promotion) and irreversible (progression) later steps in carcinogenesis, of which progression is likely to require further genotoxic events.[142,143]

Based on the foregoing considerations, *in vitro* cell transformation assays will be considered as part of a set of assays measuring genotoxic events in mammalian cells. However, it is probable that they may also involve important non-genotoxic changes in carcinogenesis and will prove to be more useful for predicting human cancer than either genotoxicity tests or rodent bioassays,[29] if the difficulties in immortalizing human cells[139,144] can be overcome, perhaps by obtaining cell lines transfected with DNA sequences for transforming growth factor α.[145] From a regulatory aspect, cell transformation assays are, at best, considered supplementary because of the uncertainty over the end-point measured, and owing to a history of unreliability.[146]

Cell transformation assays can be divided into those using primary cells and those using immortalized cell lines. Each of these subdivisions can be further divided into colony-forming assays (in agar) and assays in which foci of piled up cells in monolayer backgrounds are scored. The advantage of primary cells is that they can be used to mimic the whole process of cancer induction, including induction and promotion models, whereas transformation processes in transforming immortalized cell lines probably relate only to promotion and progression. The various cell systems commonly used are detailed below, together with key references. Methodology is given in the initial UK Environmental Mutagen Society (UKEMS) guidelines on supplementary tests[147] and by McGregor and Ashby.[146]

Primary cell assays Rat and mouse primary cells immortalize too readily (approximately 1 in 10^5 to 1 in 10^6), whilst human cells are too refractory to being transformed (less than 1 in 10^{12}). This is why Syrian hamster cells are often used: they exhibit intermediate immortalization frequencies of 1 in 10^7 (reference 139) to 1 in 10^9 (reference 140). One of the earliest effective assays of this type was the Syrian hamster embryo (SHE) assay,[148] initially using colony formation and later focus formation as end-points.[149] The reliability of this assay was improved significantly after investigations by Lubet *et al.*[150] An alternative to the SHE system is the Syrian hamster dermal (SHD) assay.[138,151]

Immortal cell line assays The baby hamster kidney (BHK) colony formation assay was an early assay using an immortal cell line.[152] This showed much promise initially, but is no longer used because other laboratories had difficulty in making the assay work reproducibly, and there were technical artefacts associated with low survival. The two currently accepted immortal cell line assays both use aneuploid mouse cell lines, Balb/c 3T3[153] and C3H/10T1/2.[154] These assays involve scoring foci as end-points and have proved reasonably reliable in use. The problem with the assays is the uncertainty about the exact processes that are being measured. It is probable that only the promotion and progression stages are detected, with the crucial immortalization stage omitted.

The principal stages of transformation tests are as follows. Exposed cells are allowed to grow in culture and assayed for their ability to exhibit loss of density (anchorage)-dependent growth, or contact inhibition. In the case of the former, the cells clone in semisolid agar, while with the latter the cells do not grow as a monolayer, but pile on top of each other in a disorganized manner to form distinct types of colonies or foci, which can be classified according to the stage of transformation reached. Thus, focus formation or growth in soft agar are the two morphological end-points scored. A compound is assumed to exhibit transforming activity if there is a significant increase in numbers of colonies or foci over vehicle controls. An exogenous metabolizing system is unnecessary with certain (usually primary) cell lines as these have sufficient endogenous activation capacity, but promutagens and procarcinogens should be used as positive controls in these cases.

Transformation assays can be useful for distinguishing promoters from initiating chemicals, and possibly for detecting non-genotoxic carcinogens. Ultimate verification of induction of the transformed phenotype can be achieved by inoculating transformants into host animals and observing for tumours. This is rarely undertaken for obvious reasons, and may often be unnecessary if a recognized assay is employed. Currently these assays do not play a major role in toxicology. The authors consider that this is likely to change, and there appear to be at least two avenues for possible development. First, it should be possible to isolate a battery of tester cells and cell lines, each of which mimics one part of the overall transformation process. Such a battery might enable the determination of which part(s) of the cancer process (if any) a pharmaceutical compound affects. Second, the development of a human cell transformation system might provide a major addition to information derived from rodent bioassays. If these two possibilities could be combined, it might be feasible to eliminate the need for carcinogenicity bioassays. Further developments, involving the use of improved cell lines, are suggested below.

6. *Human data (biomonitoring)*

Prospective cosmetic and pharmaceutical products are subjected to volunteer studies, and it would be possible in principle to assess the genotoxic effects of such exposures by undertaking non-invasive biomonitoring of blood and urine.[113] For example, peripheral lymphocytes can be scored for chromosomal damage, and urine can be analysed for mutagenic metabolites. The result from such investigations can be related to levels of compound and metabolites in body fluids, to facilitate safety assessment.[155] However, substantial amounts of inter-individual variation and other confounding factors, such as diverse exposure (dietary intake, disease and unspecified drug administration), as well as the timing of sample collection, can complicate interpretation of data. Such problems can be minimized, particularly by using each volunteer as his or her own control, and by adhering to strict sample collection times, as well as controlled diets. Biomonitoring data may contribute to clarifying the activity profiles of pharmaceuticals exhibiting divergent effects.

III. POTENTIAL NEW *IN VITRO* ASSAYS

A. Use of improved cell lines

Other types of improved cell lines are being generated, for example by introducing shuttle vectors as target DNA sequences for genotoxicity studies,[156] and also by using cells that possess stably integrated copies of a λ bacteriophage shuttle vector, containing the *lacI* gene, which can be used as a target base sequence to detect mutations, in a similar way to that used with transgenic rodent strains. Also, many different mutant mammalian cell lines with increased sensitivity to physical and chemical agents, are being generated and characterized.[157]

1. *New cell lines with targets*

The pivotal role of oncogenes and tumour suppressor genes in the process of carcinogenesis is now recognized, and assays are being developed which involve the activation of various proto-oncogenes, such as c-*myc* and c-*fos*, or the inactivation of tumour suppressor genes, especially *p53*, as additional methods to cell transformation for the characterization of potential carcinogens and tumour promoters.[158] Several phenomena, such as chromosomal deletion, insertion, point mutation, chromosomal translocation and gene amplification, are thought to be involved in altering the functions of these genes.[7] Some of these events may be caused by direct effects on targets other than DNA, and such assays may therefore prove to be useful for detecting carcinogens acting by indirect effects.

2. *Cell lines with altered metabolizing potential*

There have been various attempts to improve the sensitivity of cell lines by producing many different strains of indicator cells expressing various cloned cytochrome P450 isozymes.[5] Thus far, this approach has been more successful using mammalian cells,[159]where a variety of cell lines has been developed, possessing several different isozymes and other enzymes involved in metabolizing foreign compounds by mixed-function oxidases and other enzymes. Examples of such cell lines are human lymphoblastoid cells (AHH-1, MCL-5) and rodent fibroblasts, in which mutation at the HGPRT gene is measured. Also, several indirectly acting chemicals, requiring metabolic activation by a variety of different pathways, have been shown to induce micronuclei in MCL-5 cells.[160] More recently, human bronchial and liver epithelial cell lines have been produced by cell immortalization[161] and cDNA transfection, which retain phase II enzyme activity and cytochrome P450 inducibility and which express seven different cytochrome P450 isozymes.[162] These cell lines have been shown to be susceptible to the cytotoxic and genotoxic effects of several promutagens.

The development of such genetically engineered cell lines with high metabolizing capacity for use in detecting genotoxicity would seem to be a significant advance over the use of the standard regulatory protocol for the *Salmonella* assay. First, genotoxicity is measured in mammalian (including human) cells, and second metabolic transformation can proceed intracellularly, rather than outside the cell, as occurs when using rat liver metabolizing fractions. Thus, active metabolites can be generated closer to DNA, the target site for genotoxicity, thereby increasing the sensitivity of the assay.

IV. DATA ANALYSIS

A. Introduction

The key to successful data analysis is good experimental design. Many genotoxicity and cell transformation assays have been derived from research-based methodology, where design has not been optimized. As a consequence, the allocation of experimental units is neither optimal for determining whether there is an effect, nor best for deciding whether there is a positive concentration–response relationship. Unfortunately the design of assays for regulatory purposes is constrained by published guidelines. Therefore, we shall describe the designs as they are published, rather than as they ought to be for optimum power. First, it is always useful to conduct a range-finding assay to determine the top concentrations of test material to use in main tests. The highest concentrations should be limited by solubility, cytotoxicity and/or the highest concentration specified in regulatory guidelines. Second, it is always good scientific practice to repeat assays: the discriminatory power of two small tests is always greater than that of a single large one of equivalent size to the two small ones combined.

The manner in which tests should be repeated depends on the results of the first experiment. If a clear positive response was obtained, the test can be repeated using the same protocol, to increase confidence that the effects observed were not due to chance. Alternatively, the protocol can be changed to define the response further (e.g. trend with concentration and no-effect level). In the case of negative results on the first occasion, consideration should be given to further optimizing the protocol to be used in the second test. In this way, a second negative effect will have more meaning. In the event that a positive response is now detected, the second test should be repeated in an identical way, making three tests in all, and to allow a positive call on a weight-of-evidence approach. Such repeat testing should be distinguished from the use of duplicate assays (e.g. replicate cultures) within the same test. These are utilized to provide an indication of procedural (within-test) variation, and the results are important components of statistical analysis. Data assessment has the following logical steps:

(a) The validity of the assay must be determined.
(b) The question of whether treated groups differ from the negative control must be answered.
(c) The most difficult question – whether any observed difference is sufficient to be important in a biological sense – must be resolved.

B. Assay validity

The criteria required to establish for assay validity are:

(a) Absence of any technical problem that might invalidate the assay (e.g. contamination);
(b) Use of an adequate top concentration (see above).
(c) The expected normal responses of positive and negative controls.

The latter are best determined from the ranges of accumulated (historical) in-house laboratory data, which in turn should conform to published values. Ideally, confidence limits should be placed on laboratory data, and individual experimental results should fall within or close to these limits, usually at the 99% confidence level. Limits on group means can be set parametrically, by using distributions in the binomial family,[163,164] or by assuming a normal distribution of group means (central limit theorem), with or without data transformation. Non-parametric normal scores methodology can be used as an alternative approach, but this requires many more data than are needed for the other approaches.[164]

C. Do control and treated groups differ?

With practical experience of a particular assay, it is often clear from the data whether or not the control and treated groups differ. In such cases, statistical analysis is unnecessary.

However, where differences are small, statistical analysis is needed to determine whether negative control and treated groups are non-identical in statistical terms and/or whether there is a trend of increasing response with increasing concentration of test material. Numerous published methodologies exist for achieving this, but unfortunately some of these are flawed. However, methods described in the UKEMS book[44] *Statistical Evaluation of Mutagenicity Test Data* are generally reliable. Some general points and suggestions are found in Mitchell[165] and Mitchell *et al.*[163] Some of the more important ones are detailed below.

1. The assumptions underlying any statistical methodology should always be checked to ensure that the *in vitro* assay system in question is likely to conform with them. This should be done on theoretical considerations and/or using historical data. Suggestions in the literature that distributional matches can be carried out using within-test data should be ignored because such data are usually far too sparse for these calculations to be meaningful. When in doubt, non-parametric methodology should be used. Rank transformation, followed by parametric analysis of ranks, seems particularly useful, as it combines the generality of non-parametrics with the power of parametric analysis,[166,167] and has proved effective for genotoxicity tests with low replication within groups.[86]
2. The decision on whether to use a one- or two-sided (tailed) test should be is based on the question being asked: whether one group is greater than (one-sided) or differs from (two-sided) the other group.
3. It is crucial to correct for multiple comparisons (e.g. several concentrations, multiple end-points).
4. It is essential to correctly define the unit of analysis. For example, in treat-and-plate (make-slides) assays, it is the reaction mixture (agent, tester organism and suspending medium), and not the replicate plates or slides derived from each flask or tube, that is the unit of analysis.
5. There are two main forms of non-identity: one is based on size and consistency of response, and the other on trend of response with concentration. Both of these are useful pieces of information and, if guidelines allow, it is often useful to design an experiment to determine whether any one treated group exceeds the control (based on size and/or consistency), and then to redesign the second test to assess trend with concentration (or vice versa). Significant non-identity in test one, coupled with a significant trend in test two, gives confidence that the result is not due to chance or to an artefact, and it helps to address the question of biological importance. It should be noted that in regulatory guidelines compromise test designs are often recommended, which allow analysis for both individual group significance and trend in the same test.
6. The problem of outliers is less serious when using *in vitro* tests than *in vivo* assays. *In vitro*, an outlier is often the result of technical error, whereas *in vivo* outliers can indicate the presence of a small sensitive subgroup.[163] The solution for *in vitro* assays is to use non-parametric analysis based on ranks, parametric analysis of ranks being particularly useful (see (1)).

D. Is a response biologically important?

When it has been decided that a difference between control and treated groups is significant, the question of biological importance must be resolved. Generally, if a response is within the limits of normal (expected) variability observed in the historical database, the results can be discounted as statistically significant but not biologically important. This can be assessed by use of the historical database. With most *in vitro* assays, however, the control mean genuinely varies from test to test so that normal (expected) variability must be measured, not from confidence limits on control means, but with confidence limits on either differences between, or ratios calculated from, duplicate control data.[164]

If the response from a treated group is outside the expected range for control values, then further assessment is possible by consideration of the shape of the concentration–response curve. An exponential curve showing a geometric increase in response with geometric increases in concentration is indicative of a single-hit phenomenon without a true no-effect concentration. Conversely, a curve showing no-effect up to a given concentration, followed by an arithmetic increase in response with an arithmetic increase in concentration thereafter, is likely to indicate a threshold below which there is really no effect. Such curves often show a plateau level for maximum response.

It should be noted that it is difficult to show a statistical difference between the exponential and threshold (constrained broken stick) models. Therefore, unless a mechanism for a threshold model can be demonstrated, regulatory bodies are unlikely to accept arguments based on unproven possibilities. The worst-case scenario will always be assumed unless proof to the contrary is supplied. In view of the overall data interpretation, it may well not be worth the effort of trying to justify thresholds for *in vitro* assays (see below).

E. Data interpretation

Once it has been decided that a result is biologically important, it can be graded in terms of degree of response and potency. Three factors are relevant for undertaking this analysis:

1. Maximum size of response.
2. The slope of the steepest part of the dose–response curve.
3. The no-effect level (limited by assay sensitivity) or the threshold (true no-effect) level.

The importance of these factors is in reverse order. If the no-effect or threshold level is near or below therapeutic blood or tissue levels, then there is a clear genotoxic risk to humans based on the *in vitro* data, which is exacerbated if the concentration–response curve is steep, and if there is a high maximum response. However, it is very rare to find genotoxic activity near or below the therapeutic level, and guess-estimates have to be made as to the form of the concentration–response below the lower limit of sensitivity for the assay. A further problem in extrapolating to the *in vivo* situation arises from the possibility of test compound metabolism. *In vivo* and *in vitro* activation and detoxification can differ substantially. In the latter, the bias to phase I metabolism means that compounds are often more prone to activation (and hence to positive results) *in vitro* than *in vivo* (see Introduction).

A typical drug development programme is shown in Table 14.1 and a decision analysis diagram in Fig. 14.8. For a complete evaluation of genotoxic potential of a pharmaceutical compound the results of a full battery of *in vitro* and *in vivo* assays are needed (see Introduction). If the bacterial (Ames) assays and an *in vitro* mammalian cell cytogenetic (or mouse lymphoma $TK^{+/-}$) assay are negative, then it is considered most unlikely that the compound will be genotoxic because these assays are more (over) sensitive relative to *in vivo* assays. Nevertheless, for compounds such as pharmaceuticals with high human exposure, an

Table 14.1 Typical drug development programme.

Phase	General activity	Purpose	Genetic toxicology activity
Discovery	Identification of active compounds	Selection of compounds for development	Some companies: structural analysis and/or case-by-case *in vitro* assays
Pre-clinical development	*In vitro* and animal toxicology	Hazard identification and risk assessment for dosing to humans	*In vitro* bacterial and (1 or 2) mammalian cell assays (some companies *in vivo* assays)
Phase I Clinical	Testing in healthy volunteers	Human safety testing	Usual position of *in vivo* assays
Phase II Clinical	Small-scale clinical trials	Human safety and efficacy	
Phase III Clinical	Large-scale clinical trials	Efficacy and comparison with the competition	
Phase IV Post-registration	Additional tests required by regulators	Further safety/efficacy studies	Special studies, e.g. DNA adducts cell transformation

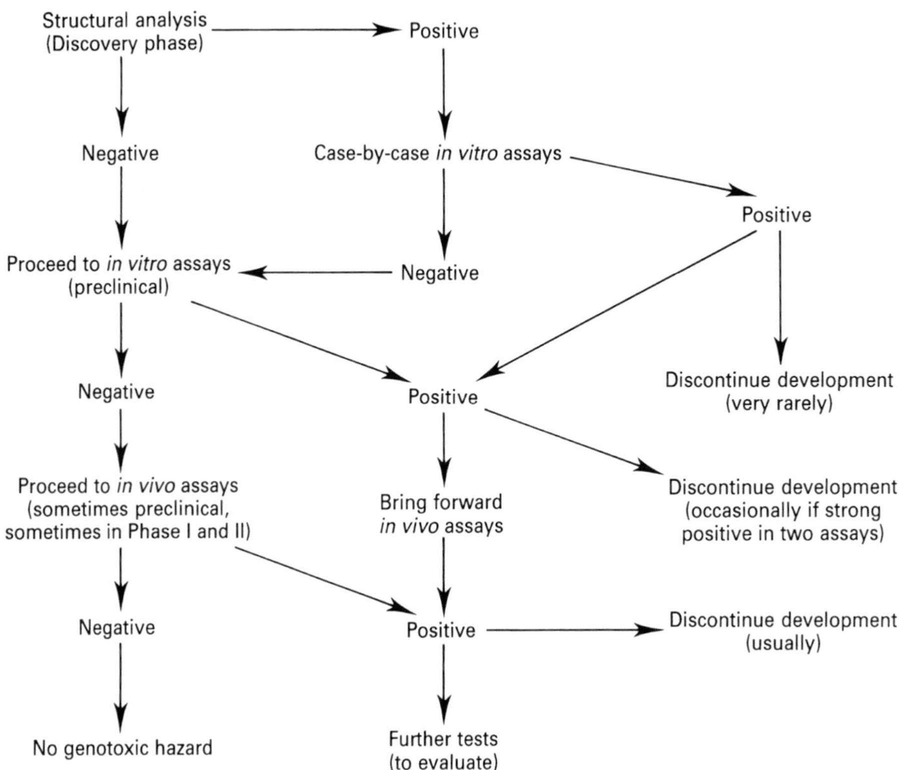

Fig. 14.8 Decision analysis for genetic toxicology.

in vivo micronucleus (or metaphase analysis) bone marrow assay is also required to eliminate the low, but finite, possibility (based on metabolic considerations) of an *in vivo*-specific genotoxin. If only one *in vitro* assay is positive, the result is likely to be a system-specific positive of no relevance to human hazard, provided there are one or two other *in vitro* assays showing no effects, and the *in vivo* bone marrow micronucleus test, and one other well-recognized *in vivo* assay in another tissue (e.g. UDS in the liver), are all negative. The major difficulty in interpretation arises when there are two clear *in vitro*-positive assays, and both *in vivo* assays are negative. The uncertainty with such definite *in vitro*-positive genotoxins is that *in vivo* effects might have been missed either because of the insensitivity of the current *in vivo* assays or because of tissue specificity.[31] It is in such cases where consideration of the shape of the *in vitro* assay concentration–response curves, and results from supplementary assays, can be crucial in making important regulatory decisions.

V. CONCLUSIONS

The main purpose of *in vitro* genotoxicity is to identify *in vivo* genotoxins. Because of the relatively high (over) sensitivity of such tests, a large number of compounds will be genotoxic *in vitro* but not *in vivo*. Therefore, negative *in vitro* genotoxicity data are very good predictors of negative *in vivo* genotoxicity. Conversely, positive *in vitro* data are not good predictors of positive *in vivo* genotoxicity. However, it should be noted that a number of the more potent *in vitro* genotoxins may be active *in vivo* but will not be identified as such owing to the limitations of current *in vivo* assays.

The use of *in vitro* assays can, therefore, go a long way towards demonstrating a lack of genotoxic hazard, but are less useful in defining the existence of such a hazard. Conversely, positive results from *in vivo* assays are indicative of a significant hazard in humans, and it seems unlikely that the use of *in vitro* assays will be able to replace *in vivo* assays for this aspect of testing of pharmaceuticals in the foreseeable future. Generally, it is very difficult to progress a pharmaceutical candidate compound that is genotoxic *in vivo*. Regulators will nearly always refuse to pass such compounds unless they possess unique pharmacological activity for the treatment of life-threatening diseases or there is good evidence of a true threshold dose well above therapeutic levels. Conversely, it is unusual for a pharmaceutical with unique *in vitro* genotoxicity (negative *in vivo*) to be rejected, unless it exhibits potent activity (especially without S9), and if it is for the alleviation of trivial complaints for which several other treatments are available. It is necessary to assess the risks and the benefits on a case-by-case basis using a weight-of-evidence approach to the risks, together with any human biomonitoring data available.[168] The importance of *in vivo* genotoxins is that they have high probability of being involved in several somatic diseases, in particular with genotoxic carcinogenicity. However, they have little relevance to non-genotoxic carcinogenicity. Although members of the latter group of carcinogens are considered far less important than their genotoxic counterparts, they are not irrelevant for human hazard. Cell transformation assays may prove useful in detecting both genotoxic and non-genotoxic carcinogens but their reliability needs to be improved, together with a better understanding of the molecular basis of the observed end-points.

Despite the plethora of available genotoxicity assays, only a few have proved to be of sufficient value and reliability, and are sufficiently well understood, to be accepted as regulatory assays. Batteries of such genotoxicity assays are now currently used for regulatory purposes, and *in vitro* assays in bacterial and mammalian cells play an important part in these batteries. In particular, they form a key element in preclinical studies in assessing safety for dosing to human volunteers. Nevertheless, supplementary tests can be useful and can provide important additional information under certain circumstances, particularly when test materials are difficult to use in conventional assays, and where equivocal data have been previously obtained.

In the future, we anticipate that *in vitro* studies will play an increasingly important role in the identification of genotoxic and carcinogenic hazard and in risk assessment. The impetus for this is likely to be derived from the development of metabolically competent tester cells in which the molecular target is identified. In particular, it seems possible that cell transformation assays may reach a point where they can replace rodent bioassays for carcinogenicity.

REFERENCES

1. Garner, R. C., Miller, E. C. and Miller, J. A. (1972) Liver microsomal metabolism of aflatoxin B1 to a reactive derivative toxic to *Salmonella typhimurium* TA1530. *Cancer Res.* **32:** 2058–2066.
2. Ames, B. N., Durston, W. E., Yamasaki, E. and Lee, F. D. (1973) Carcinogens are mutagens; a simple test system combining liver homogenates for activation and bacteria for detection. *Proc. Natl Acad. Sci. U.S.A.* **70:** 2281–2285.
3. Ames, B. N., McCann, J. and Yamasaki, E. (1975) Methods for detecting carcinogens and mutagens with the *Salmonella*/mammalian microsome mutagenicity test. *Mutat. Res.* **31:** 347–364.
4. Clive, D., Johnson, K., Spector, J., Batson, A. and Brun, M. M. (1979) Validation and characterization of the L5178Y/tk mouse lymphoma mutagen assay system. *Mutat. Res.* **59:** 61–108.

5. Combes, R. D. (1992) The *in vivo* relevance of *in vitro* genotoxicity assays incorporating enzyme activation systems. In Gibson, G. G. (ed.) *Progress in Drug Metabolism*, Vol. 13, pp. 295–321. Taylor and Francis Limited, London.
6. Elliott, B. M., Combes, R. D., Elcombe, C., Gatehouse, D., Gibson, G. G. and Wolf, C. R. (1992) Alternatives to Aroclor 1254 for genotoxicity assays. Report of the UKEMS Working Party on Enzyme Inducers. *Mutagenesis* **7:** 175–177.
7. Scrable, H. J., Sapienza, C. and Cavanee, W. K. (1990) Genetic and epigenetic losses of heterozygosity in cancer predisposition and progression. *Adv. Cancer Res.* **54:** 25–62.
8. Cohen, S. and Ellwein, L. B. (1991) Genetic errors, cell proliferation, and carcinogenesis. *Cancer Res.* **51:** 6493–6505.
9. Maronpot, R. R. (1991) Chemical carcinogenesis. In *Handbook of Toxicologic Pathology*, pp. 91–129. Academic Press, New York.
10. Parkes, J. L., Cardell, R. R., Hubbard, F. C., Hubbard, D., Meltzer, A. and Penn, A. (1991) Cultured human atherosclerotic plaque smooth muscle cells retain transforming potential and display enhanced expression of the *myc* proto-oncogene. *Am. J. Pathol.* **138:** 755–765.
11. Onraed-Dupriez, B. (1992) Athérosclérose et oncogenes. *Pathol. Biol. (Paris)* **40:** 56–65.
12. Shlomchik, M. J., Marshake-Rothstein, A., Wolfowicz, C. B., Rothstein, T. L. and Weigert, M. G. (1987) The role of clonal selection and somatic mutation in autoimmunity. *Nature* **328:** 805–811.
13. Theofilopoulos, A. N. (1995) The basis of autoimmunity: Part II genetic predisposition. *Immunol. Today* **16:** 150–158.
14. Martin, J. B. (1993) Molecular genetics of neurological diseases. *Science* **262:** 674–676.
15. Deslys, J.-P., Marcé, D. and Dormont, D. (1994) Similar genetic susceptibility in iatrogenic and sporadic Creutzfeld–Jakob disease. *J. Gen. Virol.* **75:** 23–27.
16. DeArmond, S. J. and Prusiner, S. B. (1995) Prion protein transgenes and the neuropathology in prion diseases. *Brain Pathol.* **5:** 77–89.
17. Poulton, J. (1993) Mitochondrial DNA and genetic disease. *Dev. Med. Child Neurol.* **35:** 833–840.
18. Carter, C. O. (1977) The relative contribution of mutant genes and chromosome abnormalities to genetic ill-health in man. In Scott, D., Bridges, B. A. and Sobels, F. H. (eds) *Progress in Genetic Toxicology*, pp. 1–14. Elsevier/North-Holland, Amsterdam.
19. Tweats, D. (1994) Mutagenicity. In Ballantyne, B., Marrs, T. and Turner, P. (eds) *General and Applied Toxicology*, pp. 871–936. Macmillan, London.
20. Auerbach, C. (1978) *Mutation Research*. Chapman and Hall, London.
21. Brusick, D. (ed.) (1987) Genotoxicity produced in cultured mammalian cell assays by treatment conditions. *Mutat. Res.* **189:** 1–79.
22. Ames, B. N. (1979) Identifying environmental chemicals causing mutations and cancer. *Science* **204:** 587–593.
23. Hartman, P. E. (1989) Early years of the *Salmonella* mutagen tester strains: lessons from hycanthone. *Environ. Mol. Mutagen.* **14:** 39–45.
24. Tennant, R. W., Margolin, B. H. Shelby, M. D. *et al.* (1987) Prediction of chemical carcinogenicity in rodents from *in vitro* genetic toxicity assays. *Science* **236:** 933–941.
25. Zeiger, E., Haseman, J. K., Shelby, M. D., Margolin, B. H. and Tennant, R. W. (1990) Evaluation of four *in vitro* genetic toxicity tests for predicting rodent carcinogenicity: confirmation of earlier results with 41 additional chemicals. *Environ. Mol. Mutagen.* **16S18:** 1–14.
26. Brusick, D. (1994) Genetic toxicology. In Hayes, A. W. (ed.) *Principles and Methods of Toxicology*, pp. 545–577. Raven Press, New York.
27. Ashby, J. (1986) The prospect for a simplified and internationally harmonised approach to the detection of possible human carcinogens as mutagens. *Mutagenesis* **1:** 3–16.
28. Shelby, M. D., Zeiger, E. and Tennant, R. W. (1988) Commentary on the status of short-term tests for chemical carcinogens. *Env. Mol. Mutagen.* **11:** 437–441.
29. Mitchell, I. de G. (1989) Mutagenicity/carcinogenicity association and the rationale of using genetic toxicology short-term tests for carcinogen detection. *Oncol (Life Sic Ablv)* **8:** 1–10.
30. Zeiger, E. (1990) Strategies for the use of genetic toxicity tests. *Drug. Metab. Rev.* **22:** 765–775.
31. Combes, R. D. (1995) Regulatory genotoxicity testing: a critical appraisal. *Alternatives to Laboratory Animals* **23:** 352–379.
32. Combes, R. D. (1992) Trends in genotoxicity testing. *Chemistry in Industry* **24:** 950–954.
33. DOH (Department of Health) (1989) *Guidelines for the Testing of Chemicals for Mutagenicity*. HMSO, London.
34. Bridges, B. A. (1976) Short-term screening tests for carcinogens. *Nature* **261:** 195–200.

35. Williams, G. M. (1989) Methods for evaluating chemical genotoxicity. *Annu. Rev. Pharmacol. Toxicol.* **29:** 189–211.
36. Aardema, M. J. (ed.) (1993) Updated worldwide regulatory guidelines for genotoxicity testing. Workshop Proceedings from the 1992 Environmental Mutagen Society Meeting. *Environ. Mol. Mutagen.* **21:** 1–57.
37. Madle, S. (1993) Problem of the harmonisation of philosophies for genotoxicity testing. *Mutat. Res.* **300:** 73–76.
38. Galloway, S. M. (ed.) (1994) Report of the International Workshop on Standardisation of Genotoxicity Test Procedures. *Mutat. Res.* **312:** 195–319.
39. D'Arcy, P. F. and Harron, D. W. G. (1994) *Proceedings of the Second International Conference on Harmonisation, Orlando, 1993.* Queen's University Belfast Press, Belfast.
40. Tweats, D and Scales, D. (1994) Progress with harmonisation of guidelines for human pharmaceuticals. *Toxicology and Ecotoxicology News* **1:** 113–116.
41. Speid, L. H., Lumley, C. E. and Walker, S. R. (1990) Harmonization of guidelines for toxicity testing of pharmaceuticals by 1992. *Regul. Toxicol. Pharmacol.* **12:** 179–211.
42. ASTM (American Society for Testing of Materials) (1987) Guidelines for minimal criteria of acceptability for selected short-term assays for genotoxicity. *Mutat. Res.* **189:** 81–183.
43. UKEMS Sub-committee on Guidelines for Mutagenicity Testing (1984) Dean, B. J. (ed.) *Guidelines for Mutagenicity Testing. Part II: Supplementary Tests, Mutagens in Body Fluids and Excreta, Nitrosation Products.* United Kingdom Environmental Mutagen Society, Swansea.
44. UKEMS Sub-committee on Guidelines for Mutagenicity Testing (1989) Kirkland, D. J. (ed.) *Statistical Evaluation of Mutagenicity Test Data: UKEMS Recommended Procedures.* Cambridge University Press, Cambridge.
45. UKEMS Sub-committee on Guidelines for Mutagenicity Testing (1993) Kirkland, D. J. and Fox, M. (eds) *Supplementary Mutagenicity Tests: UKEMS Recommended Procedures.* Cambridge University Press, Cambridge.
46. UKEMS Sub-committee on Guidelines for Mutagenicity Testing (1990) Kirkland, D. J. (ed.) *Basic Mutagenicity Tests: UKEMS Recommended Procedures.* Cambridge University Press, Cambridge.
47. Kilbey, B. J., Legator, M., Nicholas, W. and Ramel, C. (eds) (1984) *Handbook of Mutagenicity Test Procedures*, 2nd edn. Elsevier, Amsterdam.
48. Venitt, S. and Parry, J. M. (eds) (1984) *Mutagenicity Testing – A Practical Approach.* IRL Press, Oxford.
49. OECD (1983) *OECD Guidelines for Testing of Chemicals, Genetic Toxicology*, nos 471–485. OECD, Brussels.
50. EEC Directive (1989) Methods for the determination of toxicity: mutagenicity. No: 79/831, Annex V, Part B: B10–B14, pp. 8–49. EC, Brussels.
51. Shimada, H. (1993) Mutagenicity studies of Japanese regulatory guideline: the status quo and the point at issue. *Environmental Mutation Research Communications* **15:** 109–121.
52. MHW (Ministry of Health and Welfare, Japan) (1984) *Information on the guidelines of toxicity studies required for applications for approval to manufacture (import) drugs (Part 1).* Notification no. 118 of the Pharmaceutical Affairs Bureau, Ministry of Health and Welfare, Japan.
53. Sword, I. P. and Thomson, R. (1980) *Standard Operating Procedures* – In Vitro *Toxicology.* MTP Press, Lancaster.
54. Clare, C. (1995) Mutation assays in bacteria. In O'Hare, S. and Atterwill, C. K. (eds) In Vitro *Toxicity Testing Protocols*, pp. 297–306. Humana Press, Totowa, USA.
55. Clements, J. (1995) Gene mutation in mammalian cells. In O'Hare S. and Atterwill, C. K. (eds) In Vitro *Toxicity Testing Protocols*, pp. 277–286. Humana Press, Totowa, USA.
56. Dean, S. (1995) Measurement of unscheduled DNA synthesis *in vitro* using primary rat hepatocyte cultures. In O'Hare, S. and Atterwill, C. K. (eds) In Vitro *Toxicity Testing Protocols*, pp. 267–276. Humana Press, Totowa, USA.
57. Marshall, R. (1995) Measurement of chromosome aberrations *in vitro* using human peripheral blood lymphocytes. In O'Hare, S. and Atterwill, C. K. (eds) In Vitro *Toxicity Testing Protocols*, pp. 287–296, Humana Press, Totowa, USA.
58. Galloway, S. M., Deasy, D. A., Bean, C. L., Kraynak, A. R., Armstrong, M. J. and Bradley, M. O. (1987) Effects of high osmotic strength on chromosome aberrations, sister chromatid exchanges and DNA strand breaks, and their relation to toxicity. *Mutat. Res.* **189:** 15–25.
59. Scott, D., Danford, N. D., Dean, B. J. and Kirkland, D. J. (1990) Metaphase chromosome aberration assays. In Kirkland, D. J. (ed.) *Basic Mutagenicity Tests UKEMS Recommended Procedures*, pp. 62–86. Cambridge University Press, Cambridge.

60. Scott, D., Galloway, S. M., Marshall, R. R. *et al.* (1991) Genotoxicity under extreme culture conditions. A report from ICPEMC task group 9. *Mutat. Res.* **257:** 147–204.
61. Morita, T., Nagai, T., Fukuda, I. and Okumura, K. (1992) Clastogenicity of low pH to various cultured mammalian cells. Mutat. Res. **268:** 297–305.
62. Robinson, W. D., Green, M. H. L., Cole, J., Garner, R. C., Healy, M. J. R. and Gatehouse, D. (1989) Statistical evaluation of bacterial/mammalian fluctuation tests. In Kirkland, D. J. (ed.) *Statistical Evaluation of Mutagenicity Test Data*, pp. 102–140. Cambridge University Press, Cambridge.
63. Gatehouse, D., Rowland, I. R., Wilcox, P., Callender, R. D. and Forster, R. (1990) Bacterial mutation assays. In Kirkland, D. J. (ed.) *Basic Mutagenicity Tests: UKEMS Recommended Procedures. UKEMS Sub-committee on Guidelines for Mutagenicity Testing. Report. Part I Revised: Basic Tests*, pp. 13–61. Cambridge University Press, Cambridge.
64. Gatehouse, D. (1987) Critical features of bacterial mutation assays. *Mutagenesis* **2:** 397–409.
65. Hera, C. and Pueyo, C. (1986) Conditions for optimal use of the L-arabinose-resistance mutagenesis test with *Salmonella typhimurium. Mutagenesis* **1:** 267–273.
66. Ando, M., Shindo, Y., Fukita, M., Ozawa, S., Yamazoe, Y. and Kato, R. (1993) A new *Salmonella* tester strain expressing a hamster acetyltransferase shows high sensitivity for arylamines. *Mutat. Res.* **292:** 155–163.
67. Gee, P., Maron, D. M. and Ames, B. N. (1994) Detection and classification of mutagens: a set of base-specific *Salmonella* tester strains. *Proc. Acad. Natl Sci. U.S.A.* **91:** 11 606–11 610.
68. Rexroate, M. A., Oberly, T. J., Bewsey, B. J. and Garriott, M. L. (1995) The gradient plate assay: a modified Ames assay used as a prescreen for the identification of bacterial mutagens. *Mutat. Res.* **341:** 185–192.
69. Cole, J. Fox, M., Garner, R. C., McGregor, D. B. and Thacker, J. (1990) Gene mutation assays in culture mammalian cells. In Kirkland, D. J. (ed.) *Basic Mutagenicity Tests: UKEMS Recommended Procedures*, pp. 87–114. Cambridge University Press, Cambridge.
70. Clive, D., Caspary, W., Kirby, P. E. *et al.* (1987) Guide for performing the mouse lymphoma assay for mammalian cell mutagenicity. *Mutat. Res.* **189:** 143–156.
71. Riach, C. G., Cattanach, P. J., Howgate S. *et al.* (1990) Studies on the activities of benzo[a]pyrene, benzidine and ethyl methanesulphonate in the L5178Y $TK^{+/-}$ mouse lymphoma mutagenicity assay using standardized and non-standardized protocols. *Mutagenesis* 5 **(supplement):** 35–44.
72. Daston-Spencer, D. L., Hines, K. C. and Caspary, W. J. (1993) An *in situ* protocol for the expression of chemically-induced mutations in mammalian cells. *Mutat. Res.* **312:** 85–98.
73. Clive, D., Glover, P., Applegate, M. and Hozier, J. (1990) Molecular aspects of chemical mutagenesis in L5178Y $tk^{+/-}$ mouse lymphoma cells. *Mutagenesis* **5:** 191–197.
74. Davies, M. J., Phillips, B. J. and Rumsby, P. C. (1993) Molecular analysis of mutations at the tk locus of L5178Y mouse lymphoma cells induced by ethyl methanesulphonate and mitomycin C. *Mutat. Res.* **290:** 145–153.
75. Combes, R. D., Stopper, H. and Caspary, W. J. (1995) The use of L5178Y mouse lymphoma cells to assess the mutagenic, clastogenic and aneugenic properties of chemicals. *Mutagenesis* **10:** 403–408.
76. Brusick, D. (1987) *Principles of Genetic Toxicology*. Plenum Press, New York.
77. Aaron, C. S. and Stankowski, L. F. Jr (1989) Comparison of the AS52/XPRT and the Cho/HPRT assays: evaluation of 6 drug candidates. *Mutat. Res.* **223:** 121–128.
78. Kirkland, D. J. (1992) Chromosomal aberration test *in vitro*: problems with protocol design and interpretation of results. *Mutagenesis* **7:** 95–106.
79. Ishidate, M., Sofuni, T., Yoshikawa, K. *et al.* (1984) Primary mutagenicity screening of food additives currently used in Japan. *Fd. Chem. Toxicol.* **22:** 623–636.
80. Dean, B. J. and Danford, N. (1984) Assays for the detection of chemically induced chromosome damage in cultured mammalian cells. In Venitt, S. and Parry, J. M. (eds) *Mutagenicity Testing: A Practical Approach*, pp. 187–232. IRL Press. Oxford.
81. Preston, R. J., San Sebastian, J. R. and McFee, A. F. (1987) The *in vitro* human lymphocyte assay for assessing the clastogenicity of chemical agents. *Mutat. Res.* **189:** 175–183.
82. Tice, R., Schneider, E. L. and Rary, J. M. (1976) The utilisation of bromodeoxyuridine incorporation into DNA for the analysis of cellular kinetis. *Exp. Cell Res.* **102:** 232–236.
83. Palma, V., Tudon, H., Buenlello, L., Nava, S., Ostrosky, P. and Salamanca, F. (1993) Methods for the analysis of cellular kinetics in PHA-stimulated blood lymphocytes using BrdU incorporation. A comparative study. *Mutat. Res.* **286:** 267–273.

84. Bean, C. L. Bradt, C. I., Hill, R., Johnson, T. E., Stallworth, M. and Galloway, S. M. (1994) Chromosome aberrations: persistence of alkylation damage and modulation by O6-alkylguanine-DNA-alkyl transferase. *Mutat. Res.* **307:** 67–81.
85. Anonymous (1979) Report of the *ad hoc* committee on karyological controls of human cell substrates. *J. Biol. Standard.* **7:** 397–404.
86. Mitchell, I. de G., Lambert, T. R., Burden, M., Sunderland, J., Porter, R. L. and Carlton, J. B. (1995) Is polyploidy an important genotoxic lesion? *Mutagenesis* **10:** 79–83.
87. Piper, J. and Lundsteen, C. (1987) Human chromosome analysis by machine. *Trends Genet.* **3:** 309–313.
88. Vral, A., Verhaegen, F., Thierens, H. and de Ridder, L. (1994) The *in vitro* cytokinesis-block micronucleus assay: a detailed description of an improved slide preparation technique of micronuclei in human lymphocytes. *Mutagenesis* **9:** 439–443.
89. Reid, T., Baldini, A., Rand, T. C. and Ward, D. C. (1992) Simultaneous visualisation of seven different DNA probes by *in situ* hybridisation using combinatorial fluorescence and digital imaging microscopy. *Proc. Natl Acad. Sci. U.S.A.* **89:** 1388–1392.
90. Savage, J. K. and Simpson, P. J. (1994) FISH 'painting' patterns resulting from complex exchanges. *Mutat. Res.* **312:** 51–60.
91. Ashby, J. and Tennant, R. W. (1988) Chemical structure, *Salmonella* mutagenicity and extent of carcinogenicity as indicators of genotoxic carcinogens among 222 chemicals tested in rodents by the US NCI/NTP. *Mutat. Res.* **204:** 17–115.
92. Judson, P. N. (1994) Rule induction for systems predicting biological activity. *J. Chem. Inf. Comput. Sci.* **34:** 148–153.
93. Long, A. and Combes, R. D. (1995) Using DEREK to predict the activity of some carcinogens/mutagens found in foods. *Toxicol. In Vitro* **9:** 563–569.
94. Rosenkranz, H. S. and Klopman, G. (1990) Structural basis of carcinogenicity in rodents of genotoxicants and non-genotoxicants. *Mutat. Res.* **228:** 105–124.
95. Rosenkranz, H. S., Mitchell, C. S. and Klopman, G. (1985) Artificial intelligence and Bayesian decision theory in the prediction of chemical carcinogens. *Mutat. Res.* **150:** 1–11.
96. Benigni, R., Andreoli, C. and Giuliani, A. (1989) Quantitative structure–activity relationships: principles and applications to mutagenicity and carcinogenicity. *Mutat. Res.* **221:** 197–216.
97. Lewis, D. F. V. and Parke, D. V. (1995) The genotoxicity of benzanthracenes: a quantitative structure–activity study. *Mutat. Res.* **328:** 207–214.
98. Hansch, C., Telzer, B. R. and Zhang, L. (1995) Comparative QSAR in toxicology: examples from teratology and cancer chemotherapy of aniline mustards. *Crit. Rev. Toxicol.* **25:** 67–89.
99. Ioannides, C. and Parke, D. V. (1987) The cytochrome P-448 – a unique family of enzymes involved in chemical toxicity carcinogenesis. *Biochem. Pharmacol.* **36:** 4197–4207.
100. Lewis, D. F. V., Ioannides, C. and Parke, D. V. (1990) A prospective toxicity evaluation (COMPACT) on 40 chemicals currently being tested by the National Toxicology Program. *Mutagenesis* **5:** 433–435.
101. Ashby, J., Tennant, R. W., Zeiger, E. and Stasiewicz, S. (1989) Classification according to chemical structure, mutagenicity to *Salmonella* and level of carcinogenicity by the US National Toxicology Program. *Mutat. Res.* **223:** 73–103.
102. Ashby, J. and Tennant, R. W. (1994). Prediction of rodent carcinogenicity for 44 chemicals: results. *Mutagenesis* **9:** 7–15.
103. Combes, R. D. and Judson, P. (1995) The use of artificial intelligence systems for predicting toxicity. *Pesticide Science* **45:** 179–194.
104. Phillips, D. H. (1990) Modern methods of DNA adduct determination. In Cooper, C. S. and Grover, P. L. (eds) *Chemical Carcinogenesis and Mutagenesis*, Vol. I, pp. 503–546.
105. Dashwood, R. H. and Combes, R. D. (1987) Deficiencies in the covalent binding index (CBI) for expressing *in vivo* binding to DNA with respect to predicting chemical carcinogenicity. A proposal for a target organ binding index. *Mutat. Res.* **190:** 173–175.
106. Phillips, D. H., Cross, M. F., Kennelly, J. C., Wilcox, P. and O'Donovan, M. R. (1990) Determination of benzidine–DNA adduct formation in CHO, HeLa, L5178Y, TK6 and V79 cells. *Mutagenesis* **5 (supplement):** 67–69.
107. Wogan, G. N. (1989) Markers of exposure to carcinogens: methods for human biomonitoring. *Journal of the American College of Toxicology* **8:** 871–881.
108. Weston, A., Manchester, D. K., Povey, A. and Harris, C. C. (1989) Detection of carcinogen–macromolecular adducts in humans. *Journal of the American College of Toxicology* **8:** 913–932.

109. McKelvey-Martin, V. I., Green, M. H. L., Schmezer, P., Pool-Zobel, B. L., DeMeo, M. P. and Collins, A. (1993) The single cell gel electrophoresis assay (comet assay): a European perspective. *Mutat. Res.* **288:** 47–63.
110. Tweats, D., Bootman, J., Combes, R. D. Green, M. and Watkins, P. (1984) Assays for DNA repair in bacteria. In Dean, B. J. (ed.) *Guidelines for Mutagenicity Testing. Part II: Supplementary Tests, Mutagens in Body Fluids and Excreta, Nitrosation Products*, pp. 5–25. United Kingdom Environmental Mutagen Society, Swansea.
111. Combes, R. D. (1983) An analysis of the efficacy of bacterial DNA repair assays for predicting genotoxicity. *Mutat. Res.* **108:** 81–92.
112. Waters, R., Ashby, J., Barrett, R., Burlinson, B., Lefevre, P. and Martin, C. (1984) Unscheduled DNA synthesis. In Dean, B. J. (ed.) *Guidelines for Mutagenicity Testing. Part II: Supplementary Tests, Mutagens in Body Fluids and Excreta, Nitrosation Products*, pp. 63–87. United Kingdom Environmental Mutagen Society, Swansea.
113. Combes, R. D. (1991) Use of clinical samples for biomonitoring of genotoxic exposure. In Nimmo, W. (ed.) *Clinical Measurement in Drug Evaluation*, pp. 173–191. Wolfe Medical Publications, London.
114. Muller, K., Kasper, K. and Muller, L. (1993) An assessment of the *in vitro* hepatocyte micronucleus assay. *Mutat. Res.* **292:** 213–224.
115. Parry, E. M., Henderson, L. and Mackay, J. M. (1995) Procedures for the detection of chemically induced aneuploidy: recommendations of a UK Environmental Mutagen Society working group. *Mutagenesis* **10:** 1–14.
116. Fenech, M. and Morley, A. A. (1985) Solutions to the kinetic problem in the micronucleus assay. *Cytobios* **43:** 223–246.
117. Hennig, U. G. G., Rudd, N. L. and Hoar, D. I. (1988) Kinetochore immunofluorescence in micronuclei: a rapid method for the *in situ* detection of aneuploidy and chromosome breakage in human fibroblasts. *Mutat. Res.* **203:** 405–414.
118. Fritzenschaf, H., Kohlpoth, M., Rusche, B. and Schiffman, D. (1993) Testing of known carcinogens and noncarcinogens in the Syrian hamster embryo (SHE) micronucleus test *in vitro*; correlations with *in vivo* micronucleus formation and cell transformation. *Mutat. Res.* **319:** 47–53.
119. Stopper, H., Korber, C., Schiffman, D. and Caspary, W. J. (1993) Cell cycle dependent micronucleus formation and mitotic disturbances in mammalian cells treated with 5-azacytidine. *Mutat. Res.* **300:** 165–177.
120. Zimmermann, F. K., von Borstel, R. C., von Halle, E. S. *et al.* (1984) Testing of chemicals for genetic activity with *Saccharomyces cerevisiae*: a report of the US Environmental Protection Agency gene-tox program. *Mutat. Res.* **133:** 199–244.
121. Brooks, T. M., Kelly, D. E., Kelly, S. L., Mitchell, I. de G., Parry, J. M. and Wilcox, P. (1993) Genotoxicity studies using yeast cultures. In Kirkland, D. J. and Fox, M. (eds) *Supplementary Mutagenicity Tests: UKEMS Recommended Procedures*, pp. 10–51. Cambridge University Press, Cambridge.
122. Mehta, R. D. and von Borstel, R. C. (1981) Mutagenic activity of 42 encoded compounds in the haploid yeast reversion assay, strain XV 185-14C. In de Serres, F. J. and Ashby, J. (eds), *Progress in Mutation Research*, Vol. 1, pp. 414–423. Elsevier/North-Holland, Amsterdam.
123. Mitchell, I. de G. and Gilbert, P. J. (1991) Comparison of forward mutation at the cycloheximide, canavanine and adipic acid resistance loci in response to treatment of wild type *Saccharomyces cerevisiae* S7a with eight polycyclic aromatic compounds. *Mutagenesis* **6:** 229–236.
124. Patel, R. and Wilkie, D. (1982) Mitochondrial toxicity in *Saccharomyces cerevisiae*: a measure of carcinogenicity. *Mutat. Res.* **100:** 179–183.
125. Sengstag, C. (1994) The role of mitotic recombination in carcinogenesis. *Crit. Rev. Toxicol.* **24:** 323–353.
126. Würgler, F. E., Graf, U., Frei, H. and Juon, H. (1983) Genotoxic activity of the anti-cancer drug methotrexate in somatic cells of *Drosophila melanogaster*. *Mutat. Res.* **122:** 321–328.
127. Vogel, E. W. and Nivard, M. J. M. (1993) Performance of 181 chemicals in a *Drosophila* assay predominantly monitoring interchromosomal mitotic recombination. *Mutagenesis* **8:** 57–81.
128. Mitchell, I. de G. and Combes, R. D. (1984) Mutation tests with the fruit fly *Drosophila melanogaster*. In Venitt, S. and Parry, J. M. (eds) *Mutagenicity Testing – A Practical Approach*, pp. 149–185. IRL Press, Oxford.
129. Zimmermann, F. K. (1971) Induction of mitotic gene conversion by mutagens. *Mutat. Res.* **11:** 327–337.

130. Zimmermann, F. K., Kern, R. and Rasenberger, H. (1975) A yeast strain for simultaneous detection of induced mitotic crossing over, mitotic gene conversion and reverse mutation. *Mutat. Res.* **28:** 381–388.
131. Sharp, D. C. and Parry, J. M. (1981) Induction of mitotic gene conversion by 41 coded compounds using the yeast culture JD1. In de Serres, C. J. and Ashby J. (eds) *Progress in Mutation Research*, Vol. 1, pp. 491–501. Elsevier/North Holland, New York.
132. Parry, J. M. and Zimmermann, F. K. (1976) The detection of monosomic colonies produced by mitotic chromosome non-dysjunction in the yeast, *Saccharomyces cerevisiae. Mutat. Res.* **36:** 49–65.
133. Farber, E. (1990) Reversible and irreversible lesions in the process of cancer development. In Montesano, R., Bartsch, H. and Tomatis, L. (eds) *Molecular and Cellular Aspects of Carcinogen Screening Test*, pp. 143–151. IARC, Lyon.
134. Iversen, O. H. and Iversen, U. M. (1982) Must initiators come first? rumorigenic and carcinogenic effects on skin of 3-methylcholanthrene and TPA in various sequences. *Br. J. Cancer.* **45:** 912–919.
135. Gori, G. B. (1992) Cancer risk assessment: the science that is not. *Reg. Toxicol. Pharmacol.* **16:** 10–20.
136. Spandidos, D. A. and Anderson, M. L. M. (1987) A study of mechanisms of carcinogenesis by gene transfer of oncogenes into mammalian cells. *Mutat. Res.* **185:** 271–291.
137. Wu, S.-Q., Storer, B. E., Bookland, E. A. *et al.* Nonrandom chromosome losses in stepwise neoplastic transformation *in vitro* of human uroepithelial cells. *Cancer Res.* **51:** 3323–3326.
138. Newbold, R. F., Overell, R. W. and Connell, J. R. (1982) Induction of immortality is an early event in malignant transformation of mammalian cells by carcinogens. *Nature* **299:** 633–635.
139. Newbold, R. F., Cuthbert, A. R., Themis, M., Trott, D. A., Blair, A. G. and Li., W. (1993) Cell immortalisation as a key, rate limiting event in malignant transformation: approaches toward a molecular genetic analysis. *Toxicol. Lett.* **67:** 211–230.
140. Trott, D. A., Cuthbert, A. P., Overell, R. W., Russo, I. and Newbold, R. F. (1995) Mechanisms involved in the immortalisation of mammalian cells by ionising radiation and chemical carcinogens. *Carcinogenesis* **16:** 193–204.
141. Korsmeyer, S. J. (1995) Regulators of cell death. *Trends Genet.* **11:** 101–105.
142. Jeanteur, Ph., Theillet, C. and Pujol, H. (1990) Oncogenes, anti-oncogenes et leurs altérations dans les tumeurs humaines. *Rev. Med. Interne* **XI:** 216–220.
143. Pitot, H. C. and Dragan, Y. P. (1991) Facts and theories concerning the mechanisms of carcinogenesis. *FASEB J.* **5:** 2280–2286.
144. McCormick, A. and Campisi, J. (1991) Cellular ageing and senescence. *Curr. Opin. Cell. Biol.* **3:** 230–234.
145. Wu, J. C., Merlino, G. and Fausto, N. (1994) Establishment and characterisation of differentiated, nontransformed heptocyte cell lines derived from mice transgenic for transforming growth factor alpha. *Proc. Natl Acad. Sci. U.S.A.* **91:** 674–678.
146. McGregor, D. and Ashby, J. (1985) Summary report on the performance of the cell transformation assays. In Ashby, J., de Serres, F. J. *et al.* (eds) *Progress in Mutation Research*, Vol. 5, pp. 103–115. Elsevier Science, Amsterdam.
147. Meyer, A., McGregor, D. and Styles, J. (1984) *In vitro* cell transformation assays. In Dean, B. J. (ed.) *Report of UKEMS Sub-committee on Guidelines for Mutagenicity Tests, Part II*, pp. 123–144. UKEMS, Swansea.
148. Berwald, Y. and Sachs, L. (1965) *In vitro* transformation of normal cells to tumor cells by carcinogenic hydrocarbons. *J. Natl Cancer Inst.* **35:** 641–661.
149. Di Paolo, J. A. (1980) Quantitative *in vitro* transformation of Syrian golden hamster embryo cells with the use of frozen stored cells. *J. Natl Cancer Inst.* **64:** 1485–1489.
150. Lubet, R. A., Nims, R. W., Kiss, E., Kouri, R. E., Putman, D. L. and Schechtman, L. M. (1986) Influence of various parameters on benzo(a)pyrene enhancement of adenovirus SA7 transformation of Syrian hamster embryo cells. *Env. Mutagen.* **8:** 533–542.
151. Shiner, A. C., Newbold, R. E. and Cooper, C. S. (1988) Morphological transformation of the immortalised hamster dermal fibroblasts following treatment with simple alkylating carcinogens. *Carcinogenesis* **9:** 1701–1709.
152. Styles, J. A. (1977) A method for detecting carcinogenic organic chemicals using mammalian cells in culture. *Br. J. Cancer* **36:** 558–564.
153. Kakunaga, T. (1973) A quantitative system for assay of malignant transformation by chemical carcinogens using a clone derived from Balb 3T3. *Int. J. Cancer* **12:** 463–473.

154. Reznikoff, C. A., Bertram, J. S., Brankow, D. W. and Heidelberger, C. (1973) Quantitative and qualitative studies on chemical transformation of cloned C3H mouse embryo cells, sensitive to post confluence inhibition of cell division. *Cancer Res.* **33:** 3239–3249.
155. Combes, R. D., Anderson, D., Brooks, T., Neale, S. and Venitt, S. (1984) The detection of mutagens in urine, faeces and body fluids. In Dean, B. J. (ed.) *Guidelines for Mutagenicity Testing. Part II: Supplementary Tests, Mutagens in Body Fluids and Excreta, Nitrosation Products*, pp. 203–244. United Kingdom Environmental Mutagen Society, Swansea.
156. Yagi, T., Sato, M., Mishigori, C. and Takebe, H. (1994) Similarity in the molecular profile of mutations induced by UV light in shuttle vector plasmids propagated in mouse and human cells. *Mutagenesis* **9:** 73–77.
157. Collins, A. R. (1993) Mutant rodent cell lines sensitive to ultraviolet light, ionizing radiation and cross-linking agents: a comprehensive survey of genetic and biochemical characteristics. *Mutat. Res.* **3:** 99–118.
158. Skouv, J., Rasmussen, E. S., Frandsen, H., Forchammer, J. and Kryspin-Sorensen, I. (1995) The reducing agent dithiothreitol (DTT) increases expression of c-*myc* and c-*fos* proto-oncogenes in human cells. *Alternatives to Laboratory Animals* **23:** 497–503.
159. Crespi, C. L., Penman, B. W., Gonzalez, F. J., Gelboin, H. V., Galvin, M. and Lagenbach, R. (1993) Genetic toxicology using human cell lines expressing human P-450. *Biochem. Soc. Trans.* **21:** 1023–1028.
160. Crofton-Sleigh, C., Doherty, A., Ellard, S., Parry, E. M. and Venitt, S. (1993) Micronucleus assays using cytochalasin-blocked MCL-5 cells, a proprietary human cell line expressing five human cytochromes P-450 and microsomal hydrolase. *Mutagenesis* **8:** 363–372.
161. MacDonald, C. (1993) Development of new animal cell lines by oncogene immortalisation. *The Genetic Engineer and Biotechnologist* **13:** 121–124.
162. Pfeiffer, A., Gonzalez, F., Harris, C. C. and Mace, K. (1994) Cellular gene technology for constructing metabolically competent cells. Presentation at INVITOX Meeting, Ittigen, Switzerland, September.
163. Mitchell, I. de G., Carlton, J. B. and Gilbert, P. J. (1988) The detection and importance of outliers in the *in vivo* micronucleus assay. *Mutagenesis* **3:** 491–495.
164. Mitchell, I. de G., Rees, R. W., Gilbert, P. J. and Carlton, J. B. (1990) The use of historical data for identifying biologically unimportant but statistically significant results in genotoxicity assays. *Mutagenesis* **5:** 159–164.
165. Mitchell, I. de G. (1987) The interaction of statistical analysis, biology of dose-response and test design in assessment of genotoxicity data. *Mutagenesis* **2:** 141–145.
166. Conover, W. J. and Iman, R. L. (1982) Analysis of covariance using rank transformation. *Biometrics* **38:** 715–724.
167. Mitchell, I. de G., Amphlett, N. W. and Rees, R. W. (1994) Parametric analysis of rank transformed data for statistical assessment of genotoxicity data with examples from cultured mammalian cells. *Mutagenesis* **9:** 125–132.
168. VanParys, P. and Marsboom, R. (1985) Genetic toxicology in the pharmaceutical industry. *Fd. Chem. Toxicol* **23:** 19–22.

15

Use of Whole Embryo Cultures in *In Vitro* Teratogenicity Testing

BEAT SCHMID, RUDOLF BECHTER AND PAVEL KUCERA

I. Introduction 354
II. Application of *in vitro* systems in the pharmaceutical industry 356
III. Criteria for the suitability of an *in vitro* test 357
A. Introduction 357
B. Sensitivity versus specificity 357
C. Potency 357
D. Validation 358
IV. The choice of an appropriate *in vitro* assay 358
V. The chick embryo in an 'artificial egg' 358
A. Introduction 358
B. Materials and methods 359
1. Chicken embryos 359
2. Culture conditions 359
3. End-point measurements 359
C. Results obtained with chick embryo culture 359
1. Control experiments 359
2. Experimental studies 360
3. Comparison with other test systems 360
D. Advantages 360
E. Disadvantages 361
VI. Mammalian postimplantation whole embryo culture 363
A. Introduction 363
B. Materials and methods 363
1. Animals 363
2. Culture conditions 364
3. Treatment 364
4. End-point measurements 364
5. Statistical analysis 364
6. Methodological aspects 365
C. Results of validation studies obtained with mammalian embryo culture . . . 365
D. Advantages 365
E. Disadvantages 368
VII. Conclusions 368
References 368

IN VITRO METHODS IN PHARMACEUTICAL RESEARCH
ISBN 0-12-163390-X

I. INTRODUCTION

Chemical interference with gametes and embryonic or fetal development can cause infertility, loss of the conceptus or birth defects. The rate of human infertility is, at present, unknown. However, for the successfully fertilized ovum there is a considerable awareness that about 70% of human conceptions fail to achieve full development to birth (see Berry[1] for a bibliography). Of all human newborns, about 3% have a congenital anomaly requiring medical attention and about one-third of the anomalies can be regarded as life threatening (see Berry[2] for a bibliography). It is impossible, at present, to provide exact figures of agents that affect gametes or which contribute to the induction of abnormalities in human development. On the other hand, these side-effects create enormous social and psychological problems, and the need for techniques for the early detection of chemicals that interfere with any of the reproductive steps are thus essential. Testing in animals has represented in the past – and still represents today – an important aspect in this control.

As debate has focused on the ethics of animal experimentation, alternatives for the possible replacement or reduction in the use of animals, as well as in the refinement of existing methods (3Rs), were actively sought in the area of reproductive toxicity testing.

Examples describing reductions in animal numbers with *in vivo* tests are relatively rare, and are well summarized in the European Chemical Industry Ecology and Toxicology Centre (ECETOC) monograph of 1989.[3] Mammalian *in vivo* tests, such as the limit test, offer the advantage that entire embryonic and fetal development can be assessed, that maternal, embryonic and fetal pharmacokinetics processes are taken into consideration and that species differences can be examined. However, this approach still uses pregnant animals and involves treatment with substances that may provoke pain. Moreover, there is in many cases insufficient amounts of the new product under development available to treat animals *in vivo*.

Although reproductive toxicity testing represents an area in which many complex biological processes intervene, major activities devoted to *in vitro* studies started in the early 1980s, thus looking back to a more than 15-year history of *in vitro* alternatives. The *in vitro* assays that have been developed use viruses, invertebrates, mammalian cell lines, primary mammalian cell cultures, organ cultures, invertebrate, vertebrate and mammalian embryos, and an overview of these assays are shown in Tables 15.1–15.4. When looking at the parameters assessed in these assays, it becomes obvious that, from the reproductive cycle, systems were selected which allow the detection of embryotoxic effects. Systems that sought chemical influences on gametes, fertilization and preimplantation stages *in vitro* remained focused on mechanistic investigations. For reproductive toxicity testing the 3R principles have thus in practice been applied to the window of the early postimplantation phase. In the following sections priority had to be attributed to this fact.

Table 15.1 Viral and invertebrate systems in teratogenicity testing.

Test system	End-point	Application	References
Viruses			
Pox virus	Expression	Proposed for screening	4
Invertebrates			
Drosophila embryonic cell	Differentiation		
	Toxicity	Used for screening	5, 6
Planaria	Regeneration	Proposed for screening	7
Hydra	Regeneration		
	Toxicity	Used for screening	8–10

Table 15.2 Mammalian cells in teratogenicity testing.

Test system	End-point	Application	References
Mammalian cell lines			
Mouse ovary tumour cell	Adhesiveness Growth inhibition	Proposed for screening	11–13
Human embryonic palatal mesenchyme cell	Growth inhibition	Proposed for screening	14, 15
Neublastoma cell	Differentiation Growth inhibition	Used for screening	16
Embryonic stem cell	Differentiation Proliferation Toxicity	Used for screening	16–18
V79 cell	Cell–cell interactions	Proposed for screening	19
Primary mammalian cell cultures			
Neural tissue cell	Differentiation Growth inhibition	Used for screening	20–24
Limb-bud cell	Differentiation Growth inhibition	Used for screening	21, 25–32
Brain cell aggregate	Differentiation Cell–cell interactions Growth inhibition	Mechanistic investigations; proposed for screening	33–38

Table 15.3 Mammalian organ cultures in teratogenicity testing.

Test system	End-point	Application	References
Mammalian organ cultures			
Limb-bud cultures	Growth retardation Proliferation Malformation(?)	Mechanistic studies	39–43
Palatal shelves	Growth retardation Malformation(?)	Mechanistic studies	44, 45
Other	Differentiation Proliferation Toxicity		46–48

Table 15.4 Embryo cultures in teratogenicity testing.

Test system	End-point	Application	References
Invertebrate embryos			
Sea urchin embryo	Differentiation Lethality	Proposed for screening	49
Shrimp embryo	Differentiation Lethality	Proposed for screening	50–53
Cricket embryo	Differentiation Lethality	Proposed for screening	54
Drosophila embryo	Differentiation Lethality	Mechanistic studies and proposed for screening	55–57
Vertebrate embryos			
Chicken (*in ovo* and *in vitro*)	Differentiation Lethality Morphology	Proposed for screening and mechanistic studies	37, 58–61
Fish	Lethality Embryonic development and growth	Used for screening	62, 63
Frog (FETAX)	Morphological development of mid to late blastula embryos	Used for screening	64–66
Mammalian embryos			
Rodent Postimplantation embryos	Differentiation Retardation Lethality	Used for screening and mechanistic studies	67–72
Preimplantation embryos	Lethality	Mechanistic studies	73
Non-rodent	Differentiation Retardation Lethality	Proposed for screening and mechanistic studies	74, 75

II. APPLICATIONS OF *IN VITRO* SYSTEMS IN THE PHARMACEUTICAL INDUSTRY

During the development process of a new drug, the following major steps are involved in embryotoxicity testing:

1. Prescreening or screening of new compounds for their embryotoxic or teratogenic potential as a basis for the promotion for further development.
2. Safety evaluation before the clinical testing of a given compound in women.
3. Submission of data that allow risk assessment as a prerequisite for drug registration.
4. Mechanistic investigations when potential problems arise or adverse effects occur.

For pharmaceuticals, safety evaluation and risk assessment before human use are regulated in a defined manner, and are based on preclinical animal data. As a rule, newly developed compounds are not administered to women of childbearing potential without having defined the appropriate safety margins in animals.

Safety evaluation and risk assessment for pharmaceuticals are currently based on data collected from animal experiments, and the studies required are defined by regulatory guidelines, such as the ICH tripartite guideline[76] on the detection of toxicity to reproduction of medicinal products, established in 1993.

To fulfil the above requirements, the number of animals used is still high. At present, no risk assessments accepted by the tripartite guideline for new chemical entities are based solely on *in vitro* data. *In vitro* techniques are thus mainly used in the prescreening and screening phases, and for mechanistic investigations. The fulfilment of scientific criteria of predictability, reliability, compensatory factors and mechanisms of injury will thus determine when, and to what extent, *in vitro* methods are incorporated into the drug development process.

III. CRITERIA FOR THE SUITABILITY OF AN *IN VITRO* TEST

A. Introduction

To be of value, an alternative test in reproductive toxicity testing should ideally be predictive of toxicity to the human reproductive system; it should be reliable, reproducible, sensitive and/or specific; it should be related to concentrations of the toxicants; and it should provide a rapid response.

B. Sensitivity versus specificity

If a positive response is obtained with an *in vitro* system, there are two possible options: either the risk of a positive response does not outweigh the benefit (e.g. for a given indication area), or negative analogues are available. In both situations the chemical is generally not developed further. On the other hand, if the therapeutic principle is very important, then the chemical should be submitted with high priority to *in vivo* testing in animal studies. False-positive compounds underlie a similar selection criteria and would be filtered out without too much severe consequence, or identified in the following *in vivo* testing. False negatives, however, imply further investment in the development of the molecule and would therefore have more important consequences until the error was recognized. For these reasons, a screening model should be optimized to have a high specificity in drug development.

C. Potency

Drug screening involves, in many cases, the testing of a series of structurally related molecules. Such molecules are often congeners of compounds of an already investigated chemical class and/or therapeutic indications, so that pharmacological and toxicological knowledge is already available. In these situations, the *in vitro* test has to provide comparative data in relation to data on already existing molecules.

D. Validation

An *in vitro* system may be selected for its properties of representing a particular mechanism that is thought to be inherent to the developmental toxicity of a given molecule or a class of compounds, for example in the case of retinoids.[28,77] The same *in vitro* test may be of low predictive value for another set of chemicals as they may act via a different mechanism on the developmental process.[78] Furthermore, *in vivo* animal data on a large number of non-related chemicals often lack soundness and quality for an adequate validation of the *in vitro* data, and the selection of chemicals to be tested for a large validation study is often biased and difficult to undertake.[79] Large validation studies including a large number of non-related chemicals seem, therefore, to be of minor importance for the choice of an *in vitro* testing system in drug development. More importantly, there is a need to undertake well-designed and controlled studies in different steps to provide sufficient standardization and to improve the reliability of the system.[80]

IV. THE CHOICE OF AN APPROPRIATE *IN VITRO* ASSAY

From the wide variety of *in vitro* systems available and outlined in Tables 15.1–15.4, two basic principles can be derived: there is an increase in the complexity of the biological indicators (e.g. from cell line cultures to whole embryo cultures) and a phylogenetic evaluation in hierarchy (e.g. from hydra to humans).

A priori, as already indicated, there is no preference for a given system as long as the end-point assessed is relevant for animals and/or humans. On the other hand, within the complexity of biological systems, cell cultures using cell lines have been reported to have little success in prescreening for the embryotoxicity potential of compounds, although they were of human origin.[15] Cell systems that also allow the assessment of differentiation processes, such as embryonic stems cells, have been shown to be able to predict teratogenic potential to a greater extent.[18] If compounds interfere with yet unknown end-points, and thus the selection of a specific assay is biased, one could argue that the complex systems that are closest to humans are the best suited to provide the most reliable results. These systems then offer the additional advantage that positive outcomes can be evaluated mechanistically, thus contributing to the understanding of the relevancy of the parameter(s) assessed. These arguments led us to focus on more complex systems, such as the whole embryo culture systems in vertebrates and mammals.

V. THE CHICK EMBRYO IN AN 'ARTIFICIAL EGG'

A. Introduction

The avian embryo is easily accessible for experimentation and its development is known in great detail.[81,82] In particular, the chick embryo has been used to study the effects of toxicants.[58] However, as the agents have mostly been injected into the egg, these studies cannot provide necessary information on the concentrations inducing specific effects.

Based on extensive experience with the chick embryo in the domain of embryonal physiology,[59,83,84] a standardized system which makes it possible to expose the chick embryo *in vitro* under defined conditions has been developed and is presented below.

B. Materials and methods

The following protocol was developed and found to be suitable for the testing of chemicals.

1. *Chicken embryos*

The embryos from eggs collected from 35–70-week-old hens of a robust Warrens strain stabled in a country farm are used for *in vitro* culture.

2. *Culture conditions*

After preincubation for 20 h the eggs opened and the vitelline membrane with the attached blastoderm is excised from the yolk and transferred to an incubation chamber moulded from a transparent silicone elastomere.

The incubation medium is obtained by mixing one part of the thin albumen collected from the eggs during the explanation with one part of Tyrode solution. The compounds to be tested are dissolved in the medium or suspended in gelatin at the desired concentration. Constant volumes of culture medium are poured over the preparation, the chamber is closed, incubated at 37.5°C, and the embryo is allowed to develop for a further 3 days. The incubation medium is not changed during the incubation period. On average, 11 embryos are used per substance and concentration.

3. *End-point measurements*

Growth and morphogenesis of the skeletomotor, cardiovascular and nervous systems, and of the extraembryonic membranes and circulation, are observed and photographed under a binocular microscope at 17, 24, 42 and 66 h of incubation.

Seven quantitative and 17 qualitative criteria are used to score the development of each embryo. The parameters are introduced into a VAX computer and evaluated using the Oracle system of data analysis. The embryos are scored after 42 h for live normal, live abnormal and dead abnormal. The concentration–response curves are evaluated by covariance analysis.

C. Results obtained with chick embryo culture

1. *Control experiments*

The growth and differentiation of control embryos cultured *in vitro* closely resemble that of embryos maintained *in ovo*.[59] Blastoderms presenting normal neurulation, somitogenesis, shaping of the embryo, regular heart beats and functional blood circulation are all observed.

Spontaneous malformation is present in 10–15%, about twice the frequency of that observed *in ovo*. Typically, such malformation appears at 17 h and is characterized by a short embryonic body, missing somites, and largely open or exencephalic brain vesicles.

2. *Experimental studies*

At present, a total of 22 compounds, mostly known teratogens, have been tested with this system:[37,60] amiloride (unpublished), 6-aminonicotinamide, aspirin, cadmium chloride, caffeine, dexamethasone, dimethylsulfoxide (DMSO), diphenylhydantoin, ethanol, 4-hydroxypyridine, ketoconazole, methotrexate, methoxyacetic acid, methoxyethanol, metronidazole, phenobarbital, retinoic acid derivatives Ro-1-5488 and Ro-13-6307, saccharin, sulfadiazine, sulfanilamide and theophylline. Twelve of these compounds were assessed within the framework of a multilaboratory study using coded compounds.[37]

No harmful effects were found with amiloride (unpublished observation), ethanol and saccharin[60] even at concentrations higher than $1\,\mathrm{mmol\,l^{-1}}$. Weak or questionable teratogenic effects were found with methoxyethanol and sulfonamides.[37] The other compounds induced, within 2 days, specific patterns of growth perturbation and anomalies. These effects were concentration dependent and appeared at levels ranging from 10^{-10} to $10^{-3}\,\mathrm{mol\,l^{-1}}$ (Fig. 15.1).

Each compound has been characterized by two curves (Fig. 15.1) delimiting the living normal embryos (white area), the living abnormal ones (light grey area) and dead abnormal ones (dark grey area). These curves make it possible to determine the concentrations inducing teratogenic effects in 50% of embryos (EC_{50}) and the concentration inducing lethal effects in 50% of embryos (LC_{50}) values (Fig. 15.2). The closer these curves are, i.e. the smaller the LC_{50}–EC_{50} value is, the lower is the chance of survival of the abnormal embryo, and the compound is thus considered to exert general toxic effects (e.g. aminonicotinamide or methotrexate). On the other hand, the more the curves are apart, i.e. the larger the $LC_{50} - EC_{50}$ value is, the more specific malformations can be expected, and the compound can be considered to exert teratogenic effects (e.g. retinoids, dexamethasone or cadmium). By using this system, ranking of the compounds is possible according to their embryolethal as well as teratogenic potency (Fig. 15.2b).

3. *Comparison with other test systems*

Comparisons with other test systems, particularly to the mammalian whole embryo culture system, have been discussed in previous papers.[37,38,60] It is important to note that the tested compounds produced characteristic anomalies in chicken embryos and that the effects were obtained at concentrations similar to those found in the mammalian system. Overall, the chick culture appears to be slightly more sensitive in the sense that embryonic malformation and lethality appear at lower concentrations than, for example, in the rat embryo. This may be due to the fact that it is not surrounded by a yolk-sac membrane, and that there is a direct contact between the embryo and the compound.

D. Advantages

The test using the whole chick embryo culture is characterized by good sensitivity and reproducibility, and reveals specific, concentration-dependent patterns of response to different substances. It does not require the killing of pregnant animals for the dissection of embryos. Physicochemical conditions of the embryonic development can be controlled, and

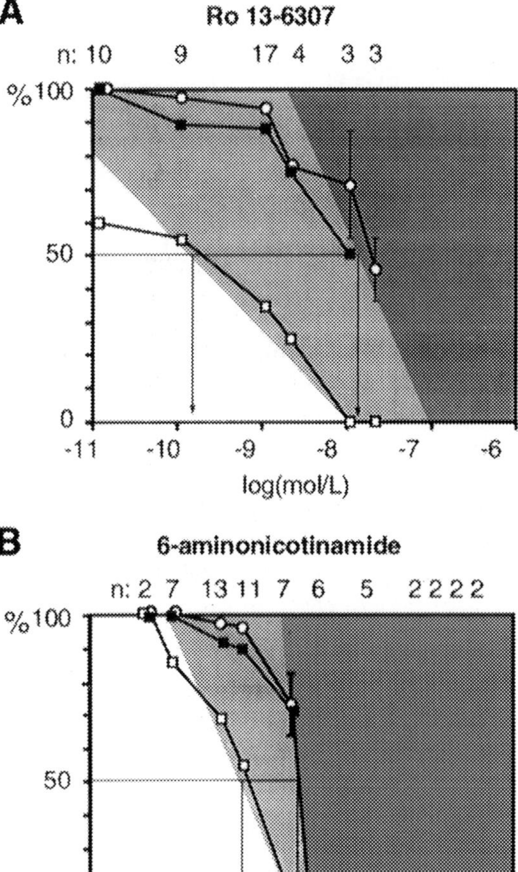

Fig. 15.1 Scoring of embryotoxicity and teratogenicity in the whole chick embryo culture. **A** and **B**: examples of the concentration–effect relationship of two known teratogens. ○, Percentage of normal growth (standard deviation is shown for values significantly different from control growth); □, percentage of normal embryos; ■, percentage of dead embryos. Areas with light grey shading indicate the range of concentrations producing living abnormal embryos. The arrows denote the EC_{50} and LC_{50}.

biochemical and physiological characterizations are possible[85,86] so that further mechanistic studies with embryotoxic agents can be carried out in the same model.

E. Disadvantages

Mammalian specific activation (e.g. addition of an S_9 fraction) cannot yet be simulated *in vitro*. Further, little information on the kinetics of compounds in chicken is available when compared with rodents and humans.

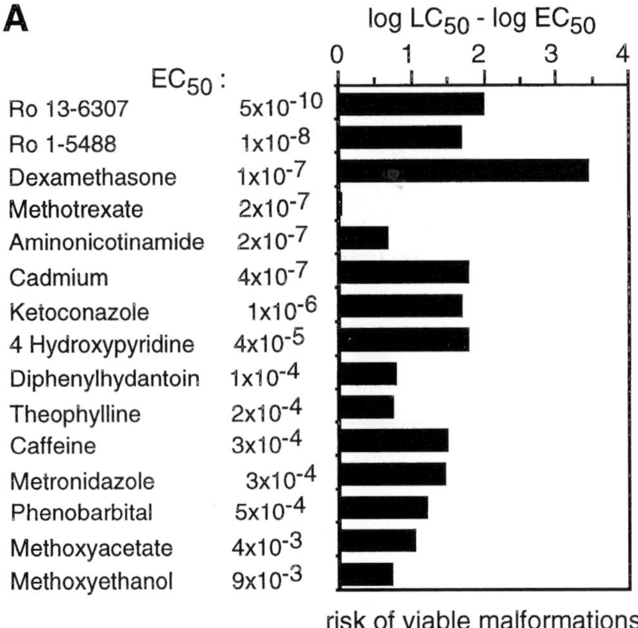

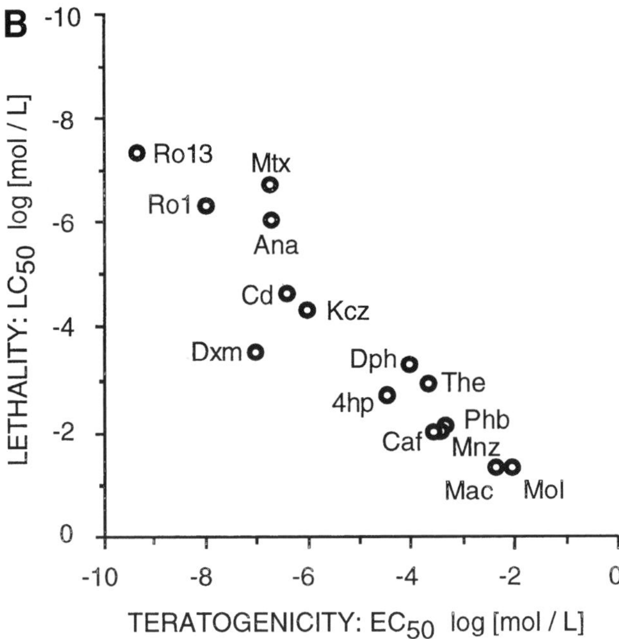

Fig. 15.2 Comparison of the teratogenic and embryotoxic potencies of 15 compounds tested in the whole chick embryo culture. A: Ranking according to teratogenic potency of known teratogens. The difference $\log LC_{50}$–$\log EC_{50}$ is taken as a criterion of the probability of producing living but abnormal embryos. B: Relationship between toxic and teratogenic potencies. Note that the culture is sensitive to a wide concentration range. Abbreviations correspond to the compounds listed in A. Non-teratogenic compounds (e.g. saccharin), although tested, are not shown.

VI. MAMMALIAN POSTIMPLANTATION WHOLE EMBRYO CULTURE

A. Introduction

Rodent and rabbit postimplantation embryos can be cultured during different stages of organogenesis.[67,75,87–89] The culture of embryos from the head-fold–early somite stage onwards was proposed for teratogenicity screening systems in the mid-1980s, using the mouse[70,90] and the rat,[69] whereas the culture of rabbit embryos has been optimized only recently.[75] Rat serum, diluted up to 50% with composition salt solutions, gave satisfactory results for normal growth and differentiation of the rat[91] and mouse[92] embryo. On the other hand, it was shown[93] that acetylsalicylic acid treatment in rat serum supplemented with 50% Waymouth medium resulted in a higher frequency of malformations occurring at lower concentrations than with pure rat serum.

Serum from cows,[71] monkeys[94] and humans[95–97] also allows satisfactory embryonic growth. Serum from rabbits diluted up to 40% has been shown to support rabbit embryonic growth *in vitro*.[75] The test compound under investigation can be added to the culture for defined culture periods[98,99] or during the entire culture. Drug metabolism can be mimicked in various ways. A liver homogenate (S_9) and appropriate co-factors have been added to the culture medium using liver from different species,[100,101] including humans.[102] Rat hepatocytes have been co-cultured with the embryo to produce metabolites concurrently in the culture medium.[103] Sequential hepatocyte–whole embryo culture, which allows the study of kinetics of toxification and detoxification *in vitro* have been reported.[104] The use of serum from animals pretreated with the test compound as culture medium also makes it possible to activate the compound metabolically and to study the effects of its metabolites on embryonic development *in vitro*.[105]

The above methodological variations can be adapted to mechanistic investigations in line with a particular problem. For the screening and prescreening of chemicals, simplified protocols have been developed, allowing a rapid assessment and reducing animal and laboratory resources to a minimum.

B. Materials and methods

The following example of a possible protocol was found to be suitable for screening and prescreening purposes.

1. *Animals*

The following rat strains have already been used successfully: the RAI strain from Ciba-Geigy (Basle, Switzerland), Han Wistar rats (Kfm: WSA; Han Ibm: WSA; Kleintierfarm Madörin, Füllinsdorf, Switzerland), Sprague Dawley COBS (CD) rats, specific pathogen free (SPF) derived nulliparous RIV:Tox rats. The animals are mated by housing one or two nulliparous females overnight with one male. Successful copulation is assessed the next day by microscopic observations of sperm in the vaginal smear, and this day is designated as day 0 of gestation.

2. *Culture conditions*

Whole rat embryos are explanted on day 9.5 of gestation. They are dissected free of maternal decidual tissue and Reichert's membrane, and embryos that have three to seven somites are used. Two or three embryos are then randomly transferred to 30 ml glass bottles containing 4 ml of heat-inactivated male rat serum. The bottles containing the embryos are gassed for 3–4 min with a mixture of 5% oxygen, 5.6% carbon dioxide and 90% nitrogen. Sixteen hours later the oxygen concentration in the mixture is increased to 10%, then to 20% 24 h later. No antibiotics are used for the preparation or during the entire culture period. The culture vessels are incubated at 37°C under continuous rotation (21 rpm) for a total of 48 h using a roller apparatus incubator (Heräus, type B5060 EK/CO2).

3. *Treatment*

Water-soluble chemicals are dissolved in Waymouth medium (Gibco, Basle, Switzerland), whereas water-insoluble compounds are normally dispersed in gelatin (0.2% final concentration). Exceptionally, the compounds are dissolved in 10 μl of absolute ethanol or DMSO as the drug vehicle. They are generally applied in a 100 μl volume, and controls receive the identical volume of the solvent administered. The highest non-toxic concentration is usually also used to test chemicals in culture medium supplemented with S_9 mix, an Aroclor 1254-induced rat liver microsomal extracts and its co-factor NADPH, in order to assess potential metabolic activation processes.

The compounds are usually added at the beginning of the culture period and remain there for 48 h. Recent investigations have shown that a 24 h exposure and culture period may not be sufficient to identify teratogenic compounds.[106] Compounds are usually tested at five concentrations, each including an average of about ten embryos. A factor of three is generally used between the individual concentrations. Two or three individual experiments are performed to screen a given compound. For rapid screening (for related analogues, for example), three embryos per concentration and one to three concentrations per analogue may suffice to provide indicative information for the selection of the most optimal drug candidate.

4. *End-point measurements*

At the end of the 48 h cumulative period, the embryos are transferred to phosphate-buffered saline (pH 7.4) and examined under a dissecting microscope. Embryonic growth and differentiation are evaluated when a beating heart and a full rotation are apparent. Otherwise the embryos are scored as 'lethal'. Crown–rump and head length measurements are taken as growth indicators, and somite numbers are used as markers of differentiation. Morphological features of the embryos are evaluated to assess the nature and extent of the abnormalities. These include: flexion, heart, fore–midbrain, and hindbrain, otic, optic and olfactory systems, branchial bars, mandibular and maxillary processes, limb buds, somites. Yolk sac vascularization and size are evaluated to assess side-effects on the extraembryonic site.

5. *Statistical analysis*

Statistical analysis of the differences between control and treated groups, with respect to parameters of growth and differentiation, are performed with the two-sided Student's *t* test (homogeneous distribution) or the *t* test of Welch (non-homogeneous distribution). The significance of an increased incidence of embryos with anomalies, compared with controls, is carried out with the Newman–Keuls multiple range test to test for statistically significant differences in embryonic parameters. The level of significance is set at $P \leq 0.05$.

6. *Methodological aspects*

Some of the methodological aspects cited below are considered important for the final interpretation of the results. For example, the solvent used may influence the outcome of the background malformation rate[107] and the exposure time may affect the sensitivity of the system.[106] The protein and drug-binding capacity of the medium have to be considered when extrapolating data to the human situation.[108]

Other methodological issues are linked to bioactivation. Van Aerts *et al.*,[109] for example, showed that bioactivation of cyclophosphamide is greatly enhanced in male rats following pretreatment with Aroclor 1254, whereas this P450 inducer has only little effect on the bioactivation of cyclophosphamide in pregnant rats.

As the scoring of embryos depends on the individual judgement of the investigator, thorough education and standardization of the morphological criteria are required.[110–112] It is important to state in this context that the criterion of general growth retardation must be clearly distinguished from that of specific malformations and embryonic lethality in terms of the concentrations affecting these parameters (for details see Figs 15.3 and 15.4). This helps to prevent generally retarded embryos (which look different from their control counterparts anyway) from being scored as malformed and the compound being classified wrongly as a 'teratogen'.

C. Results of validation studies obtained with mammalian embryo culture

Results obtained with a selected number of teratogens and non-teratogens which were assessed in the rat whole embryo culture were published as early as 1983[61] and expanded in 1988.[113,114] An interlaboratory validation study with different culture conditions[111] and selected chemicals[106] gave comparable and reproducible results. Furthermore, Cicurel and Schmid,[113,114] and Bechter *et al.*[115] reported a good correlation between *in vivo* and *in vitro* data for a series of retinoids. In an internal prospective validation study, ongoing for the past 10 years, with 14 *in vivo* teratogens and 55 *in vivo* non-teratogens (including a series of 'model' compounds), the specificity of the test system was found to be 91%, the sensitivity 86% and the overall accuracy 90%.[116]

D. Advantages

The rodent whole embryo culture system is an *in vitro* test for the detection of potentially teratogenic compounds, for the ranking of those with a positive outcome, as well as for the elucidation of mechanisms of teratogenicity. Today, the rodent whole embryo culture system is used in many laboratories and has proved to be a highly valuable, robust, screening system for the prediction of *in vivo* outcome in the course of the development of a pharmaceutical compound. It reduces the time needed for the testing of a given compound to 1–2 weeks if

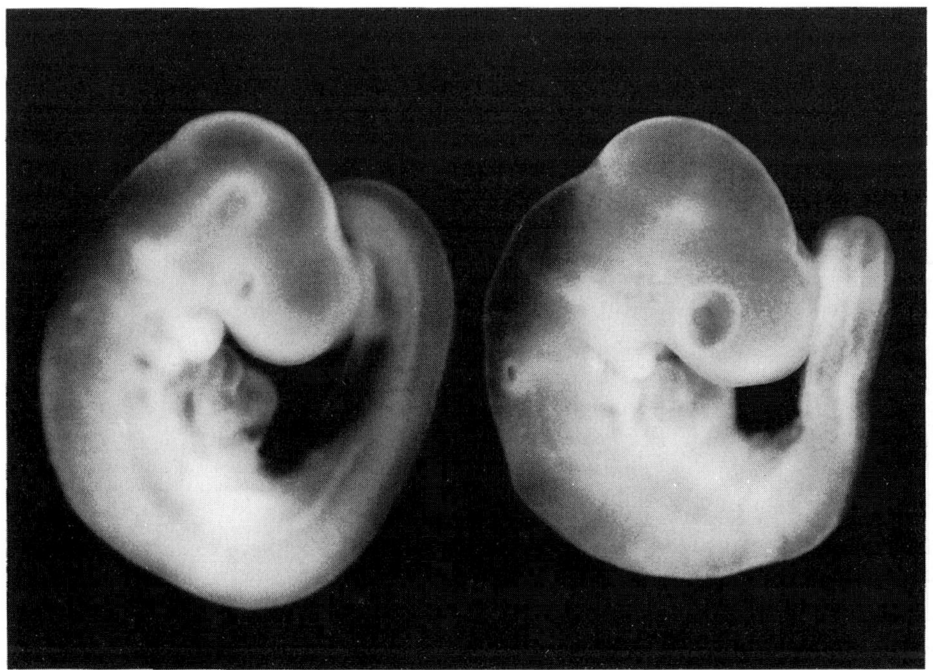

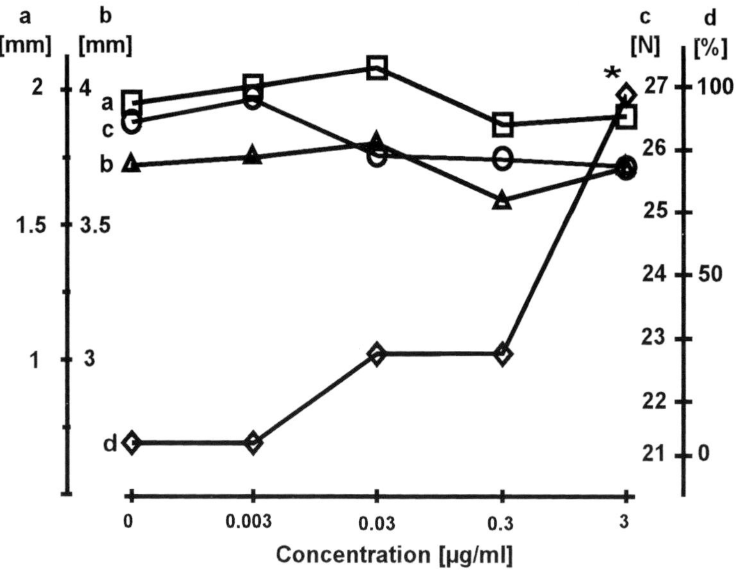

Fig. 15.3 Scoring of a compound exerting teratogenicity in the whole rat embryo culture; example of the concentration–effect relationship of a known teratogen. **a**, Crown–rump length; **b**, head length; **c**, somite number; **d**, frequency of dysmorphogenic effects.

several experiments for a compound are being carried out; eventually 2 days are sufficient if analogues are being tested or if a clear-cut result at high concentration levels has been obtained. The system allows dysmorphogenesis to be detected in many primordial organs and a distinction to be made between specific dysmorphogenic effects and adverse effects on the embryo's general growth and differentiation.

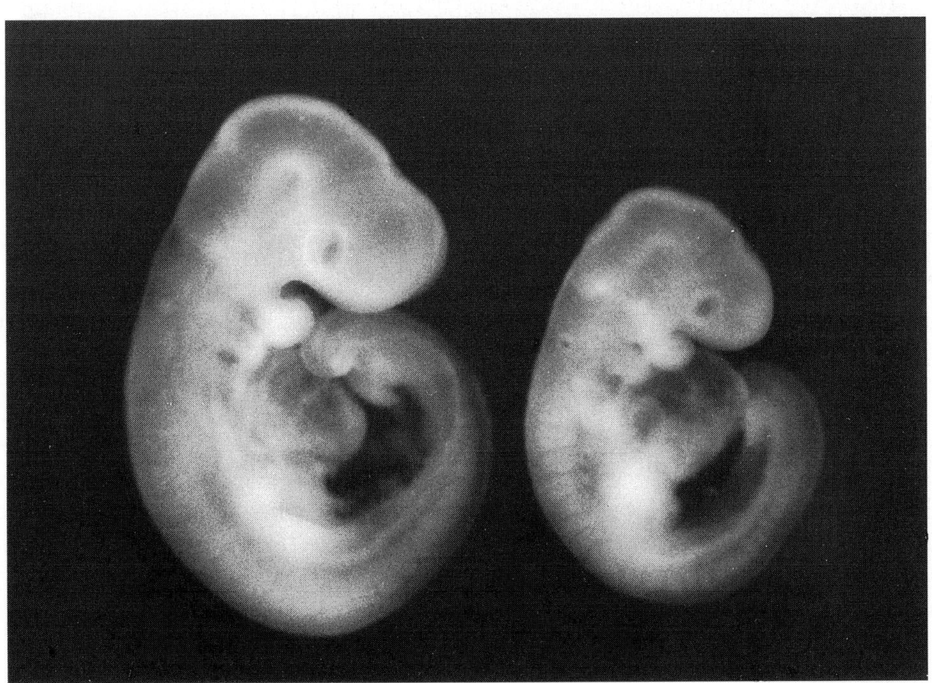

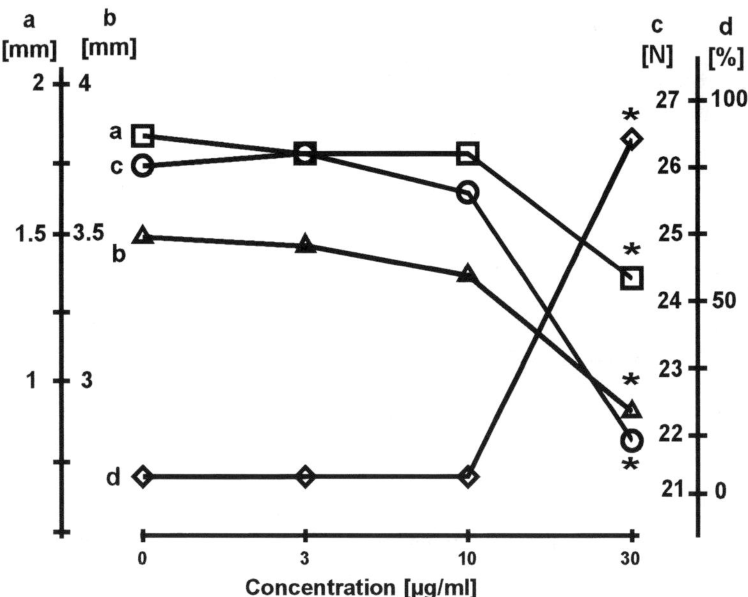

Fig. 15.4 Scoring of a compound exerting general toxicity in the whole rat embryo culture; example of the concentration–effect relationship of a non-teratogen. **a**, Crown–rump length; **b**, head length; **c**, somite number; **d**, frequency of dysmorphogenic effects.

E. Disadvantages

Although the system overviews complex biological processes, it covers a selected part of organogenesis only. The whole embryo culture requires pregnant animals for the dissection of embryos and, eventually, serum from adult rats for preparation of the culture medium.

VII. CONCLUSIONS

Within the framework of the development of pharmaceutical compounds and reproductive toxicity testing a large variety of *in vitro* tests are available today. Two *in vitro* methods are described that use whole vertebrate and mammalian embryos as indicator organisms. The tests were selected because they provide relevant answers to problems in the screening, prescreening, development and risk assessment phase of a compound. They are particularly recommended when the outcome of testing with a new molecule is uncertain and where possible interference with embryonic development is unknown. Nevertheless the choice of this method does not rule out the use of other *in vitro* short-term tests for determination of embryotoxicity in pharmaceutical development, as each test has particular merits for a given purpose.

REFERENCES

1. Berry, C. L. (1983) Reproductive toxicology. In Balls, M., Ridell, R. J. and Worden, A. (eds) *Animals and Alternatives in Toxicity Testing*, pp. 197–207. Academic Press, London.
2. Berry, C. L. (1981) Congenital malformation. In Berry, C. L. (ed.) *Paediatric Pathology*, pp. 1–31. Spinger, Heidelberg.
3. European Chemical Industry Ecology and Toxicology Centre (1989) Alternative approaches for the assessment of reproductive toxicity (with emphasis on embryotoxicity/teratogenicity). Monograph No. 12. ECETOC, Brussels.
4. Keller, S. J. and Smith, M. K. (1982) Animal virus screens for potential teratogens. I. Poxvirus morphogenesis. *Teratogenesis Carcinog. Mutagen.* **2:** 361–374.
5. Bournias-Vardiabasis, N. (1990) *Drosophila melanogaster* embryo cultures: an *in vitro* teratogen assay. *ATLA* **18:** 291–300.
6. Bournias-Vardiabasis, N., Teplitz, R. L., Chernoff, G. F. and Seecof R. L. (1983) Detection of teratogens in the *Drosophila* embryonic cell culture test: assay of 100 chemicals. *Teratology* **28:** 109–122.
7. Best, J. B. and Morita, M. (1982) Planarians as a model system for *in vitro* teratogenesis studies. *Teratogenesis Carcinog. Mutagen.* **2:** 277–291.
8. Johnson, E. M. (1980) A subvertebrate system for rapid determination of potential teratogenic hazards. *J. Environ. Pathol. Toxicol.* **4:** 153–156.
9. Johnson, E. M., Gorman, R. M., Gabel, B. E. G. and George, M. E. (1982) The *Hydra attenuata* system for detection of teratogenic hazards. *Teratogenesis Carcinog. Mutagen.* **2:** 263–276.
10. Daston, G. P., Rogers, J. M., Versteeg, D. J., Sabourin, T. D., Baines, D. and Marsh, S. S. (1991) Interspecies comparisons of A/D ratios: A/D ratios are not constant across species. *Fundam. Appl. Toxicol.* **17:** 696–722.
11. Braun, A. G. and Dailey, J. P. (1981) Thalidomide metabolite inhibits tumor cell attachment to concanavalin a coated surfaces. *Biochem. Biophys. Res. Commun.* **98:** 1029–1034.
12. Braun, A. G., Emerson, D. J. and Nichinson, B. B. (1979) Teratogenic drugs inhibit tumour cell attachment to lectin-coated surfaces. *Nature* **282:** 507–509.

13. Braun, A. G., Buckner, C. A., Emerson, D. J. and Nichinson, B. B. (1982) Quantitative correspondence between the *in vivo* and *in vitro* activity of teratogenic agents. *Proc. Natl Acad. Sci. U.S.A.* **79:** 2056–2060.
14. Pratt, R. M. and Willis, W. D. (1985) *In vitro* screening assay for teratogens using growth inhibition of human embryonic cells. *Proc. Natl Acad. Sci. U.S.A.* **82:** 5791–5794.
15. Pratt, R. M., Grove, R. I. and Willis, W. D. (1982) Prescreening for environmental teratogens using cultured mesenchymal cells from the human embryonic palate. *Teratogenesis Carcinog. Mutagen.* **2:** 313–318.
16. Mummery, C. L., Slager, H. G., van Inzen, W., Freund, E. and van den Eijnden-van Raaij, A. J. M. (1993) Regulation of growth and differentiation in early development: of mice and models. *Reprod. Toxicol.* **7:** 145–154.
17. Laschinski, G., Vogel, R. and Spielmann, H. (1991) Cytotoxicity test using blastocyst-derived euploid embryonal stem cells: a new approach to *in vitro* teratogenesis screening. *Reprod. Toxicol.* **5:** 57–64.
18. Newall, D. R. and Beedles, K. (1993) The stem-cell test – a novel *in vitro* assay for teratogenic potential. Presented at the 21st Annual Conference of the European Teratology Society, Lyon, France. *Teratology* **48:** 30A.
19. Trosko, J. E., Chang, C. C. and Netzloff, M. (1982) The role of inhibited cell-cell communication in teratogenesis. *Teratogenesis Carcinog. Mutagen.* **2:** 31–45.
20. Flint, O. P. and Boyle, F. T. (1985) An *in vitro* test for teratogens: its application in the selection of non-teratogenic triazole antifungals. In Homburger, F. (ed.) *Concepts in Toxicology*, Vol. 3, pp. 29–35. Karger, Basel.
21. Flint, O. P. and Orton, T. C. (1984) An *in vitro* assay for teratogens with cultures of rat embryo midbrain and limb bud cells. *Toxicol. Appl. Pharmacol.* **76:** 383–395.
22. Seifert, J. (1989) Teratogenesis of polychlorocycloalkane insecticides in chicken embryos resulting from their interactions at the convulsant recognition sites of the GABA (pro)receptor complex. *Bull. Environ. Contam. Toxicol.* **42:** 707–715.
23. Langille, R. M., Paulsen, D. F. and Solursh, M. (1989) Differential effects of physiological concentrations of retinoic acid *in vitro* on chondrogenesis and myogenesis in chick craniofacial mesenchyme. *Differentiation* **40:** 84–92.
24. Daston, G. P. and D'Amato, R. A. (1989) *In vitro* techniques in teratology. *Toxicol. Ind. Health* **5:** 555–585.
25. Hassell, J. R. and Horigan, E. A. (1982) Chondrogenesis: a model developmental system for measuring teratogenic potential of compounds. *Teratogenesis Carcinog. Mutagen.* **2:** 325–331.
26. Guntakatta, M., Matthews, E. J. and Rundell, J. O. (1984) Development of a mouse embryo limb bud cell culture system for the estimation of chemical teratogenic potential. *Teratogenesis Carcinog. Mutagen.* **4:** 349–364.
27. Kistler, A. (1985) Inhibition of chondrogenesis by retinoids: limb bud cell cultures as a test system to measure the teratogenic potential of compounds? In Homburger, F. (ed.) *Concepts in Toxicology*, Vol. 3, pp. 86–100. Karger, Basel.
28. Kistler, A. (1987) Limb bud cell cultures for estimating the teratogenic potential of compounds – validation of the test system with retinoids. *Arch. Toxicol.* **60:** 403–414.
29. Paulsen, D. F. and Solursh, M. (1988) Microtiter micromass cultures of limb-bud mesenchymal cells. *In Vitro Cell. Dev. Biol.* **24:** 138–147.
30. Wiger, R., Stottum, A. and Brunborg, G. (1988) Estimating chemical developmental hazard in a chicken embryo limb bud micromass system. *Pharmacol. Toxicol.* **62:** 32–37.
31. Renault, J. Y., Melcion, C. and Cordier, A. (1989) Limb bud cell culture for *in vitro* teratogen screening: validation of an improved assessment method using 51 compounds. *Teratogenesis Carcinog. Mutagen.* **9:** 83–96.
32. Uphill, P. F., Wilkins, S. R. and Allen, J. A. (1990) *In vitro* micromass teratogen test: results from a blind trial of 25 compounds. *Toxicol. In Vitro* **4:** 623–626.
33. Honegger, P. and Schilter, B. (1992) Serum-free aggregate cultures of fetal rat brain and liver cells: methodology and some practical applications in neurotoxicology. In Zbinden, G. (ed.) *The Brain in Bits and Pieces.* In Vitro *Techniques in Neurobiology, Neuropharmacology and Neurotoxicology*, pp. 51–79. MTC, Zollikon, Switzerland.
34. Honegger, P. and Schilter, B. (1995) The use of serum-free aggregating brain cell cultures in neurotoxicology. In Chang, L. W. (ed.) *Neurotoxicology, Approaches and Methods*, pp. 507–516. Academic Press, San Diego.

35. Honegger, P. and Werffeli, P. (1988) Use of aggregating cell cultures for toxicological studies. *Experientia* **44:** 817–823.
36. Honegger, P., Lenoir, D. and Favrod, P. (1979) Growth and differentiation of aggregating fetal brain cells in a serum-free defined medium. *Nature* **282:** 305–308.
37. Kucera, P., Cano, E., Honegger, P., Schilter, B., Zijlstra, J. A. and Schmid, B. (1993) Validation of whole chick embryo cultures, whole rat embryo cultures and aggregating embryonic brain cell cultures using six pairs of coded compounds. *Toxicol. In Vitro* **7:** 785–798.
38. Schmid, B. P., Honegger, P. and Kucera, P. (1993) Embryonic and fetal development: fundamental research. *Reprod. Toxicol.* **7:** 155–164.
39. Aydelotte, M. B. and Kochhar, D. M. (1972) Development of mouse limb buds in organ culture: chondrogenesis in the presence of a proline analog, L-azetidine-2-carboxylic acid. *Dev. Biol.* **28:** 191–201.
40. Neubert, D., Merker, H. J. and Tapken, S. (1974) Comparative studies on the prenatal development of mouse extremities *in vivo* and in organ culture. *Naunyn-Schmiedebergs Arch. Pharmacol.* **286:** 251–270.
41. Neubert, D., Tapken, S. and Merker, H. J. (1974) Induction of skeletal malformations in organ cultures of mammalian embryonic tissues. *Naunyn-Schmiedebergs Arch. Pharmacol.* **286:** 271–282.
42. Kochhar, D. M. (1975) The use of *in vitro* procedures in teratology. *Teratology* **11:** 273–288.
43. Ghaida, J. and Merker, H. J. (1992) Effects of cyclophosphamide and acrolein in organoid cultures of mouse limb bud cells grown in the presence of adult rat hepatocytes. *Toxicol. In Vitro* **6:** 27–40.
44. Abbott, B. D. and Buckalew, A. R. (1992) Embryonic palatal responses to teratogens in serum-free organ culture. *Teratology* **45:** 369–382.
45. Al-Obaidi, N., Kastner, U., Merker, H. J. and Klug, S. (1994) Development of a suspension organ culture of the fetal rat palate. *Arch. Toxicol.* **69:** 472–479.
46. Neubert, D. (1982) The use of culture techniques in studies on prenatal toxicity. *Pharmacol. Ther.* **18:** 397–434.
47. Faustmann, E. M. (1988) Short-term tests for teratogens. *Mutat. Res.* **205:** 355–384.
48. Whittaker, S. G., Faustmann, E. M. (1994) *In vitro* assays for developmental toxicity. In Gad, S. C. (ed.) In vitro *Toxicology*, pp. 97–122. Raven Press, New York.
49. Estus, S. and Blumer, J. L. (1989) Role of microtubule assembly in phenytoin teratogenic action in the sea urchin (arbacia punctulata) embryo. *Mol. Pharmacol.* **36:** 708–715.
50. Sleet, R. B. (1992) Brine shrimp (*Artemia*) – fish food with potential application as a prescreen to predict chemical hazard to human development. *Lab. Anim.* **21:** 26–36.
51. Sleet, R. B. and Brendel, K. (1983) Improved methods for harvesting and counting synchronous populations of *Artemia nauplii* for use in developmental toxicology. *Ecotoxicol. Environ. Safety* **7:** 435–446.
52. Sleet, R. B. and Brendel, K. (1984) A flow-through hatching and cold storage system for continuous collection of freshly hatched *Artemia nauplii. Journal of Aquariculture and Aquatic Sciences* **3:** 76–83.
53. Sleet, R. B. and Brendel, K. (1985) Homogeneous populations of *Artemia nauplii* and their potential use for *in vitro* testing in developmental toxicology. *Teratogenesis Carcinog. Mutagen.* **5:** 41–54.
54. Walton, B. T. (1983) Use of the cricket embryo (*Acheta domesticus*) as an invertebrate teratology model. *Fundam. Appl. Toxicol.* **3:** 233–236.
55. Schuler, R. L., Hardin, B. D. and Niemeier, R. W. (1982) *Drosophila* as a tool for the rapid assessment of chemicals for teratogenicity. *Teratogenesis Carcinog. Mutagen.* **2:** 293–301.
56. Schuler, R. L., Radike, M. A., Hardin, B. D. and Niemeier, R. W. (1985) Pattern of response of intact *Drosophila* to known teratogens. *J. Am. Coll. Toxicol.* **4:** 291–303.
57. Ranganathan, S., Davis, D. G. and Hood, R. D. (1987) Developmental toxicity of ethanol in *Drosophila melanogaster. Teratology* **36:** 45–49.
58. Jelinek, R. (1982) Use of chick embryo in screening for embryotoxicity. *Teratogenesis Carcinog. Mutagen.* **2:** 255–261.
59. Kucera, P. and Burnand, M. B. (1987) Routine teratogenicity that uses chick embryos *in vitro. Teratogenesis Carcinog. Mutagen.* **7:** 427–447.
60. Kucera, P. and Burnand, M. B. (1988) Teratogenicity screening in standardized chick embryo culture: effects of dexamethasone and diphenylhydantoin. *Experientia* **44:** 827–833.
61. Schmid, B. P., Trippmacher, A. and Bianchi, A. (1983) Validation of the whole-embryo culture

method for *in vitro* teratogenicity testing. In Hayes, A. W., Schnell, R. C. and Miya, T. S. (eds) *Developments in the Science and Practice of Toxicology*, pp. 563–566. Elsevier Science Publishers, Amsterdam.
62. Birge, W. J., Black, J. A., Westerman, A. G. and Ramey, B. A. (1983) Fish and amphibian embryos – a model system for evaluating teratogenicity. *Fundam. Appl. Toxicol.* **3:** 237–242.
63. Herrmann, K. (1993) Effects of the anticonvulsant drug valproic acid and related substances on the early development of the zebrafish (brachydanio rerio). *Toxicol. In Vitro* **7:** 41–54.
64. Dumont, J. N., Schultz, T. W., Buchanan, M.V. and Kao, G. L. (1983) Frog embryo teratogenesis assay: *Xenopus* (FETAX) – a short-term assay applicable to complex environmental mixtures. *Environ. Sci. Res.* **27:** 393–405.
65. Dawson, D. A. and Bantle, J. A. (1987) Development of a reconstituted water medium and preliminary validation of the frog embryo teratogenesis assay – *Xenopus* (FETAX). *J. Appl. Toxicol.* **7:** 237–244.
66. Fort, D. J., Dawson, D. A. and Bantle, J. A. (1988) Development of a metabolic activation system for the frog embryo teratogenesis assay: *Xenopus* (FETAX). *Teratogenesis Carcinog. Mutagen.* **8:** 251–263.
67. New, D. A. T. (1978) Whole embryo culture and the study of mammalian embryos during organogenesis. *Biol. Rev.* **53:** 81–122.
68. Fantel, A. G. (1982) Culture of whole rodent embryos in teratogen screening. *Teratogenesis Carcinog. Mutagen.* **2:** 231–242.
69. Schmid, B. P. (1985) Teratogenicity testing of new drugs with the postimplantation embryo culture system. In Homburger, F. (ed.) *Concepts in Toxicology*. Vol. 3, pp. 46–57. Karger, Basel.
70. Sadler, T. W., Horton, W. E. and Warner, C. W. (1982) Whole embryo culture: a screening technique for teratogens? *Teratogenesis Carcinog. Mutagen.* **2:** 243–253.
71. Klug, S., Lewandowski, C. and Neubert, D. (1985) Modification and standardization of the culture of early postimplantation embryos for toxicological studies. *Arch. Toxicol.* **58:** 84–88.
72. Bechter, R. and Schmid, B. P. (1987) Teratogenicity *in vitro* – a comparative study of four antimycotic drugs using the whole-embryo culture system. *Toxicol. In Vitro* **1:** 11–15.
73. Spielmann, H. and Eibs, H. G. (1977) Preimplantation embryos. Part I: Laboratory equipment, preparation of media, sampling and handling of the embryos. In Neubert, D., Merker, H. J. and Kwasigroch, T. E. (eds) *Methods in Prenatal Toxicology*, pp. 210–225. Georg Thieme, Stuttgart.
74. Naya, M., Kito, Y., Eto, K. and Deguchi, T. (1991) Development of rabbit whole embryo culture during organogenesis. *Congenital Anomalies* **31:** 153–156.
75. Ninomiya, H., Kishida, K., Ohno, Y., Tsurumi, K. and Eto, K. (1993) Effects of trypan blue on rat and rabbit embryos cultured *in vitro*. *Toxicol. In Vitro* **7:** 707–717.
76. ICH (1993) *International Conference on Harmonization of Technical Requirements for the Registration of Pharmaceuticals for Human Use. ICH Harmonized Tripartite Guidelines – Detection of Toxicity to Reproduction for Medicinal Products.* Endorsed by the ICH Steering Committee at Step 4 of the ICH Process, 24 June 1993.
77. Kistler, A., Tsuchiya, T., Tsuchiya, M. and Klaus, M. (1990) Teratogenicity of arotinoids (retinoids) *in vivo* and *in vitro*. *Arch. Toxicol.* **64:** 616–622.
78. Tsuchiya, T., Bürgin, H., Tsuchiya, M., Winternitz, P. and Kistler, A. (1991) Embryolethality of new herbicides is not detected by the micromass teratogen tests. *Arch. Toxicol.* **65:** 145–149.
79. Palmer, A. K. (1993) Introduction to (pre)screening methods. *Reprod. Toxicol.* **7:** 95–98.
80. Curren, R. D., Southee, J. A., Spielmann, H., Liebsch, M., Fentem, J. H. and Balls, M. (1995) The role of prevalidation in the development, validation and acceptance of alternative methods. *ATLA* **23:** 211–217.
81. Romanoff, A. (1960) *The Avian Embryo: Structural and Functional Development*. Macmillan, New York.
82. Romanoff, A. (1967) *Biochemistry of the Avian Embryo: A Quantitative Analysis of Prenatal Development*. Wiley Interscience, New York.
83. Kucera, P. and Monnet-Tschudi, F. (1987) Early functional differentiation in the chick embryonic disc: interaction between mechanical activity and extracellular matrix. *J. Cell Sci.* **S8:** 415–427.
84. Kucera, P. (1990) Physiological approach to the early embryogenesis. In Marty, H. J. (ed.) *Experimental Embryology in Aquatic Plant and Animal Organisms*, NATO ASI series, Vol. 195, pp. 377–388. Plenum Press, New York.
85. Abriel, H., Katz, U. and Kucera, P. (1994) Ion transport across the early chick embryo: II. Characterization and pH sensitivity of the transembryonic short-circuit current. *J. Membr. Biol.* **141:** 159–166.

86. Kucera, P., Abriel, H. and Katz, U. (1994) Ion transport across the early chick embryo: I. Electrical measurements, ionic fluxes and regional heterogeneity. *J. Membr. Biol.* **141:** 149–157.
87. Cockroft (1976) Comparison of *in vitro* and *in vivo* development of rat foetuses. *Dev. Biol.* **48:** 163–172.
88. Fujinaga, M. and Baden, J. M. (1992) Variation in development of rat embryos at the presomite period. *Teratology* **45:** 661–670.
89. Barber, C. V., Carda, M. B. and Fantel, A. G. (1993) A new technique for culturing rat embryos between gestation days 14 and 15. *Toxicol. In Vitro* **7:** 695–700.
90. Sadler, T. W., Warner, C. W., Tulis, S. A., Smith, M. K. and Doerger, J. (1985) Factors determining the *in vitro* response of rodent embryos to teratogens. In Homburger, F. (ed.) *Concepts in Toxicology*, Vol. 3, pp. 36–45. Karger, Basel.
91. Bechter, R., Terlouw, G. D. C., Lee, Q. P. and Juchau, M. R. (1991) Effects of QA 208-199 and its metabolite 209-668 on embryonic development *in vitro* after microinjection into the exocoelomic space or into the amniotic cavity of cultured rat conceptuses. *Teratogenesis Carcinog. Mutagen.* **11:** 185–194.
92. Sadler, T. W. (1979) Culture of early somite mouse embryos during organogenesis. *J. Embryol. Exp. Morphol.* **49:** 17–25.
93. Cicurel, L. and Schmid, B. (1986) *In Vitro* teratogenicity of acetylsalicylic acid on rat embryos: studies with various culture conditions. *Methods Find. Exp. Clin. Pharmacol.* **3:** 227–232.
94. Klein, N. W., Plenefisch, J. D., Carey, S. W. *et al.* (1982) Serum from monkeys with histories of fetal wastage causes abnormalities in cultures of whole rat embryos. *Science* **215:** 66–69.
95. Chatot, C. L., Klein, N. W., Piatek, J. and Pierro, L. J. (1980) Successful culture of rat embryos in human serum: use in the detection of teratogens. *Science* **207:** 1471–1473.
96. Van Maele-Fabry, G., Therasse, P., Lenoir, E. *et al.* (1993) Embryotoxicity of human sera from patients treated with isotretinoin. *Toxicol. In Vitro* **7:** 809–815.
97. Abir, R., Ornoy, A., Hur, H. B., Jaffe, P. and Pinus, H. (1993) IgG exchange as a means of partial correction of anomalies in rat embryos *in vitro*, induced by sera from women with recurrent abortion. *Toxicol. In Vitro* **7:** 817–826.
98. Sadler, T. W., Shum, L., Warner, C. W. and Smith, M. K. (1988) The role of pharmacokinetics in determining the response of rodent embryos to teratogens in whole-embryo culture. *Toxicol. In Vitro* **2:** 175–180.
99. Stahlmann, R., Klug, S., Foerster, M. and Neubert, D. (1993) Significance of embryo culture methods for studying the prenatal toxicity of virustatic agents. *Reprod. Toxicol.* **7:** 129–143.
100. Fantel, A. G., Greenaway, J. C., Juchau, M. R. and Shepard, T. H. (1979) Teratogenic biactivation of cyclophosphamide *in vitro*. *Life Sci.* **25:** 67–72.
101. Kitchin, K. T., Schmid, B. P. and Sanyai, M. K. (1981) Teratogenicity of cyclophosphamide in a coupled microsomal activating/embryo culture system. *Biochem. Pharmacol.* **30:** 59–64.
102. Zhao, J., Krafft, N., Terlouw, G. D. C. and Bechter, R. (1993) A model combining the whole embryo culture with human liver S-9 fraction for human teratogenic prediction. *Toxicol. In Vitro* **7:** 827–831.
103. Oglesby, L. A., Ebron-McCoy, M. T., Logsdon, T. R., Copeland, F., Beyer, P. E. and Kavlock, R. J. (1992) *In vitro* embryotoxicity of a series of para-substituted phenols: structure, activity and correlation with *in vivo* data. *Teratology* **45:** 11–33.
104. Bechter, R., Bouis, P. and Fischer, V. (1989) Primary hepatocyte culture as an activating system for xenobiotica tested in the rat whole embryo *in vitro*. In: Goldberg, A. M. and Principe, M. L. (eds) *Alternative Methods in Toxicology Vol. 7*, In Vitro *Toxicology, New Directions*, pp. 313–326. Mary Ann Liebert, New York.
105. Schmid, B. P., Trippmacher, A. and Bianchi, A. (1982) Teratogenicity induced in cultured rat embryos by the serum of procarbazine treated rats. *Toxicology* **25:** 53–60.
106. Piersma, A. H., Attenon, P., Bechter, R. *et al.* (1995) Interlaboratory evaluation of embryotoxicity in the postimplantation rat embryo culture. *Reprod. Toxicol.* **9:** 275–280.
107. Kitchin, K. T. and Ebron, M. T. (1984) Further development of rodent whole embryo culture: solvent toxicity and water insoluble compound delivery system. *Toxicology* **30:** 45–57.
108. Bechter, R. and Brouillard, J. F. (1988) The effects of different chemical forms of a test compound on embryotoxicity, distribution and metabolism *in vitro*. *Toxicol. In Vitro* **2:** 181–188.
109. Van Aerts, L. A. G. J. M., Hahné, S. J. M., Oostendorp, A. G. M. *et al.* (1993) Sex difference in aroclor 1254 induction of rat hepatocytes: consequences for *in vitro* embryotoxicity and mutagenicity of cyclophosphamide. *Toxicol. In Vitro* **7:** 769–775.

110. Brown, N. A. and Fabro, S. (1981) Quantitation of rat embryonic development *in vitro*: a morphological scoring system. *Teratology* **24:** 65–78.
111. Van Maele-Fabry, G., Picard, J. J., Attenon, P. *et al.* (1991) Interlaboratory evaluation of three culture media for postimplantation rodent embryos. *Reprod. Toxicol.* **5:** 417–426.
112. Van Maele-Fabry, G., Delhaise, F., Gofflot, F. and Picard, J. J. (1993) Developmental table of the early mouse post-implantation embryo. *Toxicol. In Vitro* **7:** 719–725.
113. Cicurel, L. and Schmid, B. P. (1988) Post-implantation embryo culture: validation with selected compounds for teratogenicity testing. *Xenobiotica* **18:** 617–624.
114. Cicurel, L. and Schmid, B. P. (1988) Postimplantation embryo culture for the assessment of the teratogenic potential and potency of compounds. *Experientia* **44:** 833–840.
115. Bechter, R., Terlouw, G. D. C., Tsuchiya, M., Tsuchiya, T. and Kistler, A. (1992) Teratogenicity of arotinoids (retinoids) in the rat whole embryo culture. *Arch. Toxicol.* **66:** 193–197.
116. Bechter, R. (1995) The validation and use of *in vitro* teratogenicity tests. *Arch. Toxicol. Suppl.* **17:** 170–191.

16

In Vitro Investigation of the Molecular Mechanisms of Hepatotoxicity

JOSÉ V. CASTELL, MARÍA JOSÉ GÓMEZ-LECHÓN, XAVIER PONSODA AND ROQUE BORT

I. Drug-induced hepatic injury 376
  A. Iatrogenic hepatitis: intrinsic and idiosyncratic toxicity 376
  B. Cell toxicity as a consequence of drug bioactivation 377
  C. Drug-induced cell death: necrosis and apoptosis 377
II. Molecular mechanisms of toxicity 378
  A. Impairment of cellular metabolism 378
    1. Alterations in the energetic balance of cells 379
    2. Effects on mitochondrial function 380
  B. Drug-induced lipid peroxidation 381
    1. Drug-derived radicals and active oxygen species 381
    2. Methods for investigating lipid peroxidation in cultured cells 382
  C. Drug-induced oxidative stress 384
    1. Drug redox cycling as cause of oxidative stress 384
    2. Glutathione and oxidative stress 385
  D. Calcium- and drug-induced cell injury 387
    1. Toxic events leading to an increase intracellular calcium level 389
    2. Consequences of sustained, increased Ca^{2+} concentration in cells . . . 389
    3. Ca^{2+} levels, GSH content, lipid peroxidation and cell viability in the course of hepatocyte injury by toxins 391
  E. Covalent binding 392
    1. Mechanisms of drug–protein adduct formation 392
    2. Covalent binding and hepatotoxicity 393
III. Immunological mechanisms of drug hepatotoxicity 395
IV. Screening for potential hepatotoxicity of new drugs 397
  A. Parameters for assessing hepatotoxicity *in vitro* 397
    1. Cytotoxicity parameters 398
    2. Metabolic parameters 398
  B. Interpretation of *in vitro* results and predictive value of *in vitro* data . . . 400
Acknowledgements 401
References 401

IN VITRO METHODS IN PHARMACEUTICAL RESEARCH
ISBN 0-12-163390-X

I. DRUG-INDUCED HEPATIC INJURY

A. Iatrogenic hepatitis: intrinsic and idiosyncratic toxicity

Substances capable of producing liver damage and, more specifically, hepatocyte damage are known as hepatotoxins. They are classified (Fig. 16.1) according to whether they exert their effects in all individuals, in a dose-dependent and hence predictable manner (intrinsic hepatotoxins), or in certain individuals, sometimes after several contacts, frequently in a non-dose-dependent and therefore unpredictable way (idiosyncratic hepatotoxins). Intrinsic toxins can directly act on cells (active hepatotoxins) or become toxic after biotransformation by hepatocytes (latent hepatotoxins).[1,2] Idiosyncratic hepatotoxicity may be the consequence either of unusual metabolism of the drug by susceptible individuals (metabolic idiosyncrasy) or of an immune-mediated response after repeated previous contacts with the drug (sensitization).[1]

The damage caused to hepatocytes can be classified as cytotoxic, genotoxic or metabolic.[3] The first type of injury is evidenced by important morphological changes in the structure of hepatocytes (vacuolization, steatosis, acidophilia, necrosis, etc.), and is accompanied by an increase in the serum level of hepatic enzymes. Cytotoxicity is a common feature of intrinsic hepatotoxins. Genotoxins are substances that produce DNA damage and show a strong tendency to act as tumour promoters inducing primary hepatocarcinomas. Finally, drugs can also alter the cellular metabolism of hepatocytes without causing cell death. This usually takes the form of alteration of the functional capacity of hepatocytes and, in particular, of the uptake, conjugation and secretion of bile acids, which, in turn, results in impaired bile flux (cholestasis) and is most frequently associated with idiosyncratic toxins.

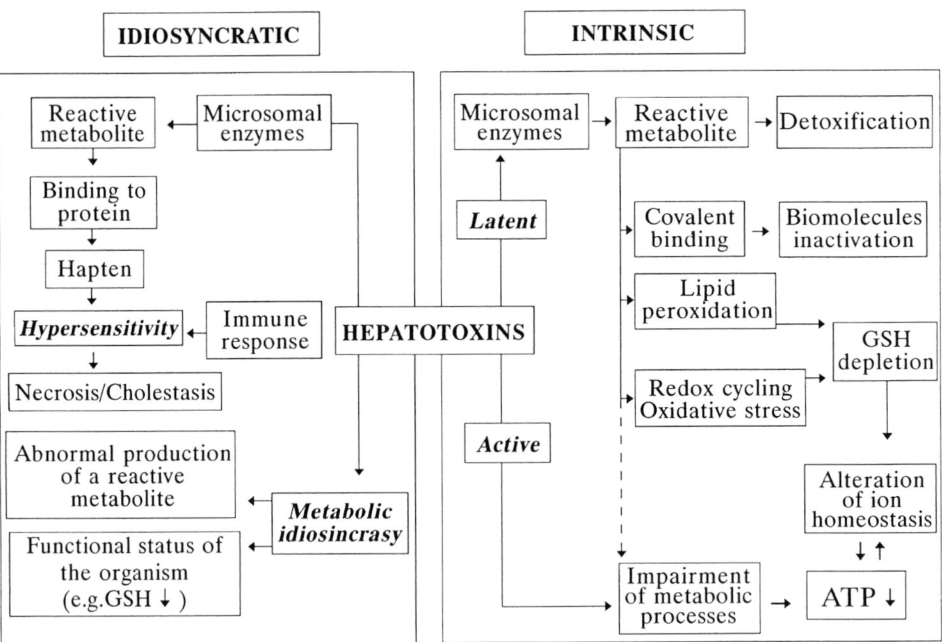

Fig. 16.1 Types of hepatotoxicity. Intrinsic hepatotoxins can elicit toxic effects in any individual. Idiosyncratic toxins act only in certain individuals, both dependently (metabolic idiosyncrasy) or independently of the dose administered (drug hypersensitivity).

B. Cell toxicity as a consequence of drug bioactivation

The liver is very active in metabolizing foreign compounds. The biotransformation of xenobiotics involves chemical modifications that facilitate their elimination from the organism. Most of them are redox reactions catalysed by a family of haemoproteins, namely, cytochrome P450-dependent mono-oxygenases.[4] The basic reaction is oxidation of the xenobiotic by one atom of molecular oxygen (hence, mono-oxygenases), while the other atom is reduced by electrons delivered by the cytochrome P450 reductase. As a result of this, new metabolites, usually more polar and reactive than the parent compound, are produced which are further conjugated with endogenous molecules (e.g. glucuronic acid, glutathione, sulfate, amino acids, etc.) to produce derivatives that are much more water soluble and usually much less toxic.[5]

Although a biotransformation sequence generally parallels a detoxification process, there are many cases in which biotransformation of a drug can cause deleterious effects on cells.[6–9] The reactions catalysed by cytochrome P450 enzymes can generate metabolites that are not only more toxic but also more reactive than the original xenobiotic. Some are potent electrophiles, or carbon-centred radicals, capable of reacting with nucleophiles, that bind covalently to macromolecules (proteins, DNA) and initiate radical chain reactions (lipid peroxidation) or cause oxidative stress.[10,11] Against these potential hazards, hepatocytes have their own defence mechanisms (enzymes, reduced glutathione (GSH), and DNA and protein repair mechanisms). Ultimately, it is the balance between bioactivation, detoxification and defence mechanisms that determines whether a reactive metabolite may elicit toxic effects.[12]

Although the large biotransforming capability of the liver allows efficient elimination of most toxic compounds from the organism, it also makes liver a target organ for drug toxicity.

C. Drug-induced cell death: necrosis and apoptosis

The mechanism of cell death can be broadly categorized into two distinct types: necrosis (pathological and accidental) and apoptosis (physiological and programmed). Necrosis is caused by a rapid collapse of the cell's internal homoeostasis, and is evidenced by alterations in cytoplasmic organelles, cell swelling leading to membrane lysis, and release of cellular content (Fig. 16.2). This is accompanied by an inflammatory response in the surrounding tissue areas.[13]

Apoptosis is a mode of cell death distinct from necrosis. It requires active RNA and protein synthesis, and is characterized by progressive condensation of the chromatin on the inner face on the nuclear membrane DNA fragmentation and cell shrinkage with subsequent loss of membrane contact with neighbouring cells, and fragmentation of the cell with formation of membrane-bound acidophilic globules (apoptotic bodies). Apoptosis is currently viewed as an equal and opposite process to mitosis, and it plays an essential role in the maintenance of renewable tissues. Most specialized cells when entering a postmitotic phase, they are sent on a one-way trip to a predictable cell death. This differentiation of cells to death is also considered a particular case of programmed cell death.[14,15]

Studies on the mechanisms of hepatotoxicity most frequently deal with a type of cell death that is commonly defined as *lytic necrosis*. However, the finding of apoptosis in chemically injured liver, together with extensive necrosis, raises the question of the participation of

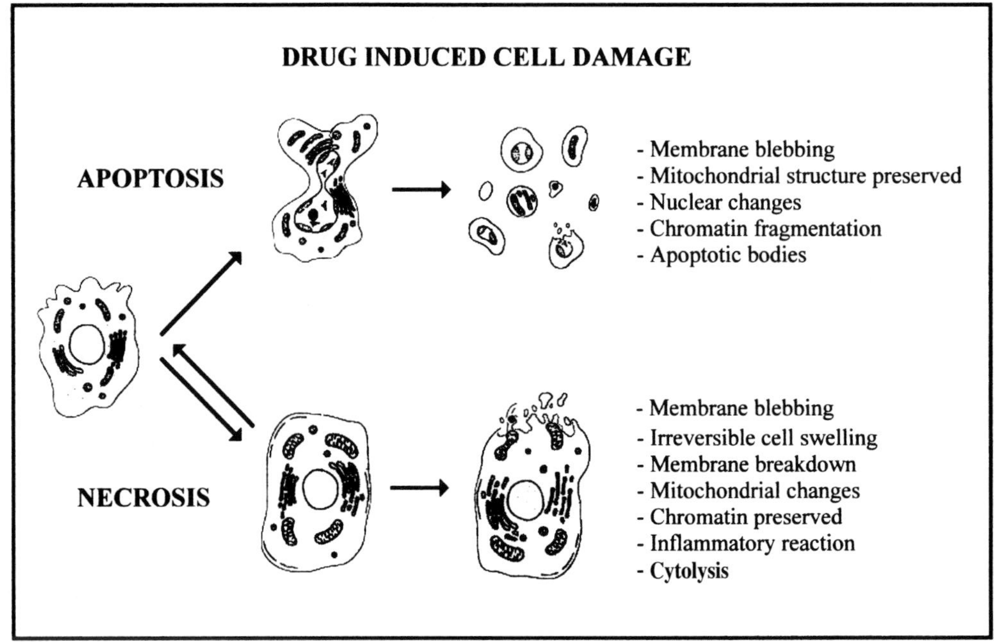

Fig. 16.2 Biochemical and morphological characteristics of drug-induced apoptosis and necrosis.

apoptosis in the mechanisms of xenobiotic liver injury.[13,16,17] The extent of apoptosis seems to be related to the concentration of the toxic agent. Moderate concentrations can apparently induce apoptosis, while higher concentrations cause cell necrosis.[18] This, however, may not be true on all occasions in the liver. For instance, soon after administration of both low and high doses of thioacetamide, apoptotic cells can be observed in the absence of signs of necrosis. Apoptosis is then followed by cell necrosis, which is associated with a strong inflammatory response. It is the severity of the necrosis rather than the extent of apoptosis that is related to the dose of thioacetamide administered.[19]

Present evidence shows that most of the agents capable of inducing death of liver cells can induce both apoptosis and necrosis, but there is little evidence that necrosis occurs in the liver in the absence of a preceding or concomitant apoptosis.[13] This raises the question of whether the mechanisms of apoptosis and necrosis are different, or whether apoptosis is simply the initial step of a process that ultimately leads to necrosis in the course of liver injury.

II. MOLECULAR MECHANISMS OF TOXICITY

A. Impairment of cellular metabolism

Different mechanisms can be invoked in drug-mediated hepatocyte injury.[20] One is alteration of cellular metabolic functions by the drug itself or by any of its stable metabolites (Fig. 16.1). Certain compounds, for instance, can act as enzyme inhibitors, impair ion transport or compete with cellular metabolites in metabolic pathways, this being the ultimate cause of hepatocyte dysfunction.

Galactosamine constitutes a classical example of a compound that acts primarily as an antimetabolite with selective toxicity for the liver.[21] This amino sugar is metabolized by enzymes of the galactose pathway, which are most abundant in the liver, to galactosamine-1-phosphate, then to UDP–galactosamine, and is finally partially epimerized to UDP–glucosamine. None of these amino sugar nucleotides is found in normal liver, but they increase after galactosamine administration. *N*-acetylated amino sugar nucleotides are present in normal liver, but again they increase considerably before the onset of galactosamine hepatitis. The result of the metabolization of galactosamine is the depletion of the UTP pool, which can drop to approximately 10% of normal values. Galactosamine-induced UTP depletion is highly selective: no reduction in the levels of ATP, GTP or CTP is normally observed.[21,22] The trapping of the uridilate moiety from UTP is associated not only with an accumulation of the UDP–sugar derivatives, but also with an increase in UMP and UDP, and with UDP–glucose and UDP–galactose deficiencies. An initial consequence of this is the decrease in RNA and protein synthesis. This is primarily the consequence of UTP (UDP–glucose and UDP–galactose) depletion rather than a direct effect of galactosamine.[23] The result of these events is a hepatitis-like process with an increase in serum markers and a decrease in liver function.

Ethionine, the ethyl analogue of methionine, is also a prototype of an active hepatotoxin.[24] The administration of ethionine produces a considerable ATP and glutathione deficiency in the liver by trapping adenosyl moieties as *S*-adenosyl-L-ethionine. This reduction in ATP results in a general inhibition of anabolic processes, among them the synthesis of very low density lipoprotein (VLDL) apoproteins which are required for the transport of triglycerides from the liver. This leads to hepatic steatosis and a decrease in the level of plasma lipids and lipoproteins. Moreover, ethylation and inhibition of RNA methylation produce deficient messenger RNAs and impaired protein synthesis.[25]

1. Alterations in the energetic balance of cells

Many hepatotoxins act indirectly by altering the energetic balance of cells, either by dramatically increasing the energy demand (increased consumption of ATP), reducing ATP production, or both.[26–28] In fact, ATP depletion is a common event in the course of cell damage which frequently precedes the irreversible stages of cell injury. The xenobiotic, for instance, can alter a normal metabolic cycle, converting it into a futile cycle with considerable dissipation of cellular energy: by reverting the ion concentration gradient across cellular membranes, ionophores considerably increase the consumption of ATP by membrane-allocated ion-pumping ATPases.[29–31]

Another example of increased energy demand constitutes the *de novo* synthesis of GSH. Under normal circumstances oxidized GSH is re-utilized after reduction by GSH reductase, a process that requires NADPH.[32,33] However, intracellular level of oxidized glutathione cannot drop beyond a certain level. If, because of the formation of a reactive metabolite, this occurs, glutathione disulfide is eliminated from the cell, thus decreasing the GSH pool, making *de novo* synthesis of this metabolite necessary and creating an important ATP demand.[34,35] A similar situation can occur if a metabolite is eliminated mainly by conjugation with GSH, and the recovery mechanisms (hydrolysis of glutamic acid and glycine from conjugates, and elimination as mercapturic acid conjugates) are overwhelmed.[33]

An energetic imbalance can also be produced if the xenobiotic or its metabolites alter ATP production in hepatocytes.[26,27,36] Hepatocytes obtain their energy basically from β-oxidation of lipids, oxidation of the carbon skeleton of amino acids and, to a much lesser extent, by glycolysis of hexose monophosphates.[37,38] Although hepatocytes can obtain ATP by anaerobic glycolysis, the bulk of ATP is produced from acetyl coenzyme A (CoA), through the Krebs' cycle and oxidative phosphorylation of NADPH in mitochondria.[38] Substances that block electron transport, depolarize mitochondria or alter the physicochemical properties of the mitochondrial membrane lead to decreased ATP production. This in turn affects almost all cellular anabolic processes as well as the service functions of hepatocytes (i.e. functions not essential to hepatocyte survival but of relevance to the homoeostasis of the organism, like gluconeogenesis, ureogenesis, bile acid transport and plasma protein synthesis). To compensate for this energy imbalance, hepatocytes can increase glycolysis, which can result in overproduction of lactic acid and acidification of the medium.

ATP measurement in cultured cells ATP can be quantified in microcultures of hepatocytes by using the bioluminescent reaction catalysed by luciferase. After incubating cells with xenobiotics, cells are homogenized in 1 ml 3% $HClO_4$ at 0°C. Acid samples are neutralized with 520 μl 1 M KOH at 4°C, and the precipitate is removed by centrifugation (5 min at 9000*g*). The supernatant is then diluted 1 in 200 with deionized distilled water and added (1 : 1 v/v) to the reaction solution (40 mM HEPES buffer, pH 7.75, containing 1.6 g ml^{-1} luciferase and 700 μM D-luciferin). Bioluminescence is then quantified in a luminescence photometer. The light produced is proportional to the ATP content of the sample in the range 20 pM to 100 μM.[39]

2. *Effects on mitochondrial function*

Mitochondria constitute an important target of drug hepatotoxicity. The high energy demand of hepatocytes confers this ATP-producing organelle a critical role in the onset of hepatic injury. Damage to mitochondria appears to be a key early event in the evolution of hepatocyte necrosis.[20] Several mechanisms can be involved in mitochondrial injury: (a) direct inhibition of mitochondrial metabolism, including electron transport and oxidative phosphorylation;[27,40,41] (b) alteration of the physicochemical properties of the mitochondrial membrane as a result of oxidative damage (i.e. mitochondrial GSH depletion[34] and lipid peroxidation[42]); (c) lipid intercalation of compounds that alter the physicochemical properties of membranes,[31,43] thus diminishing membrane potential and, hence, the driving force of ATP production; and (d) damage to mitochondrial DNA.

Mitochondrial dysfunction has immediate effects on the energetic balance of cells. A decrease in ATP production by oxidative phosphorylation tends to be compensated for by increased glycolysis and acid lactic production. Thus, if glycolytic substrates are provided to hepatocytes, irreversible cell damage (cell death) can be prevented. A typical example of this mechanism is the protective effect of fructose on liver toxicity.[44,45]

Mitochondria are also the location of many other catabolic routes that include part of the Krebs' cycle, the lipid β-oxidation enzymatic complex, as well as anabolic service functions of hepatocytes such as carbamyl phosphate synthetase, the first reaction of ureogenesis.[46] Mitochondrial damage frequently results in the cell's inability to catabolize lipids, which leads to their accumulation in hepatocytes causing microvesicular and macrovesicular steatosis.[47,48]

Some drugs may cause hepatic dysfunction because they accumulate in mitochondria and damage DNA. An interesting example is the toxicity of fialuridine, a novel nucleoside analogue shown to be effective against the hepatitis B virus. This compound showed no significant toxicity in short-term clinical trials, but when administered for several weeks had tragic consequences.[28] The compound accumulates in mitochondria, where it is incorporated into mtDNA.[49] Gradual loss of mitochondrial gene expression results in irreversible mitochondrial damage and signs of hepatocyte dysfunction.

Measurement of mitochondrial function: membrane potential and ATP production by mitochondria In addition to the succinate dehydrogenase activity (MTT test) mentioned in Chapters 3 and 9, mitochondrial integrity can be assessed by measuring the membrane potential and the ability to produce ATP. Membrane potential can be indirectly determined by measuring the distribution of the fluorescent dye rhodamine-123 cation across the mitochondrial membrane.[50] Mitochondria are isolated by homogenization and centrifugation in a sucrose gradient.[51] An aliquot of the mitochondrial suspension is diluted in buffer to a final concentration of 0.4–0.5 mg protein per ml; 200 μl aliquots are transferred to Eppendorf tubes and incubated with the xenobiotic to be tested. Finally, 1 mM glutamate, 1 mM malate, 6 mM $MgCl_2$, and rhodamine-123 (final concentration 1 μM) are added. After 15 min incubation, the Eppendorfs are centrifuged to sediment mitochondria, and the fluorescence of the upper phase and resuspended pellet is measured (excitation 505 nm, emission 523 nm). Membrane potential is related to the uptake of rhodamine by the following algorithm:[50]

$$\psi = \frac{59 \times \log[\text{rhodamine-123}]\text{intramitochondrial}}{[\text{rhodamine-123}]\text{extramitochondrial}}$$

In parallel, ATP production can be determined. The mitochondrial suspension (final concentration 0.5 mg per ml protein) is preincubated for 5 min with various concentrations of the xenobiotic to be tested. Metabolic substrates are then added (1 mM glutamate, 1 mM malate and 2.5 mM ADP in 6 mM $MgCl_2$, final concentration). Aliquots (100 μl) are taken at regular intervals and dropped on 1 ml cold 3% $HClO_4$, neutralized, centrifuged and, after appropriate dilution, the ATP concentration is measured with the luciferin–luciferase assay, as described above.[39]

B. Drug-induced lipid peroxidation

Lipid peroxidation is also a common event in toxic phenomena. It is a free radical-mediated process that leads to oxidative degradation of the lipids present in cell membranes (triglycerides, phospholipids, unsaturated fatty acids, cholesterol, etc.).[52,53] Although this occurs to a limited extent in aerobic organisms as a consequence of cellular oxidation, external factors (e.g. ionizing radiation, UV light[53]) and xenobiotic metabolism by cytochrome P450-dependent enzymes can augment this process so that it escapes cell control. Lipid peroxidation is easily propagated to other unsaturated molecules when oxygen is present. The oxidation of lipids continues with the formation of a wide range of degradation products (e.g. hydroperoxides, aldehydes, including malondialdehyde, and ketones) until the lipid has been degraded totally.[54] The first consequence of this process is a profound alteration in the physicochemical properties of the membrane and in the functionality of membrane-allocated enzyme activities.[55]

Lipid radicals, as well as most lipid degradation products, are chemically very reactive and, if not detoxified or removed from the cell by endogenous mechanisms, cause additional cellular damage such as enzyme inactivation, protein–protein cross-linking and DNA damage.[56,57]

1. *Drug-derived radicals and active oxygen species*

Lipid peroxidation is a mechanism of cell injury by chemicals,[58–60] where drug radicals generated during P450 metabolism often act as initiators. For example, in the course of halogenated hydrocarbon metabolism (Cl_3C, Cl_4C), carbon-centred radicals[61] capable of initiating lipid peroxidation and are formed by halogen abstraction by the haem group of cytochromes.[62,63]

Another classical example is the metabolism of compounds like paraquat and diquat which undergo one-electron redox cycling reactions, generating continuously drug-derived radicals[64,65] and superoxide anion which becomes dismuted to H_2O and H_2O_2. The latter, by the Fenton–Harber–Weiss reaction, can yield $OH^{\cdot}$ radicals which, in turn are able to promote new lipid radicals by H abstraction. Lipid radicals can react with molecular oxygen to yield unstable hydroperoxides that suffer homolytic breakdown, generating new radicals.

Cells use several strategies to protect themselves from uncontrolled lipid peroxidation: (a) inactivation of active oxygen species; (b) trapping of eventually formed radicals; (c) inhibition of the radical chain propagation; and (d) repair of damaged lipids. Superoxide dismutase, catalase and glutathione peroxidase, together with reduced glutathione (GSH) are the most efficient cellular agents against oxygen species and radicals. Natural antioxidants, such as vitamin E present in biological membranes, act by inhibiting the propagation step of lipid peroxidation.[66,67] Lipid hydroperoxides are substrates of glutathione peroxidase. Using 2 mol of GSH, this enzyme reduces the –OOH group to an alcohol. However, for this enzyme to act efficiently, a minimal level of reduced glutathione needs to be present in cells.

Lipid peroxidation can be the direct consequence of drug-derived radical formation, or may appear concomitantly after previous GSH depletion as the result of the cell's inability to protect itself from active oxygen species generated during cellular oxidative metabolism.[33,68] Lipid peroxidation often precedes irreversible cell damage, being an early cause of cell death.[33,63,69]

An indirect way to assess the role of lipid peroxidation in the mechanism of cell injury is to evaluate the effects of the xenobiotic in the presence or absence of antioxidant agents like *N,N′*-diphenylphenylenediamine, vitamin E and promethazine.[58,69–71] However, it is not always possible to draw conclusions about what occurs first in the course of cell injury. Even in cases in where lipid peroxidation has been shown not to be the critical step in causing cell death, there is evidence showing that peroxidation can act synergistically with other damaging mechanisms to amplify liver injury.[70]

2. *Methods for investigating lipid peroxidation in cultured cells*

Several procedures for quantifying lipid peroxidation have been developed. They are based on the detection of intermediates, reactants or end-products of lipid peroxidation. Currently, the decrease in polyunsaturated fatty acids, oxygen consumption, chemiluminescence, formation of conjugated dienes, lipid hydroperoxides, detection of aldehydes (e.g. malondialdehyde) and formation of ethane, pentane, etc. are used to monitor lipid oxidation (for a review see Cheeseman[72]). Most procedures require sophisticated or expensive equipment and have a low sensitivity for *in vitro* research. The two fluorimetric procedures here described have shown good results when used with cell microcultures.

Fluorimetric measurement of lipid peroxidation with thiobarbituric acid Malondialdehyde (MDA) is one of the end-products of lipid peroxidation. The major problem with direct determination of MDA is the low recovery and separation from other interfering compounds frequently present in samples.[73] Reaction with thiobarbituric acid (TBA) has been one of the most widely used assays for measuring lipid peroxidation. It is an indirect method that detects degradation products of lipids (aldehydes and malondialdehyde). Two molecules of TBA react with one molecule of malondialdehyde to generate a chromophore that absorbs at

532–535 nm. The absorbance of the reaction product is referred to that of malondialdehyde *bis*-(dimethylacetal) adduct ($\varepsilon = 150 \times 10^3$ M^{-1} l). The results obtained with this method and ethane production are coincidental in most cases[59,74] and, although the sensitivity is low, it correlates well with chemiluminescence and ethane and pentane production.[75]

The MDA–TBA adduct is also fluorescent, and this property can be used to increase the sensitivity of the method used in *in vitro* assays. We have adapted the original procedure[76] for use with microplates:

1. Culture medium is collected and centrifuged to remove dead cells.
2. Prepare a standard curve 0–1000 pmol of malondialdehyde *bis*-(dimethylacetal) in culture medium (final volume 250 μl).
3. Add to problems and standard tubes: 100 μl 7% sodium dodecyl sulfate solution; 1 ml 0.1 N HCl solution; 150 μl 1% phosphotungstic acid solution; and finally 500 μl 0.67% TBA solution, and mix.
4. Maintain the tubes in a boiling bath for 60 min in the dark. Then cool the tubes in a cold-water bath.
5. Add 1 ml *n*-butanol to tubes, shake vigorously and centrifuge (10 min at 3000 rpm).
6. Transfer the *n*-butanol layer to microplates and read fluorescence (515 nm excitation, 553 nm emission).

There might be some interference when measuring MDA–TBA adducts in culture medium. Glucose, an aldehyde like MDA, can react with thiobarbituric acid to produce a chromophore that absorbs at 535 nm. Because the concentration of glucose in culture medium is significant (10 mM), interference of glucose needs to be taken into account. The emission maximum of TBA–MDA complex is 552 nm, but the use of narrow-band optical filters centred at 590 ± 35 nm can minimize interferences.[77]

Determination of lipid hydroperoxides with glutathione peroxidase The method is based on the enzymatic reduction of lipid hydroperoxides. The enzyme glutathione peroxidase catalyses the reaction:

$$\text{R–OOH} + 2\text{GSH} \xrightarrow{\text{GSH-Px}} \text{R–OH} + \text{H}_2\text{O} + \text{GSSG}$$

After incubating a peroxide-containing sample with an excess of GSH in the presence of the enzyme, the amount of remaining GSH is quantified by the fluorimetric reaction with *o*-phthaldialdehyde. Atmospheric oxygen interferes in the reaction by increasing non-enzymatic GSH consumption. Consequently, solutions need to be vacuum-degassed and purged with nitrogen to remove oxygen traces before use. Pipetting and transfer of samples to microtitre plates should be carried out under inert atmosphere whenever possible (e.g. inside a plastic bag inflated with nitrogen).

1. Up to 20 nmol peroxides in a maximal volume of 140 μl can be assayed per well in a 96-microwell plate.
2. Add 50 nmol GSH (50 μl of a 1 M solution of GSH in 50 mM phosphate buffer, pH 7.2) to each well.
3. Dilute the required amount of glutathione peroxidase in phosphate buffer and add 50 μl to each well with a multichannel pipette (final assay concentration 0.5 units ml^{-1}).
4. Seal the 96-well plate with adhesive plastic tape under inert atmosphere and incubate for 30 min at room temperature (25°C).

5. Add 10 μl to each well of an *o*-phthaldialdehyde solution (10 mg ml^{-1} in methanol). Shake the plate gently and seal it again under inert atmosphere. Leave in the dark at 25°C for an additional 30 min.
6. Read fluorescence with a microplate fluorescence reader (Cyfofluor® 2350, Millipore; 340 nm excitation, 420 nm emission).

Consumed GSH is proportional to the amount of hydroperoxide present in the sample. Titrated hydrogen peroxide or *t*-butyl hydroperoxide solutions can be used as reference compounds.

C. Drug-induced oxidative stress

The term oxidative stress is defined as a disturbance in the pro-oxidant–antioxidant balance of a cell (for a review see Sies[78] and Spiteller[79]). In active aerobic cells, oxidative challenge occurs as a consequence of the oxidation of substrates taking place in the cell to produce ATP, but this alone does not constitute oxidative stress. Likewise, a decrease in the antioxidant elements of a cell because of nutritional or physiological changes does not constitute oxidative stress. However, when, as a result of the presence of a xenobiotic, there is increased formation of active oxygen species accompanied by an absolute loss of GSH equivalents, the cell reaches a state in which the balance is altered in favour of oxidative damage.[78] The immediate result is increased lipid peroxidation, alteration of membrane functionality and, indirectly, the inability of the cell to generate its own energy or to maintain the ionic homoeostasis.

1. *Drug redox cycling as cause of oxidative stress*

Certain drugs can easily alter the balance between the normal oxidative challenge and cell mechanisms for antioxidant defence. The most active substances in eliciting oxidative stress are compounds able to undergo repeated oxidation and reduction cycles within the cell.[80]

A representative example of this type of toxins are quinones (Fig. 16.3), which cause cell injury by two mechanisms. First, quinones are electrophiles able to react with nucleophiles such as the thiol group of GSH and proteins. Because GSH plays a key protective role within the cell, depletion of GSH renders the cell more sensitive to physiologically generated oxygen active species. Second, a number of flavoproteins (e.g. cytochrome P450 reductase) catalyse the reduction of quinones to semiquinones by NAD(P)H. Semiquinones can be detoxified by reaction with nucleophiles (GSH), but they can also react spontaneously with molecular oxygen in a one-electron oxidation process to regenerate the parent quinone and superoxide anion. Superoxide dismutase produces H_2O_2, which by the Harber–Weiss–Fenton reaction generates oxygen-derived radicals and related species (OH, $O_2^{\cdot -}$, $^1O_2$). The quinone can be reduced again, and becomes trapped in a series of redox cycles. The stoichiometric balance of the whole redox cycling is the continuous one-electron reduction of molecular oxygen by cellular NADPH (Fig 16.3). The consequences are that: (a) a larger amount of reactive oxygen species is produced; (b) reduced thiol and nicotinamide nucleotide pools are depleted; and (c) the loss of protective thiols (GSH) renders macromolecules susceptible to alkylation and arylation by the drug and to oxygen species generated by physiological oxidative reactions.[32,81–83]

Other compounds that can participate in redoxcycles are chatecols, pyridinium derivatives (paraquat, diquat, etc), *N*-nitrosoureas, aromatic nitro and nitroso compounds.[80,84–88]

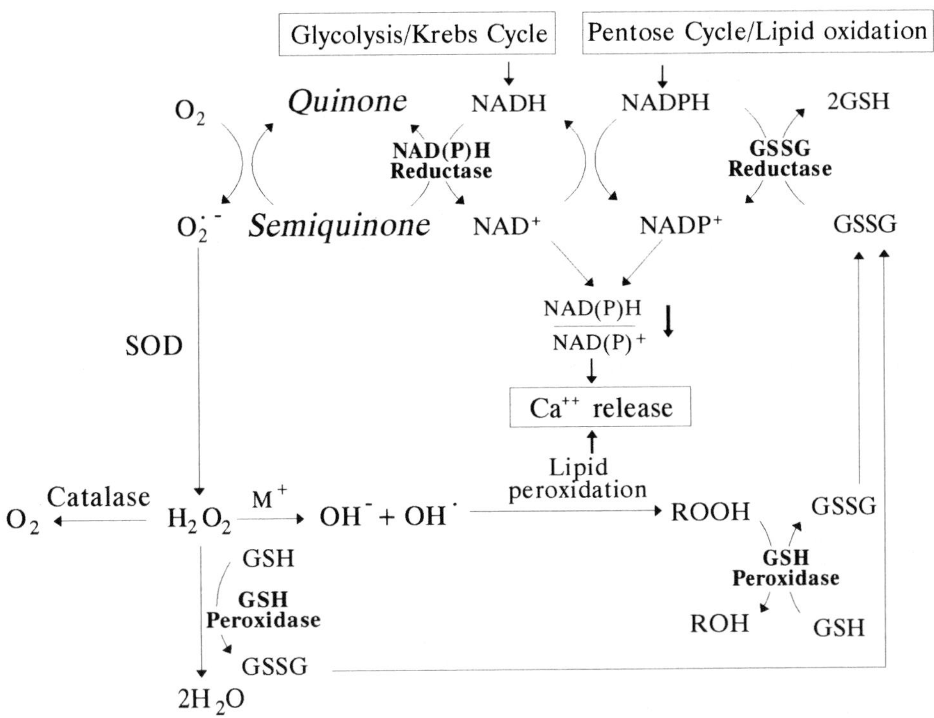

Fig. 16.3 Drug redox cycling and oxidative stress. Quinones can be partially reduced by reductases with NADPH consumption. The semiquinone can react readily with molecular oxygen in a one-electron oxidation, thereby regenerating the parent quinone. This redox cycling causes the continuous production of reactive oxygen species (superoxide anion), and depletion of GSH and nicotinamide nucleotide pools, with a concomitant increase in lipid peroxidation and Ca^{2+} release. GSH, reduced glutathione; GSSG, glutathione disulfide; SOD, superoxide dismutase.

2. *Glutathione and oxidative stress*

Cellular glutathione (GSH) is a strong nucleophile present in living cells that protects cells against the damage produced by a variety of electrophiles (free radicals, oxidants, etc.)[89]. In addition, GSH serves as an essential co-factor of the enzyme glutathione peroxidase, which removes hydroperoxides formed during oxidative processes. Finally, another defence system involving the tripeptide GSH is the conjugation and inactivation of reactive metabolites produced during cytochrome P450-dependent oxidation of foreign compounds by glutathione *S*-transferases.[11,33,90]

Cellular glutathione can decrease for several reasons: (a) oxidation to GSSG; (b) conjugation with metabolites or endogenous proteins; and (c) reduced *de novo* synthesis. Oxidized glutathione (Fig. 16.3) is reduced back to GSH via the glutathione reductase pathway.[33] This process requires the consumption of NADPH and, indirectly, NADH.[91] GSSG is toxic to the intracellular milieu, and when glutathione reductase is overwhelmed and GSSG accumulates beyond a critical level, it is exported and lost from the cell. GSH can also be lost from cells by conjugation to metabolites. Conjugates are further processed in other tissues (e.g. kidney) to recover glutamate and glycine. The resulting mercapturic acid derivatives are eliminated in the urine.[92] In both cases, GSH is irreversibly lost and can be replaced only by *ex novo* synthesis.[93]

One of the consequences of GSH depletion can be the modification of the sulphydryl (SH) groups of target proteins, which are the most susceptible nucleophilic centres to arylating and oxidizing species.[32] Oxidative stress produces *S*-thiolation of proteins, presumably by thiol/disulfide exchange, and this phenomenon has been shown to occur with several xenobiotics.[94] Dethiolation of proteins depends on the reaction between the modified protein and one or more reduced thiols. Two mechanisms of dethiolation have been identified, both ultimately requiring GSH and enzymatic reduction by NADPH. One involves GSH and glutathione reductase, and the other thioredoxin and thioredoxin reductase, a thiol reductant showing a broad specificity for reduction of disulfides.[33,94]

Except in the case of drugs acting as specific inhibitors of glutathione synthesis,[95] the most common pathway of glutathione depletion in drug toxicity is excessive consumption of GSH without recovery. Severe and sustained deficiency of glutathione leaves cells and tissues vulnerable to active oxygen species, radicals and electrophilic metabolites, derived or not from the drug. This causes progressive and irreversible deterioration of cell structures and macromolecules, and finally cell death. GSH levels are of great relevance in toxicological terms, for they can modulate the cytotoxicity of a xenobiotic, the extent of oxidative stress, and ultimately cell survival.[32]

Mitochondria constitute a second reservoir of GSH in cells capable of preventing the effects of oxidants generated during oxidative phosphorylation on sensitive thiol groups.[96] Certain proteins are highly sensitive to changes in the cellular thiol and energetic status of the cell, among them Ca^{2+}-dependent ATPases, which serve as membrane-bound pumps to maintain cytoplasmic Ca^{2+} at low levels.[81,97] Because mitochondria have no catalase, they rely totally on GSH peroxidase, and hence on GSH, to detoxify hydroperoxides. Experimental evidence in isolated mitochondria incubated with *tert*-butyl hydroperoxide have shown that, although the GSH/GSSG balance drastically decreases, no GSSG efflux or loss of total GSH equivalents occurs, suggesting that no transport system for GSSG out of mitochondria exists. Consequently, all GSSG formed must be reduced *in situ*, and only by mitochondrial metabolism. This makes mitochondria particularly susceptible to xenobiotics.[33,98,99]

Fluorimetric quantification of reduced GSH in cultures Both oxidized and reduced glutathione in cells can be measured enzymatically[100] or detected by high-performance liquid chromatography,[101,102] but both methods lack the sensitivity needed for use in microcultures. Flow cytometry, on the other hand,[103] requires sophisticated equipment and is applicable only to cells. A procedure based on the reaction of thiols with o-phthaldialdehyde (OPD) in deproteinated samples shows good specificity and sensitivity towards GSH.[104] The resulting adduct possesses a strong fluorescence that makes this method sensitive enough to measure GSH in microcultures (50–5000 pmol per well).

1. Wash plates. Detach cells by scraping and homogenize by ultrasound with 5% trichloroacetic acid (TCA) containing 2 mM ethylene diamine tetra-acetic acid (EDTA). Centrifuge the plates for 30 min at 3000 rpm.
2. Transfer aliquots of 50 μl (triplicated) to 96-well microtitre plates.
3. Add 15 μl 1 M NaOH to neutralize the acid supernatant.
4. Add 175 μl 0.1 M sodium phosphate buffer, pH 8, containing 5 mM EDTA and add 10 litre of OPD (stock solution 10 mg ml^{-1} in methanol for spectroscopy). Keep the plate for 15–20 min at room temperature in the dark.
5. Read fluorescence at 350 nm excitation, 420 nm emission.

Measurement of glutathione in intact cultured hepatocytes Bimanes are essentially non-fluorescent thiol reagents[105] that yield bright blue fluorescent adducts. Monobromobimane reacts readily with thiols, whereas the reaction of monochlorobimane is much slower. However, the reaction of monochlorobimane with GSH is efficiently catalysed by cellular GSH-*S*-transferases, and the resulting GSH–bimane conjugate is also highly fluorescent. This allows derivatization of cellular GSH inside cells under conditions in which other thiol groups do not contribute significantly to cellular fluorescence.[106] Comparison of GSH measurement by flow cytometry and by enzymatic methods has shown excellent correlation between both assays in several types of cells.[103]

The following procedure can be used to measure GSH levels in cultured hepatocytes using fluorescence microplate readers.

1. Wash the cell monolayers with warm phosphate-buffered saline (PBS).
2. Add to each well 100 μl 20 μM monochlorobimane in Krebs–Henseleit buffer (stock solution 1 mM in ethanol).
3. Incubate at room temperature for 5 min in the dark.
4. Read fluorescence at 390 nm excitation, 460 emission.

Known amounts of GSH are allowed to react with monochlorobimane for 1 h in the dark, and are used as standards. Alternatively, a few units of GSH *S*-transferase can be added to reduce incubation time.

D. Calcium- and drug-induced cell injury

Intracellular calcium plays a fundamental role as a regulator of many enzymes and as an effector for hormones and growth factors controlling a wide variety of physiological processes. Moreover, intracellular calcium is also involved in many pathological and toxicological processes where it accumulates in dying cells.[82,83,107–111]

The cytosolic free Ca^{2+} concentration in mammalian cells is very low (approximately 0.1 μM) compared with the concentration of Ca^{2+} in extracellular fluids (1–2 mM). The major pathways for Ca^{2+} entry into cells are voltage-dependent channels, gated by the electrical potential across the plasma membrane (types L, T and N), and receptor-operated channels.[112] While the existence of the former is still controversial in liver cells, experimental evidence has been reported in favour of the latter.[113]

Under normal circumstances, the passive influx of Ca^{2+} is balanced by an active Ca^{2+} extrusion by an outward-directed membrane Ca^{2+}-ATPase. Other Ca^{2+} extrusion mechanisms occur in cells associated with the influx of Na^+ by membrane pumps acting as Na^+-driven antiports[114,115] (Fig. 16.4).

The cytosolic Ca^{2+} concentration is also controlled by active sequestration into intracellular stores. In hepatocytes, the mitochondria and the endoplasmic reticulum constitute major reservoirs of Ca^{2+} both of which are involved in xenobiotic-induced cytotoxicity.[116] In mitochondria, a specific carrier protein located in the inner membrane is responsible for the inward translocation of Ca^{2+}. The driving force for Ca^{2+} uptake is the electrochemical gradient across the inner membrane generated during oxidative phosphorylation.[114,117] In the endoplasmic reticulum, the uptake of Ca^{2+} is carried out by a Ca^{2+} ATPase pump, analogous to that of the sarcoplasmic reticulum of muscle.[118] In summary, intracellular Ca^{2+} homoeostasis is normally maintained by the concerted operation of cellular transport and compartmentation systems. This equilibrium can be altered in the course of the toxic phenomena.

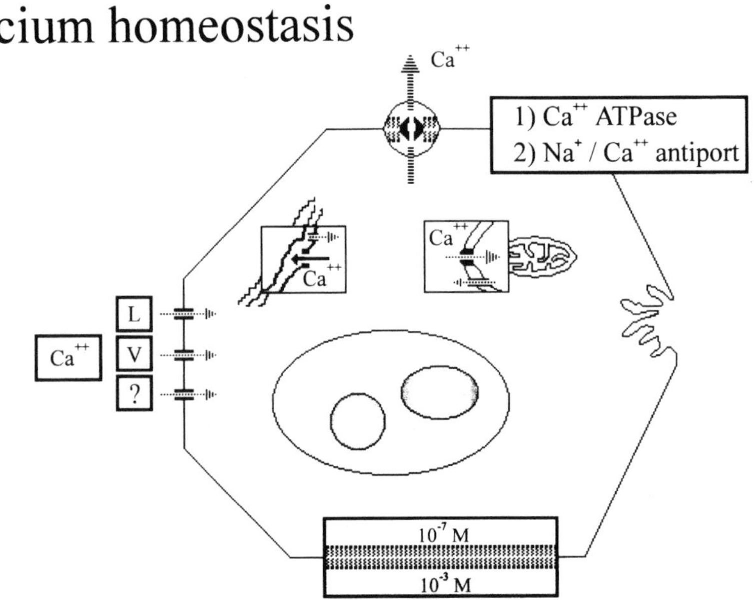

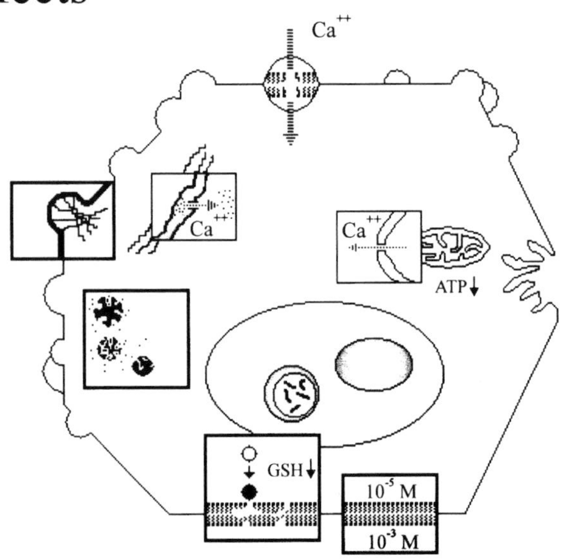

Fig. 16.4 Homoeostasis of cellular Ca^{2+} in hepatocytes and the consequences of its alteration in injured cells. The major pathways for Ca^{2+} entry into cells (upper panel) are voltage-dependent channels (V) and ligand-operated channels (L) The existence of the former is controversial in liver cells, but experimental evidence has been reported in favour of the latter. In hepatocytes, the mitochondria and endoplasmic reticulum constitute the major reservoirs of Ca^{2+}. Cytosolic Ca^{2+} concentration is controlled by active sequestration into intracellular stores. A sustained increase in cytosolic Ca^{2+} levels (lower panel) results in activation of enzymes (phospholipases, non-lysosomal proteases, endonucleases) and membrane blebbing, which ultimately cause cell death.

1. *Toxic events leading to an increased intracellular calcium level*

Toxins can alter Ca^{2+} homoeostasis by increasing the external influx, release from intracellular stores, impair Ca^{2+} uptake by organelles or extrusion to the external medium. Compounds are known to cause the collapse of the transmembrane potential,[119] but most toxic xenobiotics act indirectly by modifying membrane properties, inactivating enzymes or reducing the energy availability.

Free SH groups play a critical role in the catalytic mechanism of many enzymes, among them the Ca^{2+}-ATPases responsible for maintaining ionic homoeostasis in the cell.[115,120] Consequently, depletion of intracellular GSH and subsequent protein thiolation or oxidation of SH groups (Fig. 16.5) are generally associated with alterations in Ca^{2+} homoeostasis.[107,121] Concomitantly, lipid peroxidation of mitochondria may also induce Ca^{2+} release before morphological alterations become apparent.[122] The mechanisms can involve both physicochemical changes of the lipid bilayer where pumps are allocated, or depletion of GSH and modification of the enzymes.

Several mechanisms in the course of toxic phenomena may lead to an increased and sustained concentration of cytosolic calcium. For instance, quinones inducing oxidative stress (e.g. menadione[107]) cause an imbalance between increased formation of active oxygen species and an absolute loss of GSH equivalents. The Ca^{2+} concentration increase which is observed in hepatocytes can be related to three different causes: (a) decreased GSH, and protein modification; (b) a major demand of NADPH; and (c) decreased ATP production (Fig. 16.5).

2. *Consequences of sustained, increased Ca^{2+} concentration in cells*

As a consequence of the toxic action of xenobiotics, a sustained rise in cytosolic Ca^{2+} levels can occur. This situation clearly differs from the physiological rapid, and transient increase observed in response to hormones[110,111,113] and is almost invariably associated with cell toxicity and death (for a review see Nicotera *et al.*[83]).

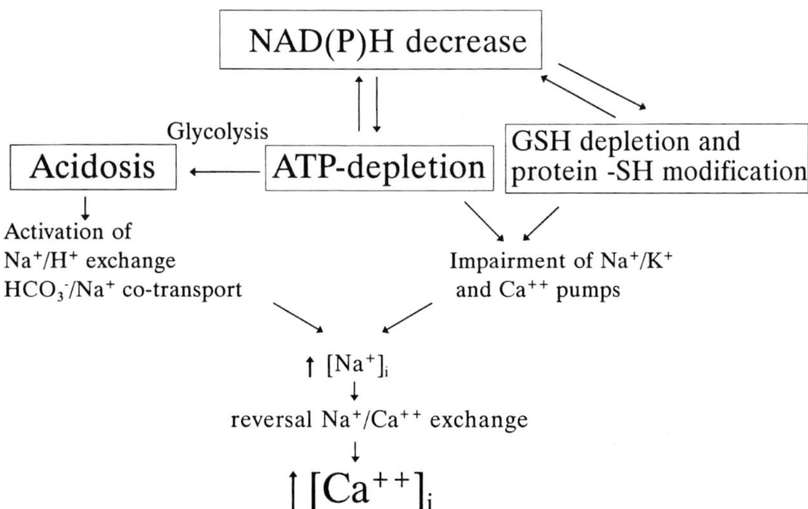

Fig. 16.5 Biochemical events leading to sustained increases in cytosolic Ca^{2+} concentration. Several biochemical events can lead to a sustained increase in cytosolic levels of Ca^{2+}. A decrease in GSH and protein SH- modification of Ca^{2+}-ATPases, ATP depletion and metabolic acidosis result in the inability of cells to pump Ca^{2+} from the cytosol.

An immediate consequence of raised cytosolic Ca^{2+} levels is plasma membrane blebbing (Fig. 16.4), a phenomenon caused by the disruption of the cytoskeletal organization and/or cleavage of critical anchoring cytoskeletal proteins which are regulated by intracellular Ca^{2+} and Ca^{2+}-dependent proteases. However, this is not the only mechanism responsible for chemically induced cytoskeletal damage, which also involves other Ca^{2+}-independent mechanisms (e.g. ATP depletion[83]).

An increase in cytosolic free Ca^{2+} concentration may also result in activation of phospholipases and non-lysosomal proteases, which can cause irreparable damage and functional injury to cell components.[111,123] Moreover, a sustained increase in the cytosolic Ca^{2+} concentration causes endonuclease activation and extensive DNA fragmentation, similar to that observed in apoptosis.[16,123] The alteration of Ca^{2+} homoeostasis parallels other ion concentration changes, decreasing ATP production because of disruption of mitochondrial membrane potential.[113,124] Decreased ATP levels render inactive the otherwise intact ATP-dependent pumps, thus causing rapid increases in cytosolic Na^{+} levels and loss of intracellular K^{+}.[125]

Measurement of intracellular free Ca^{2+} levels in cultured hepatocytes A new generation of fluorescent dyes (quin-2, fura-2, indo-1 and fluo-3) have made the measurement of intracellular free Ca^{2+} concentration easier, requiring simple laboratory instrumentation. Fluo-3 can be non-disruptively loaded into cells by using the corresponding acetoxymethyl (AM) ester, which is cleaved by cytosolic esterases to generate the free dye now trapped in the cytosol.[126–128] Fluo-3-AM is non-fluorescent until hydrolysed by cell esterases and complexed with Ca^{2+}. Fluo-3 has good spectroscopic qualities: a 40-fold enhancement of fluorescence upon Ca^{2+} binding and good photostability. Alkali metal complexes are weakly fluorescent. Fluorescence can be measured in cell suspensions and monolayers attached to a coverslip with a conventional fluorimeter. Other more sophisticated techniques include flow cytometry[61,129] and quantitative epifluorescence microscopy.[130,131]

We have adapted the fluo-3 technique to the specific needs of *in vitro* assays by using microcultures and microplate fluorimeters capable of quantifying both soluble and monolayer-associated fluorescence directly in the culture plates.[77,132]

1. Incubate hepatocytes for 30 min at 37°C in culture medium with 5 μmM fluo-3-AM (from a stock solution of 1 mM in DMSO) and 0.075% (w/v) Pluronic F-127 (1/200 dilution from the stock solution).
2. Shift cells to HEPES-buffered medium and incubate for an additional 5 min to complete ester hydrolysis.
3. Wash the cells twice with the same buffer, add medium and monitor fluorescence with a multiwell fluorimeter (excitation 485 ± 22 nm, emission 530 ± 30 nm).
4. Once a stable fluorescence baseline has been reached, add toxic substances to be tested to selected wells. Monitor fluorescence at regular times. To correct readings for extracellular fluorescence interference due to dye leakage, the medium ($\pm$toxic substance) is replaced before each fluorescence scan.
5. Lysate cells with 20 μM digitonin (8 mM stock solution in DMSO) in a medium containing 2 mM $CaCl_2$ (4 min) and read fluorescence (F_{max}).
6. Add 10 mM Ethylene glycol-bis (β-aminoethyl ether) (EGTA) (100 mM stock solution in 0.3 M NaOH) to quench Ca^{2+} and read fluorescence (F_{min}).

For any recorded fluorescence (F), the concentration of Ca^{2+} can be calculated by the following algorithm:

$$[Ca^{2+}]_i = K_d[(F - F_{min})/(F_{max} - F)]$$

assuming a value of K_d of 400 nM for the dissociation constant of the fluo-3–Ca^{2+} complex.[132,133]

Under the experimental conditions mentioned above, the leakage of fluo-3 out of the cell is less than 5–10% within 30 min of incubation, and cell viability is not altered.[77] If longer incubation times with the toxic substance are needed, it is recommended that fluo-3-AM be added shortly before Ca^{2+} measurement.

3. *Ca^{2+} levels, GSH content, lipid peroxidation and cell viability in the course of hepatocyte injury by toxins*

Glutathione levels, lipid peroxidation, ATP content and Ca^{2+} levels are biochemical parameters that are interdependent and become altered preceding cellular death. However, their time course may differ depending on the precise mechanism of toxicity involved. This is illustrated by the toxicity of cocaine to hepatocytes.[134] Biotransformation of cocaine in the liver proceeds mainly via hydrolytic cleavage of the ester bond, producing stable non-toxic metabolites (benzoyl ecgonine). However, a small fraction of the drug is oxidated to *N*-hydroxynorcocaine via a nitrosonium ion generated by cytochrome P450 and flavin adenine dinucleotide (FAD) mono-oxygenases.[135] This metabolite participates in a redox cycling process, generating superoxide anion, depleting GSH and causing lipid peroxidation.[136]

On incubating hepatocytes with cocaine, a series of sequential biochemical events occurs. Based on them, two different pathways for cocaine hepatotoxicity have been proposed:[132] (a) in non-induced hepatocytes the major biochemical alteration preceding cell death is the non-transient rise in cytosolic Ca^{2+} levels, presumably due to a direct interference with Ca^{2+} pumps (Fig. 16.6A); no major changes in GSH or lipid peroxidation are observed; and (b) in phenobarbital-induced hepatocytes, the larger oxidative metabolism of the drug produces rapid and extensive GSH depletion, is followed by increased lipid peroxidation; both phenomena precede cell death. The increase in Ca^{2+} concentration became noticeable when cell viability starts to decrease (Fig. 16.6B).

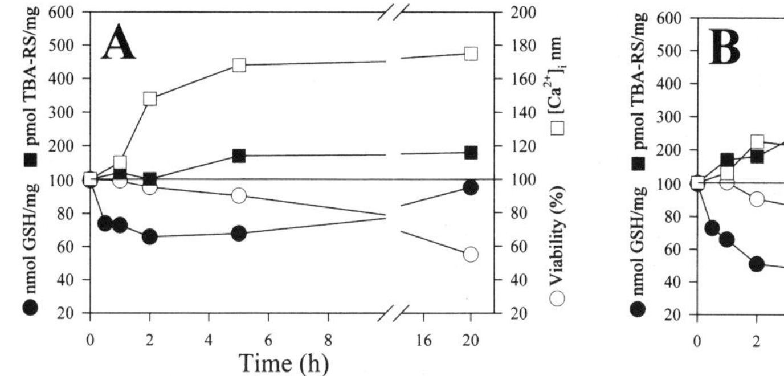

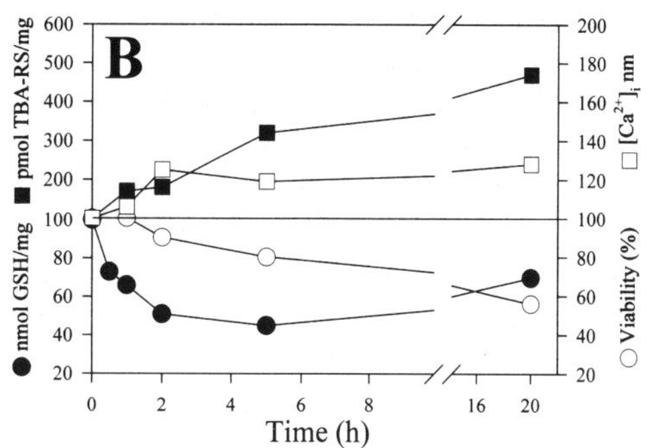

Fig. 16.6 Time course changes of cytosolic Ca^{2+}, GSH and lipid peroxidation in hepatocytes incubated with cocaine. Control (A) and phenobarbital-induced (B) hepatocytes were incubated with a toxic concentration of cocaine. In non-induced hepatocytes (A) the increase in cytosolic Ca^{2+} concentration was the parameter that preceded cell death. In contrast, in phenobarbital-induced hepatocytes (B) the greater oxidative metabolism of the drug caused a rapid and important depletion of GSH which was followed by lipid peroxidation and later by an increase in Ca^{2+} concentration.

E. Covalent binding

Biotransformation of xenobiotics can also result in the formation of chemical intermediates capable of reacting with cell macromolecules, forming stable drug adducts.[137,138] DNA, RNA and proteins are among the most frequent targets of drug binding. The term covalent binding is used to describe the irreversible binding of a drug to a macromolecule. This irreversibility is assessed by the resistance of the label to stringent washing with both polar and non-polar solvents, and does not preclude the chemical nature of the bond between drug and the macromolecule.

Proteins constitute the most frequent targets of drug covalent binding. Depending both on the site of generation and on the nature and reactivity of the intermediate, differences in the subcellular localization of protein adducts may occur. For instance, endoplasmic reticulum drug adducts are often generated, a fact that probably reflects the proximity of the site of bioactivation (cytochrome; CYP) and of binding.[139] Drug–protein adducts have also been identified in plasma membrane.[138] This finding could be the consequence of either a membrane-located bioactivation (CYP has been reported to be expressed in plasma membrane too[140,141]), or the transport of a cytosolic drug-modified protein to the membrane.

Few critical proteins in hepatocytes have been identified as specific targets of drug covalent binding. CYPs giving rise to reactive metabolites are among the most frequently identified protein targets,[139,142–146] although other enzymes, (e.g. Ca^{2+}-ATPase, carboxyl esterase, GSH transferase) have also been reported to be specific targets of drug binding.[139,147–149] Covalent binding of halothane[150–153] and diclofenac[149,153] have been studied in detail, and the presence of several protein bands bearing the trifluoroacetyl or diclofenac moiety have been identified in hepatocytes.

1. *Mechanisms of drug–protein adduct formation*

The extent of drug binding depends on the mechanisms of bioactivation of the drug, the reactivity of the resulting metabolite, and the cellular mechanism of defence. Because of their capability to participate in many different biotransformation reactions, CYP isozymes are usually involved in reactions leading to covalent binding. Electrophiles, generated as a result of oxidative reactions, radicals and conjugates can react with nucleophilic functional groups of proteins to form stable bonds. Unsaturated carbonyl compounds (e.g. α, β unsaturated ketones) and aldehydes constitute two of the most frequently occurring reactive groups capable of reacting with proteins through a Michael-type reaction or Schiff's base formation. *o*-quinones are α, β unsaturated ketones that not only can participate in redox cycling processes, but can also readily react with amino groups in proteins.[138]

Halogenated compounds (CCl_4, halothane, etc.) represent a major class of protein-binding compounds. For this type of compound it has been postulated that the generation of C-centred radicals after halogen abstraction by the haem group of cytochromes or haemoglobin is the major mechanism involved in covalent binding.[154]

Epoxides are highly reactive metabolites that are decomposed by epoxide hydrolases. However, the formation of aromatic polycyclic epoxides by CYP 1A1/2, which are not good substrates for epoxide hydrolase, seems to be the explanation behind the binding of methylcholanthrene 7,8-diol, 9,8-oxide to DNA and proteins (for a review see Hindson and Roberts).[138]

Glucuronides constitute another group of reactive metabolites able to bind macromolecules covalently. Conjugation of a drug that contains a free carboxyl group with glucuronic acid yields acyl glucuronides that are unstable towards other –OH or $-NH_2$ groups. In the first case, a transacylation with displacement of the glucuronic acid moiety results in binding of the drug to the protein. A second possibility involves an internal transacylation with displacement of the drug moiety from the C-1 OH of glucuronic acid to another OH position on the ring. The resulting hemicetal can now bind to $-NH_2$ groups of the protein, via ring opening and generation of a Schiff's base.[155,156]

2. *Covalent binding and hepatotoxicity*

In spite of the fact that many hepatotoxins are metabolized to reactive intermediates that can covalently bind to macromolecules, the relationship between covalent binding and tissue injury has proven difficult to ascertain in many cases. Quite frequently covalent binding is a concomitant process that cannot be experimentally dissociated from toxicity, and in only a few cases does it result in well-defined type of cell injury. On the other hand, it is widely agreed that covalent binding is a frequent prerequisite for triggering an immune response.

Covalent binding is dependent on the proportion of the chemical converted into a reactive metabolite, the half-life of the reactive intermediate, and its ability to react with cell macromolecules, e.g. proteins and nucleic acids.[157] For a certain subset of drugs (acetaminophen, bromobenzene), there is a clear correlation between the extent of covalent binding to proteins and the severity of hepatocyte injury.[139,146] Modulation of P450-dependent metabolism of the drug by enzyme induction of inhibition has been shown to correlate well with the extent of covalent binding and liver damage. However, with other xenobiotics, there is a lack of correlation with hepatotoxicity. This is the case with bromophenol, which is able to bind covalently to hepatocytes, yet does not result in liver damage.[139] The paracetamol analogue *N*-acetyl-m-aminophenol also shows this discrepancy as it forms reactive metabolites that bind to hepatocyte proteins but is not hepatotoxic.[158]

Finally, in a few cases, covalent binding is inversely correlated with the extent of hepatotoxicity. Diclofenac has been reported to cause hepatotoxicity in humans.[159] This compound is metabolized to produce glucoronide conjugates as well as oxidized metabolites. Binding of the drug to proteins takes place mainly via transacylation of diclofenac glucuronide to form diclofenac adducts with proteins.[156] This process does not *per se* cause cytotoxicity. On the other hand, metabolism of diclofenac by P450 produces toxic metabolites that ultimately cause cell injury.[160] These two metabolic routes coexist. Thus, the more diclofenac is metabolized by P450, the less it becomes available for covalent binding through the formation of the glucuronide. In contrast, inhibition of CYP2C metabolism reduces cytotoxicity, increasing diclofenac conjugation and covalent binding.[153]

Procedure for measuring covalent binding of drugs in cultured hepatocytes Measurement of drug covalent binding to cell macromolecules is not difficult and can be done by the use of either radiochemical or immunological techniques. Each method has its advantages and disadvantages. The major disadvantage of radiochemical methods is the difficulty in differentiating between binding of the drug or metabolites.[161] The drawback of immunoassay techniques is that it may not quantify all drug adducts formed because of the antibody's epitope selectivity.

Covalent binding can be examined in cultures by measuring the non-extractable radioactivity of cells exposed to the radiolabelled drug. Specific radioactivity in the 50–100 MBq $mmol^{-1}$ range is, in most cases, adequate.

1. Incubate cells (6 cm plates) with the radioactive drug (10–100 μCi) for an appropriate time.
2. Wash the plates three times with 3 ml cold PBS.
3. Scrape cells from culture plates with a rubber policeman, in 1 ml cold PBS.
4. Add 5 ml ice-cold methanol per ml homogenate (15 min, 4°C).
5. Centrifuge samples to pellet the precipitates (10 000*g*, 10 min, 4°C). Supernatants are discharged.
6. Wash pellets sequentially by repeated vortexing and centrifugation with 2 ml ice-cold methanol (twice), ethanol (twice). Additional washes of pellets with acetonitrile, ethyl acetate, urea, etc. can be performed depending on the solubility of the unbound compound.
7. Dry pellets under a nitrogen stream.
8. Dissolve pellets in 0.5 ml 10% SDS and 0.5 ml 0.8 M NaOH. Transfer an aliquot of the solubilized pellet into scintillation vials containing 5–10 ml adequate scintillation solution. Shake vigorously. Determine the radioactivity of the sample.
9. Determine the protein content in another aliquot of the solubilized pellet.

Identification of drug–protein adducts by immunological methods Antibodies directed at the drug can help to identify the formation of drug–protein adducts. This requires very sensitive visualization methods and antibodies capable of recognizing the drug epitope once it has bound to protein. Obviously the preparation of suitable antibodies may be problematic if the binding mechanism of the drug is not known. An example of this procedure is the identification of diclofenac–protein adducts in hepatocytes incubated with the drug (Fig. 16.7). As previously mentioned, drug binding seems to proceed in part by amide formation between diclofenac and amino groups of the protein, and in part with the formation of Schiff's bases of the glucuronic conjugated and amino groups of proteins.[155,156] Identification of drug–protein adducts can be achieved in both cases by using antibodies against diclofenac epitope.

1. Incubate hepatocytes for 24 h with 100–300 μM diclofenac .
2. Scrap, homogenize cells and obtain the S9 fraction containing microsomes by centrifugation (10 min at 15 000*g*).
3. Separate proteins (*c.*100 g) by polyacrylamide gel electrophoresis (12.5% T, 5% C), under denaturing conditions (SDS, 2-mercaptoethanol).
4. Blot proteins electrophoretically to a polyvinyl diisopropil fluoride (PVDF) membrane.
5. Incubate the membrane for 1 h at 25°C with 10% skimmed milk in PBS to saturate unspecific binding sites. Wash the membrane (six times) with PBS containing 0.05% Tween-20.
6. Incubate for 2–16 h with affinity-purified antibody conveniently diluted in PBS–Tween and 3% skimmed milk.
7. Wash the membrane (six times) with PBS–Tween, and incubate for 1–2 h with peroxidase-labelled goat anti-rabbit immunoglobulin G diluted in PBS–Tween and 3% skimmed milk.
8. Repeatedly wash the membrane and incubate for 1 min with luminol (commercially available from Amersham, UK) prior exposure to a photographic film.

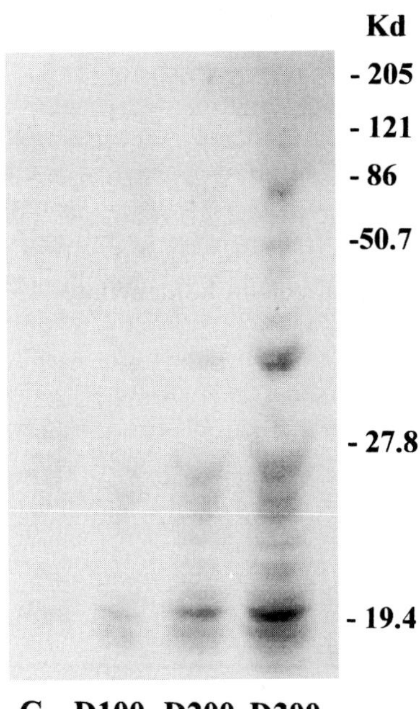

Fig. 16.7 Binding of diclofenac to hepatocyte proteins. Rat hepatocytes were incubated with 100–300 μM diclofenac for 24 h. The S9 fraction was obtained and separated by SDS–PAGE. Proteins were transferred to nitrocellulose paper and sequentially incubated with rabbit IgG anti-diclofenac and peroxidase-labelled goat IgG anti-rabbit IgG. Incubation of blots with luminol and exposure to a photographic film allowed visualization of drug–protein adducts.

The immunocomplexes are visualized by the luminescence reaction of peroxidase with luminol.[162,163] After incubation, the membrane is drained, wrapped in a plastic film and immediately laid on photographic film for 1–5 min. The membrane can then be repeatedly exposed to several films.

III. IMMUNOLOGICAL MECHANISMS OF DRUG HEPATOTOXICITY

Certain types of drug-induced hepatitis show clinical features characteristic of a hypersensitivity reaction against the drug. Allergic hepatitis is a type of idiosyncratic toxicity that occurs in certain individuals after previous exposure and sensitization to the drug (see Fig. 16.1). This phenomenon is unpredictable, dose independent and difficult to anticipate with animal models. Several immune-mediated mechanisms (Fig. 16.8) seem to be involved in the damage to hepatocytes, which becomes clinically evident as necrosis (cytolytic hepatitis with increased serum markers), cholestasis (with minor signs of necrosis) or both (mixed hepatitis).[3]

Drugs are small organic molecules unable to elicit an immune response unless they are bound to a macromolecule (hapten). Thus, covalent binding of the drug (or any metabolite) to proteins becomes a necessary stage of the mechanism but it cannot by itself trigger the immune response (Fig. 16.8). The next step is the accessibility of the neoantigen to immune surveillance. Different mechanisms can be envisaged to explain this process: (a) the drug could bind to the CYP that has interacted with the drug; this adduct would be transported to

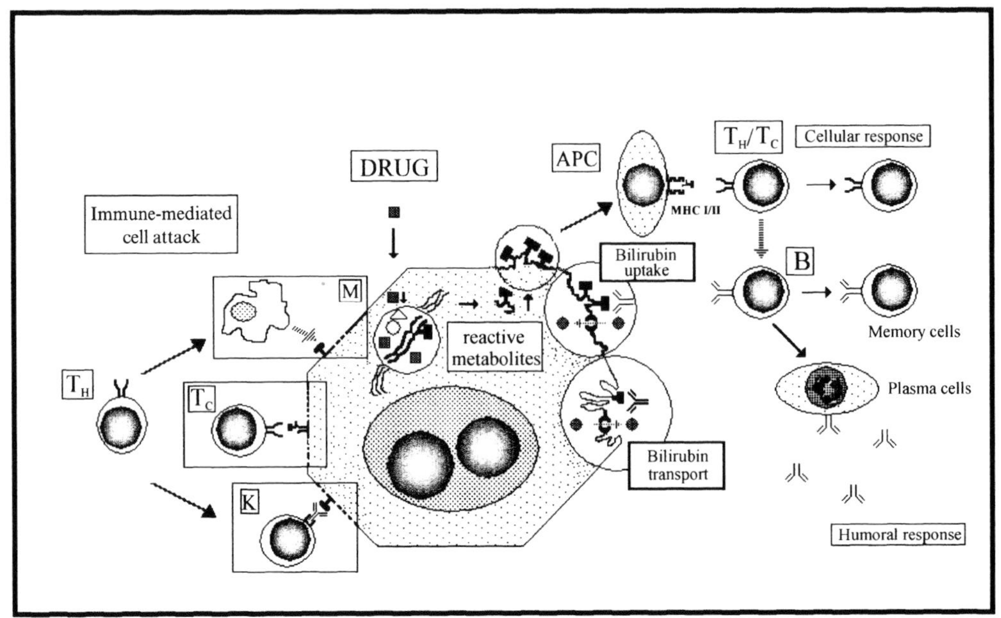

Fig. 16.8 Key events in the course of allergic hepatitis. In the course of drug bioactivation, reactive metabolites can bind to hepatocyte proteins. Recognition of these neoantigens by the immune system raises humoral and cellular responses directed to the drug. Both elements participate in hepatocyte injury, causing necrosis and/or cholestasis.

the cell membrane and become exposed to the external surface;[164] (b) the reactive metabolite has a long enough half-life to allow it to react with membrane proteins or proteins that would be transported to the membrane; (c) because CYP activities have been demonstrated in the plasma membrane of hepatocytes, they could locally catalyse bioactivation reactions, leading to the formation of drug–protein adducts in the cell membrane.[140,141]

The immune response in allergic hepatitis has a humoral and a cellular component.[165,166] From the review of a significant number of clinical cases of allergic hepatitis, Homberg *et al.*[165] found that four types of response can be established: (a) a lack of antibodies against hepatic or drug antigens; (b) the presence of autoantibodies (anti-mitochondrion, anti-nucleus, anti-smooth muscle); (c) antibodies directed against isoforms of CYP; and (d) drug-directed antibodies.

Antibodies directed against autoantigens have been well documented in the case of patients with halothane hepatitis.[167,168] Antibodies directed against CYPs have also been reported.[169] In only a few cases has it been possible to demonstrate patient's drug-directed antibodies acting on human hepatocytes. In a recent paper,[170] antibodies against erythromycin were demonstrated in a patient suffering from acute drug-induced hepatic cholestasis. The antibodies were able to recognize erythromycin that became covalently bound to human hepatocytes after incubation of cells with the antibiotic. Little is known about the linkage between circulating antibodies and the observed liver dysfunction. Antibodies are large macromolecules and do not readily enter the cell. Instead they may bind to haptenized hepatocyte membranes, thus altering their physicochemical properties and, indirectly, the functionality of membrane-allocated proteins (e.g. enzymes, ion pumps), ion transport and ultimately bile production.

T-lymphocyte sensitization to drugs (or metabolites) is also considered to be a mechanism involved in allergic hepatitis.[166] The existence of sensitized T-cell clones could be demonstrated in sensitized patients by means of an *in vitro* test. This is based on a proliferation assay using peripheral lymphocytes of patients which are incubated with the suspected drug and/or its metabolites, and a prostaglandin inhibitor. With this combined approach, positive responses for the suspected drug was demonstrated in approximately 80% of patients.[171,172]

IV. SCREENING FOR POTENTIAL HEPATOTOXICITY OF NEW DRUGS

When a new pharmaceutical is being developed, potential hepatotoxic effects are examined as part of the normal battery of assays to which compounds are routinely subjected. This is currently done in experimental animals, assuming they are a good model for humans. However, the fact that in some cases toxic effects on humans were not discovered until the first clinical trials because of significant interspecies drug metabolism differences has stimulated the use of human-derived cells for the detection of potential hepatotoxicity at early stages of drug development.[173,174]

Cellular models show ideal advantages for preliminary screening of hepatic effects and drug metabolism studies: they are applicable at first stages of drug development; only a small amount of the compound is needed for the assays; they can be of help in selecting the best animal model for metabolic and pharmacokinetic studies and, if human hepatocytes are used, they can provide a specific and direct information about potential effects of the compound on the human liver. Moreover, drug-drug interactions can be easily investigated under conditions that would be ethically unacceptable with human beings.[175,176]

A. Parameters for assessing hepatotoxicity *in vitro*

A first step when investigating the *in vitro* hepatotoxicity of a compound is to discern whether the observed toxicity is hepatocyte specific. Assessing cytotoxicity (cell viability, cell survival, morphology, enzyme leakage, etc.) is a simple first approach to this problem.[177,178] By comparing the concentration–toxicity curves of the compound (a) in fully competent primary cultured hepatocytes, (b) in non-hepatic cells (e.g. fibroblasts), and (c) in non-metabolizing hepatocytes (e.g. well-differentiated human hepatomas HepG2 that lack cytochrome P450), it is possible to ascertain whether the compound elicits toxic effects preferentially on hepatocytes, or whether bioactivation (metabolization) of the xenobiotic is required for there to be cellular damage.[1]

Cytotoxicity end-points represent a first approach to assessing cytotoxicity,[178] but evaluation of these parameters alone may leave out of consideration xenobiotics that impair cell function without causing cell death. This may not be critical for the hepatocyte itself, but can be of toxicological significance for the whole organism.[179–182] By examining the effects on hepatocyte-specific metabolism (e.g. gluconeogenesis, ureogenesis, plasma protein synthesis), it is possible to determine whether relevant hepatic specific functions become altered by the presence of a xenobiotic. In general, metabolic parameters are more sensitive to the toxic effect of hepatotoxins than cytotoxicity indicators. In particular, a decrease in plasma protein synthesis is one of earliest and most sensitive indicators of cellular damage in hepatocytes.[1]

The question of how many toxicity end-point parameters need to be assessed to identify a potential hepatotoxic compound is worth discussing. In most cases, the different quantitative cytotoxic parameters currently used give equivalent information on the toxicity of a compound. For a first screening of cytotoxicity it normally suffices to determine only one parameter. However, the use of several markers can provide additional information, for example as to whether the damage affects only cell membranes (e.g. lactate dehydrogenase (LDH) leakage) or also involves subcellular structures (GPT, succinate dehydrogenase or ATP production for mitochondrial damage; ATP-mediated neutral red uptake for lysosomes).

Metabolic parameters can give answers to specific questions, like whether the ability of the hepatocyte to render glucose from serum lactate is impaired or not by a given drug, whether the rate of conversion of ammonia into urea is decreased, or whether the synthesis or metabolism of lipids is altered by the presence of a xenobiotic. Although many metabolic pathways ultimately have in common the requirement of ATP, and an energy imbalance will affect many of them, inhibition of one function does not preclude alteration of others. Quite frequently hepatotoxins show preferential effects on the inhibition of a certain hepatocyte functions.[183–189] Consequently, to be fully confident of the possible implications that a compound might have for hepatocytes *in vivo*, it may be necessary to examine several relevant metabolic functions. For most screening purposes it is sufficient to monitor the production of the final product of a metabolic route (e.g. urea produced from ammonia, glucose produced from lactate) to gain an estimation about the potential effects of the drug, before undertaking a more precise investigation of the mechanisms of toxicity.

1. *Cytotoxicity parameters*

Damage to cells by xenobiotics commonly results in an early alteration of cell membrane permeability. Consequently, leakage of cytoplasmic enzymes into the culture medium is a first-choice parameter for a rapid and sensitive evaluation of cytotoxicity. Among cytosolic enzymes, LDH is a very good marker because the hepatic isoenzyme (type V) is quite stable in culture conditions, allowing reproducible measurements in culture supernatants after 12–24 h incubation.[190] Leakage of enzymes associated with organelles (mitochondrial activities glutamate oxaloacetate transaminase and glutamate pyruvate transaminase can also be used. The neutral red test and the MTT test[191] used often for cytotoxicity assessment in cells give also satisfactory results with hepatocytes.[192,193] These techniques have been presented in detail elsewhere in this book. Other less frequently used cytotoxicity parameters are inhibition of cell attachment, cell extension, monolayer formation and cell survival.[1,179]

Experiments on cytotoxicity are ultimately aimed at determining the maximal non-toxic concentration of a drug, i.e. the highest concentration compatible with cell survival (Fig. 16.9). This is estimated from the lowest concentration causing a significant cytotoxicity (usually IC_{10}[192–194]).

2. *Metabolic parameters*

Several metabolic parameters that are representative of the most characteristic functions of the liver can be used to evaluate the potential toxic effects of xenobiotics. Gluconeogenesis,[183,185,186] glycogen metabolism,[186,195] ureogenesis,[183,187] plasma protein synthesis[176,183,185] and synthesis of VLDL[186,196] have been used in hepatocyte *in vitro* studies and shown to be of value in the identification of potential hepatotoxins.

Of the above-mentioned parameters, gluconeogenesis and glycogen synthesis constitute two characteristic liver functions that can easily be monitored in culture.[197]

In vitro Screening of hepatotoxicity of drugs

1) Determination of basal / hepatic cytotoxicity

Hepatocyte	Hepatoma	Non-hepatic cell	Type of toxin
+	+	+	Non-hepatic specific
+	-	-	Hepatic specific (latent)
+	+	-	Hepatic specific (active)

Determination of Maximal Non-Toxic Concentration (MNTC)

2) Effects on cellular metabolism

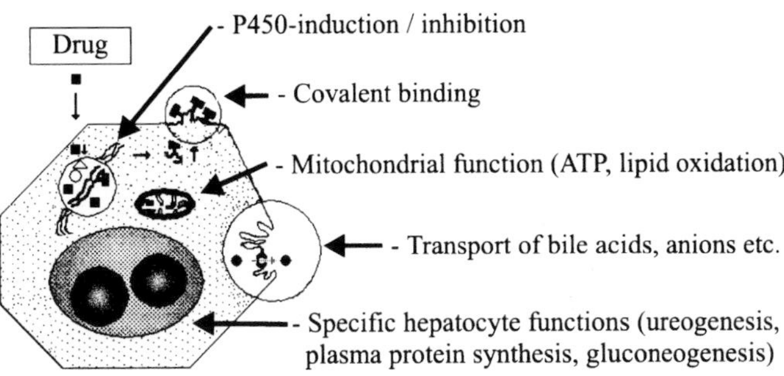

3) In vitro extrapolation / Risk assessment

- Relevance of the metabolic function altered
- Reversibility
- Biokinetic modelling
- Toxicity risk

T_R	Reversibility	P450 induction	
<1	+	-	LOW
<1	-	+/-	Further studies
≥1	+	+/-	Requested
≥1	-	+	HIGH

Fig. 16.9 Stepwise *in vitro* screening for potential hepatotoxicity of drugs. A first step is to discern whether toxicity is hepatocyte specific, and to determine the maximal non-cytotoxic concentration from concentration curves. This should be followed by analysis of xenobiotic effects on specific hepatocyte functions and CYP induction. Interpretation of results should take into account the relevance and reversibility of the metabolic alteration and the *in vitro* and *in vivo* concentrations.

Evaluation of gluconeogenesis in cultured hepatocytes Hepatocytes have the ability to produce glucose from lactate, amino acids, glycerol and other sugars. This process requires ATP and is readily impaired by toxic xenobiotics. In absence of glycogen, glucose produced by cells and released to culture medium is an indicator of the gluconeogenic capability of cells. Assay needs to be performed in Krebs–Henseleit solution and the glucose produced is enzymatically quantified by the reaction of glucose oxidase. Previous glycogen depletion is required in the case of human hepatocytes, but not in 24-h rat hepatocytes.[198]

1. Hepatocytes are incubated with xenobiotics at variable concentrations and times.
2. To deplete cellular glycogen add glucagon (final concentration 10^{-7}M) to each well and incubate cells for 2 h.
3. Carefully rinse plates with PBS and shift to glucose-free Krebs–Ringer solution containing 10 mM lactate (or other gluconeogenic precursor).
4. Remove aliquots (40 μl) of culture medium at regular intervals (0–2 h) and place in microtitre wells.
5. Add to wells 200 μl of a solution containing 1 mg ml^{-1} 2,2′-Azinobis (3-ethylbenzthiazoline sulfonic acid) (ABTS), 10 units ml^{-1} glucose oxidase and 0.8 units ml^{-1} peroxidase in 100 mM phosphate buffer pH 7.2.
6. Incubate for 30–40 min at room temperature. Read plates at 405 nm using a 490 nm filter as reference. Determine cellular protein. Results are expressed as nanomoles of glucose per milligram of cellular protein.

Glycogen determination in microcultures of hepatocytes Glycogen can be quantified in cultured cells after extraction, precipitation, acid hydrolysis and reaction of the resulting glucose.[183] A new method[197] has been recently developed that combines enzymatic hydrolysis of glycogen, and enzymatic quantitation of glucose and is suitable for microcultures.

1. After incubating cells with the drugs, rinse plates three times with PBS (100 μl), and freeze–thaw the plates to break the cells.
2. Cellular glycogen is enzymatically hydrolysed *in situ* by adding 100 μl of glucoamylase (2500 mU/ml) to each well in 0.2 M sodium acetate buffer pH 4.8, and incubated for 2 h at 4°C with gentle shaking.
3. Centrifuge plates at 2500 rpm for 10 min and transfer 40 μl aliquots to another 96-well plate.
4. Neutralize samples with 10 μl 0.25 MM NaOH and quantify glucose by the colorimetric reaction of glucose oxidase, peroxidase and ABTS as described above.

Results are expressed as nanomoles of glucose per microgram of DNA, estimated fluorimetrically by staining with the dye Hoescht 33528.

B. Interpretation of *in vitro* results and predictive value of *in vitro* data

The ultimate goal of *in vitro* experiments is to generate the type of scientific information needed to identify compounds that are potentially toxic to humans. For this purpose, not only the design of experiments but also the interpretation of results are essential. A first aspect of this problem is the sensitivity of the biological model (and that of each individual end-point parameter used) in discriminating among compounds and drugs acting on the basic functions of any cell or, more specifically, of hepatocytes.

A second point is the metabolic relevance of the observed alteration and its reversion upon withdrawal of the xenobiotic from the incubation medium.[1,181] Certain hepatocyte functions might be transiently altered but this may lack *in vivo* significance if the cell rapidly recovers upon biotransformation or elimination of the xenobiotic.

A final point is the influence of *in vivo* pharmacokinetics on the toxicity of the compound. In *in vitro* experiments, xenobiotics are kept in culture plates at a constant concentration during the incubation time. This contrasts with what occurs *in vivo*, where the concentration of the drug reaches a maximum and decreases thereafter in a characteristic concentration–time curve. Whenever possible, this circumstance should be taken into account in the experimental design of *in vitro* experiments. This is, however, technically complex for reproduction *in vitro*. A simplified procedure to bring the *in vivo* situation closer to *in vitro* experimental conditions is to incubate the cell for a time and concentration equivalent to the *in vivo* AUC (area under the concentration–time curve), experimentally determined or estimated by physiologically based pharmacokinetic models.[199]

A simplified way of estimating the relative potential hepatotoxicity of a drug within a homologous series of compounds is to compare the concentration of the drug reaching the liver *in vivo* with that causing toxic effects *in vitro*. The toxicity risk (T_R) is then defined as the quotient of both magnitudes. The larger the value of T_R (close to 1 or even greater), the greater the toxicity risk will be for a given drug.

For drugs having a first-pass effect, T_R calculated on the basis of peripheral blood levels can be misleading. Differences in the concentration in portal and peripheral blood can be very large. For example, the portal or hepatic concentration could be so high as to elicit hepatocyte damage *in vitro*, while the peripheral blood concentration, even after repeated dosage, can be lower that the IC_{10}.[186,188,200] From the *in vitro* data it can be reasonably assumed that, if a drug reaches the liver at a concentration and for a time that is toxic *in vitro*, it is highly probable that this compound will show toxic effects *in vivo*.[1]

An *in vitro* assay cannot give a straightforward answer about whether a certain compound will or will not be hepatotoxic in humans. It is also simplistic to attempt to make predictions based on simple cytotoxic end-point parameters without investigating the effects of the compound on hepatocyte metabolism. However, skilful interpretation of the scientific information generated in experiments using human-derived cells can be of great value in making decisions during the development of new pharmaceuticals.

ACKNOWLEDGEMENTS

The authors acknowledge the financial support of the European Union (Biomed I, Project Nr. BMH1-1097 and AIR, Project Nr. CT93-0860) the Spanish Fondo de Investigaciones Sanitarias (Project Nr. 94/1084) and The ALIVE Foundation.

REFERENCES

1. Castell, J. V. and Gómez-Lechón, M. J. (1992) The *in vitro* evaluation of the potential risk of hepatotoxicity of drugs. In Castell, J. V. and Gómez-Lechón, M. J. (eds) In Vitro *Alternatives to Animal Pharmaco-toxicology*, pp. 179–204. Farmaindustria, Barcelona.
2. Hinson, J. A., Pumford, N. R. and Nelson, S. D. (1994) The role of metabolic activation in drug toxicity. *Drug Metab. Rev.* **26:** 395–412.

3. Meeks, R. G., Harrison, S. D. and Bull, R. J. (eds) (1991) *Hepatotoxicology*. CRC Press, Boca Raton, Florida.
4. Testa, B. (1995) The metabolism of drugs and other xenobiotics. In Testa, B. and Caldwell, J. (eds) *Biochemistry of Redox Reactions*, pp. 410–428. Academic Press, New York.
5. Hodgson, E. and Levi, P. E. (1987) *A Textbook of Modern Toxicology*. Elsevier Science, Amsterdam.
6. Pessayre, D. (1986) Drug metabolism in the liver. In Fillastre, J. P. (ed.) *Hepatotoxicity of Drugs*, pp. 39–62. Editions INSERM, Rouen.
7. King, L. J. (1987) Metabolism and mechanisms of toxicity: an overview. In Benford, D. J., Bridges, J. W. and Gibson, G. G. (eds) *Drug Metabolism from Molecules to Man*, pp. 657–668. Taylor and Francis, London.
8. Zimmerman, H. J. and Ishak, K. G. (1995) General aspects of drug-induced liver diseases. *Gastroenterol. Clin. North Am.* **24:** 739–758.
9. DeLeve, L. D. and Kaplowitz, N. (1995) Mechanisms of drug-induced liver diseases. *Gastroenterol. Clin. North Am.* **24:** 787–810.
10. Kaplowitz, N., Aw, T. Y., Simon, F. R. and Stolz, A. (1986) Drug-induced hepatotoxicity. *Ann. Intern. Med.* **104:** 826–839.
11. Ross, D. (1988) Glutathione, free radicals and chemotherapeutic agents. Mechanisms of free radical induced toxicity and glutathione dependent protection. *Pharmacol. Ther.* **37:** 231–249.
12. Okey, A. B., Roberts, E. A., Harper, P. A. and Denison, M. S. (1986) Induction of drug-metabolizing enzymes: mechanisms and consequences. *Clin. Biochem.* **19:** 132–136.
13. Columbano, A. (1995) Cell death: current difficulties in discriminating apoptosis from necrosis in the context of pathological processes *in vivo*. *J. Cell. Biochem.* **58:** 181–190.
14. Bowen, I. D. (1993) Apoptosis or programmed cell death? *Cell Biol. Int.* **17:** 365–380.
15. Cohen, J. J. (1994) Apoptosis: physiological dell death. *J. Lab. Clin. Med.* **124:** 761–765.
16. Bellomo, G., Perotti, M., Taddei, F. *et al.* (1992) Tumor necrosis factor-alpha induces apoptosis in mammary adenocarcinoma cells by an increase in intranuclear free Ca^{2+} concentration and DNA fragmentation. *Cancer Res.* **52:** 1342–1346.
17. Alison, M. R. and Sarraf, C. (1995) Apoptosis: regulation and relevance to toxicology. *Hum. Exp. Toxicol.* **14:** 234–247.
18. Bonfoco, E., Kranic, D., Ankarcrona, M., Nicotera, P. L. and Liptom, S. A. (1995) Apoptosis and necrosis: two distinct events induced, respectively, by mild and intense insults with *N*-methyl-D-aspartate or nitric oxide/superoxide in cortical cell cultures. *Proc. Natl Acad. Sci. U.S.A.* **92:** 7162–7166.
19. Ledda-Columbano, G. M., Coni, P., Curto, M. *et al.* (1991) Induction of two different modes of cell death, apoptosis and necrosis, in rat liver after single dose of thioacetamide. *Am. J. Pathol.* **139:** 1009–1089.
20. Rosser, B. G. and Gores, G. J. (1995) Liver cell necrosis: cellular mechanisms and clinical implications. *Gastroenterology* **108:** 252–275.
21. Decker, K. and Keppler, D. (1974) Galactosamine hepatitis: key role of nucleotide deficiency period in the pathogenesis of cell injury and cell death. *Rev. Biochem. Pharmacol.* **71:** 78–106.
22. Roig, T., De-Oliveira, J. R., Bartrons, R. and Bermudez, J. (1994) Fructose 12,6-biphosphate protects against D-galactosamine toxicity in isolated rat hepatocytes. *Am. J. Physiol.* **266:** C172–C1728.
23. Anukarahanonta, T., Shinozuka, H. and Farber, E. (1973) Inhibition of protein synthesis in rat liver by D-galactosamine. *Res. Commun. Chem. Pathol. Pharmacol.* **5:** 481–491.
24. Zimmerman, H. J. (1976) Indirect hepatotoxins – cytotoxic. In Zimmerman, H. J. (ed.) *Hepatotoxicity. The Adverse Effects of Drugs and Other Chemicals on the Liver*, pp. 220–258. Appleton Century Crofts, New York.
25. Farber, E. (1967) Ethionine fatty liver. *Lipid Res.* **5:** 119–127.
26. Dubin, M., Carrizo, P. H., Biscardi, A. M. *et al.* (1994) Effect of 5-nitroindole on adenylate energy charge, oxidative phosphorylation and lipid peroxidation in rat hepatocytes. *Biochem. Pharmacol.* **48:** 1483–1492.
27. Nieminen, A. L., Saylor, A. K., Herman, B. and Lamasters, J. J. (1994) ATP depletion rather than mitochondrial depolarization mediates hepatocyte killing after metabolic inhibition. *Am. J. Physiol.* **267:** C67–C74.
28. Swartz, M. N. (1995) Mitochondrial toxicity: new adverse drug effects. *N. Engl. J. Med.* **333:** 1146–1148.

29. Miyoshi, H., Tamaki, M., Harada, K. *et al.* (1992) Uncoupling action of antibiotic sporaviridins with rat liver mitochondria. *Biosci. Biotechnol. Biochem.* **56:** 1776–1779.
30. Drahota, Z., Mares, V., Rauchova, H., Saf, P. and Kalous. (1995) Inhibition of mitochondrial ATPase by dicarbopolyborate, a new enzyme inhibitor. *J. Bioenerg. Biomembr.* **26:** 583–586.
31. Palmeira, C. M., Moreno, A. J. and Madeira, V. M. (1995) Mitochondrial bioenergetics is affected by the herbicide paraquat. *Biochem. Biophys. Acta* **1229:** 187–192.
32. Boobis, A. R., Duncan, J., Fawthrop, J. and Davies, D. S. (1989) Mechanisms of cell death. *Trends Pharmacol. Sci.* **10:** 275–280.
33. Reed, J. D. (1990) Glutathione: toxicological implications. *Ann. Rev. Pharmacol. Toxicol.* **30:** 603–631.
34. Shan, X., Jones, D. P., Hashmi, M. and Anders, M. W. (1993) Selective depletion of mitochondrial glutathione concentrations by (*R,S*)-3-hydroxy-4-pentenoate potentiates oxidative cell death. *Chem. Res. Toxicol.* **6:** 75–81.
35. Sood, C. and O'Brien, P. J. (1993) Molecular mechanisms of chloroacetaldehyde-induced cytotoxicity in isolated hepatocytes. *Biochem. Pharmacol.* **46:** 1621–1626.
36. Deschamps, D., DeBeco, V., Fishc, C. *et al.* (1994) Inhibition by perhexiline of oxidative phosphorylation and the beta-oxidation of fatty acids: possible role of pseudoalcoholic liver lesions. *Hepatology* **19:** 948–961.
37. Seifer, S. and Englard, S. (1982) Energy metabolism. In Arias, I. M., Popper, H., Schachter, D. and Shafritz, D. A. (eds) *The Liver: Biology and Pathobiology*, pp. 219–250. Raven Press, New York.
38. Alberts, B., Bray, D., Lewis, J., Raff, M., Roberts, K. and Watson, J. D. (1989) Energy conversion: mitochondria and chloroplasts. In Alberts, B., Bray, D., Lewis, J., Raff, M., Roberts, K. and Watson, J. D. (eds) *Molecular Biology of the Cell*, pp. 342–401. Gerland Publishing, New York.
39. De Luca, M. and McElroy, W. D. (1978) Purification and properties of firefly luciferase. *Methods Enzymol.* **57:** 3–14.
40. Berson, A., Schmets, L., Fisch, C. *et al.* (1994) Inhibition by nilutamide of the mitochondrial respiratory chain and ATP formation. Possible contribution to the adverse effects of this antiandrogen. *J. Pharmacol. Exp. Ther.* **270:** 167–176.
41. Donnelly, P. J., Walker, R. M. and Racz, W. J. (1994) Inhibition of mitochondrial respiration *in vivo* as an early event in acetaminophen-induced hepatotoxicity. *Arch. Toxicol.* **68:** 110–118.
42. Nieminen, A. L., Saylor, A. K., Tesfai, S. A., Herman, B. and Lemasters, J. J. (1995) Contribution of the mitochondrial permeability transition to lethal injury after exposure of hepatocytes to *t*-butylhydroperoxide. *Biochem. J.* **307:** 99–106.
43. Botla, R., Spivey, J. R., Aguilar, H. *et al.* (1995) Ursodeoxycholate (UDCA) inhibits the mitochondrial membrane permeability transition induced by glycochenodeoxycholate: a mechanism of UDCA cytoprotection. *J. Pharmacol. Exp. Ther.* **272:** 930–938.
44. Silva, J. M., McGirr, L. and O'Brien, P. J. (1991) Prevention of nitrofurantoin-induced cytotoxicity in isolated hepatocytes by fructose. *Arch. Biochem. Biophys.* **289:** 313–318.
45. Imberti, R., Nieminen, A. L., Herman, B. and Lemasters, J. J. (1993) Mitochondrial and glycolytic dysfunction in lethal injury to hepatocytes in *t*-butylhydroperoxide: protection by fructose, cyclosporin A and trifluoperazine. *J. Pharmacol. Exp. Ther.* **265:** 392–400.
46. Powers, S. G. and Meister, A. (1982) Urea synthesis and ammonia metabolism. In Arias, I. M., Popper, H., Schachter, D. and Shafritz, D. A. (eds) *The Liver: Biology and Pathobiology*, pp. 251–264. Raven Press, New York.
47. Fromenty, B., Grimbert, S., Mansouri, A. *et al.* (1995) Hepatic mitochondrial DNA deletion in alcoholics: association with microvesicular steatosis. *Gastroenterology* **108:** 193–200.
48. Krahenbuhl, S., Mang, G., Kupferschmid, H. *et al.* (1995) Plasma and hepatic carnitine and coenzyme A pools in a patient with fatal valproate induced hepatotoxicity. *Gut* **37:** 140–143.
49. Richardson, F. C., Engelhardt, J. A. and Bowsher, R. R. (1994) Fialuridine accumulates in DNA of dogs, monkeys and rats following long-term oral administration. *Proc. Natl Acad. Sci. U.S.A.* **91:** 1200–1237.
50. Emaus, R. K., Grunwald, R. and Lemasters, J. J. (1986) Rhodamine 123 as a probe of transmembrane potential in isolated rat-liver mitochondria: spectral and metabolic properties. *Biochem. Biophys. Acta* **850:** 436–448.
51. Lemasters, J. J., Grunwald, R. and Emaus, R. K. (1984) Thermodynamic limits to the ATP/site stoichiometries of oxidative phosphorylation by rat liver mitochondria. *J. Biol. Chem.* **259:** 3058-3063.
52. Porter, N. A. (1984) Chemistry of lipid peroxidation. *Methods Enzymol.* **105:** 273–282. Academic Press, Orlando.

53. Rice-Evans, C. A., Diplock, A. T. and Symons, M. C. R. (1991) Mechanisms of radical production. In Burdon, R. H. and Knippenberg, P. H. (eds) *Laboratory Techniques in Biochemistry and Molecular Biology. Techniques in Free Radical Rersearch*, pp. 19–50. Elsevier, Amsterdam.
54. Esterbauer, H. (1982) Aldehydic products of lipid peroxidation. In McBrien, D. C. H. and Slater, T. F. (eds) *Free Radicals, Lipid Peroxidation and Cancer*, pp. 101–128. Academic Press, New York.
55. Ross, D. (1989) Mechanistic toxicology: a radical perspective. *J. Pharm. Pharmacol.* **41:** 505–511.
56. Vaca, C. E., Wilhelm, J. and Harms-Rindgdahl, M. (1988) Studies on lipid peroxidation in rat liver nuclei and isolated nuclear membranes. *Biochim. Biophys. Acta* **958:** 375–387.
57. Zollner, H., Shaur, R. J. and Esterbauer, H. (1991) Biological activities of 4-hydroxyalkenals. In Sies, H. (ed.) *Oxidative Stress. Oxidants and Antioxidants.* Academic Press, London.
58. Stacey, N. H. and Klaassen, C. D. (1981) Inhibition of lipid peroxidation without prevention of cellular injury in isolated rat hepatocytes. *Toxicol. Appl. Pharmacol.* **58:** 8–18.
59. Stacey, N. H. and Kappus, H. (1982) Comparison of methods of assessment of metal-induced lipid peroxidation in isolated rat hepatocytes. *J. Toxicol. Environ. Health* **9:** 277–285.
60. Buc-Calderon, P., Latour, I. and Roberfroid, M. (1991) Biochemical changes in isolated hepatocytes exposed to *tert*-butyl hydroperoxide: implications for its cytotoxicity. *Cell Biol. Toxicol.* **7:** 129–143.
61. Davies, T. A., Bernardo, J., Lazzari, K. *et al.* (1991) Cytosolic calcium determination: a fluorometric technique. *J. Nutr. Biochem.* **2:** 102–106.
62. Brault, D., Neta, P. and Patterson, L. K. (1985) The lipid peroxidation model for halogenated hydrocarbon toxicity. Kinetics of peroxyl radical processes involving fatty acids and Fe(III) porphyrins. *Chem. Biol. Interact.* **54:** 289–297.
63. Biasi, F., Albano, E., Chiarpotto, E. *et al.* (1991) *In vivo* and *in vitro* evidence concerning the role of lipid peroxidation in the mechanism of hepatocyte death due to carbon tetrachloride. *Cell Biochem. Funct.* **9:** 111–118.
64. Shu, H., Talcott, R. E., Rice, S. A. and Wei, E. T. (1979) Lipid peroxidation and paraquat toxicity. *Biochem. Pharmacol.* **28:** 327–331.
65. Eklöw-Lastbom, L., Rossi, L., Thor, H. and Orrenius, S. (1986) Effects of oxidative stress caused by hypoxia and diquat. A study in isolated hepatocytes. *Free Radic. Res. Comm.* **2:** 57–68.
66. Sokol, R. J., Deberaux, M. W., Traber, M. G. and Shikes, R. H. (1989) Copper toxicity and lipid peroxidation in isolated rat hepatocytes: effect of vitamin E_1. *Pediatr. Res.* **25:** 55–62.
67. Comporti, M., Maellaro, E., Del-Bello, B. and Casini, A. F. (1991) Glutathione depletion: its effects on other antioxidant systems and hepatocellular damage. *Xenobiotica* **2:** 1067–1076.
68. Maellaro, E., Casini, A. F., Del-Bello, B. and Comporti, M. (1990) Lipid peroxidation and antioxidant systems in the liver injury produced by glutathione depleting agents. *Biochem. Pharmacol.* **39:** 1513–1521.
69. Poli, G., Chiarpotto, E., Albano, E. *et al.* (1986) Iron overload: experimental approach using rat hepatocytes in single cell suspensions. In Dianzani, M. U. and Gentillini, P. (eds) *Chronic Liver Disease, Frontiers in Gastrointestinal Research*, Vol. 9, pp. 38–49. Karger, Basel.
70. Poli, G., Albano, E. and Dianzani, M. U. (1987) The role of lipid peroxidation in liver damage. *Chem. Phys. Lipids* **45:** 117–142.
71. Danni, O., Chiarpotto, E., Aragno, M. *et al.* (1991) Lipid peroxidation and irreversible cell damage: synergism between carbon tetrachloride and 1,2-dibromoethane in isolated rat hepatocytes. *Toxicol. Appl. Pharmacol.* **110:** 216–222.
72. Cheeseman, K. H. (1990) Methods of measuring lipid peroxidation in biological systems: an overview. In Crates de Paulet, A., Douste-Blazy, L. and Paoletti, R. (eds) *Free Radicals, Lipoproteins and Membrane Lipids*, pp. 143–152. Plenum Press, New York.
73. Bird, R. P. and Draper, H. H. (1984) Comparative studies on different methods of malonaldehyde determination. *Methods Enzymol.* **105:** 299–305.
74. Wendel, A. and Reiter, R. (1984) *In vitro* assesment of hepatic lipid peroxidation by malondialdehyde or ethane determination. In Bors, W., Saran, M. and Tait, D. (eds) *Oxygen Radicals in Chemistry and Biology*, pp. 345–349. Walter de Gruyter, Berlin.
75. Smith, M. T., Thor, H., Hartzell, P. and Orrenius, S. (1982) The measurement of lipid peroxidation in isolated hepatocytes. *Biochem. Pharmacol.* **31:** 19–26.
76. Masugi, F. and Nakamura, T. (1977) Measurement of thiobarbituric acid value in liver homogenate solubilized with sodium dodecyl sulphate and variation of the values affected by vitamin E and drugs. *Vitamins* **51:** 21–29.

77. Jover, R., Ponsoda, X. and Castell, J. V. (1992) *In vitro* investigation of the molecular mechanisms of toxicity. In Castell, J. V. and Gómez-Lechón, M. J. (eds) In vitro *Alternatives to Animal Pharmaco-toxicology*, pp. 293–328. Farmaindustria, Madrid.
78. Sies, H. (1991) Oxidative stress: introduction. In Seis, H. (ed.) *Oxidative Stress. Oxidants and Antioxidants*. Academic Press, London.
79. Spiteller, G. (1993) Review on the chemistry of oxidative stress. *J. Lipid Mediat.* **7:** 199–221.
80. Klohn, P. C., Massalha, H. and Neumann, H. G. (1995) A metabolite of carcinogenic 2-acetylaminofluorene, 2-nitrofluorene, induces redox-cycling in mitochondria. *Biochim. Biophys. Acta* **1229:** 363–372.
81. Bellomo, G., Mirabelli, F., Richelmi, P. and Orrenius, S. (1983) Critical role of sulfhydryl groups in the ATP-dependent Ca^{2+}-sequestration by the plasma membrane fraction from rat liver. *FEBS Lett.* **163:** 136–139.
82. Bellomo, G., Jewell, S. A., Smith, M. T., Thor H. and Orrenius, S. (1983) Perturbation of Ca^{2+} homeostasis during hepatocyte injury. In Keppler, D., Popper, H., Bianchi, L. and Reutter, W. (eds) *Mechanisms of Hepatocyte Injury and Death*, pp. 119–128. MTP Press Limited, Lancaster, UK.
83. Nicotera, P., Bellomo, G. and Orrenius, S. (1992) Calcium-mediated mechanisms in chemically induce cell death. *Annu. Rev. Pharmacol. Toxicol.* **32:** 449–470.
84. Mason, R. P. (1990) Redox-cycling of radical anion metabolites of toxic chemicals and drugs and the Marcus theory of electron transfer. *Environ. Health Perspect.* **87:** 237–243.
85. Sreider, C. M., Grinblat, L. and Stoppani, A. O. (1990) Catalysis of nitrofuran redox-cycling and superoxide anion production by heart lipoamide dehydrogenase. *Biochem. Pharmacol.* **40:** 1849–1857.
86. Adam, A., Smith, L. L. and Cohen, G. M. (1990) An assessment of the role of cycling in mediating the toxicity of paraquat and nitrofurantoin. *Environ. Health Perspect.* **85:** 113–117.
87. Nunoshiba, T. and Temple, B. (1993) Potent intracellular oxidative stress exerted by the carcinogen 4-nitroquinoline-*N*-oxide. *Cancer Res.* **53:** 3250–3252.
88. Silva, J. M., Khan, S. and O'Brien, P. J. (1993) Molecular mechanisms of nitrofurantoin-induced hepatocyte toxicity in aerobic versus hypoxic conditions. *Arch. Biochem. Biophys.* **305:** 362–369.
89. Poli, G. (1993) Liver damage due to free radicals. *Br. Med. Bull.* **49:** 604–620.
90. Meister, A. (1982) Glutathione. In Arias, I. M., Popper, H., Schachter, D. and Shafritz, D. A. (eds) *The Liver: Biology and Pathobiology*, pp. 297–308. Raven Press, New York.
91. Kehrer, J. P. and Lund, G. (1994) Cellular reducing equivalents and oxidative stress. *Free Radic. Biol. Med.* **17:** 65–75.
92. Lash, L. H. (1994) Role of renal metabolism in risk to toxic chemicals. *Environ. Health Perspect.* **190:** 75–79.
93. Deneke, S. M. and Fanburg, B. L. (1989) Regulation of cellular glutathion. *Am. J. Physiol.* **257:** L163–L173.
94. Thomas, J. A. and Park, E. M. (1988) Oxy radical-initiated *S*-thiolation and enzymic dethiolation. *Basic Life Sci.* **49:** 365–368.
95. Runnegar, M. T., Kong, S. M., Zhong, Y. Z. and Lu, S. C. (1995) Inhibition of reduced glutathione synthesis by cyanobacterial alkaloid cylindrospermopsin in cultured rat hepatocytes. *Biochem. Pharmacol.* **42:** 219–225,.
96. Vignais, P. M. and Vignais, P. V. (1973) Fucsin, an inhibitor of mitochondrial SH-dependent transport-linked functions. *Biochem. Biophys. Acta* **325:** 357–374.
97. Beatrice, M. C., Stiers, D. L. and Pfeiffer, D. R. (1984) The role of glutathione in the retention of Ca^{2+} by liver mitochondria. *J. Biol. Chem.* **259:** 1279–1287.
98. Siliprandi, N., Siliprandi, D., Bindoli, A. and Toninellos, A. (1978) Effect of oxidation of glutathione and membrane thiol groups on mitochondrial functions. In Sies, H. and Wendel, A. (eds) *Functions of Glutathione in Liver and Kidney*, pp. 127–138. Springer, Berlin.
99. Kosower, N. S. and Kosower, E. M. (1983) Glutathione and cell membrane thiol status. In Larsson, A., Orrenius, S., Holmgren, A. and Mannervick, B. (eds) *Functions of Glutathione: Biochemical, Physiological, Toxicological and Clinical Aspects*, pp. 307–315. Raven Press, New York.
100. Griffiths, O. W. (1985) Glutathione and glutathione disulphide. In Bergmeyer, J., Bergmeyer, H. U. and Grabl, M. (eds) *Methods of Enzymatic Analysis*, Vol. III, pp. 521–529. VCH Verlagsgesellchaft, Weinheim.

101. Awasthi, S., Ahmad, F., Sharma, R. and Ahmad, H. (1992) Reverse-phase chromatographic method for specific determination of glutathione in cultured malignant cells. *J. Cromatogr. Biomed. Appl.* **584:** 167–173.
102. Slordal, L. Andersen, A., Dajani, L. and Warren, D. J. (1993) A simple HPLC method for the determination of cellular glutathione. *Pharmacol. Toxicol.* **73:** 124–126.
103. Shrieve, D. C., Bump, E. A. and Rice, G. C. (1988) Heterogeneity of cellular glutathione among cells derived from a murine fibrosarcoma or a human renal cell carcinoma detected by flow cytometric analysis. *J. Biol. Chem.* **263:** 14 107–14 114.
104. Hissin, P.J. and Hilf, R. A. (1976) A fluorimetric method for determination of oxidized and reduced glutathione in tissues. *Anal. Biochem.* **74:** 214–226.
105. Kosower, N. S., Kosower, E. M., Newton, G. L. and Ranney, A. M. (1979) Bimane fluorescent labels: labeling of normal human red blood cells under physiological conditions. *Proc. Natl Acad. Sci. U.S.A.* **76:** 3382–3386.
106. Rice, G. C., Bump, E. A., Shrieve, D. C., Lee, W. and Kovacs, M. (1986) Quantitative analysis of cellular glutathione by flow cytometry utilizing monochlorobimane: some applications to radiation and drug resistance *in vitro* and *in vivo*. *Cancer Res.* **46:** 6105–6110.
107. Bellomo, G. and Orrenius, S. (1985) Altered thiol and calcium homeostasis in oxidative injury. *Hepatology* **5:** 876–882.
108. Farber, J. L. (1983) The role of calcium in liver cell death. In Keppler, D., Popper, H., Bianchi, L. and Reutter, W. (eds) *Mechanisms of Hepatocyte Injury and Death*, pp. 111–118. MTP Press, Lancaster, UK.
109. Fleckenstein, A., Frey, M. and Fleckenstein-Grun, G. (1983) Cellular injury by cytosolic calcium overload and its prevention by calcium antagonists – a new principle of tissue protection. In Keppler, D., Popper, H., Bianchi, L. and Reutter, W. (eds) *Mechanisms of Hepatocyte Injury and Death*, pp. 321–335. MTP Press, Lancaster, UK.
110. Orrenius, S., McConkey, D. J., Bellomo, G. and Nicotera, P. (1989) Role of Ca^{2+} in toxic cell killing. *TIPS* **10:** 281–284.
111. Orrenius, S., McConkey, D. J. and Nicotera, P. (1989) Role of calcium in oxidative cell injury. In Fiskum, G. (ed.) *Cell Calcium Metabolism. Physiology, Biochemistry, Pharmacology and Clinical Implications*, pp. 441–450. Plenum Press, New York.
112. Spedding, M. and Paoletti, R. (1992) Classification of calcium channels and the sites of action of drugs modifying channel function. *Pharmacol. Rev.* **44:** 363–376.
113. Kass, G. E., Nicotera, P., Llopis, J. and Orrenius, S. (1991) Hepatic calcium netabolism: physiological and toxicological aspects. In Grunnet, N. and Quistorff, B. (eds) *Regulation of Hepatic Function*, pp. 344–354. Alfred Benzon Symposium 30, Munksgaard, Copenhagen.
114. Kraus-Friedmann, N. (1990) Calcium sequestration in liver cells. *Cell. Calcium* **11:** 625–640.
115. Clapham, D. E. (1995) Calcium signaling. *Cell* **80:** 259–268.
116. Orrenius, S. and Nicotera, P. (1986) Studies of Ca^{2+}-mediated toxicity in hepatocytes. *Klin. Wochenschr.* **64:** 138–141.
117. Weis, M., Kass, G. E. N., Orrenius, S. and Moldéus, P. (1992) *N*-acetyl-para-benzoquinone imine induces Ca^{2+} release from mitochondria by stimulating pyridine nucleotide hydrolysis. *J. Biol. Chem.* **267:** 804–809.
118. Gerok, W., Heilmann, C. and Spamer, C. (1990) Regulation of intracellular calcium by endoplasmic reticulum of hepatocytes. *Intracellular Calcium Regulation* **17:** 139–162.
119. Kutty, R. K., Singh, Y. and Krishna, G. (1989) Maitotoxin-induced liver cell death involving loss of cell ATP following influx of calcium. *Toxicol. Appl. Pharmacol.* **101:** 1–10.
120. Scherer, N. M. and Deamer, D. W. (1986) Oxidative stress impairs the function of sarcoplasmic reticulum by oxidation of sulphydryl groups in the Ca^{2+}-ATPase. *Arch. Biochem. Biophys.* **246:** 589–601.
121. Moore, M., Thor, H., Moore, G., Nelson, S., Moldéus, P. and Orrenius, S. (1985) The toxicity of acetaminophen and *N*-acetyl-*p*-benzoquinone imine in isolated hepatocytes is associated with thiol depletion and increased cytosolic Ca^{2+}. *J. Biol. Chem.* **260:** 13 035–13 040.
122. Masini, A., Trenti, T., Ceccarelli, D. and Muscatello, V. (1987) The effect of a ferric iron complex on isolated rat-liver mitochondria. III. Mechanistic aspects of iron-induced calcium efflux. *Biochim. Biophys. Acta* **891:** 150–156.
123. Shen, W., Kamendulis, L. M., Ray, S. D. and Corcoran, G. B. (1992) Acetaminophen-induced cytotoxicity in cultured mouse hepatocytes: effects of Ca^{2+}-endonuclease, DNA repair and glutathione depletion inhibitors on DNA fragmentation and cell death. *Toxicol. Appl. Pharmacol.* **112:** 32–40.

124. Kass, G. E. N., Bellomo, G., Juedes, M. J. and Orrenius, S. (1993) Toxic effects of calcium on mitochondria. *Methods Toxicol.* **2:** 378–388.
125. Carini, R., Bellomo, G., Benedetti, A. *et al.* (1995) Alteration of Na^+ homeostasis as a critical step in the development of reversible hepatocyte injury after adenosine triphosphate depletion. *Hepatology* **21:** 1089–1098.
126. Tsien, R. Y., Pozzan, T. and Rink, T. J. (1984) Measuring and manipulating cytosolic Ca^{2+} with trapped indicators. *TIBS* **9:** 263–266.
127. Malgaroli, A., Milani, D., Meldolesi, J. and Pozzan, T. (1987) Fura-2 measurement of cytosolic free Ca^{2+} in monolayers and suspensions of various types of animal cells. *J. Cell Biol.* **105:** 2145–2155.
128. Kao, J. P. Y., Harootunian, A. T. and Tsien, R. Y. (1989) Photochemically generated cytosolic calcium pulses and their detection by fluo-3. *J. Biol. Chem.* **264:** 8179–8184.
129. Vandenberghe, P. A. and Ceuppens, J. L. (1990) Flow cytometric measurement of cytoplasmic free calcium in human peripheral blood T lymphocytes with fluo-3, a new fluorescent calcium indicator. *J. Immunol. Methods* **127:** 197–205.
130. Tsien, R. Y. and Poenie, M. (1986) Fluorescence ratio imaging: a new window into intracellular ionic signaling. *TIBS* **11:** 450–455.
131. Waybill, M. M., Yelamarty, R. V., Zhang, Y. L. *et al.* (1991) Nuclear calcium gradients in cultured rat hepatocytes. *Am. J. Physiol.* **261:** E49–E57.
132. Jover, R., Ponsoda, X., Gómez-Lechón, M. J. and Castell, J. V. (1993) Cocaine hepatotoxicity: two different toxicity mechanisms for phenobarbital-induced and non-induced rat hepatocytes. *Biochem. Pharmacol.* **46:** 1967–1974.
133. Minta, A., Kao, J. P. and Tsier, R. Y. (1989) Fluorescent indicators for cytosolic calcium based on rhodamine and fluorescein chronophores. *J. Biol. Chem.* **264:** 8171–8178.
134. Kloss, M. W., Rosen, G. M. and Rauckman, E. J. (1984) Cocaine-mediated hepatotoxicity: a critical review. *Biochem. Pharmacol.* **33:** 169–173.
135. Roberts, S. M., Harbison, R. D. and James, R. C. (1991) Human microsomal *N*-oxidative metabolism of cocaine. *Drug Metab. Dispos.* **19:** 1046–1051.
136. Mallat, A. and Dhumeaux, D. (1991) Cocaine and the liver. *J. Hepatol.* **12:** 275–278.
137. Nelson, S. D. and Pearson, P. G. (1990) Covalent and noncovalent interactions in acute lethal cell injury caused by chemicals. *Annu. Rev. Pharmacol. Toxicol.* **30:** 169–195.
138. Hinson, J. A. and Roberts, D. W. (1992) Role of covalent and noncovalent interactions in cell toxicity: effects on proteins. *Annu. Rev. Pharmacol. Toxicol.* **32:** 471–510.
139. Boelsterli, U. A. (1993) Specific targets of covalent drug–protein interactions in hepatocytes and their toxicological significance in drug-induced liver injury. *Drug Metabol. Rev.* **25:** 395–451.
140. Loeper, J., Descatoire, V., Maurice, M. *et al.* (1989) Presence of functional cytochrome P-450 on isolated rat hepatocyte plasma membrane. *Hepatology* **11:** 850–858.
141. Loeper, J., Descatoire, V., Maurice, M. *et al.* (1993) Cytochromes P-450 in human hepatocyte plasma membrane: recognition by several autoantibodies. *Gastroenterology* **104:** 203–216.
142. Boelsterli, U. A., Lanzotti, A., Goldlin, C. and Oertle, M. (1992) Identification of cytochrome P-450IIB1 as cocaine-bioactivating isoform in rat hepatic microsomes and in cultured rat hepatocytes. *Drug Metab. Dispos.* **20:** 96–101.
143. Bourdi, M., Tinel, M., Beaune, P. H. and Pessayre, D. (1994) Interactions of dihydralazine with cytochromes P4501A: possible explanation for the appearance of anti-cytochrome P4501A2 autoantibodies. *Mol. Pharmacol.* **45:** 1287–1295.
144. Lecoeur, S., Bonierbale, E., Challine, D. *et al.* (1994) Specificity of *in vitro* covalent binding of tienilic acid metabolites to human liver microsomes in relationship to the type of hepatotoxicity: comparison with two directly hepatotoxic drugs. *Chem. Res. Toxicol.* **7:** 434–442.
145. Mani, C., Pearce, R., Parkinson, A. and Kupfer, D. (1994) Involvement of cytochrome P4503A in catalysis to tamoxifen activation and covalent binding to rat and human liver microsomes. *Carcinogenesis* **15:** 2715–2720.
146. Holtzman, J. L. (1995) The role of covalent binding to microsomal proteins in the hepatotoxicity of acetaminophen. *Drug Metab. Rev.* **27:** 277–297.
147. Satoh, H., Martin, B. M., Schulick, A. H. *et al.* (1989) Human anti-endoplasmic reticulum antibodies in sera of patients with halothane-induced hepatitis are directed against a trifluoroacetylated carboxylesterase. *Proc. Natl Acad. Sci. U.S.A.* **86:** 322–326.
148. Brown, A. P., Hastings, K. L., Gandolfi, A. J. *et al.* (1992) Formation and identification of protein adducts to cytosolic proteins in guinea pig liver slices exposed to halothane. *Toxicology* **73:** 281–295.

149. Kenna, J. G., Knight, T. L. and Pelt F. N. (1993) Immunity to halothane metabolite-modified proteins in halothane hepatitis. *Ann. N.Y. Acad. Sci.* **685:** 646–661.
150. Urban, G. and Dekant, W. (1994) Metabolism of 1,1-dichloro-2,2,2-trifluoroethene in rats. *Xenobiotica* **24:** 881–892.
151. Van Pelt, F. N. and Kenna, J. G. (1994) Formation of trifluoroacetylated protein antigens in cultured rat hepatocytes exposed to halothane *in vitro. Biochem. Pharmacol.* **48:** 461–471.
152. Lind, R. C., Gandolfi, A. J. B. and Hall, P. D. (1995) Biotransformation and hepatotoxicity of HCFC-123 in the guinea pig: potentiation of hepatic injury by prior glutathione depletion. *Toxicol. Appl. Pharmacol.* **134:** 175–181.
153. Kretz-Rommel, A. and Boelsterli, U. A. (1994) Mechanism of covalent adduct formation of diclofenac in rat hepatic microsomal proteins. Retention of the glucuronic acid moiety in the adduct. *Drug Metab. Dispos.* **22:** 956–961.
154. Davies, H. W., Satoh, H., Schulick, R. and Pohl, L. R. (1985) Immunochemical identification of an irreversible bound heme-derived adduct to cytochrome P-450 following CCl_4 pretreatment of rats. *Biochem. Pharmacol.* **34:** 32 006–32 006.
155. Pumford, N. R., Myers, T. G., Davila J. C. *et al.* (1993) Immunochemical detection of liver protein adducts of the nonsteroidal antiinflamatory drug diclofenac. *Chem. Res. Toxicol.* **6:** 147–150.
156. Hargus, S. J., Amouzedeh, H. R., Pumford, N. R. *et al.* (1994) Metabolic activation and immunochemical localization of liver protein adducts on the nonsteroidal anti-inflammatory drug diclofenac. *Chem. Res. Toxicol.* **7:** 575–582.
157. Gillette, J. R. (1987) Significance of covalent binding of chemically reactive metabolites of foreign compounds to proteins and lipids. In Kocsis, J. J., Jollow, D. J., Witmer, C. M., Nelson, J. O. and Snyder, R. (eds) *Biological Reactive Intermediates III*, pp. 63–82. Plenum Press, New York.
158. Beierschmitt, W. P., Brady, J. T., Bartolone, J. B. *et al.* (1989) Selective protein arylation and the age dependency of acetominophen hepatotoxicity in mice. *Toxicol. Appl. Pharmacol.* **98:** 517–529.
159. Banks, A. T., Zimmerman, H. J., Ishak, K. J. and Harter, J. G. (1995) Diclofenac-associated hepatotoxicity: analysis of 180 cases reported in the Food and Drug Administration as adverse reactions. *Hepatology* **22:** 820–827.
160. Ponsoda, X., Bort, R., Jover, R., Gómez-Lechón, M. J. and Castell, J. V. (1995) Molecular mechanisms of diclofenac hepatotoxicity: cell injury is associated to the metabolism of the drug and is preluded by a decrease in ATP levels. *Toxicol. In Vitro* **9:** 439–444.
161. Gillette, J. R. and Pohl, L. R. (1977) A prospective on covalent binding and toxicity. *J. Toxicol. Environ. Health.* **2:** 849–871.
162. Roswell, D. F. and White, E. H. (1978) The chemiluminescence of luminol and related hydrazydes. *Methods Enzymol.* **57:** 409–423.
163. Kaufmann, S. H., Ewing, Ch. M. and Shaper, J. H. (1987) The erasable Western blot. *Anal. Biochem.* **161:** 89–95.
164. Robin, M. A., Maratrat, M., Loeper, J. *et al.* (1995) Cytochrome P4502B follows a vesicular route to the plasma membrane in cultured rat hepatocytes. *Gastroenterology* **108:** 1110–1123.
165. Homberg, J. C. N., Abauf, S., Helmy-Khalil, M. *et al.* (1985) Drug induced hepatitis associated with anticytoplasmic organelle autoantibodies. *Hepatology* **5:** 722–727.
166. Tsutsui, H., Terano, Y., Sakagami, C. *et al.* (1992) Drug-specific T cells derived from patients with drug-induced allergic hepatitis. *J. Immunol.* **149:** 706–716.
167. Smith, G. C., Kenna, J. G., Harrison, D. J., Tew, D. and Wolf, C. R. (1993) Autoantibodies to hepatic microsomal carboxylesterase in halothane hepatitis. *Lancet* **342:** 963–964.
168. Martin, J. L., Kenna, J. G., Martin, B. M. *et al.* (1993) Halothane hepatitis patients have serum antibodies that react with protein disulfide isomerase. *Hepatology* **18:** 858–863.
169. Beaune, P., Pessayre, D., Dansette, P. *et al.* (1994) Autoantibodies against cytochromes P450: role in human disease. *Adv. Pharmacol.* **30:** 199–245.
170. Gómez-Lechón, M. J., Carrasquer, J., Berenguer, J. and Castell, J. V. (1996) Evidence of antibodies to erythromycin in serum of a patient following an episode of acute drug-induced hepatitis. *Clin. Exp. Allergy* (in press).
171. Maria, V. A. J. and Victorino, R. (1994) Lymphocyte proliferative response to drugs: analysis of the value of a 24-well lymphocyte culture system. Toxicol. In Vitro **5:** *1041–1044.*
172. Maria, V. A. J., Pinto, L. and Vitorino, R. M. M. (1994) Lymphocyte reactivity to *ex-vivo* drug antigens in drug-induced hepatitis. *J. Hepatol.* **21:** 151–158.

173. Guillouzo, A., Morel, F., Fardel, O. and Meunier, B. (1993) Use of human hepatocyte cultures for drug metabolism studies. *Toxicology* **82:** 209–219.
174. Skett, P., Tyson, C., Guillouzo, A. and Maier, P. (1995) Report of the international workshop on the use of human *in vitro* liver preparations to study drug metabolism in drug development, Utrecht, The Netherlands, 6–8 September 1994. *Biochem. Pharmacol.* **17:** 280–285.
175. Jover, R., Ponsoda, X., Gómez-Lechón, M. J. *et al.* (1991) Potentiation of cocaine hepatotoxicity by ethanol in human hepatocytes. *Toxicol. Appl. Pharmacol.* **107:** 526–534.
176. Ponsoda, X., Jover, R., Castell, J. V. and Gómez-Lechón, M. J. (1992) Potentiation of cocaine hepatotoxicity in human hepatocytes by ethanol. *Toxicol. In Vitro.* **6:** 155–158.
177. Gad, C. S. (ed.) (1994) In Vitro *Toxicology*. Raven Press, New York.
178. Barile, F. (1994) In Vitro *Cytotoxicology. Mechanisms and Methods*. CRC Press, Boca Raton, Florida.
179. Castell, J. V. and Gómez-Lechón, M. J. (1987) The use of cultured hepatocytes to assess the hepatotoxicity of xenobiotics. In Plaa, G. and Erill, S. (eds) *Interactions of Drugs and Chemicals in Industrial Societies*, pp. 135–149. Elsevier, Amsterdam.
180. Gómez-Lechón, M. J., Montoya, A., Lopez, P. *et al.* (1988) The potential use of cultured hepatocytes in predicting the hepatotoxicity of xenobiotics. *Xenobiotica* **18:** 725–735.
181. Gómez-Lechón, M. J., Larrauri, A., Donato, T. *et al.* (1988) Predictive value of the *in vitro* tests for hepatotoxicity of xenobiotics. In Guillouzo, A. (ed.) *Liver Cells and Drugs*, Vol. 164, pp. 371–377. Colloque INSERM, John Libbey Eurotext, Paris.
182. Gómez-Lechón, M. J., Ponsoda, X., Jover, R. *et al.* (1990) Hepatocitos humanos en cultivo: un modelo para la predicción del riesgo potencial de hepatotoxicidad de medicamentos. *Rev. Toxicol.* **7:** 241–248.
183. Castell, J. V., Montoya, A., Larrauri, A. *et al.* (1985) Effects of benorylate and impacine on the metabolism of cultured hepatocytes. *Xenobiotica* **15:** 743–749.
184. Castell, J. V., Gómez-Lechón, M. J., Miranda, M. A. and Morera, I. (1987) Toxic effects of the photoproducts of chlorpromazine on cultured hepatocytes. *Hepatology* **7:** 349–354.
185. Castell, J. V., Larrauri, A. and Gómez-Lechón, M. J. (1988) A study of the relative hepatotoxicity *in vitro* of the non-steroidal antiinflammatory drugs ibuprofen, flurbiprofen and butibufen. *Xenobiotica* **18:** 737–745.
186. Donato, M. T., Goethals, F., Gómez-Lechón, M. J. *et al.* (1992) Toxicity of the antitumoral drug datelliptium in hepatic cells: use of models *in vitro* for the prediction of toxicity *in vivo*. *Toxicol. In Vitro* **6:** 295–302.
187. Masanet, J., Gómez-Lechón, M. J. and Castell, J. V. (1988) Hepatic toxicity of paraquat assessed in primary culture of rat hepatocytes. *Toxicol. In Vitro* **2:** 275–282.
188. Gómez-Lechón, M.J., Ponsoda, X., Jover, R. *et al.* (1989) Hepatotoxicity of the opioids morphine, heroin, meperidin and methadone to cultured human hepatocytes. *Mol. Toxicol.* **1:** 453–463.
189. Larrauri, A., Fabra, R., Gómez-Lechón, M. J., Trullenque, R. and Castell, J. V. (1989) Toxicity of paracetamol in human hepatocytes. Comparison of the protective effects of sulfhydryl compounds acting as glutathione precursors. *Mol. Toxicol.* **1:** 301–311.
190. Ponsoda, X., Jover, R., Castell, J. V. and Gómez-Lechón, M. J. (1991) Measurement of intracellular LDH activity in 96-well cultures: a rapid and automated assay for cytotoxicity studies. *J. Tissue Culture Methods* **13:** 21–24.
191. Borenfreund, E., Babich, H. and Martín-Alguacil, N. (1988) Comparison of two *in vitro* cytotoxicity assays. The neutral red (NR) and tetrazolium (MTT) test. *Toxicol. In Vitro* **2:** 1–6.
192. Ekwall, B., Bondeson, I., Castell, J. V. *et al.* (1989) Cytotoxicity evaluation for the first ten MEIC chemicals: acute lethal toxicity in man predicted by cytotoxicity in five cellular assays and by oral LD_{50} in rodents. *ATLA* **17:** 83–100.
193. Ekwall, B., Gómez-Lechón, M. J., Hellberg, S. *et al.* (1990) Preliminary results from the Scandinavian Multicenter Evaluation of *In Vitro* Cytotoxicity (MEIC). *Toxicol. In Vitro* **4:** 688–691.
194. Jover, R., Ponsoda, X., Castell, J. V. and Gómez-Lechón, M. J. (1992) Evaluation of the cytotoxicity of ten chemicals on human cultured hepatocytes: predictability of human toxicity and comparison with rodent cellular systems. *Toxicol. In Vitro* **6:** 47–52.
195. Krack, G., Gravier, O., Roberfroid, M. and Mercier, M. (1980) Interference of chemicals with glycogen metabolism in isolated hepatocytes. *Toxicology* **18:** 213–233.
196. Deboyser, D., Goethals, F., Krack, G. and Roberfroid, M. (1989) Investigation into the mechanisms of tetracycline-induced steatosis. Study in isolated hepatocytes. *Toxicol. Appl. Pharmacol.* **97:** 473–479.

197. Gómez-Lechón, M. J., Ponsoda, X. and Castell, J. V. (1996) A microassay for measuring glycogen in 96-well cultured cells. *Anal. Biochem.* **236**: 296–301.
198. López, M. P., Gómez-Lechón, M. J. and Castell, J. V. (1988) Active glycolysis and glycogenolysis in early stages of primary cultured hepatocytes. Role of AMP and fructose 2,6-biphosphate. *In Vitro Cell. Dev. Biol.* **24**: 511–517.
199. Krishnan, K. and Andersen, M. E. (1994) Physiologically based pharmacokinetic modeling in toxicology. In Hayes, A. W. (ed.) *Principles and Methods of Toxicology*, pp. 149–188. Raven Press, New York.
200. Ponsoda, X., Jover, R., Gómez-Lechón, M. J., Fabra, R., Trullenque, R. and Castell, J. V. (1991) The effects of buprenorphine on the metabolism of human hepatocytes. *Toxicol. In Vitro* **3**: 219–224.

17

Biotransformation of Drugs by Hepatocytes

ANDRÉ GUILLOUZO

I. Introduction 411
II. Conditions for maintenance of liver-specific functions and for cell growth in hepatocyte cultures 412
A. Factors influencing *in vitro* survival and function of hepatocytes 413
1. Composition of the nutrient medium 413
2. Use of matrix proteins as a substratum 414
3. Interactions with other cells 414
B. Factors influencing hepatocyte growth *in vitro* 415
C. Comments 416
III. Expression of drug-metabolizing enzymes in cultured hepatocytes 416
IV. Response of drug-metabolizing enzymes to inducers and inhibitors 419
V. Drug biotransformation capacity of isolated hepatocytes 422
VI. Conclusions 425
Acknowledgements 426
References 426

I. INTRODUCTION

Studies on the metabolism of a drug candidate are required during the early stages of the development process. They are usually carried out *in vivo* using animal models such as rat, dog and monkey. However, over the past 10 years *in vitro* liver preparations have been increasingly used for studying drug metabolism. Intact cell models offer the advantage of containing the whole drug-metabolizing enzyme equipment of the liver. Thus isolated hepatocytes are attracting much attention because they represent the only model that potentially fully mimics the *in vivo* situation over several days. However, phenotypic changes leading to the loss of liver-specific characteristics rapidly occur, the extent being dependent on the culture conditions used. This explains why attention is still paid to the development of techniques for prolonged hepatocyte cultures reproducing *in vivo* metabolism.

IN VITRO METHODS IN PHARMACEUTICAL RESEARCH
ISBN 0-12-163390-X

In this chapter, the strategies presently proposed for long-term hepatocyte cultures are considered before discussing maintenance of phase I and II enzyme activities and their response to inducers or inhibitors, and the use of hepatocytes *in vitro* for biotransformation studies.

II. CONDITIONS FOR MAINTENANCE OF LIVER-SPECIFIC FUNCTIONS AND FOR CELL GROWTH IN HEPATOCYTE CULTURES

Although the preparation of isolated hepatocytes by the two-step collagenase perfusion method is now a routine procedure in many laboratories,[1–2] it must be borne in mind that the source of human material is erratic and unpredictable. Moreover, its use is associated with problems of technical safety and ethics, and this material must be treated as biohazardous; ideally, possible infection of the donor by hepatitis viruses and/or human immunodeficiency virus should be screened before handling. Most human liver cell populations are obtained by disruption of waste tissue pieces resected for primary or secondary hepatomas or other liver diseases. In addition, resected tissue samples must be preserved under minimum warm ischaemia, not exceeding 20–30 min; otherwise they must be flushed with cold Euro–Collins solution and stored at 0–4°C for less than 4–6 h before liver dissociation. Obviously functional alterations can occur during transient storage of liver samples and during tissue dissociation, so exacerbating individual variations related to intrinsic and/or environmental factors. Therefore it is critical to assess the quality of any human liver cell preparation in order to interpret the results correctly.[3]

Isolated hepatocytes can be used either immediately or after storage. As with human tissue, the availability of liver samples from large mammals such as monkey and dog is limited, so short-term preservation at 0–4°C or long preservation by freezing the freshly isolated hepatocytes is desirable. Over recent years, several protocols for hypothermic preservation and cryopreservation of isolated hepatocytes have been proposed.[4]

Survival of isolated hepatocytes in suspension does not exceed a few hours and thus restricts their use in drug metabolism studies. Early experiments showed that rat hepatocytes rapidly lost specific functions when plated on plastic or collagen-coated dishes.[5,6] Thus, the total cytochrome P450 (CYP) content declined to 10–30% its initial value after 2–3 days. However, not all the CYP enzymes declined similarly.[7]

Under conventional culture conditions, in addition to the early decrease in various liver-specific functions, hepatocytes show limited survival, not exceeding a few days, do not divide and can express fetal-like functions after 2 or 3 days.[6] In fact, expression of a set of genes is already altered during liver disruption, as shown for c-*fos*[8] and several CYPs[9] in rat hepatocytes. Other genes are overexpressed early after cell seeding (e.g. c-*myc*[8] and laminin B2[10]), and the level of many other transcripts is rapidly decreased. Consequently in all *in vitro* situations, hepatocytes are in G1 phase and somewhat altered phenotypically. Perturbations are further differently exacerbated depending on the culture conditions used. Surprisingly functional P-glycoprotein is overexpressed in rat hepatocytes after 2–3 days of culture.[11] The functional instability of hepatocytes in primary culture differs with species origin; thus human hepatocytes are more stable than their rodent counterparts[12] (Fig. 17.1).

Various culture conditions were introduced to improve both survival and function of hepatocytes *in vitro* and three groups of factors were rapidly considered to be important: (1) the composition of the nutrient medium; (2) the matrix supporting the cells; and

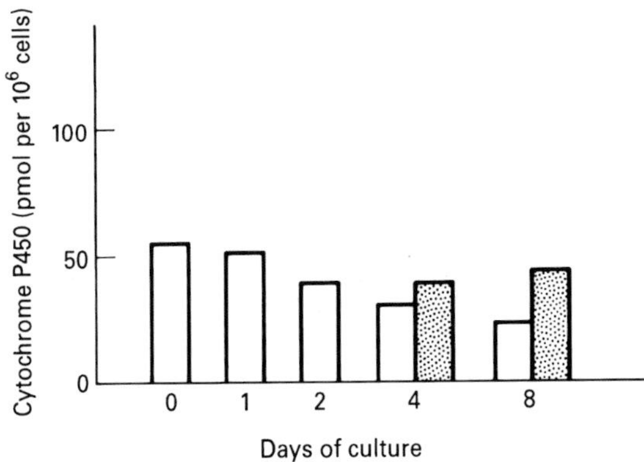

Fig. 17.1 Cytochrome P450 content of adult human hepatocytes cultured alone (□) or with rat liver epithelial cells (▩) for various times. The results are expressed as pmoles per 10^6 hepatocytes. From Guillouzo *et al.*[12]

(3) interactions with other cells. Culture conditions that support limited hepatocyte growth have also been defined. Several reviews[13,14] and books[1,15,16] have already been devoted to these different aspects, and only the main conclusions and recent progress will be considered here.

A. Factors influencing *in vitro* survival and function of hepatocytes

1. *Composition of the nutrient medium*

A wide variety of culture media has been tested. However, no 'hepatocyte medium' has yet been defined. According to Skett,[17] the definition of a medium that mimics the *in vivo* medium in which the cells are bathed has been attempted only on a empirical basis and a more ordered, rational approach is necessary. Nevertheless, many supplements have been reported to prevent or delay the rapid decline in liver-specific functions; they include hormones, nicotinamide, phenobarbital and metyrapone.

Among the many hormones tested, insulin and glucocorticoids have received particular attention. Corticosteroids have various beneficial effects, but not all have the same efficiency. Dexamethasone and hydrocortisone are used most frequently. Pichard *et al.*[18] have reported that dexamethasone and prednisone but not prednisolone, or methyl prednisolone, affect the oxidation of cyclosporin in primary human hepatocyte cultures. Nicotinamide was thought to be efficient by completely restoring the loss of NAD, which reaches 60% in rat hepatocytes during the first 24 h of culture. However, isonicotinamide, an isomer that is not converted to NAD(P) or NAD(P)H, also favours maintenance of liver functions.[19] Dimethylsulfoxide (DMSO) is very effective for prolonged survival and function of hepatocytes, but must be used at a concentration as high as 2%.[20] The peroxisome proliferator nafenopin, added at 50 μM to primary rat hepatocyte cultures, was recently shown to suppress apoptosis and to increase cell viability by up to 6 weeks.[21] These authors detected apoptotic cells as early as 24 h after isolation, which represented 0.5–1% of the total cell number on each of the following 8 days, the usual survival time in the absence of nafenopin.

Obviously, some supplements to the classical culture media improve hepatocyte survival and function. As an example, the use of a serum-free modified Chee's medium permits the induction of CYP 2B1/2 by phenobarbital in rat hepatocytes;[22] however, some early phenotypic changes cannot be prevented.

2. *Use of matrix proteins as a substratum*

Different extracellular matrix substrates have been tested, and most have little, if any, effect on hepatocyte function *in vitro*. It is recognized that only extracellular matrix proteins that allow the cells to retain their globular shape appear to be efficient. This was achieved with matrigel, a multicomponent extracellular matrix formed of basement membrane proteins and derived from a mouse sarcoma.[23] Various functions are stabilized for some days, but qualitative changes in CYP expression have been observed.[24] In addition, matrigel is contaminated by transferrin,[25] growth factors and cytokines,[26] and relatively large amounts of murine proteins can leak out during culture.[27] Matrigel cannot be replaced by one of its components or a reconstituted gel from the different components mixed in appropriate amounts.[10,27]

Another method is to culture hepatocytes between two layers of matrix proteins, either two layers of collagen,[28,29] or one layer of collagen and one layer of matrigel.[30] A variant has been designed by Koebe *et al.*[31] which consists in seeding hepatocytes in a collagen solution. At 37°C, hepatocytes forming a monolayer become entrapped in a gel. All these conditions allow prolonged survival and function of hepatocytes. Further studies are, however, required to determine whether a large spectrum of liver-specific functions is well preserved and whether total cellular DNA and/or protein are easily measured in these systems.

Individual hepatocytes can also be entrapped in a gel. Freshly isolated hepatocytes from various species including humans can be immobilized in an alginate gel without loss of viability. They do not aggregate but survive for a few days, exhibiting various functions at levels close to those measured in cells maintained in conventional monolayers, as shown for the formation of bilirubin mono- and di-conjugates in rat hepatocytes by Fremond *et al.*[32]

3. *Interactions with other cells*

The liver is composed of many cell types, and both homotypic and heterotypic interactions may influence liver-specific functions. Such interactions have been analysed in both monolayer and three-dimensional cultures.

Monolayer cultures When placed in pure culture, hepatocytes reaggregate but intercellular communication via gap junctions and transcriptional activity of specific genes disappear within a few hours. Although various functions are dependent on cell density, hepatocytes have comparable life spans and exhibit phenotypic changes whatever the cell density, indicating that homotypic changes are not critical for the maintenance of specific functions *in vitro*.[33]

The first attempts to co-culture hepatocytes with other cell types, such as sinusoidal cells and human fibroblasts, showed only limited improvement in hepatocyte survival and function. A considerable step forward in long-term maintenance of differentiated hepatocytes was made by Guguen-Guillouzo *et al.*[34] who mixed rat hepatocytes with another rat liver epithelial cell type, probably derived from primitive biliary cells. In this system hepatocytes could survive for several weeks and retained various functions, including production of plasma proteins and expression of various phase I and II drug-metabolizing enzymes. The rat liver epithelial cells are undifferentiated cells; they express limited hepatic functions: only one CYP (i.e. CYP 2E1) appears to be functional.[35] Hepatocytes can be selectively detached by collagenase treatment, allowing data to be expressed per milligram of hepatocyte protein or DNA.[36] It was further found that these rat liver epithelial cells interact with both immature and mature hepatocytes from various species including humans.[37,38] In co-culture, hepatocytes retain functional gap junctions and transcribe specific genes at higher values (still representing 20–40% of initial values) than those measured in parenchymal cells cultured in the presence of 2% DMSO or on matrigel. The presence of corticosteroids and direct cell–cell contacts are requested. The maintenance of differentiated functions is associated with early deposition of matrix proteins primarily between the two cell types.[33] Co-cultured hepatocytes, except those from pig,[39] do not divide. More recently, liver endothelial cells and non-hepatic cells such as 3T3 cells and established cell lines have also been reported to enhance hepatocyte function.[40–42]

Interactions between hepatocytes and other cell types probably involve a common mechanism, the primary target being an integral plasma membrane glycoprotein expressed on both cells.[43] The importance of plasma membrane protein(s) is further supported by studies showing that addition of crude plasma membrane preparations improves hepatocyte function.[44]

Three-dimensional cultures When hepatocytes are cultured in aggregates ('spheroids'), liver-specific functions are better preserved and survival is increased,[45,46] suggesting that in this system homotypic interactions are efficient. This may be explained by maintenance of the cuboidal shape of cells in this system. However, some drawbacks also exist: central cells frequently die and the number of hepatocytes per aggregate cannot be estimated precisely. The spheroids can also contain non-parenchymal cells, but whether these cells influence hepatocyte function as in monolayer culture has not yet been evaluated.

A new approach was recently described for the preparation of three-dimensional cultures. The cells were allowed to attach and reaggregate on woven capillary membranes coated with a biomatrix. In this system, pig hepatocytes were shown to survive and function (albumin production, lidocaine metabolism) for several weeks.[47]

B. Factors influencing hepatocyte growth *in vitro*

It is well established that adult hepatocytes can undergo limited proliferation when cultured at low density in the presence of growth factors.[48] A high percentage of rat hepatocytes synthesize DNA and divide in the presence of epidermal growth factor (EGF), insulin and pyruvate. The proportion is higher when hepatocyte growth factor (HGF) is used instead of EGF. Maximum DNA synthesis occurs 72 h after seeding in rat hepatocytes whereas, depending on the study, the peak occurs at 48 h,[49] 72 h (personal observation) or 96 h[50] in human hepatocytes. In fact, liver disruption and hepatocyte isolation result in a transition from G0 to G1 phase and, when placed in standard culture, the cells remain blocked in the G1 phase in the absence of mitogens, at what has been called the transitional point. Mitogens are needed for the cells to cross this transitional point and entering S phase.[51] Most studies on rat hepatocytes suggest these cells can divide only once or twice. However, Mitaka *et al.*[52] reported that a few cells undergo four cycles in the presence of EGF and isonicotinamide. Hepatocyte proliferation is accompanied by changes in liver-specific function, such as production of plasma proteins.[50]

C. Comments

Although exogenous factors, extracellular matrix proteins and cell–cell interactions are efficient in maintaining differentiated hepatocytes *in vitro* and their effects can be additive to a certain extent, they cannot fully prevent phenotypic changes, particularly those associated with hepatocyte isolation and plating, even by using the most sophisticated culture conditions.[53] In addition, oxygen tension may also affect hepatic functions.[54,55]

Obviously, there is a link between cellular architecture and maintenance of differentiated functions *in vitro*. Functions are better preserved when hepatocytes retain a cuboidal morphology. Only a few studies[56] have reported that transcription of specific genes is still active in spread parenchymal cells. This observation was made with albumin and it must be pointed out that expression of this protein is not particularly sensitive to environmental changes.

Although recent progress has been made in understanding the behaviour of adult hepatocytes in an *in vitro* environment, the co-culture system designed in our laboratory more than 12 years ago[34] appears to remain the most powerful system for long-term maintenance of hepatocytes expressing various specific functions.[57]

The choice of culture conditions must depend on the study to be performed. It is essential to keep in mind that expression of data can be more difficult when sophisticated culture conditions are used (e.g. presence or release of exogenous matrix proteins).

III. EXPRESSION OF DRUG-METABOLIZING ENZYMES IN CULTURED HEPATOCYTES

The rapid decline in total CYP content and various CYP-related enzymes observed in rat hepatocytes cultured under standard conditions led authors to question the suitability of this model for drug metabolism and toxicity studies. Fortunately, by using the most sophisticated culture conditions, as described above, most constitutive and inducible drug-metabolizing enzymes have been demonstrated in primary rat hepatocytes. Even expression of phenobarbital-inducible rat CYP 2B1/2 genes, or their orthologous mouse CYPs 2b9 and 2b10 genes, can be detected by adding nicotinamide to the medium,[58] using matrigel as a support[59] or the co-culture system.[60] However, compared with the values measured *in vivo* both phase I and II enzymes are present in different relative amounts and they respond differently to experimental conditions in culture.[61,62]

In addition, respective levels of messenger RNA (mRNA) and protein can vary. As an example, in mouse hepatocytes cultured in the presence of nicotinamide, mRNAs encoding CYP 2b9 and 2b10 are expressed but at levels far lower than those *in vivo*, whereas protein content was similar.[58] It must be remembered that considerable variability in CYP mRNA levels can be observed, even among rat parenchymal liver cell preparations.[59]

As reported by Padgham and Paine,[9] the abundance of most CYP mRNAs is altered shortly after isolation in rat hepatocytes. A two- to threefold increase was observed in the mRNAs encoding CYP 1A2, 2B1/2, 3A1/2 and 4A1, while CYP2C11 mRNA declined by 50%. As the hepatocytes attached, mRNAs encoding CYPs 2C11, 2C13, 2E1, 3A1, 3A2 and 4A1 continuously declined, while CYPs 1A2, 2A1/2 and 2B1/2 mRNAs were temporarily stabilized for about 2 h at a reduced level before declining further. The loss of CYP 1A2 and 2B1/2 mRNAs paralleled the loss of mRNAs encoding CAAT enhancer binding protein α

(C/EBP-α) and hepatocyte nuclear factor 1 (HNF-1).[63] Changes are also observed in phase II enzymes. Thus, the level of glutathione *S*-transferase (GST) α rapidly decreased in rat hepatocytes after seeding and reincreased later on. GST-μ remained relatively stable and GST-π became detectable after 2–3 days.[53,64]

The extent of variation and the maintenance of drug-metabolizing enzyme activities depend on the culture conditions, as discussed above. Thus, total cytochrome P450 was found to be higher and closer to the initial value in human hepatocyte co-cultures than in corresponding pure culture (Fig. 17.1). Another example is shown with GST activity, as described by Vandenberghe *et al.*[53,64] Both mRNA levels and enzyme activities were better and longer preserved in rat hepatocyte co-cultures than in pure cultures.

In vitro stability of phase I and II enzymes show species differences under similar culture conditions. In human hepatocytes CYP-related enzymes are more stable than in rodent cells.[12] However, marked transient changes in CYP mRNA levels can be observed. A strong decrease during the first 24–48 h of culture followed by a later increase is common.[65,66]

Sex change in CYP phenotype has been reported by growth hormone treatment of rat hepatocytes.[67]

Consequently it is critical to determine the drug-metabolizing enzymatic capability in each model system and to refer to *in vivo* values. Comparison may be easy for rodent hepatocytes, but it is much more difficult for human hepatocytes. Indeed, it is well established that marked interindividual variations are frequent in humans and that the conditions of resection, preservation and dissociation of human liver fragments may induce additional changes. In humans, genetic polymorphism exists for various enzymes, including several CYPs, GST M1 and θ and *N*-acetyltransferase-2, and can be of critical importance. Recently, we demonstrated that only individuals expressing GST M1 (which is absent in about 50% of the population) are capable of conjugating the carcinogenic aflatoxin B1-8,9 epoxide with glutathione.[68] We believe it is critical to measure a set of phase I and II enzymes, and to compare their values with the mean values previously obtained from a number of other cell populations (Table 17.1).

The level of expression of many drug-metabolizing enzymes in liver parenchymal cells differs depending on their location within the lobule. In particular, CYPs are frequently preferentially distributed in perivenous hepatocytes.[70,71] Rat periportal and perivenous hepatocytes isolated by the digitonin–collagenase technique maintain their different patterns of phase I and II enzyme activities during short-term cultivation.[72]

Other studies have been conducted to determine whether drug-metabolizing enzyme activities are preserved after hepatocyte storage. Adult hepatocytes can be stored for a short period (24–48 h) at 0–4°C[73] or extended periods by cryopreservation.[74] After storage, a fraction of viable cells can attach to plastic; they represent about 50% of the corresponding fresh cells. They express drug-metabolizing activities at levels close to those measured in unstored counterparts (Table 17.2). In thawed hepatocytes, an increase or decrease has been observed, but the changes did not exceed two- to threefold, thereby remaining in the range of individual variation observed *in vivo*.[74,75] In some studies, cytosolic enzymes were found to be more decreased.[75] Compared with their fresh counterparts, thawed hepatocytes show earlier functional disturbances in conventional culture; however, when placed in co-culture they recover after a few days and exhibit specific functions at levels close to those expressed in co-cultures of fresh hepatocytes.[76]

The cryopreservation method represents a unique way to establish a bank of hepatocytes from human and large mammals, and to study isolated hepatocytes from different donors in parallel, or to use the same population at different time periods. It is thus theoretically possible to investigate the metabolism of a new drug in parenchymal cell populations from both extensive and slow drug metabolizers.

Table 17.1 Drug-metabolizing enzyme activities in human hepatocytes.[69]

Substrate (reaction)	Enzyme activity		
	Range	Mean	n
Ethoxyresorufin* (de-ethylation)	0.2–8	3.0	19
Phenacetin† (de-ethylation)	0.1–25	4.7	25
Pentoxyresorufin* (dealkylation)	0.1–5	0.7	19
Mephenytoin† (hydroxylation)	0.1–2	0.7	6
Dextrometorphan† (demethylation)	0.1–2	0.5	6
Nifedipine† (oxidation)	0.5–13	5.3	8
Lauric acid† (hydroxylation)	0.3–2	0.8	7
Paracetamol†			
Glucuroconjugation	0.3–16	4.1	26
Sulfoconjugation	0.1–14	3.6	27
1-chloro-2,4-dinitrobenzene‡ (conjugation with glutathione)	0.05–0.5	0.2	14
Procainamide† (*N*-acetyl transferase)	0.1–7	1.1	32

Activities were measured 16–48 h after hepatocyte seeding. n, Number of tested cell populations from different donors.

* Nanomol metabolites formed per h per mg cellular protein; † picomol metabolites formed per min per mg cellular protein; ‡ units per mg cellular protein.

Table 17.2 Drug-metabolizing enzyme activities in fresh and cryopreserved human hepatocytes.[74]

Patient no.	Age (yrs)	Sex	Cells	Drug-metabolizing enzyme activity*			
				Phenacetin de-ethylation	Procainamide *N*-acetylation	Paracetamol sulfoconjugation	Paracetamol glucuronidation
1	58	F	Non-frozen	1.6	1.0	2.0	3.9
			Thawed	1.5	1.1	4.3	6.1
2	52	F	Non-frozen	6.2	1.8	2.0	4.7
			Thawed	4.4	2.0	3.4	5.1
3	50	M	Non-frozen	2.1	0.4	10.3	6.9
			Thawed	3.1	0.9	6.2	4.2
4	59	M	Non-frozen	2.2	1.2	ND	ND
			Thawed	0.6	2.8	ND	6.6
5	65	F	Non-frozen	8.6	0.6	2.6	3.2
			Thawed	4.3	0.8	6.0	ND

* Substrates were added after 24 h of culture and incubation lasted for 20 h. Values are expressed as nanomoles of metabolites formed per hour and per 10^6 seeded viable cells; they represent mean values of duplicate experiments. Intra-assay variation did not exceed 10%. ND, not determined.

IV. RESPONSE OF DRUG-METABOLIZING ENZYMES TO INDUCERS AND INHIBITORS

The response of the main drug-metabolizing enzymes to inducers in primary hepatocytes has been extensively analysed, and it appears that, even when an enzyme is markedly decreased it can still respond to inducers (Table 17.3). Both phase I and II enzymes remain capable of responding to inducers after 1–3 days of treatment. Only for a few enzymes, which are either expressed in low amounts or particularly unstable, are sophisticated culture conditions required to demonstrate inducibility. However, the extent of induction may greatly vary among liver cell populations and with culture conditions. A typical example is given by PB-inducible CYP 2Bs. The extent of induction is dependent on culture conditions. Sidhu *et al.*[30] found that PB-inducible CYP 2B1/2 and 3A1 mRNAs were stimulated by 10^{-7} M dexamethasone but the effects varied in a medium-specific manner. Inducibility of CYP 2B1/2 is retained in perivenous hepatocytes after isolation by the digitonin–collagenase perfusion method.[77]

When liver parenchymal cells are cultured in conditions that favour maintenance of liver-specific functions, the response of drug-metabolizing enzymes to inducers is retained longer than in conventional culture and its extent is often higher.[24,60,62,78]

The CYP 1A family has been found to be markedly induced by 3-methylcholanthrene,[65] omeprazole[79] and dihydralazine[80] at the level of mRNA, protein and related enzyme activities (i.e. ethoxyresorufin-O-de-ethylase) (Table 17.4). Ethanol (90 mM) increases both CYP 2E1 protein (7.7-fold over control) and chlorzoxazone 6-hydroxylation, which is supported mainly by this CYP (2.7-fold over control) without significant alterations in CYP 2E1 mRNAs.[82] CYP2C involved in the metabolism of mephenytoin was found to be increased after treatment by phenobarbital and rifampicin.[65] Various compounds are inducers of the CYP 3A family, including dexamethasone, rifampicin, troleandomycin, phenobarbital and lovostatin.[18,65,83,84] CYP 3A4 and 3A5 are co-inducible but not coordinately regulated in human hepatocytes.[84]

Recently, Donato *et al.*[85] examined a set of CYP-dependent enzymes and their response to various inducers in primary hepatocytes. The inducers tested were 3-methylcholanthrene

Table 17.3 Lauric acid hydroxylase activity in cultured rat hepatocytes.[62]

	Activity (pmol per min per mg protein)
Control	
Freshly isolated hepatocytes	220 (100%) ($n=2$)
4 h control culture	157 (71%) ($n=2$)
3 day control culture	107 ± 5 (48%) ($n=4$)
Treatment	
DMSO	122 ± 10 (55%) ($n=4$)
Ethanol	240 ± 23 (109%) ($n=4$)
Clofibrate	1205 ± 17 (545%) ($n=4$)
Ethanol plus clofibrate	1860 ± 48 (845%) ($n=4$)

Lauric acid hydroxylase activity in homogenates of rat hepatocytes after 3 days of treatment with 90 mM ethanol, 1 mM clofibrate, both compounds (30 mM ethanol plus 1 mM clofibrate) or 0.5% DMSO (clofibrate vehicle). Values in parentheses represent percentage of freshly isolated hepatocyte values when $n=4$. Values are expressed as mean ± SD.

Table 17.4 Effect of 3′ methylcholanthrene on ethoxyresorufin-O-de-ethylase activity in human hepatocyte primary cultures from four donors.[81]

Human liver cell preparation	Culture condition	Enzyme activity (pmol per mg protein per min)		
		Day 1	Day 2	Day 3
HL1	Control	ND	0.86 ± 0.15	1.21 ± 0.27
	3-MC	ND	56.89 ± 7.29	50.31 ± 6.69
HL2	Control	1.57 ± 0.19	0.68 ± 0.4	0.33 ± 0.05
	3-MC	18.32 ± 5.40	13.60 ± 3.0	10.36 ± 0.76
HL3	Control	0.73 ± 0.06	1.40 ± 0.18	0.83 ± 0.08
	3-MC	12.05 ± 1.2	12.26 ± 0.75	6.85 ± 2.82
HL4	Control	ND	0.92 ± 0.14	0.82 ± 0.24
	3-MC	ND	28.05 ± 5.63	25.74 ± 2.98

3-MC, cultures exposed to 5 μM 3′-methylcholanthrene for 1, 2 or 3 days. ND, not determined.

(3-MC), ethanol, dexamethasone, clofibric acid and isosafrole. 3-MC and isosafrole preferentially induced ethoxyresorufin-O-de-ethylase (EROD) and ethanol *p*-nitophenol hydrolase activity, while other inducers had a moderate effect on several enzymes. These results support and extend previous observations.

In vivo/*in vitro* differences can be observed. As an example, several authors have observed an increase in EROD activity in rat hepatocytes exposed *in vitro* to phenobarbital.[30,86]

The induction of CYPs and other drug-metabolizing enzymes can also be demonstrated by quantitation of specific metabolites. Thus caffeine biotransformation was found to be increased in primary human hepatocytes after treatment by 3-MC, whereas phenobarbital was ineffective,[87] in agreement with the involvement of CYP 1A in its metabolism. Some drugs induce their own metabolism, as shown for dihydralazine, which is an inducer of CYP 1A2.[80]

Studies on phase II enzymes are much more limited.[88] A recent study from our laboratory[89] on the effects of 3-MC, phenobarbital, 1,2-dithiole-3-thione and its 5-(2-pyrazinyl)-4 methyl derivative, oltipraz, on GST enzymes in primary rat hepatocyte cultures showed responses close to those observed *in vivo*. Each type of inducer elicited a different response. In culture, 3-MC had a rapid effect on GST-α mRNAs (starting within 2 h of its addition) and also increased GST subunit 7 mRNA. Dithiole thiones induced both subunit 1b and 7 mRNAs after 4 h and, to a much lower extent, subunit 3 mRNA after 72 h. *In vivo*, 3-MC was found to induce significantly both subunits 1b and 7 mRNAs, while oltipraz increased significantly subunits 1b, 3 and 7 mRNA levels (Fig. 17.2). Results obtained in mRNA studies were confirmed by high-performance liquid chromatography (HPLC) analysis of GST subunits, which also demonstrated an induction of subunit 10 (of which the mRNA was not realized).

In cultured human hepatocytes, GST-α is also induced by 3-MC, phenobarbital and oltipraz.[91] Inducibility of this GST class has been recovered in dog, monkey and human hepatocytes after freezing.[92]

Dramatic interspecies differences in CYP induction can be observed that mimic the *in vivo* situation. Rifampicin is a potent inducer of CYP3A in human hepatocytes,[65] but it does not affect this CYP in rat hepatocytes. By contrast, phenobarbital and clofibric acid, which are potent inducers of CYP 2B1/2 and CYP 4A1 in rat hepatocytes, have limited effects in human hepatocytes.

Drug-metabolizing enzymes can also be downregulated in cultured hepatocytes. Over recent years, cultured hepatocytes have been used to show that cytokines are capable of

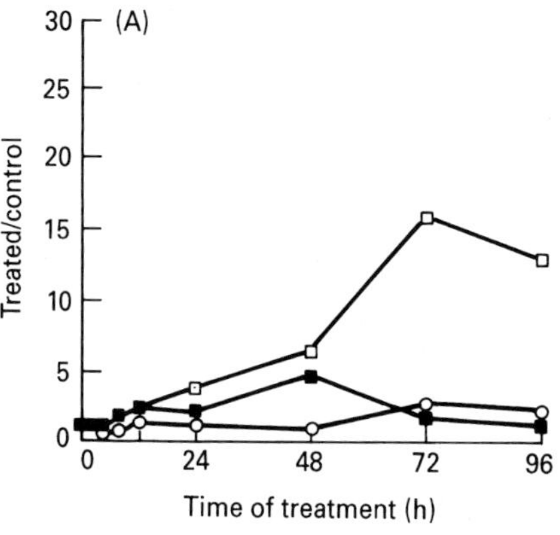

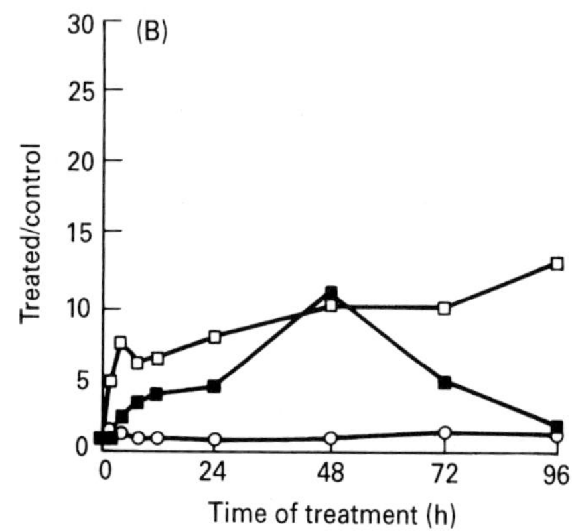

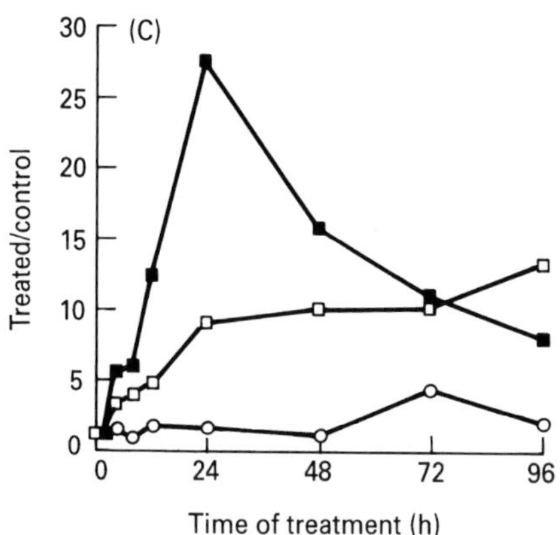

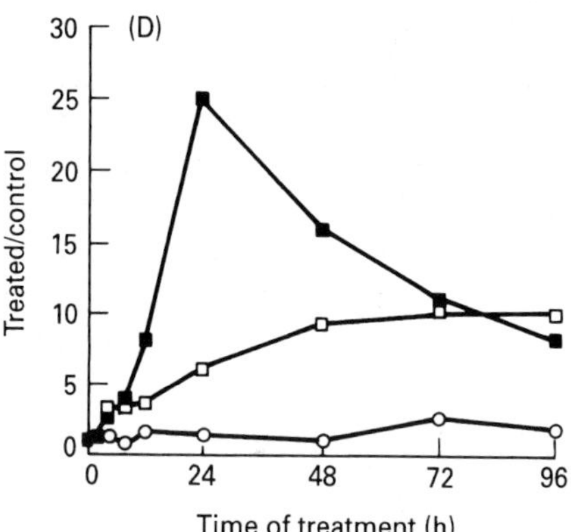

Fig. 17.2 Effects of (A) phenobarbital, (B) 3-methylcholanthrene, (C) 1,2-dithiole-3-thione (D3T) and (D) oltipraz on the levels of GST subunit 1 (□), GST subunits 3–4 (○) and GST subunit 7 (■) mRNAs in cultured hepatocytes. Total RNA was extracted from control and treated cells and then analysed on Northern blots hybridized with complementary DNA (cDNA) for GST subunits 1, 3–4 and 7, as described in experimental procedures. Filters were reprobed with cDNA specific for glyceraldehyde phosphodehydrogenase (GAPDH) as a control, which provides a positive control for RNA loading. Data are from one experiment, repeated twice with similar results. From Langouët *et al.*[89]

directly modulating CYP-related enzymes. We have examined the role of five cytokines (interleukin (IL) 1β, IL-4, IL-6, tumour necrosis factor (TNF) α and interferon (INF) γ) on the expression of CYP 1A2, CYP2C, CYP2E1, CYP3A and epoxide hydrolase in primary human hepatocyte cultures.[66] After a day's exposure to the cytokines, different effects were observed. IL-1, IL-6 and TNF-α were the most potent cytokines: they inhibited both mRNA levels and enzyme activities, typically by at least 40%, whatever the cytokine and enzyme tested. INF-γ also suppressed CYP1A2 and CYP2E1. IL-4 has unique effects, as it increased CYP2E1 up to fivefold and did not significantly affect EROD and nifedipine oxidation activities, which are supported by CYP1A and CYP3A respectively. IL-4 is classified as an anti-inflammatory mediator; its ability to inhibit C-reactive protein production and induction of haptoglobin by IL-6 in human hepatocytes[93] supports this assumption. Recently, we found that IL-4 also specifically increased GST-α.[90] In another study we found that transforming growth factor (TGF) β1 similarly inhibited basal CYP1A expression and, in addition, completely blocked induction of this CYP by 3-MC in primary human hepatocytes.[81]

Rodent hepatocytes in primary culture are also sensitive to cytokines. IL-1 was found to inhibit basal EROD and pentoxyresorufin-O-de-ethylase (PROD) activities and to block their induction by phenobarbital in a dose-dependent fashion in primary rat hepatocytes;[86] it also suppresses 3-MC-mediated induction of CYP1A in these cells.[94] TGF-β has been reported to exert the same suppressing effect in cultured mouse hepatocytes.[95]

V. DRUG BIOTRANSFORMATION CAPACITY OF ISOLATED HEPATOCYTES

Cultured hepatocytes and/or liver slices are now widely used for drug metabolism studies. Since our initial work on ketotifen metabolism,[96] a number of studies have been performed on isolated human hepatocytes to determine drug metabolic rates, identify drug metabolites formed in humans, predict interspecies differences, and establish *in vivo/in vitro* correlations.[69] It is now well agreed that there is a good qualitative *in vivo/in vitro* correlation and that interspecies variations are retained *in vitro* whether metabolites are formed by phase I or II reactions.

However, it must be remembered that experimental conditions can affect the results and, consequently, must be well defined. The choice of concentration(s) of the drug to be tested is important. The plasma drug concentrations are helpful but they are not known at the early stages of drug development. Moreover, various drugs have extensive first-pass metabolism and/or biliary excretion, and consequently hepatocyte concentration can be quite different from plasma concentration. It is advisable to consider physicochemical properties and cytotoxicity of the drug and to test a few concentrations over a wide range; this allows it to be determined whether major variations in drug metabolism profiles occur as a function of drug concentration and the detection of low- and high-affinity components. Some metabolic pathways can be missing with too low a concentration, while cellular toxicity can be observed with high concentrations.

The extent and duration of the biotransformation capacity of cultured hepatocytes depend on culture conditions and origin of the cells. Conventional cultures are usually suitable. However, release of phase II metabolites is sometimes greatly delayed (8–10 h or more) and minor metabolites can remain undetectable until 24 or 48 h of incubation.[97] Particularly for rodent hepatocytes, which are metabolically unstable, experimental conditions that favour transient maintenance of phase I and II enzymes are desirable.

Metabolic rates and profiles are roughly retained in primary human hepatocytes for several days. Even after 5 days, both phase I and II reactions, including sulfation, are still active,[96,98] and this can also be observed when the drug is added daily, if no major induction or inhibition of metabolic pathways occurs.[97] Exposure of human hepatocytes to drugs beyond a few hours may be useful as these cells frequently metabolize drugs to a lesser extent than their rat counterparts.[99–101]

Drug metabolic studies can be performed for much longer than 5–7 days by using the co-culture model. Thus ketotifen, which is metabolized to two major metabolites in humans (reduced ketotifen and a glucuronide) was reduced in only 8 days in pure human hepatocytes while glucuronidation was still high in corresponding co-cultures. Glucuronides remained detectable for 21 days in co-cultures.[96] Similar longer biotransformation in co-cultures was

Table 17.5 Metabolism of fluperlapine in normal human hepatocytes maintained either in pure culture or in co-culture: percentage of parent drug and its metabolites.[98]

	Pure culture		Co-culture	
	8 h	5 days	5 days	8 days
Parent drug	12.1	3.7	6.8	12.4
Metabolite				
8 (*N*-oxide)	28.1	33.4	30.1	33.6
10 (sulfate)	5.4	3.1	1.7	1.5
16 (sulfate)	13.4	8.6	13.2	6.0
21 (glucuronide)	5.1	7.7	9.2	9.0
22 (*N*-demethylated)	13.7	10.7	6.4	12.4
23 (sulfate)	4.3	5.7	4.8	3.6
25 (sulfate)	3.6	2.3	2.1	1.9
Unknown	14.3	28.8	25.7	19.6

Cultures were incubated with [^{14}C]fluperlapine for 24 h. Quantification of metabolites and parent drug was based on the integrated area of radioactive peaks obtained after analysis by HPLC.

observed for pindolol and fluperlapine.[98] As shown for fluperlapine in Table 17.5, the relative proportion of metabolites, including sulfate conjugates, remained more or less unchanged during at least 8 days in co-culture. Metabolic rates are also maintained at higher levels in co-cultured hepatocytes. The difference is much more pronounced when biotransformation is low; it can reach twofold or more, as shown for theophylline and caffeine in co-cultured human hepatocytes.[87]

A number of studies have demonstrated that most of the metabolites (if not all) produced *in vivo* are usually recovered *in vitro*, indicating that primary hepatocytes represent a good model for predicting the metabolic pathways of new drugs. Even stereoselective metabolism is preserved.[102] On the other hand, quantitative differences are common. It cannot be ignored that, in this *in vitro* system, drugs come into direct contact with hepatocytes, that metabolites accumulate in the medium because of the absence of clearance, and that some drugs are metabolized to a significant extent in non-hepatic tissues, particularly in the kidney.

Clearly the data summarized above indicate that the primary hepatocyte model has some limitations and that results must be evaluated correctly. Nevertheless, it is now established that various types of information can be obtained on the metabolism of a drug by using primary hepatocyte cultures: kinetic parameters, interspecies metabolism profile, prediction of inhibition or induction of drug metabolic pathways, prediction of drug–drug interactions and mechanisms of drug toxicity.

By testing a range of concentrations *in vitro*, kinetic parameters such as the Michaelis–Menten constant (K_m) and the maximal reaction velocity (V_{max}) of a drug can be estimated. Biphasic kinetics are observed when different CYPs are involved in metabolism.

Analysis of interspecies drug metabolic profiles is of major importance in the early stages of the development process. A number of studies have demonstrated that species differences found *in vitro* are qualitatively similar to those found *in vivo* with a large variety of compounds, such as ketotifen,[99] amphetamine,[103] diazepam,[104] anthracyclines,[105] minaprine[106] and tosufloxacin[107] (Table 17.6). However, large quantitative differences may exist between *in vitro* and *in vivo* values.[108]

Primary hepatocyte cultures represent a unique *in vitro* model for investigating drug induction, as at least 2–3 days of exposure are usually required. As examples, omeprazole[79] and dihydralazine[80] have been shown to induce CYP1A2 in human hepatocytes at levels

Table 17.6 Metabolism of tosufloxacin in cultured hepatocytes from rat, dog, monkey and humans.[107]

Species	Parent drug	Glucuronide of parent drug	*N*-acetyl metabolite (M_2)	Glucuronides of *N*-acetyl metabolites	Hydroxy metabolite (M_1)
Rat	71	3	26	ND	ND
Dog	90	10	ND	ND	ND
Monkey	63	ND	37	ND	ND
Human	100	ND	ND	ND	ND

Cells were incubated with tosufloxacin at 10 $\mu g\,ml^{-1}$ for 24 h. Values are means of duplicates, expressed as percentages of total drug and metabolites recovered. The percentages of recovery from the initial dose were 70–81% irrespective of the species. Intra-assay variability did not exceed 10%. ND, not detected.

close to those obtained with 3′-MC treatment. Drug inhibitors can also be identified; the results are usually similar to those obtained by using microsomes.[18]

Detailed knowledge of the different enzymes involved in the biotransformation of a new drug is now frequently required by regulatory agencies. Indeed, if two drugs are metabolized by, or interact with, the same CYP, drug interactions can occur. Determination of the CYP enzymes involved is made by various means: use of selective inhibitors or inducers, measurement of CYP-dependent mono-oxygenase activities and immunoinhibition analysis with specific antibodies. Such studies can be made with isolated hepatocytes as well as microsomes and heterologous cells expressing specific CYPs. When working on human liver cell populations, it is essential to consider case histories, metabolic profiles and CYP-dependent enzyme activities in order to interpret the data correctly. Expression of the CYP (or one of the CYPs) involved in biotransformation can have a genetic polymorphism. Drug interaction with cyclosporin A metabolism at the level of CYP3A has been extensively analysed. Exposure of human hepatocytes to various concentrations of erythromycin estolate results in a dose-dependent inhibition of cyclosporin metabolism, both compounds being transformed by CYP3A.[109] More recently, Pichard *et al.*[83] have analysed the effects of 59 compounds on the metabolism of cyclosporin by primary human hepatocytes and identified various new inducers and inhibitors (Table 17.7).

A number of compounds induce cytotoxicity and/or genotoxicity in the liver after biotransformation. Hepatocyte cultures offer a good approach for establishing a correlation between drug metabolism and toxicity, and for determining which metabolites are involved.[4,13] Although they are mostly used for investigating predictable hepatotoxins, hepatocyte cultures can also be of interest in the study of idiosyncrasy-dependent

Table 17.7 Cyclosporin A drug interactions in primary human hepatocyte cultures.[83]

Inhibitor	Inducer	Drugs that do not interact
Triacetyloleandomycin*	Rifampicin	Isoniazid
Erythromycin*	Phenobarbital	Valproic acid
Ketoconazole	Phenytoin	Omeprazole
Nifedipine*	Dexamethasone	Aspirin
Nicardipine	Phenylbutazone	Debrisoquine
Cortisol*	Sulfinpyrazone	Pefloxacin
Progesterone*		Paracetamol
		Furosemide

* Specific CYP3A substrate.

unpredictable drugs. We have provided some evidence that hepatocyte cultures represent a valuable model for detecting circulating antibodies in the serum of patients with drug-induced hepatitis, characterizing the antigens recognized by these antibodies and identifying drug metabolites involved in the formation of neoantigens. Siproudhis *et al.*[110] showed that normal human hepatocytes exposed *in vitro* to clometacin, a drug responsible for immunologically induced hepatitis, were consistently damaged after further incubation with serum from patients with clometacin-induced hepatitis in the presence of autologous lymphoid cells. Exposure of human hepatocytes to halothane resulted in the formation of novel antigens which could be detected either by a rabbit antitrifluoroacetyl antiserum or by serum from patients with halothane hepatitis.[111] It is well demonstrated that this anaesthetic is converted by CYP-dependent mono-oxygenases to a reactive intermediate, trifluoroacetyl halide, capable of covalently binding to hepatocyte proteins, and rarely this is followed (approximately 1 in 35 000 patients) by an immune response.

VI. CONCLUSIONS

The importance of *in vitro* liver preparations for studying drug biotransformation is now well established. Among these different models, isolated hepatocytes appear to be quite powerful (Table 17.8). This system provides early knowledge on kinetic parameters, metabolic profile and possible interactions with other drugs. From these data it is possible to select the most appropriate second animal species for toxicological studies and to obtain information on the behaviour of a drug in humans before its administration to healthy volunteers.

The major problems presently encountered are the erratic and unpredictable availability of human samples, interindividual functional variations in human cell populations, and early phenotypic changes and limited growth capacity in primary hepatocyte cultures. However, whichever species is considered, no hepatic cell line capable of expressing most of the liver-specific functions has yet been established.[4]

Table 17.8 Applications of human *in vitro* liver preparations in pharmacotoxicological studies.

	In vitro liver preparation*			
Assay	Slices	Suspended hepatocytes	Cultured hepatocytes	Microsomes
Metabolic profile	+	+	+	−
Comparative interspecies metabolism	+	+	−	−
Kinetic studies	±	+	+	+
Drug–drug interactions	±	+	+	+
Induction studies	−	−	+	−
Drug screening	±	+‡	+	−
Mechanistic studies	+	+‡	+	−
UDS test†	±	±	+	−

* Isolated organs not included because of the lack of availability; † unscheduled DNA synthesis; ‡ short-term study.
±, Possible; +, currently used; −, not suitable.

ACKNOWLEDGEMENTS

The author wishes to thank Mrs Annie Vannier for typing the manuscript. Personal studies described in this chapter were supported by INSERM, the Association pour la Recherche Contre le Cancer (ARC) et le Comité d'Ille et Vilaine de la Ligue Française contre le Cancer.

REFERENCES

1. Berry, M. N., Edwards, A. M. and Barritt, G. J. (eds) (1991) Isolated hepatocytes: preparation, properties and applications. In *Laboratory Techniques in Biochemistry and Molecular Biology*, Vol. 21, pp. 1–439. Elsevier, Amsterdam.
2. Guguen-Guillouzo, C. (1992) Isolation and culture of animal and human hepatocytes. In Freshney, R. I. (ed.) *Culture of Epithelial Cells*. Vol. 1, pp. 197–223. Alan R. Liss, Glasgow.
3. Skett, P., Tyson, C., Guillouzo, A. and Maier, P. (1995) Report on the international workshop on the use of human *in vitro* liver preparations to study drug metabolism in drug development. *Biochem. Pharmacol.* **50:** 280–285.
4. Guillouzo, A. (1995) Hépatotoxicité *in vitro*. In Adolphe, M., Guillouzo, A. and Marano, F. (eds) *Toxicologie Cellulaire* In Vitro, pp. 69–120. Les Editions INSERM, Paris.
5. Bissell, D. M. and Guzelian, P. S. (1980) Phenotypic stability of adult rat hepatocytes in primary monolayer culture. *Ann. N.Y. Acad. Sci.* **77:** 4831–4835.
6. Guguen-Guillouzo, C. and Guillouzo, A. (1983) Modulation of functional activities in cultured rat hepatocytes. *Mol. Cell. Biochem.* **53/54:** 35–56.
7. Steward, A. R., Dannan, G. A., Guzelian, P. S. and Guengerich, F. P. (1985) Changes in the concentration of seven forms of cytochrome P-450 in primary cultures of adult rat hepatocytes. *Mol. Pharmacol.* **27:** 125–132.
8. Etienne, P. L., Baffet, G., Desvergne, B., Boisnard-Rissel, M., Glaise, D. and Guguen-Guillouzo, C. (1988) Transient expression of c-*fos* and constant expression of c-*myc* in freshly isolated and cultured normal adult rat hepatocytes. *Oncogene Res.* **3:** 255–262.
9. Padgham, C. R. W. and Paine, A. J. (1993) Altered expression of cytochrome P-450 mRNAs and potentially of other transcripts encoding key hepatic functions, are triggered during the isolation of rat hepatocytes. *Biochem. J.* **289:** 621–624.
10. Levavasseur, F., Mayer, U., Guillouzo, A. and Clément, B. (1994) Influence of nidogen complexed or not with laminin on attachment, spreading and albumin and laminin B2 mRNA levels of rat hepatocytes. *J. Cell. Physiol.* **161:** 257–266.
11. Fardel, O., Ratanasavanh, D., Loyer, P., Ketterer, B. and Guillouzo, A. (1992) Overexpression of the multidrug resistance gene product in adult rat hepatocytes during primary culture. *Eur. J. Biochem.* **205:** 847–852.
12. Guillouzo, A., Beaune, P., Gascoin, M. N. *et al.* (1985) Maintenance of cytochrome P-450 in cultured adult human hepatocytes. *Biochem. Pharmacol.* **34:** 2991–2995.
13. Guillouzo, A. (1992) Hepatotoxicity. In Frazier, J. M. (ed.) In Vitro *Toxicity Testing. Applications to Safety Evaluation*, pp. 45–83. Marcel Dekker, New York.
14. Guillouzo, A., Morel, F., Ratanasavanh, D., Chesné, C. and Guguen-Guillouzo, C. (1990) Long-term culture of functional hepatocytes. *Toxicol. In Vitro* **4:** 415–427.
15. Guillouzo, A. and Guguen-Guillouzo, C. (eds.) (1986) *In Isolated and Cultured Hepatocytes*. Les Editions INSERM, Paris, John Libbey Eurotext, London.
16. Castell, J. V. and Gómez-Lechón, M. J. (eds) (1992) In Vitro *Alternatives to Animals*. Farmaindustria, Madrid.
17. Skett, P. (1994) Problems in using isolated and cultured hepatocytes for xenobiotic metabolism/metabolism based toxicity testing solutions. *Toxicol. In Vitro* **8:** 491–504.
18. Pichard, L., Favre, I., Daujat, M., Domergue, J., Joyeux, H. and Maurel, P. (1992) Effects of glucocorticoids on the expression of cytochromes P-450 and on cyclosporin A oxidase activity in primary cultures of human hepatocytes. *Mol. Pharmacol.* **41:** 1047–1055.

19. Paine, A. J. (1990) The maintenance of cytochrome P-450 in rat hepatocyte culture: some applications of liver cell cultures to the study of drug metabolism, toxicity and the induction of the P-450 system. *Chem. Biol. Interact.* **74:** 1–31.
20. Isom, H. C., Secott, T., Georgoff, I., Woodworth, C. and Mummaw, J. (1985) Maintenance of differentiated rat hepatocytes in primary culture. *Proc. Natl Acad. Sci. U.S.A.* **82:** 3252–3256.
21. Bayly, A. C., Roberts, R. A. and Dive, C. (1994) Suppression of liver cell apoptosis *in vitro* by the non-genotoxic hepatocarcinogen and peroxisome proliferator nafenopin. *J. Cell Biol.* **125:** 197–203.
22. Waxman, D. J., Morrisey, J. J., Naik, S. and Jaureguy, H. O. (1990) Phenobarbital induction of cytochromes P-450. *Biochem.* J. **271:** 113–119.
23. Bissell, D. M., Arenson D. M., Maher, J. J. and Roll, F. J. (1987) Support of cultured hepatocytes by a laminin-rich gel. *J. Clin. Invest.* **79:** 801–812.
24. Schuetz, E. G., Li, D., Omieciski, C. J. *et al.* (1988) Regulation of gene expression in adult rat hepatocytes cultured on a basement membrane matrix. *J. Cell. Physiol.* **134:** 309–323.
25. Dirami, G., Papadopoulos, V., Kleinman, H. K., Defreese, D. C., Musto, N. A. and Dyn, M. (1995) Identification of transferrin and inhibin-like proteins in matrigel. *In Vitro Cell Dev. Biol.* **31:** 409–411.
26. Vukicevic, S., Kleinman, H. K., Luyten, F. P., Roberts, A. B., Roche, N. S. and Reddi, A. H. (1992) Identification of multiple active growth factors in basement membrane matrigel suggests caution in interpretation of cellular activity related to extracellular matrix components. *Exp. Cell Res.* **202:** 1–8.
27. Te Velde, A. A., Ladiges, N. C. J. J., Flendrig, L. M. and Chamuleau, R. A. F. M. (1995) Functional activity of isolated pig hepatocytes attached to different extracellular matrix substrates. Implication for application of pig hepatocytes in a bioartificial liver. *J. Hepatol.* **23:** 184–192.
28. Dunn, J. C. Y., Tompkins, R. G. and Yarmuch, M. L. (1992) Hepatocytes in collagen sandwich: evidence for transcriptional and translational regulation. *J. Cell Biol.* **116:** 1043–1053.
29. Bader, A., Zech, K., Crome, O. *et al.* (1994) Use of organotypical cultures of primary hepatocytes to analyse drug biotransformation in man and animals. *Xenobiotica* **24:** 623–633.
30. Sidhu, J. S., Farin, F. M. and Omiecinski, C. J. (1993) Influence of extracellular matrix overlay on phenobarbital mediated induction of CYP2B1, 2B2 and 3A1 genes in primary adult rat hepatocyte culture. *Arch. Biochem. Biophys.* **301:** 103–113.
31. Koebe, H. G., Pahernik, S., Eyer, P. and Schildberg, F. (1994) Collagen gel immobilization: a useful cell culture technique for long-term metabolic studies on human hepatocytes. *Xenobiotica* **24:** 95–107.
32. Frémond, B., Malandain, C., Guyomard, C., Chesné, C., Guillouzo, A. and Campion, J. P. (1993) Correction of bilirubin conjugation in the Gunn rat using hepatocytes immobilized in alginate gel beads as an extracorporeal bioartificial liver. *Cell Transplant.* **2:** 453–460.
33. Guguen-Guillouzo, C. (1986) Role of homotypic and heterotypic cell interactions in expression of specific functions by cultured hepatocytes. In Guillouzo, A. and Guguen-Guillouzo, C. (eds) *Isolated and Cultured Hepatocytes*, pp. 259–283. Les Editions INSERM, Paris, John Libbey Eurotext, London.
34. Guguen-Guillouzo, C., Clément, B., Baffet, G. *et al.* (1983) Maintenance and reversibility of active albumin secretion by adult rat hepatocytes co-cultured with another liver epithelial cell type. *Exp. Cell Res.* **143:** 47–54.
35. Lerche, C., Le Jossic, Fautrel, A. *et al.* (1996) Rat liver epithelial cells express functional cytochrome P-450 2E1. *Carcinogenesis* **17:** 1101–1106.
36. Fraslin, J. M., Kneip, B., Vaulont, S., Glaise, D., Munnich, A. and Guguen-Guillouzo, C. (1985) Dependence of hepatocyte specific gene expression on cell–cell interactions in primary culture. *EMBO J.* **4:** 2484–2491.
37. Clément, B., Guguen-Guillouzo, C., Campion, J. P., Glaise, D., Bourel, M. and Guillouzo, A. (1984) Long-term cocultures of adult human hepatocytes with rat liver epithelial cells: modulation of active albumin secretion and accumulation of extracellular material. *Hepatology* **4:** 373–380.
38. Guguen-Guillouzo, C., Clément, B., Lescoat, G., Glaise, D. and Guillouzo, A. (1984) Modulation of human fetal hepatocyte survival and differentiation by interactions with a rat liver epithelial cell line. *Dev. Biol.* **105:** 211–220.
39. Wegner, H., Schareck, W., Bayer-Helms, H. and Gebhardt, R. (1992) Different proliferative

potential of rat and pig hepatocytes in primary culture and coculture. *Eur. J. Cell Biol.* **58:** 411–417.

40. Donato, M. T., Castell, J. V. and Gómez-Lechón, M. J. (1990) Prolonged expression of biotransformation activities of rat hepatocytes co-cultured with established cell lines. *Toxicol. In Vitro* **4:** 461–466.
41. Mendoza-Figueroa, T., Hernandez, A., Lopez, M. L. and Kuharcuch, W. (1988) Intracytoplasmic triglyceride accumulation produced by dexamethasone in adult rat hepatocytes cultivated on 3T3 cells. *Toxicology* **52:** 273–286.
42. Morin, O. and Normand, C. (1986) Long-term maintenance of hepatocyte functional activity in co-culture: requirements for sinusoidal endothelial cells and dexamethasone. *J. Cell. Physiol.* **129:** 103–110.
43. Corlu, A., Kneip, B., Lhadi, C. *et al.* (1991) A plasma membrane protein is involved in cell contact-mediated regulation of tissue-specific genes in adult hepatocytes. *J. Cell. Biol.* **115:** 505–515.
44. Saad, B., Scholl, F. A., Thomas, H., Schawalder, H. *et al.* (1993) Crude liver membrane fractions and extracellular matrix components as substrata regulate differentially the preservation and inducibility of cytochrome P-450 isoenzymes in cultured rat hepatocytes. *Eur. J. Biochem.* **213:** 805–814.
45. Landry, J., Bernier, D., Quellet, Goyette, R. and Marceau, N. (1985) Spheroidal aggregate culture of rat liver cells: histotypic reorganization, biomatrix deposition and maintenance of functional activities. *J. Cell Biol.* **101:** 914–923.
46. Tong, J. Z., De Lagausie, P., Furlan, V., Cresteil, T., Bernard, O. and Alvarez, F. (1992) Long-term culture of adult rat hepatocyte spheroids. *Exp. Cell Res.* **200:** 326–332.
47. Gerlach, J. C. and Neuhans, P. (1994) Culture model for primary hepatocytes. *In Vitro Cell Dev. Biol.* **30A:** 640–642.
48. MacGowan, J. A. (1986) Hepatocyte proliferation in culture. In Guillouzo, A. and Guguen-Guillouzo, C. (eds) *Isolated and Cultured Hepatocytes*, pp. 13–38. Les Editions INSERM and John Libbey Eurotext, Paris.
49. Blanc, P., Etienne, H., Daujat, M. *et al.* (1992) Mitotic responsiveness of cultured adult human hepatocytes to epidermal growth factor, transforming growth factor alpha and human serum. *Gastroenterology* **102:** 1340–1350.
50. Gómez-Lechón, M., Castell, J., Guillen, I. *et al.* (1995) Effects of hepatocyte growth factor on the growth and metabolism of human hepatocytes in primary culture. *Hepatology* **21:** 1248–1254.
51. Loyer, P., Cariou, S., Glaise, D., Bilodeau, M., Baffet, G. and Guguen-Guillouzo, C. (1996) Growth factor-dependence of entry and progression through g1 and s phases of adult rat hepatocytes *in vitro*. *J. Biol. Chem.* **271:** 11 484–11 492.
52. Mitaka, T., Sattler, C. A., Sattler, G. L., Sargent, L. M. and Pitot, H. C. (1991) Multiple cell cycles occur in rat hepatocytes cultured in the presence of nicotinamide and epidermal growth factor. *Hepatology* **13:** 21–30.
53. Vandenberghe, Y., Morel, F., Pemble, S. *et al.* (1990) Changes in expression of mRNA coding for glutathione *S*-transferase subunits 1–2 and 7 in cultured rat hepatocytes. *Mol. Pharmacol.* **37:** 372–376.
54. Saad, B., Thomas, H., Schawalder, H., Waechter, F. and Maier, P. (1994) Oxygen tension, insulin and glucagon affect the preservation and induction of cytochrome P-450 isoforms in cultured rat hepatocytes. *Toxicol. Appl. Pharmacol.* **126:** 372–379.
55. Wodey, E., Fautrel, A., Rissel, M., Tanguy, M., Guillouzo, A. and Mallédant, Y. (1993) Halothane-induced cytotoxicity to rat centrilobular hepatocytes in primary culture is not increased under low oxygen concentration. *Anesthesiology* **79:** 1296–1303.
56. Caron, J. M. (1990) Induction of albumin gene transcription in hepatocytes by extracellular matrix proteins. *Mol. Cell. Biol.* **10:** 1239–1243.
57. Blaauboer, B. J., Boobis, A. E., Castell, J. V. *et al.* (1994) The practical applicability of hepatocyte cultures in routine testing. *ATLA* **22:** 231–241.
58. Nemoto, N., Sukurai, J. and Funae, Y. (1995) Maintenance of phenobarbital-inducible Cyp2b gene expression in C57BL/6 mouse hepatocytes in primary culture as spheroids. *Arch. Biochem. Biophys.* **316:** 362–369.
59. Kocarek, T. A., Schuetz, E. G. and Guzelian, P. S. (1993) Expression of multiple forms of cytochrome P-450 mRNAs in primary cultures of rat hepatocytes maintained on matrigel. *Mol. Pharmacol.* **43:** 328–334.
60. Akrawi, M., Rogiers, V., Vandenberghe, Y. *et al.* (1993) Maintenance and induction in

cocultured rat hepatocytes of components of the cytochrome P-450 mediated monooxygenase. *Biochem. Pharmacol.* **45:** 1583–1591.

61. Forster, U., Luippold, G. and Schwarz, L. R. (1986) Induction of monooxygenase and UDP-glucuronosyltransferase activities in primary cultures of rat hepatocytes. *Drug Metab. Dispos.* **14:** 353–360.
62. Perrot, N., Chesné, C., De Waziers, I., Conner, J., Beaune, P. and Guillouzo, A. (1991) Effects of ethanol and clofibrate on expression of cytochrome P-450 enzymes and epoxide hydrolase in cultures and cocultures of rat hepatocytes. *Eur. J. Biochem.* **200:** 255–262.
63. Padgham, C. R. W., Boyle, C. C., Wang, X. J., Raleigh, S. M., Wright, M. C. and Paine, A. J. (1993) Alteration of transcription factor mRNAs during the isolation and culture of rat hepatocytes suggests the activation of a proliferative mode underlies their de-differentiation. *Biochem. Biophys. Res. Commun.* **197:** 599–605.
64. Vandenberghe, Y., Ratanasavanh, D., Glaise, D. and Guillouzo, A. (1988) Influence of medium composition and culture conditions on glutathione *S*-transferase activity in adult rat hepatocytes during culture. *In Vitro Cell Develop. Biol.* **24:** 281–288.
65. Morel, F., Beaune, P., Ratanasavanh, D. *et al.* (1990) Expression of cytochrome P-450 enzymes in cultured human hepatocytes. *Eur. J. Biochem.* **191:** 437–444.
66. Abdel-Razzak, Z., Loyer, P., Fautrel, A. *et al.* (1993) Cytokines down-regulate expression of major cytochrome P-450 enzymes in adult human hepatocytes in primary culture. *Mol. Pharmacol.* **44:** 707–715.
67. Guzelian, P. S., Li, D., Schuetz, E. G. *et al.* (1988) Sex change in cytochrome P-450 phenotype by growth hormone treatment of adult rat hepatocytes maintained in a culture system on matrigel. *Proc. Natl Acad. Sci. U.S.A.* **85:** 9783–9787.
68. Langouët, S., Coles, B., Morel, F. *et al.* (1995) Inhibition of CYP1A2 and CYP3A4 by oltipraz results in reduction of aflatoxin b1 metabolism in human hepatocytes in primary culture. *Cancer Res.* **55:** 5574–5579.
69. Guillouzo, A. and Chesné, C. (1996) Xenobiotic metabolism in epithelial cell cultures. In Shaw, A. J. (ed.) *Cell Culture Models of Epithelial Tissues: A Practical Approach*, pp. 67–85. Oxford University Press, Oxford.
70. Baron, J., Redick, J. A. and Guengerich, F. P. (1981) An immunohistochemical study on the localizations and distributions of phenobarbital- and 3-methylcholanthrene-inducible cytochromes P-450 within the livers of untreated rats. *J. Biol. Chem.* **256:** 5931–5937.
71. Ratanasavanh, D., Beaune, P., Morel, F., Flinois, J. P., Guengerich, F. P. and Guillouzo, A. (1991) Intralobular distribution and quantitation of cytochrome P-450 enzymes in human liver as a function of age. *Hepatology* **13:** 1142–1151.
72. Gebhardt, R., Alber, J., Wegner, H. and Mecke, D. (1994) Different drug metabolizing capacities in cultured periportal and pericentral hepatocytes. *Biochem. Pharmacol.* **4:** 466–761.
73. Poullain, M. G., Fautrel, A., Guyomard, C., Chesné, C., Grislain, L. and Guillouzo, A. (1992) Viability and primary culture of rat hepatocytes after hypothermic preservation: the superiority of the Leibovitz medium over the UW solution for cold storage. *Hepatology* **15:** 97–106.
74. Chesné, C., Guyomard, C., Fautrel, A. *et al.* (1993) Viability and function in primary culture of adult hepatocytes from various animal species and human beings after cryopreservation. *Hepatology* **18:** 406–414.
75. Diener, B., Traisier, M., Arand, M. *et al.* (1994) Xenobiotic metabolizing enzyme activities in isolated and cryopreserved human liver parenchymal cells. *Toxicol. In Vitro* **8:** 1161–1166.
76. Chesné, C., Gripon, G. and Guillouzo, A. (1988) Primary culture of cryopreserved rat hepatocytes. In Guillouzo, A. (ed.) *Liver Cells and Drugs*, Vol. 164, pp. 343–350. Les Editions INSERM, Paris, John Libbey Eurotext, London.
77. Bars, R. G., Bell, D. R., Elcombe, G. R., Oinonen, T., Jalava, T. and Lindros, K. O. (1992) Zone-specific inducibility of cytochrome P-450 2B1/2 is retained in isolated perivenous hepatocytes. *Biochem. J.* **282:** 635–638.
78. Souilinna, E. M. and Pitkaranta, T. (1986) Effect of culture age on drug metabolizing enzymes and their induction in primary culture of rat hepatocytes. *Biochem. Pharmacol.* **35:** 2241–2245.
79. Diaz, D., Fabre, I., Daujat, M. *et al* (1990) Omeprazole is an aryl hydrocarbon-like inducer of human hepatic cytochrome P-450. *Gastroenterology,* **99:** 737–747.
80. Bourdi, M., Gautier, J. C., Mircheva, J. *et al.* (1992) Anti-liver microsomes autoantibodies and dihydralazine-induced hepatitis: specificity of autoantibodies and inductive capacity of the drug. *Mol. Pharmacol.* **42:** 280–285.
81. Abdel-Razzak, Z., Corcos, L., Fautrel, A., Campion, J. P. and Guillouzo, A. (1994) Transforming

growth factor-β1 down-regulates basal and polycyclic aromatic hydrocarbon-induced cytochromes P-450 1A1 and 1A2 in adult human hepatocytes in primary culture. *Mol. Pharmacol.* **46:** 1100–1110.
82. Carrière, V., Goasduff, T., Ratanasavanh, D. *et al.* (1993) Both cytochromes P-450 2E1 and 1A1 are involved in the metabolism of chlorzoxazone. *Chem. Res. Toxicol.* **6:** 852–857.
83. Pichard, L., Fabre, G., Domergue, J., Saint Aubert, B., Mourad, G. and Maurel, P., (1990) Cyclosporin A drug interactions. Screening for inducers and inhibitors of cytochrome P-450 (cyclosporin A oxidase) in primary cultures of human hepatocytes and liver microsomes. *Drug Metab. Dispos.* **18:** 595–606.
84. Schuetz, E. G., Schuetz, J. D., Strom, S. C. *et al.* (1993) Regulation of human liver cytochromes P-450 in family 3A in primary and continuous culture of human hepatocytes. *Hepatology* **18:** 1254–1262.
85. Donato, T., Castell, J. V. and Gómez-Lechón M. J. (1995) Effect of model inducers on cytochrome P-450 activities of human hepatocytes in primary culture. *Drug Metab. Dispos.* **23:** 553–558.
86. Abdel-Razzak, Z., Corcos, L., Fautrel, A. and Guillouzo, A. (1995) Interleukin-1β antagonizes phenobarbital induction of several major cytochromes P-450 in adult rat hepatocytes in primary culture. *FEBS Lett.* **366:** 159–164.
87. Ratanasavanh, D., Berthou, F., Dreano, Y., Mondine, P., Guillouzo, A. and Riché, C. (1990) Methylcholanthrene but not phenobarbital enhances caffeine and theophylline metabolism in cultured adult human hepatocytes. *Biochem. Pharmacol.* **39:** 85–94.
88. Grant, M. H. and Hawksworth, G. M. (1986) The activity of UDP-glucuronyl-transferase, sulfotransferase and glutathione-*S*-transferase in primary cultures of rat hepatocytes. *Biochem. Pharmacol.* **35:** 2979–2982.
89. Langouët, S., Morel, F., Meyer, D. J. *et al.* (1996) A comparison of the effect of inducers on the expression of glutathione *S*-transferases in the liver of the intact rat and in hepatocytes in primary culture. *Hepatology* **43:** 881–887.
90. Langouët, S., Corcos, L., Abdel-Razzak, Z., Loyer, P., Ketterer, B. and Guillouzo, A. (1995) Up-regulation of glutathione *S*-transferases alpha by interleukin 4 in human hepatocytes in primary culture. *Biochem. Biophys. Res. Commun.* **216:** 793–800.
91. Morel, F., Fardel, O., Meyer, D. J. *et al.* (1993) Preferential increase of glutathione *S*-transferase class alpha transcripts in cultured human hepatocytes by phenobarbital, 3-methylcholanthrene and dithiolethiones. *Cancer Res.* **53:** 230–234.
92. Nicolas, F., Langouët, S., De Sousa, G., Placidi, M., Rahmani, R. and Guillouzo, A. (1994) Expression and regulation of glutathione *S*-transferase and cytochrome P-450 1A transcripts in cultured hepatocytes from dog, monkey and man after cryopreservation. *14th European Workshop on Drug Metabolism*, Paris, 3–8 July 1994.
93. Loyer, P., Ilyin, G., Abdel-Razzak, Z. *et al.* (1993) Interleukin 4 inhibits the production of some acute-phase proteins by human hepatocytes in primary culture. *FEBS Lett.* **336:** 215–220.
94. Barker, C. W., Fagan, J. B. and Pasco, D. S. (1992) Interleukin-1b suppresses the induction of P450 1A1 and P450 1A2 in isolated hepatocytes. *J. Biol. Chem.* **267:** 6389–6395.
95. Höhne, M., Becker-Rabbenstein, V., Kahl, G. F. and Taniguchi, H. (1990) Regulation of cytochrome P-450 CYP1a1 gene expression and proto-oncogene expression by growth factors in primary hepatocytes. *FEBS Lett.* **273:** 219–222.
96. Bégué, J. M., Le Bigot, J. F., Guguen-Guillouzo, C., Kiechel, J. R. and Guillouzo, A. (1983) Cultured human adult hepatocytes: a new model for drug metabolism studies. *Biochem. Pharmacol.* **3:** 1643–1646.
97. Bégué, J. M., Koch, P., Maurer, G. and Guillouzo, A. (1993) Maintenance of the biotransformation capacity by cultured human hepatocytes after several daily exposures to drugs. *Toxicol. In Vitro* **227:** 493–498.
98. Guillouzo, A., Bégué, J. M., Maurer, G. and Koch, P. (1988) Identification of metabolic pathways of pindolol and fluperlapine in adult human hepatocyte cultures. *Xenobiotica* **18:** 131–139.
99. Le Bigot, J. F., Bégué, J. M., Kiechel, J. R. and Guillouzo, A. (1987) Species differences in metabolism of ketotifen in rat, rabbit and man: demonstration of similar pathways *in vivo* and in cultured hepatocytes. *Life Sci.* **40:** 883–890.
100. Lee, K., Vandenberghe, Y., Herin, M. *et al.* (1994) Comparative metabolism of SC-42867 and SC-51089, two PGE_2 antagonists, in rat and human hepatocyte cultures. *Xenobiotica* **24:** 25–36.
101. Sandker, G. W., Vos, R. M. E., Delbressine, L. P. C., Slooff, M. J. H., Meijer, D. K. F. and Groothuis, G. M. M. (1994) Metabolism of three pharmacologically active drugs in isolated

human and rat hepatocytes: analysis of interspecies variability and comparison with metabolism *in vivo*. *Xenobiotica* **24**: 143–155.

102. Le Corre, P., Ratanasavanh, D., Chevanne, F. *et al.* (1991) *In vitro* assessment of stereoselective hepatic metabolism of disopyramide in humans – comparison with *in vivo* data. *Chirality* **3**: 405–411.
103. Green, C. E., Levalley, S. E. and Tyson, C. A. (1986) Comparison of amphetamine metabolism using isolated hepatocytes from five species including human. *J. Pharmacol. Exp. Ther.* **237**: 931–936.
104. Chenery, R. J., Ayrton, A., Oldham, H. G. *et al.* (1987) Diazepam metabolism in cultured hepatocytes from rat, rabbit, dog, guinea pig and man. *Drug Metab. Dispos.* **15**: 312–317.
105. Le Bot, M. A., Bégué, J. M., Kernaleguen, D. *et al.* (1988) Different cytotoxicity and metabolism of doxorubicin, daunorubicin, epirubicin, esorubicin and idarubicin in cultured human and rat hepatocytes. *Biochem. Pharmacol.* **37**: 3691–3700.
106. Lacarelle, B., Marre, F., Durand, A., Davi, H. and Rahmani, R. (1991) Metabolism of minaprine in human and animal hepatocytes and liver microsomes – prediction of metabolism *in vivo*. *Xenobiotica* **21**: 317–329.
107. Dauphin, J. F., Gravière, C., Bouzard, D., Rohou, S., Chesné, C. and Guillouzo, A. (1993) Comparative metabolism of tosufloxacin and BMY 43748 in hepatocytes from rat, dog, monkey and man. *Toxicol. In Vitro* **7**: 499–503.
108. Grislain, L., Ratanasavanh, D., Moquard, M. T. *et al.* (1988) Primary cultures of rat and human hepatocytes as a model system for the evaluation of cytotoxicity and metabolic pathways of a new drug S-3341. In Guillouzo, A. (ed.) *Liver Cells and Drugs*, pp. 357–363. Les Editions INSERM, Paris, John Libbey Eurotext, London.
109. Rahmani, R., Richard, B., Fabre, G. and Cano, J. P. (1988) Extrapolation of preclinical pharmacokinetic data to therapeutic drug use. *Xenobiotica* **18**: 71–88.
110. Siproudhis, L., Beaugrand, M., Malledant, Y., Brissot, P., Guguen-Guillouzo, C. and Guillouzo, A. (1991) Use of adult human hepatocytes in primary culture for the study of clometacin-induced immunoallergic hepatitis. *Toxicol. In Vitro* **5**: 529–534.
111. Ilyin, G.P., Rissel, M., Mallédant, Y., Tanguy, M. and Guillouzo, A. (1994) Human hepatocytes express trifluoroacetylated neoantigens after *in vitro* exposure to halothane. *Biochem. Pharmacol.* **48**: 561–567.

18

Drug Metabolism and Carcinogen Activation Studies with Human Genetically Engineered Cells

KATHERINE MACÉ, ELIZABETH A. OFFORD AND ANDREA M. A. PFEIFER

I. Introduction 433
II. CYP450 expression in human tissues 434
III. Human cellular models 437
A. Vaccinia virus expression system 437
B. Human lymphoblast cell system 438
C. Human bronchial epithelial cell system 440
IV. Potential applications 445
V. Current techniques for toxicological testing 445
VI. Present limitations and outlook 447
A. CYP450 expression and response 447
B. Organ specificity 448
C. Future trends 448
Acknowledgements 449
References 449

I. INTRODUCTION

Assuring the safety of pharmaceuticals, food additives, agrochemicals and cosmetics has required extensive toxicity testing involving large numbers of animals. Therefore, development and application of predictive *in vitro* methods is becoming an important issue in pharmacotoxicological testing due to public concern and legislatory interest in reducing animal experiments. Drug metabolism can be evaluated with a wide variety of *in vitro* systems, ranging from perfused organs, tissue slices or homogenates, short- and long-term isolated cell culture, subcellular fractions (cytosols and microsomes) to purified enzymes (e.g. cytochrome P450, glutathione *S*-transferase (GST)).

IN VITRO METHODS IN PHARMACEUTICAL RESEARCH
ISBN 0-12-163390-X

In recent years, the use of explant cultures, epithelial cells isolated from various normal human tissues together with epidemiological data have contributed significantly to the knowledge of mechanisms of toxicity and have improved the predictive value of laboratory animal studies for extrapolation to humans.[1–6] Studies of carcinogen metabolism in cultured cells derived from normal human tissues closely reflect the *in vivo* situation and provide insight into the problem of tissue specificity in chemical carcinogenesis. However, the limited access to human tissue and the short life span of primary cells make it difficult to use such an approach for routine testing in toxicology.

Established cell lines with an indefinite life span are an interesting alternative to human tissue and primary cells. However, most of these cell lines have no or limited metabolic capacity, primarily due to the absence of phase I enzyme expression. This lack of metabolic competence can be compensated by exogenous activation systems (S9 or microsomal preparations). Caution is nevertheless required with such a system because reactive intermediates are generated outside of the target cell in which the genetic end-point is measured. To overcome this limitation, metabolism-competent cell systems have been recently developed by the application of gene transfer techniques. To date, various human cytochrome P450 (CYP450) complementary DNAs (cDNAs) have been introduced into mammalian cell lines (Table 18.1). In contrast to transient expression systems, cell lines with stably expressed CYP450 allow the measurement of toxicological end-points in the same cells in which the metabolism occurs. Moreover, the use of a panel of cell lines expressing individual CYP450 permits the identification of the cytochrome(s) involved in the metabolism of a given drug.

Table 18.1 summarizes the different mammalian cell systems used for cDNA-directed expression of human CYP450s. Here we will focus primarily on three genetically engineered human cell systems for human CYP450 expression: the transient vaccinia virus expression system in the human hepatoma HepG2 cell line,[35] the Epstein–Barr virus (EBV) system in the human B lymphoblastoid cell line (AHH-1 TK + / −)[36] and our own methodology using a cytomegalovirus promoter system in human simian virus 40 (SV40)-immortalized epithelial bronchial cells (BEAS-2B).[16] The scientific basis of their establishment, their practical application to toxicological and pharmaceutical problems and a critical analysis of their advantages and limitations will be discussed.

II. CYP450 EXPRESSION IN HUMAN TISSUES

In the past, numerous studies were performed to characterize drug-metabolizing enzymes in animals and, more specially, in rodents. In view of the finding that important species differences exist, the necessity to identify CYP450 forms in human tissues and to develop cellular models containing these CYP450s has become evident. Establishment of genetically engineered cell systems for human CYP450 expression has become feasible as a result of the availability of an increasing number of human CYP450 cDNAs. At least 20 human CYP450 cDNAs have been isolated and characterized.[37] *In vivo*, the CYP450 enzymes are abundant in liver, and some forms are also expressed in extrahepatic tissues (Table 18.2). A few isoenzymes, such as CYP2F1 and 4B1, are expressed in lung but are not found in liver, whereas CYP1A2, 2A6, 2B6, 2C, 2D6, 2E1 and 3A account for 80% of hepatic CYP450.[74] A recent study on the characterization of CYP450 level and activity in a large number of human liver samples showed that CYP3A (about 30% of total CYP450) and 2C (about 20%) enzymes were the major forms.[74] High levels of CYP1A2 (about 13%) and 2E1 (about 7%) could be determined, whereas CYP2A (about 4%), 2D6 (about 2%) and 2B6 (<1%) were the minor CYP450 forms (Fig. 18.1).

Table 18.1 Mammalian cell systems used for cDNA-directed transient and stable expression of human CYP450s.

CYP450	Cell type	Expression system	Reference
CYP1A1	AHH-1	EBV-HSVTK vector	7, 8
	COS	*SV40 vector*	9, 10
	NIH-3T3	Retrovirus	11
	V79	SV40 promoter–vector	12
	XPA, GM	MTT promoter–vector	13
CYP1A2	AHH-1	EBV-HSVTK vector	14, 15
	BEAS-2B	CMV promoter–vector	16
	COS	*SV40 vector*	9, 10
	Hepa-1c1	SV40 promoter–vector	17
	HepG2	*Vaccinia virus*	18–23
	NIH-3T3	Retrovirus	11
	V79	SV40 promoter–vector	24, 25
CYP2A6	AHH-1	EBV-HSVTK vector	14, 26, 27
	AS52	Retroviral vector	28
	BEAS-2B	CMV promoter–vector	K. Macé *et al.* (unpublished results)
	C3H/10T1/2	Retrovirus	29
	HepG2	*Vaccinia virus*	19–23
	NIH-3T3, RLE	Retrovirus	30
CYP2B6	BEAS-2B	CMV promoter–vector	K. Macé *et al.* (unpublished results)
	HepG2	*Vaccinia virus*	19–23
CYP2C8	HepG2	*Vaccinia virus*	19–23
CYP2C9	BEAS-2B	CMV promoter–vector	K. Macé *et al.* (unpublished results)
	HepG2	*Vaccinia virus*	19–23
	NIH-3T3	Retrovirus	11
CYP2D6	AHH-1	EBV-HSVTK vector	31, 32
	BEAS-2B	CMV promoter–vector	K. Macé *et al.* (unpublished results)
	HepG2	*Vaccinia virus*	19–23
	NIH-3T3	Retrovirus	11
CYP2E1	AHH-1	EBV-HSVTK vector	
	BEAS-2B	CMV promoter–vector	K. Macé *et al.* (unpublished results)
	HepG2	*Vaccinia virus*	19–23
	NIH-3T3, RLE	Retrovirus	33
	NIH-3T3	Retrovirus	11
CYP2F1	BEAS-2B	CMV promoter–vector	K. Macé *et al.* (unpublished results)
	HepG2	*Vaccinia virus*	19–23
CYP3A4	AHH-1	EBV-HSVTK vector	14
	BEAS-2B	CMV promoter–vector	K. Macé *et al.* (unpublished results)
	CHL	SRa promoter–vector	34
	COS	*SV40 vector*	10
	Hep G2	*Vaccinia virus*	19–23
	NIH-3T3	Retrovirus	11
CYP3A5	COS	*SV40 vector*	10
	Hep G2	*Vaccinia virus*	19–23
CYP4B1	Hep G2	*Vaccinia virus*	19–23

Transient expression systems are indicated in italics. AHH-1, human lymphoblastoid cell line; AS52, Chinese hamster ovary cell line; BEAS-2B, human bronchial epithelial cell line; C3H/10T1/2, mouse fibroblast cell line; CHL, Chinese hamster fibroblast cell line; COS, African green monkey kidney cell line; GM, human fibroblasts; Hepa-1c1, mouse hepatoma cell line; HepG2, human hepatoma cell line; NIH-3T3, mouse embryo cell line; V79, Chinese hamster lung cell line; XPA, DNA repair-deficient human fibroblasts.

Table 18.2 Tissue distribution of human CYP450s.

Family	Member	Tissue	Detection§	Reference
CYP1A	1A1*	Liver	mRNA	38, 39
		Lung	Protein	40, 41
		Lymphocytes	Protein	42
		Placenta	Protein	42, 43
		Skin	Protein	44
	1A2	Liver	Protein	45
CYP1B	1B1†	Skin	mRNA	46
		Kidney	mRNA	46
		Lung	mRNA	46
		Intestinal tract	mRNA	46
CYP2A	2A6	Liver	Protein	47–49
CYP2B	2B6	Liver	Protein	50
CYP2C	2C8	Liver	Protein	51–53
		Intestine	Protein¶	
	2C9/10‡	Liver	Protein	51–53
		Intestine	Protein¶	
	2C17	Liver	mRNA	51
	2C18	Liver	mRNA	51, 54
	2C19	Liver	mRNA	51, 52
CYP2D	2D6	Liver	Protein	55, 56
		Intestine	Protein	53
		Bladder	mRNA	57
		Kidney	Protein	58
CYP2E	2E1	Liver	Protein	59–61
		Intestine	Protein	53
		Lung	Protein	62
CYP2F	2F1	Lung	mRNA	63
CYP3A	3A3/4‡	Liver	Protein	64
		Intestine	Protein	65, 66
		Colon	mRNA	65, 66
		Skin	mRNA	67
	3A5	Liver	Protein	68–70
		Skin	mRNA	67
		Colon	mRNA	66
	3A7	Liver (fetal)	Protein	71
		Placenta	Protein	72
		Endometrium	Protein	72
CYP4B	4B1	Lung	mRNA	73
		Colon	mRNA	66

* CYP1A1 expression seems to be associated with inducer exposure; † CYP1B1 mRNA expression has been detected in several other tissues such as brain, heart, spleen, thymus, prostate, testis, ovary and leucocytes; ‡ CYP450 coded by two different genes not distinguishable by immunochemical studies; § P450 expression directly demonstrated by protein or mRNA analysis; ¶ protein detected by a polyclonal anti-human CYP2C8-10.

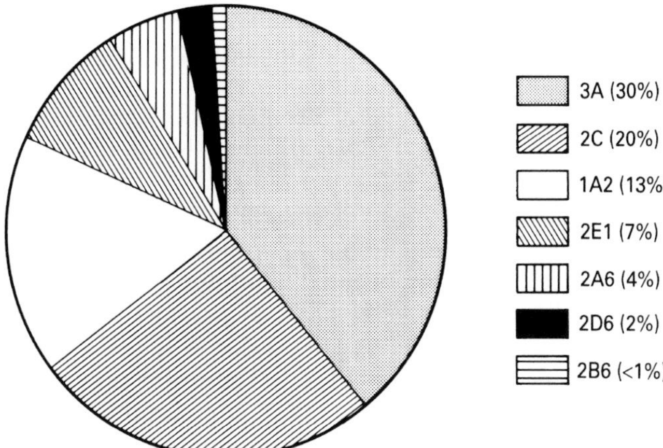

Fig. 18.1 Relative proportion of CYP450 known to be involved in xenobiotic metabolism. The level of individual forms of CYP450 were determined immunochemically from 60 human microsome samples. Data from Shimada *et al.*[74]

III. HUMAN CELLULAR MODELS

A. Vaccinia virus expression system

A number of cDNAs have been efficiently expressed in a wide variety of eukaryotic cells using vaccinia virus vectors. This transient expression system has a number of useful characteristics, including the capacity for cloning large fragments of foreign DNA (>20 000 base pairs (bp)), a wide host range and a high level of protein synthesis. The general procedure for construction of recombinant viruses and their use in producing CYP450s has been described by Gonzalez *et al.*[75] Twelve forms of human CYP450 have been expressed in the human hepatoma HepG2 cell line (Table 18.1) and applied to the metabolism of various drugs. The oxidation of warfarin has recently been studied with vaccinia virus-expressed CYP450s.[21] This drug is used clinically as an anticoagulant but high interdividual variability exists regarding the dose required for optimal effect. *In vitro* studies using human liver microsomes suggested that one or more CYP450s could hydroxylate the therapeutically active *S* enantiomer of warfarin at the C7 position to an *in vivo* inactive metabolite.[76] Among 11 vaccinia virus-expressed CYP450s, Rettie *et al.* showed that CYP2C9 was the major CYP450 responsible for 7-hydroxylation of *S*-warfarin, while CYP1A2 and CYP3A4 exhibited approximately 4- and 12-fold lower rates of metabolism, respectively. No significant *S*-warfarin 7-hydroxylation could be detected with CYP2A6, 2B7, 2C8, 2D6, 2E1, 2F1, 3A5 and 4B1.[21] This study illustrates the potential of *in vitro* studies using cDNA-expressed CYP450s to determine which isoenzyme is involved in human drug metabolism and to predict certain risk groups with unusual (polymorphic) metabolism patterns. Additionally, *in vitro* drug metabolism data can contribute to the identification of drug interactions (e.g. inhibition or induction of the specific CYP450 by other drugs) as well as to the explanation of the high degree of variability in clinical response to drugs (interindividual differences in CYP450 expression).

The panel of vaccinia virus-expressed CYP450s has also been used to determine which P450s are responsible for the activation of the human carcinogen aflatoxin B_1 (AFB_1).[19] Determination of DNA adduct formation in AFB_1-treated HepG2 cells previously infected with recombinant virus revealed that CYP1A2, 2A6, 2B6, 3A3 and 3A4 are able to activate

AFB_1. Comparison of these *in vitro* data with the known profile of CYP450 expression in liver (Fig. 18.1) suggests that CYP3A and 1A2 are the principal isoenzymes involved in AFB_1 activation in humans.

This virus expression system exhibits several advantages for drug metabolism studies. It is capable of producing a large amount of CYP450 within 24 h and, due to the wide host range of the virus, can be used in various cell types. HepG2 cells, although derived from a hepatocarcinoma, are interesting as host cells because they express high amounts of NADPH-P450 oxidoreductase and cytochrome b5 required for maximal CYP450 activity. In absence of specific inducers they do not have detectable levels of endogenous CYP450. Moreover, the HepG2 cells express several phase II enzymes including GST-α, epoxide hydrolase, UDP-glucuronyl transferases (UDP-GTs),[77,78] phenolsulfotransferases,[79] *N*-acetyl transferase (NAT) type 1, but not NAT-2.[80] The major drawback of this system is that infection of host cells with vaccinia virus results in cytopathic effects, hindering stable recombinant protein expression. Host protein expression is rapidly suppressed, limiting the participation of other important drug-metabolizing enzymes such as phase II enzymes. In addition, a transient expression system is unsuitable for applications in genetic toxicology such as mutagenesis and transformation studies, which require stable expression of CYP450 in non-transformed cell lines. However, alternatives for mutagenesis studies have been developed where the typical S9 fractions used as an extracellular activation system in the Ames test have been replaced by cell lysates from vaccinia virus-infected cells.[19]

B. Human lymphoblast cell system

To establish cell lines containing a stable endogenous activation system, CYP450 cDNAs have been transfected into human B-lymphoblastoid AHH-1 cells.[81] The methods for the development of this CYP450-expressing cell system have been widely described.[36,81] Vectors that contain the EBV origin of replication (OriP), the promoter of herpes simplex virus thymidine kinase gene (HSVtk) and sequences conferring resistance to hygromycin B or 1-histidinol have been used. The interaction between the EBV OriP sequence and the EBV nuclear antigen (EBNA-1) gene product allows extrachromosomal replication of the vector in EBV-transformed cells.[82] As the transfected vector is not integrated into the cellular genome, continuous selection for the respective selection marker is required for stability of expression.[36,82] By transfecting different CYP450-expressing EBV vectors, Crespi *et al.*[36] have established a panel of human lymphoblastoid cells exhibiting high CYP450 expression (1.0–160 pmol per mg microsomal protein). Variation in the level of CYP450 expression is dependent on the number of transcriptional cassettes per vector molecule transfected into the cells.[36] The AHH-1 host cells have a low basal level of CYP1A1 expression, which can be induced with appropriate polycyclic aromatic hydrocarbon inducers.[83] Moreover, this cell line exhibits GST activity (4.7 nmol per 10^6 cells per min) and forms limited amounts of glucuronide conjugates, but does not show detectable epoxide hydrolase activity.[83,84] This cell system has been used widely for both drug metabolism and procarcinogen activation studies. For example, the anticancer drug cyclophosphamide and its isomeric analogue, ifosphamide, require metabolism to generate pharmacologically active, cytotoxic species.[85] Identification of specific human CYP450s involved in the metabolism of cyclophosphamide and ifosphamide would allow prediction of interdividual variability and potential drug interactions that might compromise therapeutic efficiency. A four- to ninefold interdividual variation in the 4-hydroxylation of these oxazaphosphorines was observed with a panel of human liver microsomes and evidence for the involvement of multiple CYP450s was established.[86] The use of microsomal preparations from CYP450-expressing AHH-1 cell lines indicated that CYP2A6, 2B6, 2C8, 2C9 and 3A4 were catalytically competent in hydroxylating cyclophosphamide and ifosphamide, whereas CYP1A1, 1A2, 2D6 and 2E1 did not exhibit detectable activities. In human liver microsomes, inhibition studies using selective inhibitors and specific antibodies confirmed that CYP2B and CYP3A preferentially activate cyclophosphamide and ifosphamide, respectively.[86] CYP2A6 was found to play only a minor role in the activation of these drugs in human liver microsomes. This result is probably due to the low content of CYP2A6 in liver samples[74] (Fig. 18.1). This study clearly illustrates the advantages of using the combination of human liver microsome preparations which contain multiple CYP450s and cells genetically engineered to express an individual CYP450. Single CYP450-expressing cell models are useful to define which CYP450s are involved in the metabolism of the studied drug, and the relevance of this finding can be confirmed by subsequent analysis with human liver microsomes.

Table 18.3 summarizes the genetic toxicology studies performed on different promutagens in the CYP450-expressing AHH-1 cells. AFB_1 activation by cells containing CYP1A1, CYP1A2, CYP2A6 or CYP3A4 cDNA has been analysed by measuring cytotoxicity, DNA adduct formation and mutagenicity as end-points.[8,14] After correction for the differences in P450 content, the results indicate that CYP1A2 is 3-, 30- and 40-fold more effective in the activation of AFB_1 than CYP3A4, 2A6 and 1A1, respectively. Based on these observations, as well as their relatively low expression, CYP2A6 and 1A1 would have a limited role in AFB_1-induced hepatocarcinogenesis. On the other hand, a controversy exists concerning the relative involvement of CYP1A2 and CYP3A4 in the activation of AFB_1 to genotoxic species. Several studies have reported that CYP3A4 is the primary human liver CYP450 involved in AFB_1 epoxidation.[87,88] However, it has been shown recently[89] that CYP1A2 is the high-affinity P450 enzyme for AFB_1 bioactivation whereas CYP3A4 appears to have a relatively low affinity for AFB_1. Indeed, although CYP3A enzymes are the major CYP450 forms expressed in the liver, the CYP1A2 activation pathway seems to be particularly important for low doses of AFB_1. Therefore this isoform could be an important determinant of AFB_1-induced hepatocarcinogenesis where low exposure levels are involved.

Table 18.3 Mutational studies performed in CYP450-expressing AHH-1 cells.

CYP450	Promutagens	Reference
CYP1A1	AAF, AFB_1	7, 8
	B(a)P, CCP, NNK	8
CYP1A2	AFB_1	14, 15
	NNK	31
CYP2A6	B(a)P, DMN	27
	NNK	31
	DEN, DMN	26
	AFB_1	14
CYP2D6	NNA, NNN, NNK	31
	NNK	32
CYP2E1	DEN, DMN	26
	NNK	31
CYP3A4	AFB_1	14

AAF, 2-acetylaminofluorene; AFB_1, aflatoxin B_1; B(a)P, benzo(*a*)pyrene; CCP, cyclopenta(*a,d*)pyrene; DEN, diethylnitrosamine; DMN, dimethylnitrosamine; NNA, 1-(*N*-methyl-*N*-nitro)-1-(3-pyridyl)-4-butanol; NNK, 4-(methylnitrosamino)-1-(3-pyridyl)-1-butanone; NNN, *N*-nitrosonornicotine.

Among the tobacco-specific nitrosamines, 4-(methylnitrosamino)-1-(3-pyridyl)-1-butanone (NNK) is the most potent carcinogen in experimental animals and has been linked to tobacco-related cancers in humans.[90] Numerous studies have been performed to identify which CYP450(s) is responsible for NNK activation. Yamazaki *et al.*[91] have shown, by measuring DNA damage in a bacterial tester strain *Salmonella typhimurium* in presence of human liver microsomes, that CYP2A6, 2E1 and to a lesser extent CYP1A2 are major catalysts for NNK metabolic activation. On the other hand, CYP3A4, 2D6 and 2C do not appear to be extensively involved in NNK activation.[91] However, these data are not entirely in agreement with studies performed with transient or stable CYP450 expression systems, where CYP1A2 seemed to be the most active CYP450 for NNK activation.[31,92] Indeed, Smith *et al.*[92] showed that, among 12 forms of P450 expressed in HepG2 cells, CYP1A2 had by far the highest capacity to catalyse the oxidation of NNK. The formation of keto alcohol is also catalysed by CYP2A6, 2B6, 2E1, 2F1 and 3A5, whereas CYP2C9, 2D6, 3A4 and 4B1 do not seem to be involved in NNK metabolism. Mutation studies on the CYP450-expressing AHH-1 cells revealed that the sensitivity of the cell lines to NNK is CYP1A2 = CYP1A1 = CYP2A6 > CYP2E1 = CYP2D6.[8,31,32] Although epidemiological studies have linked the extensive debrisoquine metabolic phenotype of the CYP2D6 gene to increased lung cancer risk in smokers,[93,94] the *in vitro* observations suggested no or a minor role for CYP2D6 in NNK activation. On the other hand, CYP1A1, 1A2, 2A6 and 2E1 could be the major enzymes involved in the metabolism of NNK in human tissue. Interestingly, CYP1A1 was shown to be very efficient in activating NNK to mutagenic species.[8] As a strong association has been observed between active cigarette smoking and CYP1A1 gene expression in normal human lung tissue,[95,96] this isoenzyme appears to be an important factor in the aetiology of lung cancer in smokers.

One major advantage of the lymphoblastoid cell system is its applicability in mutagenicity testing of different classes of carcinogens (Table 18.3). Mutation rates can be determined by assessing mutations at the *hprt* and thymidine kinase loci,[84] micronucleus assays[97] and sister chromatid exchange.[98] Unfortunately, the CYP450-expressing systems employing EBV vectors can be efficiently used only in EBNA-1 positive cells such as EBV-transformed lymphoblastoid cell lines.

C. Human bronchial epithelial cell system

As most human tumours arise from epithelial cells and many carcinogens exhibit organ specificity, the establishment of metabolically competent epithelial cells from various tissues may yield valuable tools for toxicity testing. For this purpose we have chosen the SV40 T-antigen immortalized human bronchial epithelial cells (BEAS-2B)[99] as a host for the stable transfection of CYP450 cDNAs. BEAS-2B cells retain many characteristics of normal cell growth and differentiation such as a growth inhibitory response to transforming growth factor (TGF) β_1 and prove to be a useful model to study activated proto-oncogenes and inactivated tumour suppressor genes in human carcinogenesis.[100–103] In addition, BEAS-2B cells xenotransplanted into de-epithelialized rat trachea demonstrate changes similar to those occurring during human lung carcinogenesis *in vivo* upon exposure to individual and complex mixtures of chemical carcinogens.[104,105] Expression of CYP450s, including CYP1A2, CYP3A, 2E1, 2B6, 2A6 and 2D6, was undetectable by reverse transcriptase-polymerase chain reaction (RT-PCR) analysis. Nevertheless, as for most cultured cell lines, BEAS-2B cells exhibit polycyclic aromatic hydrocarbon-induced CYP1A1 activity.[106] The expression of oxidant defence enzymes such as catalase, glutathione peroxidase and superoxide dismutase was retained in BEAS-2B cells at levels similar to those of normal primary bronchial cells.[16] In addition, this cell line expresses epoxide hydrolase,[16] quinone reductase and GST-π.[106] After testing several promoters for their ability to direct transcription in the BEAS-2B cells, the cytomegalovirus (CMV) promoter was selected as it showed the strongest activity.[16] Therefore, CYP450 cDNAs were cloned into the plasmid pCMVneo which contains the CMV promoter, the selectable neomycin (*neo*) gene conferring G418 resistance and the polyadenylation site from the rabbit β-globin gene (Fig. 18.2). The general procedure for the establishment of BEAS-2B cells stably expressing human CYP450 enzymes is described in Fig. 18.3. Briefly, the CYP450-expressing pCMVneo vectors are introduced into the cells by liposome-mediated transfection.[16] Some 48 h later, the cells are selected for G418 resistance and subsequently cloned. After culture expansion, the different clones are analysed for CYP450 expression by Western blot analysis (Fig. 18.4). Although the polyclonal population always exhibits a high level of protein expression, cell cloning is an essential step because about 20–50% of clones showed low or no expression, probably as a result of plasmid recombination. Immunofluorescence of CYP450-expressing clones shows CYP450 staining in 100% of the cells (Fig. 18.5). A useful property of BEAS-2B cells is the possibility of determining catalytic activities in intact cultured cells (Table 18.4).

Carcinogen activation can be studied easily in the CYP450-expressing BEAS-2B cells by direct measurement of toxicological relevant end-points such as cytotoxicity, DNA adduct formation and mutagenesis. Cytotoxicity tests including colony-forming efficiency (CFE) and hexosaminidase have been evaluated on CYP1A2-expressing cells treated by AFB_1. The hexosaminidase assay[107] appears to be faster and cheaper but less sensitive than the CFE assay. CYP1A2-expressing cells treated with AFB_1 for 24 h showed a CD_{50} value (AFB_1 dose resulting in 50% cytotoxicity) of 6 ng ml^{-1} in the CFE assay. The cytotoxic response was accompanied by the formation of the DNA adduct AFB_1-N^7-guanine,[16] which is the major

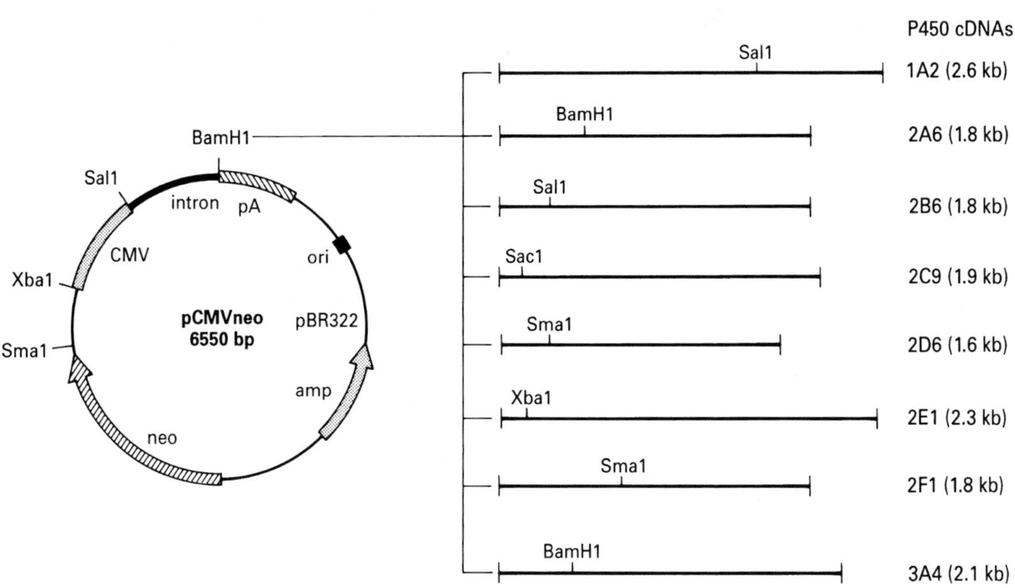

Fig. 18.2 Schematic map of the CYP450-expressing pCMV vectors. CYP450 cDNAs were cloned into the BamHI cloning site of the pCMVneo vector. The neomycin (*neo*) gene confers G418 resistance. amp, Ampicillin resistance gene; ori, origin of replication; pA, polyadenylation site from the rabbit β-globin gene; CMV, cytomegalovirus promoter.

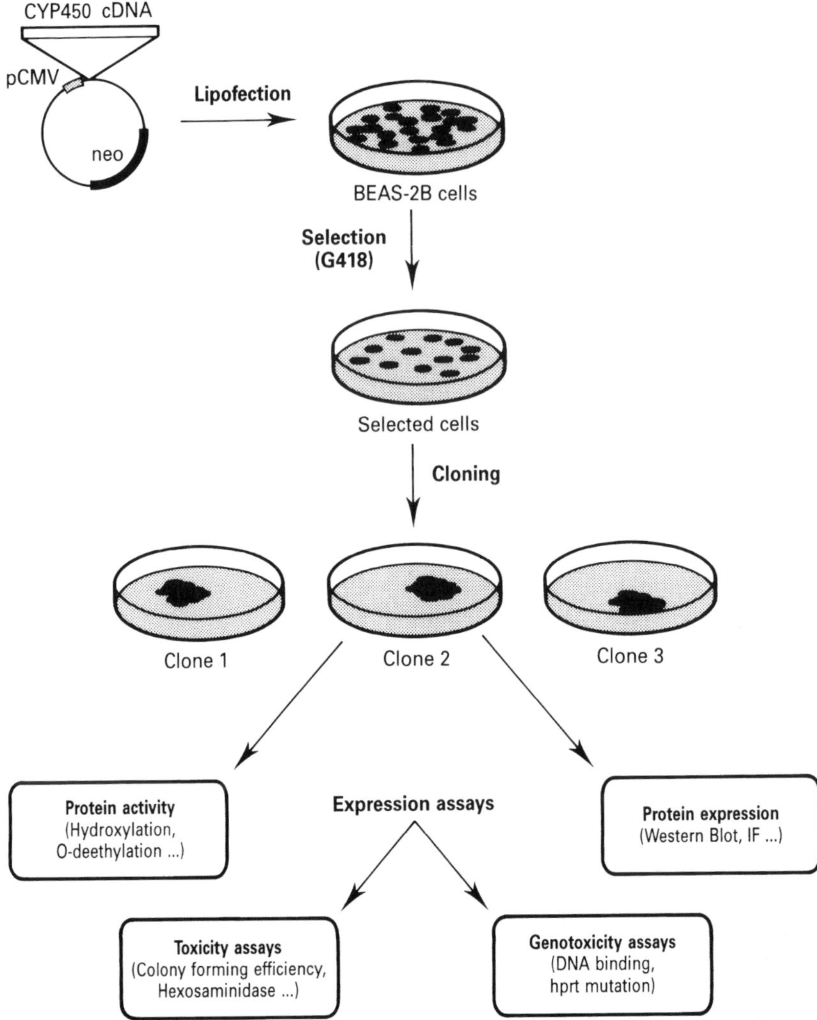

Fig. 18.3 General procedure for the establishment of BEAS-2B cells with stable expression of CYP450 enzymes. The CYP450-expressing pCMV vectors were introduced into the BEAS-2B cells by liposome-mediated transfection. After 48 h the cells were selected for G418 resistance and subsequently cloned. The different clones were analysed for the expression and activity of CYP450 enzymes. High CYP450-expressing cells were chosen for additional analysis such as toxicity and genotoxicity assays.

genotoxic lesion found in human tissues[108] and a biomarker for AFB_1 exposure.[5] The mutagenic effect of AFB_1 treatment was evaluated at the *hprt* locus in control and CYP1A2-expressing cells. AFB_1 was found to induce a sevenfold increase in the mutant fraction of CYP1A2 cells without a significant effect on the control cells (Fig. 18.6). The level of cytotoxic and genotoxic effects of AFB_1 in the CYP1A2-expressing cells is comparable with that previously reported by Crespi *et al.*[14] with CYP1A2-AHH-1 cells.

The BEAS-2B cell model is useful not only for carcinogen activation studies but also for studying compounds with anticarcinogenic effects. Many dietary phytochemicals found in teas, spices and herbs have such properties.[109] We have shown that rosemary extract very efficiently inhibits benzo(*a*)pyrene–DNA adduct formation by strongly inhibiting CYP1A1

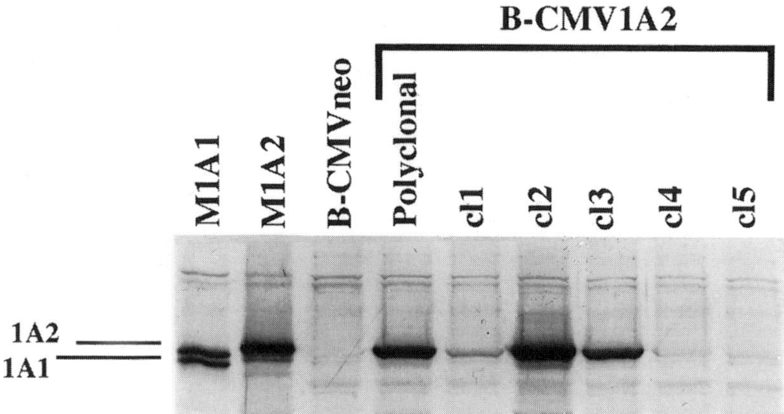

Fig. 18.4 Western blot analysis of several clones derived from CYP1A2-transfected cells. 10 μg of microsomes from human CYP1A1 (M1A1)- and CYP1A2 (M1A2)-expressing AHH-1 cells (Gentest, Woburn, MA) or 20 μg of cell lysates were subjected to electrophoresis. Immunodetection was performed as described previously.[16] B-CMVneo (control cells) and B-CMV1A2 were derived from BEAS-2B cells transfected with the respective pCMV plasmids.

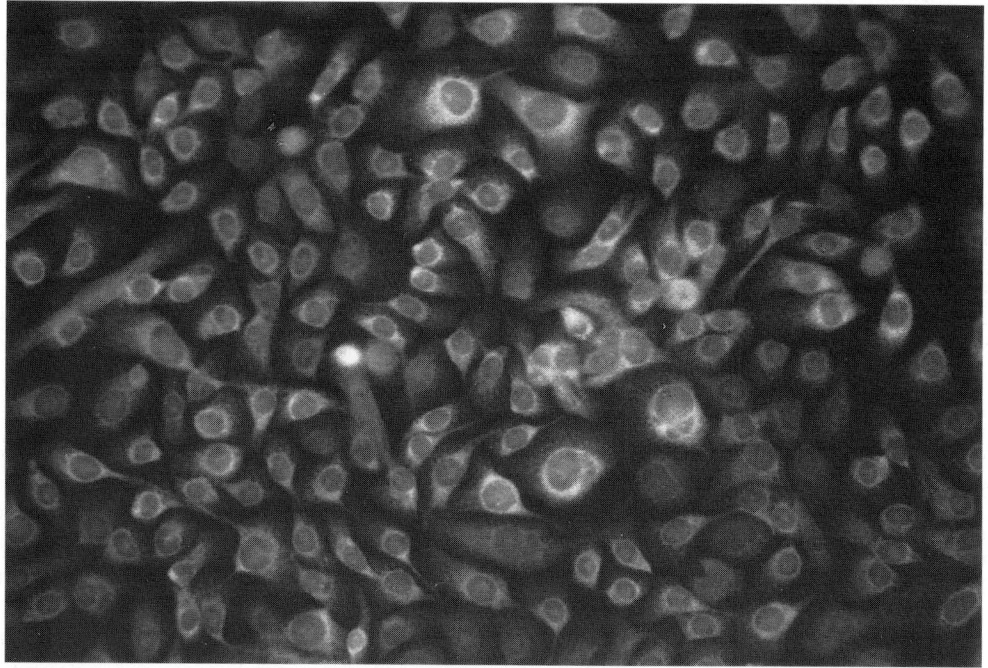

Fig. 18.5 Indirect immunofluorescence on CYP1A2-expressing BEAS-2B cells (B-CMV1A2 cl2). A rabbit anti-rat CYP1A (kindly provided by F. Gonzalez) was used as the first antibody. No immunostaining could be detected in control cells.

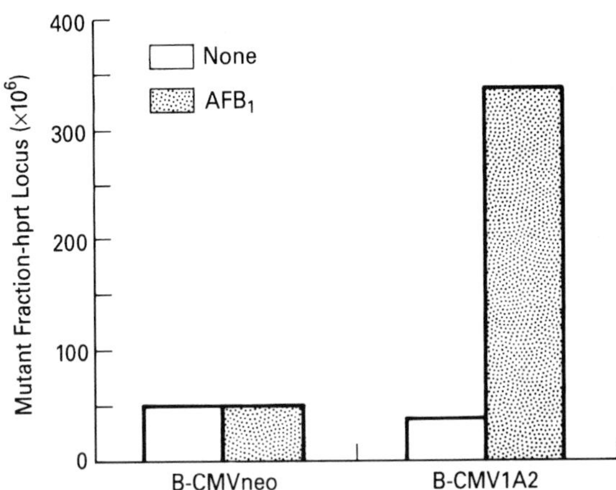

Fig. 18.6 Mutagenicity of AFB_1 at the *hprt* locus. 10^6 BEAS-2B cells (about 10^4 cells per cm^2) were exposed to 100 ng ml^{-1} AFB_1 for 24 h. Seven days later, $hprt^-$ selection was achieved by culturing 10^5 cells (10^3 cells per cm^2) in the presence of 17.5 ng ml^{-1} 6-thioguanine (6-TG). Colonies were stained and counted after 2 weeks of selection. The mutant fraction was calculated as the ratio between the plating efficiency in the selective (6-TG) versus non-selective medium. B-CMVneo cells correspond to BEAS-2B cells transfected with pCMVneo vector (control cells). B-CMV1A2 cells correspond to cells transfected with the recombinant pCMV1A2 vector.

activity. Similarly, aflatoxin B_1–DNA adduct formation in CYP1A2-expressing BEAS-2B cells is strongly inhibited by rosemary extract. Both benzo(*a*)pyrene and AFB_1 are detoxified by GST. We have shown that rosemary extract not only inhibits CYP450 activity but it also induces the expression of the phase II enzyme, GST.[106] Therefore, the CYP450-expressing BEAS-2B cell system represents an interesting model for screening other dietary components, suspected to exhibit health beneficial effects.

Table 18.4 Catalytic activities of various CYP450-expressing BEAS-2B cells.

CYP450 expressed	Activity*	
CYP1A2	EROD	19.3 ± 3.4
	MROD	50.7 ± 7.2
CYP2A6	CH	305 ± 79
CYP2B6	BROD	17.9 ± 4.4
CYP2D6	DXM	145 ± 5
CYP2E1	CHZ	76.9 ± 4.0
CYP3A4	TH	17.5 ± 1.9

* Activity (pmol per min per mg total protein) were measured in intact cell cultures. MROD and BROD, methoxy and benzoxyresorufin O-de-ethylase activity, respectively; CH, coumarin hydroxylase activity; DXM, dextromethorphan O-demethylase activity; CHZ, chlorzoxazone 6-hydroxylase activity; TH, testosterone 6β-hydroxylase activity; EROD, ethoxyresorufin O-de-ethylase activity.

The CYP450-expressing BEAS-2B cells system has several practical and functional properties that gives it a strong potential for exploitation in predictive pharmacotoxicological screening and risk assessment. BEAS-2B cells are non-tumorigenic up to a very high passage number[99,103,110] and are therefore suitable for transformation assays. These cells are of epithelial origin and are derived from a target organ for human carcinogens. In addition, BEAS-2B cells grow under defined serum-free conditions, eliminating potential interactions of test compounds with unknown factors in serum, test variability due to different serum batches and uncontrolled influences on cell proliferation by serum.[111] They form monolayers which facilitate cytotoxicity, mutagenicity and transformation assays. The advantages of the BEAS-2B cells, i.e. functional phase II enzymes, stable CYP450 expression, *in situ* metabolism and activation of drugs and carcinogens, imply that this model may be useful for more predictive human risk assessment.

IV. POTENTIAL APPLICATIONS

The use of CYP450-expressing human cell systems for identifying isoenzymes responsible for drug metabolism and procarcinogen activation is now widely recognized. These models represent sensitive systems and allow rapid screening for biotransformation, cytototoxicity and genotoxicity.

Because of interspecies differences in the expression of phase I and II enzymes, the development of sensitive and specific human *in vitro* models is an essential step for relevant risk extrapolation from animal studies to humans. Although such *in vitro* models cannot completely replace the *in vivo* metabolism and pharmacokinetic studies, they provide important insight into specific metabolic pathways and bioconversion mechanisms. A better understanding of the molecular and cellular mechanisms of drug metabolism and chemical-induced toxicity in human models allows a more relevant choice of animal species for *in vivo* studies and the appropriate end-point to be considered for a better human risk assessment. Besides improving toxicological predictions, these metabolically competent human systems can considerably reduce the use of animals. Prescreening of the cytotoxic and genotoxic potential of new drugs or compounds in human cell systems can rapidly eliminate undesirable candidates and avoid further animal experimentation.

In situ assays with living cells have several advantages over assays performed on subcellular fractions such as microsomes for pharmacotoxicological studies. The compounds can be added directly to the medium of the cell cultures and may be easily extracted after a desired incubation time. The absence of extraction steps for microsomal preparations increases the reproducibility and reliability of the assays. *In situ* approaches are more physiological, avoid the addition of NADPH-generating systems and the problem of enzymatic stability. They allow long-term toxicological studies, such as transformation assays, facilitate the correlation of drug metabolism with cellular indices of toxicity and permit the measurement of genetic end-points in the target cells where the reactive intermediates are generated.

V. CURRENT TECHNIQUES FOR TOXICOLOGICAL TESTING

The usefulness of the *in vitro* cell systems in toxicological studies depends not only on the metabolic competence of the cellular models but also on the relevance of the assays used for measuring toxicity and genotoxicity end-points.

Several techniques for assessing the acute cytotoxicity of chemical agents in cell culture systems are available. Among them, the colony-forming efficiency assay[16] is the most sensitive and reliable method for monitoring viable cell number. However, this method is time- and cost-consuming when many samples have to be analysed. Colorimetric and fluorimetric assays miniaturized into 24- or 96-well plates reduce medium and plastic costs and permit the rapid analysis of many samples. Two major classes of cytotoxicity assays are used routinely. The assays monitoring (1) plasma membrane integrity by measuring, for example, lactate dehydrogenase activity[112] or the incorporation of fluorescent dyes (BCECF-AM, propidium iodide)[113,114] and (2) the damage of subcellular structures by measuring lysosomal activity (neutral red assay, hexosaminidase activity)[107,115] or mitochondrial activity (MTT, rhodamine-123).[116,117] Different markers can be used at the same time, providing additional information on the cytotoxic mechanisms.[113,114] More specific end-points can also be measured, such as the tight junction integrity by using sodium fluorescein.[118] More recently, new cytotoxicity assays have been developed based on the evaluation of the transcriptional responses of several stress gene promoter–CAT fusion constructs. The CAT-Tox assay (Xenometrix, Boulder, Colorado) using HepG2 cells stably transfected with stress promoter– or response element–CAT fusion constructs, including *fos*, metallothionine, GST, heat shock protein (HSP) 70 or cAMP response element (CRE), xenobiotic response element (XRE), nuclear factor-κB (NFκB), allows a direct rapid screening of the molecular mechanism of a variety of toxic agents.[119]

The major end-points of short-term genotoxicity assays include chromosomal aberrations, primary DNA damage and gene mutations. The available tests detecting chromosome breaks include the sister chromatid exchange (SCE) and the micronucleus assays, which have been established with different cellular models.[120,121] The micronucleus test has been recently used for monitoring the clastogenic effects of numerous promutagens including mycotoxins, aromatic amines, nitrosamines and heterocyclic amines, in cells expressing several CYP450s.[97] The detection of micronucleus formation in these genetically engineered cells appears to be a rapid and sensitive screening method for measuring genotoxicity activity *in vitro*.

A battery of tests has been established for evaluating DNA damage. These tests can be divided schematically into two groups: one measuring DNA strand breaks and the other monitoring DNA adduct formation. Of all the procedures for measuring DNA strand breaks there is increasing interest in the Comet assay, which appears to be a sensitive and rapid method for DNA damage analysis, applicable to any eukaryotic cells (for a review see Fairbain *et al.*[122]). The advantage of this assay, which provides direct determination of the extent of DNA strand breaks in individual cells, is the possibility of determining whether all cells within a population demonstrate the same level of damage.

In the past decade several methods for assessing and quantifying DNA adducts have been developed for *in vivo* and *in vitro* studies. Three distinct approaches utilizing ^{32}P-postlabelling, immunoassays or gas chromatography-mass spectrometry (GC/MS) technologies are used.[123,124] The major advantages of these methodologies are their sensitivity (one DNA adduct per 10^6–10^{10} normal nucleotides) and the possibility to compare directly DNA adduct formation in human and *in vitro* experimental systems. A major limitation of these systems is that they require knowledge of the structural identity of the carcinogen–base adducts for the generation of appropriate standards. In addition these methodologies are too sophisticated for rapid screening analysis. An easier but less informative evaluation of carcinogen-induced damage can be achieved with radiolabelled compounds followed by scintillation counting.[106,125]

Numerous laboratories have directed considerable effort to optimize and simplify the assays measuring chemical-induced mutations. Among them the HPRT-variant short-term assay,[126] which uses the hypoxanthine phosphoribosyl transferase (*hprt*) gene as an endogenous marker for monitoring genotoxic damage, is the most extensively used rapid screening test. The mutagenicity of several chemical classes, including mycotoxins, polycyclic aromatic hydrocarbons, nitrosamines and aromatic amines, have been studied at the *hprt* locus of the CYP450-expressing AHH-1 cells.[81] Selection of HPRT-specific mutations has been applied to different human cells such as lymphocytes,[127,128] fibroblasts,[129] uroepithelial cells,[130] epidermal keratinocytes[131] and bronchial epithelial cells,[132] but this mutation assay is not applicable to all available cell lines.

Shuttle vectors which can replicate in both eukaryotic and prokaryotic cells are powerful tools for the study of the rearrangement and mutagenesis of DNA in cellular systems. The shuttle vector is introduced into the eukaryotic cells where it replicates extrachromosomally and, after treatment by chemical mutagens, the vector can be rescued and transferred to bacteria for mutational analysis of the marker gene. The use of bacterial *lacZ′* fragment as a reporter gene allows a rapid determination of mutation frequency. This approach has been used to study the occurrence of AFB_1-mediated mutations in cell lines transiently expressing rat CYP1A2[133] or human CYP3A4[11] and can easily be applied to different cell lines. The major drawback of this system is perhaps its lack of relevance with the biological situation. As the vector is expressed extrachromosomally, the extent and location of modifications in the marker gene might not reflect the mutational events occurring on a chromosomal gene.

Mutations in the tumour suppressor gene *p53* are common in human cancer, and exposure to ultraviolet light, cigarette smoke and AFB_1 has been found to lead to specific *p53* mutation spectra.[134] Restriction fragment length polymorphism (RFLP)/PCR or 'fish-RFLP/PCR' assays allowing sensitive mutation analysis at specific codons of the *p53* exons have been developed.[132,135] These techniques have recently been used to show that AFB_1 exposure of a metabolically competent cellular system leads to the induction of G : C to T : A transversions at the third position of codon 249 of the *p53* gene.[135] This type of mutation has previously been observed in human hepatocellular carcinomas from regions with a high level of AFB_1 exposure.[136] Mutational analysis of oncogenes or tumour suppressor genes, in human cellular models, clearly constitutes a powerful approach for studying initiation and promotion steps of chemically induced cancers. However, the complexity of the available techniques does not yet permit their use in the screening of numerous compounds, although they are useful to confirm the relevance of rapid assays such as HPRT and shuttle vector mutational analysis.

VI. PRESENT LIMITATIONS AND OUTLOOK

A. CYP450 expression and response

Interpretation of pharmacotoxicological data with the engineered cell lines needs some consideration. *In vitro* systems are devoid of many of the variables that occur *in vivo*. They cannot mimic the complex interactions of other cell types, blood flow, immune, endocrine and nervous systems, and do not reflect the normal systemic mechanisms such as absorption, penetration, distribution and excretion. Moreover, most of the available cellular models still require further characterization of endogenous phase II enzyme expression, which may explain differences between these and other *in vitro* assays using subcellular fractions (e.g. microsomes). The inability of these systems to evaluate potential effects of drugs or food components on CYP450 transcriptional induction (except for CYP1A1) or inhibition should be taken into account as expression in the engineered cell lines is directed by heterologous promoters. Interactions between different CYP450 isoenzymes during drug metabolism cannot be studied in cell systems exhibiting individual CYP450 expression. However, this will be overcome by the establishment of cell lines expressing multiple CYP450s. The introduction of a human lymphoblastoid cell line expressing four transfected CYP450 and one microsomal epoxide hydrolase cDNAs is the first step in this direction.[97,137] The difficulty of multiple CYP450-expressing cell systems resides in obtaining relevant CYP450 activity in relation to human tissue such as liver (Fig. 18.1). One approach to 'tissue-like' CYP450 expression could be the use of plasmids with different promoters allowing low, medium and high levels of protein expression. For example, CYP3A4- and CYP2A6-coding cDNA could be directed by a strong and a weak promoter, respectively.

B. Organ specificity

Another limitation of these human cellular models is the absence of a panel of cell lines for target-organ toxicity studies. For this purpose one focus of our developmental effort is the establishment of metabolically competent cells derived from various toxicologically relevant organs, such as the lung, liver, colon, skin, buccal mucosa, eye and kidney, to examine possible tissue-specific toxicity. Our current approach consists of the immortalization of primary cultures by SV40 T-antigen gene introduction through retroviral infection.[138,139] Cells immortalized with SV40 large T-antigen may show reduced differentiation and altered tissue-specific functions, including enzymes responsible for the activation of carcinogens, and genetic instability.[140,141] However, SV40 T-antigen immortalized cell lines have been established which maintain differentiated functions and have a relatively stable karyotype.[138,142,143] Moreover, the maintenance of differentiation can be influenced by medium composition, growth factor supplements and the state of differentiation of the primary cell type.[142,144,145] Therefore, immortalization offers a feasible approach to the development of functional human cell lines, especially as deficiencies in metabolism can be restored by genetic manipulation. Several SV40 T-antigen immortalized human cell lines have been already established, including bronchial (BEAS-2B),[99] liver (THLE),[138,139] corneal (CEPI) (A. M. A. Pfeifer, unpublished results), buccal (SVpgC2a),[146] and colonic (HCEC) (S. Blum unpublished results) epithelial cells. We have recently used the pCMV-CYP450 vector system to increase the metabolic competence of the immortalized liver epithelial cell line (THLE). This panel of CYP450-expressing liver cell lines constitutes promising human cellular models for pharmacotoxicological testing as they are non-tumorigenic, show endogenous expression of the phase II enzymes, exhibit liver-like CYP450 expression and are suitable for cytotoxicity and genotoxicity assays (K. Macé, unpublished results).

C. Future trends

Considerable progress has been made in drug metabolism studies by the development of cellular models expressing CYP450s. The enormous potential of cultured cells for drug screening/metabolism and toxicological evaluation can be further increased by selective expression of human phase II enzymes. First steps in this direction have recently been made by using recombinant cell lines stably expressing sulfotransferases or glucuronyltransferases.[79,147,148]

The future of genetically engineered cell lines should focus on the establishment of cellular models with 'tissue-like' phase I and II metabolism. Additional emphasis should be laid on the validation of these models and the creation of databases, which is the prerequisite of an integrated approach to better toxicological risk assessment consisting of animal *in vivo* and *in vitro* studies, human *in vitro* systems and epidemiological studies.

ACKNOWLEDGEMENTS

The authors gratefully acknowledge Drs Maria Gómez-Lechón, Isabelle de Waziers and François Berthou for measurement of the testosterone 6β-hydroxylase, dextromethorphan O-demethylase and chlorzoxazone 6-hydroxylase activities, respectively. We also would like to thank Drs F Gonzalez and B Vogelstein for providing us CYP450 cDNAs and the pCMV neo vector, respectively.

REFERENCES

1. Abbott, P. J. (1992) Carcinogenic chemicals in food: evaluating the health risk. *Fd. Chem. Toxicol.* **30:** 327–333.
2. Autrup, H., Grafstrom, R. C., Brugh, M. *et al.* (1982) Comparison of benzo(a)pyrene metabolism in bronchus, esophagus, colon and duodenum from the same individual. *Cancer Res.* **42:** 934–938.
3. Brash, D. E., Mark, G. E., Farrell, M. P. and Harris, C. C. (1987) Overview of human cells in genetic research: altered phenotypes in human cells caused by transferred genes. *Somat. Cell Mol. Genet.* **13:** 429–440.
4. Grafstrom, R. C. (1990) Carcinogenesis studies in human epithelial tissues and cells *in vitro*: emphasis on serum-free culture conditions and transformation studies. *Acta Physiol. Scand. Suppl.* **592:** 93–133.
5. Groopman, J. D., Wild, C. P., Hasler, J., Junshi, C., Wogan, G. N. and Kensler, T. W. (1993) Molecular epidemiology of aflatoxin exposures: validation of aflatoxin-N^7-guanine levels in urine as a biomarker in experimental rat models and humans. *Environ. Health Perspect.* **99:** 107–113.
6. Harris, C. C. (1987) Human tissues and cells in carcinogenesis research. *Cancer Res.* **47:** 1–10.
7. Crespi, C. L., Langenbach, R., Tudo, K., Chen, Y.-T. and Davies, R. L. (1989) Transfection of a human cytochrome P-450 gene into the human lymphoblastoid cell line, AHH-1 and use of the recombinant cell line in gene mutation assays. *Carcinogenesis* **10:** 295–301.
8. Penman, B. W., Chen, L., Gelboin, H. V., Gonzalez, F. J. and Crespi, C. L. (1994) Development of a human lymphoblastoid cell line constitutively expressing human CYP1A1 cDNA: substrate specificity with model substrates and promutagens. *Carcinogenesis* **15:** 1931–1937.
9. McManus, M. E., Burgess, W. M., Veronese, M. E., Huggett, A., Quattrochi, L. C. and Tukey, R. H. (1990) Metabolism of 2-acetylaminofluorene and benzo(a)pyrene and activation of food-derivated heterocyclic amine mutagens by human cytochrome P-450. *Cancer Res.* **50:** 3367–3376.
10. Roberts-Thomson, S. J., McManus, M. E., Tukey, R. H. and Gonzalez, F. F. (1993) The catalytic activity of four expressed human cytochrome P450s towards benzo(a)pyrene and the isomers of its proximate carcinogen. *Biochem. Biophys. Res. Commun.* **192:** 1373–1379.
11. de Groene, E. M., Hassing, I. G. A., Blom, M. J., Seiner, W., Finf-Gremmels, J. and Horbach, G. J. M. J. (1996) Development of human cytochrome P450-expressing cell lines: application in mutagenicity testing of Ochratoxin A. *Cancer Res.* **56:** 299–304.

12. Schmalix, W. A., Maser, H., Kiefer, F. *et al.* (1993) Stable expression of human cytochrome P4501A1 cDNA in V79 chinese hamster cells and metabolic activation of benzo(a)pyrene. *Exp. Mol. Pathol.* **248:** 251–261.
13. States, J. C., Quan, T., Hines, R. N., Novak, R. F. and Runge-Morris, M. (1993) Expression of human cytochrome P450 1A1 in DNA repair deficient and proficient human fibroblasts stably transformed with an inducible expression vector. *Carcinogenesis* **14:** 1643–1649.
14. Crespi, C. L., Penman, B. W., Steimel, D. T., Gelboin, H. V. and Gonzalez, F. J. (1991) The development of human cell line stably expressing human CYP3A4: role in the metabolic activation of aflatoxin B_1 and comparison to CYP1A2 and CYP2A3. *Carcinogenesis* **12:** 355–359.
15. Crespi, C. L., Steimel, D. T., Aoyama, T., Gelboin, H. V. and Gonzalez, F. J. (1990) Stable expression of human cytochrome P450IA2 cDNA in a human lymphoblastoid cell line: role of the enzyme in the metabolic activation of aflatoxin B_1. *Mol. Carcinog.* **3:** 5–8.
16. Macé, K., Gonzalez, F. J., McConnell, I. R. *et al.* (1994) Activation of promutagens in a human bronchial epithelial cell line stably expressing human cytochrome P450 1A2. *Mol. Carcinog.* **11:** 65–73.
17. Puga, A., Raychaudhuri, B., Salata, K., Zhang, Y.-H. and Nebert, D. (1990) Stable expression of mouse cyp1A1 and human CYP1A2 cDNAs transfected into mouse hepatoma cells lacking detectable P450 enzyme activity. *DNA Cell Biol.* **9:** 425–436.
18. Aoyama, T., Gonzalez, F. J. and Gelboin, H. V. (1989) Human cDNA expressed cytochrome P450IA2: mutagen activation and substrate specificity. *Mol. Carcinog.* **2:** 192–198.
19. Aoyama, T., Yamano, S., Guzelian, P. S. and Gelboin, H. V. (1990) Five of 12 forms of vaccinia virus-expressed human hepatic cytochrome P450 metabolically activate aflatoxin B_1. *Proc. Natl Acad. Sci. U.S.A.* **87:** 4790–4793.
20. Czerwinski, M., McLemore, L. T., Philpot, R. M. *et al.* (1991) Metabolic activation of 4-ipomeanol by complementary DNA-expressed human cytochromes P-450: evidence for species-specific metabolism. *Cancer Res.* **51:** 4636–4638.
21. Rettie, A. E., Korzekwa, K. R., Kunze, K. L. *et al.* (1992) Hydroxylation of warfarin by human cDNA-expressed cytochrome P-450: a role for P-4502C9 in the etiology of (s)-warfarin–drug interactions. *Chem. Res. Toxicol.* **5:** 54–59.
22. Thornton-Manning, J. R., Ruangyuttikarn, W., Gonzalez, F. J. and Yost, G. S. (1991) Metabolic activation of the pneumotoxin, 3-methylindole, by vaccinia-expressed cytochrome P450s. *Biochem. Biophys. Res. Commun.* **181:** 100–107.
23. Waxman, D. J., Lapenson, D. P., Aoyama, T., Gelboin, H. V., Gonzalez, F. J. and Korzekwa, K. (1991) Steroid hormone hydroxylase specificities of eleven cDNA-expressed human cytochromes P450s. *Arch. Biochem. Biophys.* **290:** 160–166.
24. Fuhr, U., Doehmer, J., Battula, N. *et al.* (1992) Biotransformation of caffeine and theophylline in mammalian cell lines genetically engineered for expression of single cytochrome P450 isoforms. *Biochem. Pharmacol.* **43:** 225–235.
25. Wölfel, C., Heinrich-Hirsch, B., Seidel, A. *et al.* (1992) Genetically engineered V79 chinese hamster cells for stable expression of human cytochrome P4501A2. *Eur. J. Pharmacol.* **228:** 95–102.
26. Crespi, C. L., Penman, B. W., Leakey, J. A. E. *et al.* (1990) Human cytochrome P450IIA3: cDNA sequence, role of the enzyme in the metabolic activation of promutagens, comparison to nitrosamine activation by human cytochrome P450IIE1. *Carcinogenesis* **11:** 1293–1300.
27. Davies, R. L., Crespi, C. L., Rudo, K., Turne, T. R. and Langenbach, R. (1989) Development of a human cell line by selection and drug-metabolizing gene transfection with increased capacity to activate promutagens. *Carcinogenesis* **10:** 885–891.
28. Tiano, H. F., Wang, R.-L., Hosokawa, M., Crespi, C., Tindall, K. R. and Langenbach, R. (1994) Human CYP2A6 activation of 4-(methylnitrosamino)-1-(3-pyridyl)-1-butanone (NNK): mutational specificity in the *gpt* gene of AS52 cells. *Carcinogenesis* **15:** 2859–2866.
29. Tiano, H. F., Hosokawa, M., Chulada, P. C. *et al.* (1993) Retroviral mediated expression of human cytochrome P450 2A6 in C3H/10T1/2 cells confers transformability by 4-(methylnitosamino)-1-(3-pyridyl)-1-butanone (NNK). *Carcinogenesis* **14:** 1421–1427.
30. Salompää, P., Hakkala, J., Pasanen, M. *et al.* (1993) Retrovirus-mediated stable expression of human CYP2A6 in mammalian cells. *Eur. J. Pharmacol.* **248:** 95–102.
31. Crespi, C. L., Penman, B. W., Gelboin, H. V. and Gonzalez, F. J. (1991) A tobacco smoke-derived nitrosamine, 4-(methylnitrosamino)-1-(3-pyridyl)-1-butanone, is activated by multiple human

cytochrome P450s including the polymorphic human cytochrome P4502D6. *Carcinogenesis* **12:** 1197–1201.
32. Penman, B. W., Reece, J., Smith, T. *et al.* (1993) Characterization of a human cell line expressing high levels of cDNA-derived CYP2D6. *Pharmacogenetics* **3:** 28–39.
33. Nouso, K., Thorgeirsson, S. S. and Battula, N. (1992) Stable expression of human cytochrome P450IIE1 in mammalian cells: metabolic activation of nitrosodimethylamine and formation of adducts with cellular DNA. *Cancer Res.* **52:** 1796–1800.
34. Hashimoto, H., Nakagawa, T., Yokoi, T., Sawada, M., Itoh, S. and Kamataki, T. (1995) Fetus-specific CYP3A7 and adult-specific CYP3A4 expressed in chinese hamsters CHL cells have similar capacity to activate carcinogenic mycotoxins. *Cancer Res.* **55:** 787–791.
35. Gonzalez, F. J., Aoyama, T. and Gelboin, H. V. (1991) Expression of mammalian cytochrome P450 using vaccinia virus. *Methods Enzymol.* **206:** 85–92.
36. Crespi, C. L., Langenbach, R. and Penman, B. W. (1993) Human cell lines, derived from AHH-1 TK+/− human lymphoblasts, genetically engineered for expression of cytochromes P450. *Toxicology* **82:** 89–104.
37. Gonzalez, F. J. (1992) Human cytochromes P450: problems and prospects. *TiPS* **13:** 346–352.
38. Hakkola, J., Pasanen, M., Purkunen, R. *et al.* (1994) Expression of xenobiotic-metabolizing cytochrome P450 forms in human adult and fetal liver. *Biochem. Pharmacol.* **48:** 59–64.
39. McKinnon, R. A., Hall, P., Quattrochi, L. C., Tukey, R. H. and McManus, M. E. (1991) Localization of CYP1A1 and CYP1A2 messenger RNA in normal human liver and in hepatocellular carcinoma by *in situ* hybridization. *Hepatology* **14:** 848–856.
40. Anttila, S., Hietanen, E., Vainio, H. *et al.* (1991) Smoking and peripheral type of cancer are related to high levels of pulmonary cytochrome P450IA in lung cancer patients. *Inst. J. Cancer* **47:** 681–685.
41. Shimada, T., Yun, C.-O., Yamazaki, H., Gautier, J.-C., Beaune, P. H. and Guengerich, F. P. (1992) Characterization of human lung microsomal cytochrome P-450 1A1 and its role in the oxidation of chemical carcinogens. *Mol. Pharmacol.* **41:** 856–864.
42. Song, B.-J., Gelboin, H. V. and Park, S. S. (1985) Monoclonal antibody-directed radioimmunoassay detects cytochrome P-450 in human placenta and lymphocytes. *Science* **228:** 490–492.
43. Wong, T. K., Domin, B. A., Bent, P. E., Blanton, T. E., Anderson, M. W. and Philpot, R. M. (1986) Correlation of placental microsomal activities with protein detected by antibodies to rabbit cytochrome P-450 isoenzyme 6 in preparations from human exposed to polychlrorinated biphenyls, quaterphenyls and dibenzofurans. *Cancer Res.* **46:** 999–1004.
44. Vecchini, F., Macé, K., Magdalou, J., Mahe, Y., Bernard, B. A. and Shroot, B. (1995) Constitutive and inducible expression of drug metabolizing enzymes in cultured human keratinocytes. *Br. J. Dermatol.* **132:** 14–22.
45. Wrighton, S. A., Campanile, C., Thomas, P. E. *et al.* (1986) Identification of a human liver cytochrome P-450 homologous to the major isosafrole-inducible cytochrome P-450 in the rat. *Mol. Pharmacol.* **29:** 405–410.
46. Sutter, T. R., Tang, Y. M., Hayes, C. L. *et al.* (1994) Complete cDNA sequence of a human dioxin-inducible mRNA identifies a new gene subfamily of cytochrome P450 that maps to chromosome 2. *J. Biol. Chem.* **269:** 13 092–13 099.
47. Maurice, M., Emiliani, S., Dalet-Beluche, I., Derancourt, J. and Lange, R. (1991) Isolation and characterization of a cytochrome P450 of the IIA subfamily from human liver microsomes. *Eur. J. Biochem.* **200:** 511–517.
48. Yamano, S., Tatsuno, J. and Gonzalez, F. J. (1990) The CYP2A3 gene product catalyzes coumarin 7-hydroxylation in human liver microsomes. *Biochemistry* **29:** 1322–1329.
49. Yun, C.-H., Shimada, T. and Guengerich, F. P. (1991) Purification and characterization of human liver microsomal cytochrome P-450 2A6. *Mol. Pharmacol.* **40:** 679–685.
50. Mimura, M., Baba, T., Yamazaki, H. *et al.* (1993) Characterization of cytochrome P450 2B6 in human liver microsomes. *Drug Metab. Dispos.* **21:** 1048–1056.
51. Romkes, M., Faletto, M. B., Blaisdell, J. A., Raucy, J. L. and Goldstein, J. A. (1991) Cloning and expression of complementary DNAs for multiple members of the human cytochrome P450IIC subfamily. *Biochemistry* **30:** 3247–3255.
52. Wrighton, S. A., Stevens, J. C., Becker, G. W. and VandenBranden, M. (1993) Isolation and characterization of human liver cytochrome P450 2C19: correlation between 2C19 and s-mephenytoin 4/-hydroxylation. *Arch. Biochem. Biophys.* **306:** 240–245.

53. de Waziers, I., Cugnenc, P. H., Yang, C. S., Leroux, J. P. and Beaune, P. H. (1990) Cytochrome P450 isoenzymes, epoxide hydrolase and glutathione transferases in rat and human hepatic and extrahepatic tissues. *J. Pharmacol. Exp. Ther.* **253:** 387–394.
54. Furuya, H., Meyer, U. A., Gelboin, H. V. and Gonzalez, F. J. (1991) Polymerase chain reaction-directed identification, cloning and quantification of human CYP2C18 mRNA. *Mol. Pharmacol.* **40:** 375–382.
55. Distlerath, L. M., Reilly, P. E. B., Martin, M. V., Davis, G. G., Wilkinson, G. R. and Guengerich, F. P. (1985) Purification and characterization of the human liver cytochromes P-450 involved in debrisoquine 4-hydroxylation and phenacetin *O*-deethylation, two prototypes for genetic polymorphism in oxidative drug metabolism. *J. Biol. Chem.* **260:** 9057–9067.
56. Gut, J., Catin, T., Dayers, P., Kronbach, T., Zanger, U. and Meyer, U. A. (1986) Debrisoquine/sparteine-type polymorphism of drug oxidation. *J. Biol. Chem.* **261:** 11 734–11 743.
57. Romkes-Sparks, M., Mnuskin, A., Chern, B.-D. *et al.* (1994) Correlation of polymorphic expression of CYP2D6 mRNA in bladder mucosa and tumor tissue to *in vivo* debrisoquine hydroxylase activity. *Carcinogenesis* **15:** 1955–1961.
58. Rizzeto, M., Swana, G. and Doniach, D. (1973) Microsomal antibodies in active chronic hepatitis and other disorders. *Clin. Exp. Immunol.* **15:** 331–344.
59. Tsutsumi, M., Lasker, J. M., Shimizu, M., Rosman, A. S. and Lieber, C. S. (1989) The intralobular distribution of ethanol-inducible P450IIE1 in rat and human liver. *Hepatology* **10:** 437–446.
60. Umeno, M., McBride, O. W., Yang, C. S., Gelboin, H. V. and Gonzalez, F. J. (1988) Human ethanol-inducible P450IIE1: complete gene sequence promoter, characterization, chromosome mapping and cDNA-directed expression. *Biochemistry* **27:** 9006–9013.
61. Wrighton, S. A., Thomas, P. E., Ryan, D. E. and Levin, W. (1987) Purification and characterization of ethanol-inducible human hepatic cytochrome P-450HLj. *Arch. Biochem. Biophys.* **258:** 292–297.
62. Wheeler, C. W., Wrighton, S. A. and Guenthner, T. M. (1992) Detection of human lung cytochromes P450 that are immunochemically related to cytochrome P450IIE1 and cytochrome P450IIIA. *Biochem. Pharmacol.* **44:** 183–186.
63. Nhamburo, P. T., Kimura, S., McBride, O. W., Kozak, C. A., Gelboin, H. V. and Gonzalez, F. J. (1990) The human CYP2F subfamily: identification of a cDNA coding for a new cytochrome P450 expressed in lung, cDNA-directed expression and chromosome mapping. *Biochemistry* **29:** 5491–5499.
64. Guengerich, F. P., Martin, M. V., Beaune, P., Kremers, P., Wolff, T. and Waxman, D. J. (1986) Characterization of the rat and human microsomal cytochrome P450 forms involved in nifedipine oxidation, a prototype for genetic polymorphism in oxidative drug metabolism. *J. Biol. Chem.* **261:** 5051–5060.
65. McKinnon, R. A., Burgess, W. M., de la M Hall, P., Roberts-Thomson, S. J., Gonzalez, F. J. and McManus, M. E. (1995) Characterisation of CYP3A gene subfamily expression in human gastrointestinal tissues. *Gut* **36:** 259–267.
66. McKinnon, R. A., Burgess, W. M., Gonzalez, F. J. and McManus, M. E. (1993) Metabolic differences in colon mucosa cells. *Mutat. Res.* **290:** 27–33.
67. Li, X. Y., Duell, E., Oin, L., Watkins, P. B. and Voorhees, J. J. (1994) Cytochrome P450 3A5 is the major 3A subfamily member expressed in normal human skin *in vivo*. *J. Invest. Dermatol.* **102:** 624.
68. Aoyama, T., Yamano, S., Waxman, D. J. *et al.* (1989) Cytochrome P-450 hPCN3, a novel cytochrome P-450 IIIA gene product that is differentially expressed in adult human liver: cDNA and deduced amino acid sequence and distinct specificities of cDNA-expressed hPCN1 and hPCN3 for the metabolism of steroid hormones and cyclosporine. *J. Biol. Chem.* **264:** 10 388–10 395.
69. Wrighton, S. A., Brian, W. R., Sari, M.-A. *et al.* (1990) Studies on the expression and metabolic capabilities of human liver cytochrome P450IIIA5 (HLp3). *Mol. Pharmacol.* **38:** 207–213.
70. Wrighton, S. A., Ring, B. J., Watkins, P. B. and VandenBranden, M. (1989) Identification of a polymorphically expressed member of the human cytochrome P-450III family. *J. Biol. Chem.* **36:** 97–105.
71. Kitada, M., Kato, T., Ohmori, S. *et al.* (1992) Immunochemical characterization and toxicological significance of P-450HFLb purified from human fetal livers. *Biochem. Biophys. Acta* **1117:** 301–305.
72. Schuetz, J. D., Kauma, S. and Guzelian, P. S. (1993) Identification of the fetal liver cytochrome CYP3A7 in human endometrium and placenta. *J. Clin. Invest.* **92:** 1018–1024.

73. Nhamburo, P. T., Gonzalez, F. J., McBride, O. W., Gelboin, H. V. and Kimura, S. (1989) Identification of a new P450 expressed in human lung: complete cDNA sequence, cDNA-directed expression and chromosome mapping. *Biochemistry* **28:** 8060–8066.
74. Shimada, T., Yamazaki, H., Mimura, M., Inui, Y. and Guengerich, F. P. (1994) Interindividual variations in human liver cytochrome P-450 enzymes involved in the oxidation of drugs, carcinogens and toxic chemicals: studies with liver microsomes of 30 Japanese and 30 Caucasians. *J. Pharmacol. Exp. Ther.* **270:** 414–423.
75. Gonzalez, F. J., Crespi, C. L. and Gelboin, H. V. (1991) cDNA-expressed human cytochrome P450s: a new age of molecular toxicology and human risk assessment. *Mutat. Res.* **247:** 113–127.
76. Rettie, A. E., Eddy, A. C., Heimark, L. D., Gibaldi, M. and Tragger, W. F. (1989) Characteristics of warfarin hydroxylation catalyzed by human liver microsomes. *Drug Metab. Dispos.* **253:** 7813–7820.
77. Castro, V. M., Söserstöm, M., Carlberg, I., Widersten, M., Platz, A. and Mannervik, B. (1990) Differences among human tumor cell lines in the expression of glutathione transferases and other glutathione-linked enzymes. *Carcinogenesis* **11:** 1569–1576.
78. Grant, M. H., Duthie, S. J., Gray, A. G. and Burke, M. D. (1988) Mixed function oxidase and UDP-glucuronyltransferase activities in the human Hep G2 hepatoma cell line. *Biochem. Pharmacol.* **37:** 4111–4116.
79. Walle, T., Walle, U. K., Shwed, J. A., Thornburg, K. R., Mathis, C. E. and Pesola, G. R. (1994) Human phenolsulfotransferases: chiral substrates and expression in Hep G2 cells. *Chem. Biol. Interact.* **92:** 47–55.
80. Coroneos, E. and Sim, E. (1993) Arylamine *N*-acetyltransferase activity in human cultured cell lines. *Biochem. J.* **294:** 481–486.
81. Langenbach, R., Smith, P. B. and Crespi, C. (1992) Recombinant DNA approaches for the development of metabolic systems used in *in vitro* toxicology. *Mutat. Res.* **277:** 251–275.
82. Yates, J. L., Warren, N. and Sugden, B. (1985) Stable replication of plasmids derived from Epstein–Barr virus in various mammalian cells. *Nature* **313:** 812–815.
83. Crespi, C. L., Seixas, G. M., Turner, T. R., Ryan, C. G. and Penman, B. W. (1985) Mutagenicity of 1,2-dichloroethane and 1,2-dibromoethane in two human lymphoblastoid cell lines. *Mutat. Res.* **142:** 133–140.
84. Crespi, C. L., Altman, J. F. and Marletta, M. A. (1985) Xenobiotic metabolism and mutation in a human lymphoblastoid cell line. *Chem. Biol. Interact.* **53:** 257–272.
85. Sladek, N. E. (1988) Metabolism of oxazaphosphorines. *Pharmacol. Ther.* **37:** 301–355.
86. Chang, T. K. H., Weber, G. F., Crespi, C. L. and Waxman, D. J. (1993) Differential activation of cyclophosphamide and ifosphamide by cytochromes P450-2B and 3A in human liver microsomes. *Cancer Res.* **53:** 5629–5637.
87. Guengerich, F. P. (1991) Oxidation of toxic and carcinogenic chemicals by human cytochrome P-450 enzymes. *Chem. Res. Toxicol.* **4:** 391–407.
88. Shimada, T. and Guengerich, F. P. (1989) Evidence for cytochrome P-450NF, the nifedipine oxidase, being the principal enzyme involved in the bioactivation of aflatoxins in human liver. *Proc. Natl Acad. Sci. U.S.A.* **86:** 462–465.
89. Gallagher, E. P., Wienkers, L. C., Stapleton, P. L., Kunze, K. L. and Eaton, D. L. (1994) Role of human microsomal and human complementary DNA-expressed cytochromes P4501A2 and P4503A4 in the bioactivation of aflatoxin B_1. *Cancer Res.* **54:** 101–108.
90. Hecht, S. S. and Hoffmann, D. (1988) Tobacco-specific nitrosamines, an important group of carcinogens in tobacco and tobacco smoke. *Carcinogenesis* **9:** 875–884.
91. Yamazaki, H., Inui, Y., Yun, C.-H., Guengerich, F. P. and Shimada, T. (1992) Cytochrome P450 2E1 and 2A6 enzymes as major catalysts for metabolic activation of *N*-nitrosodialkylamines and tobacco-related nitrosamines in human liver microsomes. *Carcinogenesis* **13:** 1789–1794.
92. Smith, T. J., Guo, Z. G., Gonzalez, F. J., Guengerich, P., Stoner, G. D. and Yang, C. S. (1992) Metabolism of 4-(methylnitrosamino)-1-(3-pyridyl)-1-butanone in human lung and liver microsomes and cytochromes P-450 expressed in hepatoma cells. *Cancer Res.* **52:** 1757–1763.
93. Ayesh, R., Idle, J. R., Ritchie, J. C., Crothers, M. J. and Hetzel, M. R. (1984) Metabolic oxidation phenotypes as markers for susceptibility to lung cancer. *Nature* **312:** 169–170.
94. Caporaso, N., Hayes, R. B., Dosemeci, J. *et al.* (1989) Lung cancer risk, occupational exposure and the debrisoquine metabolic phenotype. *Cancer Res.* **49:** 3675–3679.
95. McLemore, T. L., Adelberg, S., Liu, M. C. *et al.* (1990) Expression of CYP4501A1 gene in patients with lung cancer: evidence for cigarette smoke-induced gene expression in normal lung

tissue and for altered gene regulation in primary pulmonary carcinomas. *J. Natl Cancer Inst.* **82:** 1333–1339.

96. Petruzzelli, S., Camus, A.-M., Carrozzi, L. *et al.* (1988) Long-lasting effects of tobacco smoking on pulmonary drug-metabolizing enzymes: a case–control study on lung cancer patients. *Cancer Res.* **48:** 4695–4700.
97. Crofton-Sleigh, C., Doherty, A., Ellard, S., Parry, J. M. and Vennit, S. (1993) Micronucleus assays using cytochalasin-blocked MCL-5 cells, a proprietary human cell line expressing five human cytochromes P-450 microsomal epoxide hydrolase. *Mutagenesis* **8:** 363–372.
98. Tohda, H., Horaguchi, K., Takahashi, K., Oikawa, A. and Matsushima, T. (1980) Epstein–Barr virus-transformed human lymphoblastoid cells for study of sister chromatid exchange and their evaluation as a test system. *Cancer Res.* **40:** 4775–4780.
99. Reddel, R. R., Ke, Y., Gerwin, B. I. *et al.* (1988) Transformation of human bronchial epithelial cells by infection with SV40 or adenovirus-12 SV40 hybrid virus, or transfection via strontium phosphate coprecipitation with a plasmid containing SV40 early region genes. *Cancer Res.* **48:** 1904–1909.
100. Amstad, P., Reddel, R. R., Pfeifer, A., Malan-Shibley, L., Mark, G. E. and Harris, C. C. (1988) Neoplastic transformation of a human bronchial epithelial cell line by a recombinant retrovirus encoding viral harvey *ras. Mol. Carcinog.* **1:** 151–160.
101. Gerwin, B. L., Spillare, E., Forrester, K. *et al.* (1992) Mutant p53 can induce tumorigenic conversion of human bronchial epithelial cells and reduce their responsiveness to a negative growth factor, transforming growth factor b_1. *Proc. Natl Acad. Sci. U.S.A.* **89:** 2759–2763.
102. Pfeifer, A., Lechner, J. F., Masui, T., Reddel, R. R., Mark, G. E. and Harris, C. C. (1989) Control of growth and squamous differentiation in normal human bronchial epithelial cells by chemical and biological modifiers and transferred genes. *Environ. Health. Perspect.* **80:** 209–220.
103. Pfeifer, A., Mark, G. E., Malan-Shibley, L., Graziano, S. L., Amstad, P. and Harris, C. C. (1989) Cooperation of c-*ras-1* and c-*myc* protooncogenes in the neoplastic transformation of SV40 T-antigen immortalized human bronchial epithelial cells. *Proc. Natl Acad. Sci. U.S.A.* **86:** 10 075–10 079.
104. Iiazasa, T., Momiki, S., Bauer, B. *et al.* (1993) Invasive tumors derived from xenotransplanted, immortalized human cells after *in vivo* exposure to chemical carcinogenesis. *Carcinogenesis* **14:** 1789–1794.
105. Klein-Szanto, A. J. P., Iizasa, T., Momiki, S. *et al.* (1992) A tobacco-specific *N*-nitrosamine or cigarette smoke condensate causes neoplastic transformation of xenotransplanted human bronchial epithelial cells. *Proc. Natl Acad. Sci. U.S.A.* **89:** 6693–6697.
106. Offord, E. A., Macé, K., Ruffieux, C., Malnoë, A. and Pfeifer, A. M. A. (1995) Rosemary components inhibit benzo(a)pyrene-induced genotoxicity in human bronchial cells. *Carcinogenesis,* **16:** 2057–2062.
107. Landegren, U. (1984) Measurement of cell numbers by means of the endogenous enzyme hexosaminidase. Applications to detection of lymphokines and cell surface antigens. *J. Immunol. Methods* **67:** 379–388.
108. Autrup, H., Essigmann, J. M., Croy, R. G., Trump, B. F., Wogan, G. N. and Harris, C. C. (1979) Metabolism of aflatoxin B_1 and identification of the major aflatoxin B_1-DNA adducts formed in cultured human bronchus and colon. *Cancer Res.* **39:** 694–698.
109. Ho, C.-T., Ferraro, T., Chen, Q., Rosen, R. T. and Huang, M.-T. (1994) Phytochemicals in teas and rosemary and their cancer-preventive properties. In Ho, C.-T., Osawa, T., Huang, M.-T. and Rosen, R. T. (eds) *Food Phytochemicals for Cancer Prevention II*, pp. 2–19. American Chemical Society, Washington, D.C.
110. Ura, H., Bonfil, R. D., Reich, R. *et al.* (1989) Expression of type IV collagenase and procollagen genes and its correlation with the tumorigenic, invasive and metastatic abilities of oncogene-transformed human bronchial epithelial cells. *Cancer Res.* **49:** 4615–4621.
111. Ke, Y., Gerwin, B. I., Ruskie, S. E., Pfeifer, A. M. A., Harris, C. C. and Lechner, J. F. (1990) Cell density governs the ability of human bronchial epithelial cells to recognize serum and transforming growth factor beta-1 as squamous differentiation-inducing agents. *Am. J. Pathol.* **137:** 833–843.
112. Decker, T. and Lohmann-Matthes, M.-L. (1988) A quick and simple method for quantitation of lactate dehydrogenase release in measurements of cellular cytotoxicity and tumor necrosis factor (TNF) activity. *J. Immunol. Methods* **115:** 61–69.
113. Essig-Marcello, J. S. and Van Buskirk, R. G. (1990) A double-label *in situ* cytotoxicity assay using the fluorescent probes neutral red and BCEFC-AM. *In Vitro Toxicol.* **3:** 219–227.

114. Soclum, H. K., Tòth, K., Li, L., Chang, S.-G., Hoffman, R. B. and Rustum, Y. M. (1992) Long-term passage of human tissues *in vitro* as three-dimensional histolines. *In Vitro Cell. Dev. Biol.* **28A:** 573–577.
115. Borenfreund, E. and Puerner, J. A. (1984) A simple quantitative procedure using monolayer cultures for cytotoxicity assays. *J. Tissue Culture Methods* **9:** 7–9.
116. Lachowiez, R. M., Clayton, B., Thallman, K., Dix, J. and Van Buskirk, R. G. (1989) Rhodamine 123 as a probe of *in vitro* toxicity in MDCK cells. *Cytotechnology* **2:** 203–211.
117. Mossmann, T. (1983) A simple quantitative procedure using monolayer cultures for cytotoxicity assays. *J. Immunol. Methods* **65:** 55–63.
118. Tchao, R. (1988) Transepithelial permeability of fluorescein *in vitro* as an assay to determining eye irritants. *Prog. In Vitro Toxicol.* **6:** 271–283.
119. Todd, M. D., Lee, M. J. and Williams, J. L. (1995) The CAT-Tox (L) assay: a sensitive and specific measure of stress-induced transcription in transformed human liver cells. *Fundamental Appl. Toxicol.* **28:** 118–128.
120. Heddle, J. A., Hite, M., Kirkhart, B. *et al.* (1983) The induction of micronuclei as a measure of genotoxicity. A report of the U.S. Environmental Protection Agency Gene-Tox Program. *Mutat. Res.* **123:** 61–118.
121. Tucker, J. D., Auletta, A., Cimino, M. C. *et al.* (1993) Sister-chromatid exchange: second report of the Gene-Tox program. *Mutat. Res.* **297:** 101–180.
122. Fairbain, D. W., Olive, P. L. and O'Neill, K. L. (1995) The comet assay: a comprehensive review. *Mutat. Res.* **339:** 37–59.
123. Beach, A. C. and Gupta, R. C. (1992) Human biomonitoring and the ^{32}P-postlabeling assay. *Carcinogenesis* **13:** 1053–1074.
124. Kaderlik, R. K., Lin, D.-X., Lang, N. P. and Kadlubar, F. F. (1992) Advantages and limitations of laboratory methods for measurement of carcinogen–DNA adducts for epidemiological studies. *Toxicol. Lett.* **64/65:** 469–475.
125. Sharma, S., Stutzman, J. D., Kelloff, G. J. and Steele, V. E. (1994) Screening potential chemopreventive agents using biochemical markers of carcinogenesis. *Cancer Res.* **54:** 5848–5855.
126. Strauss, G. H. and Albertini, R. J. (1979) Enumeration of 6-thioguanine-resistant peripheral blood lymphocytes in man as a potential test for somatic cell mutations arising *in vivo. Mutat. Res.* **61:** 353–379.
127. Crespi, C. and Thilly, W. G. (1984) Assay for gene mutation in human lymphoblast line, AHH-1, competent for xenobiotic metabolism. *Mutat. Res.* **128:** 221–230.
128. Furth, E. E., Thilly, W. G., Penman, B. W., Liber, H. L. and Rand, W. M. (1981) Quantitative assay for mutation in diploid human lymphoblasts using microtiter plates. *Anal. Biochem.* **110:** 1–8.
129. Johnson, G. G. and Littlefield, J. W. (1979) Assay of hypoxanthine–guanine phosporibosyl-transferase in human fibroblast lysates: inactivation of nucleotidase. *Anal. Biochem.* **92:** 403–410.
130. Bookland, E. A., Reznikoff, C. A., Lindstrom, M. and Swaminathan, S. (1992) Induction of thioguanine-resistant mutations in human uroepithelial cells by 4-aminobiphenyl and its *n*-hydroxy derivatives. *Cancer Res.* **52:** 1615–1621.
131. Allen-Hoffmann, B. L. and Rheinwald, J. G. (1984) Polycyclic aromatic hydrocarbon mutagenesis of human epidermal keratinocytes in culture. *Proc. Natl Acad. Sci. U.S.A.* **81:** 7802–7806.
132. Felley-Bosco, E., Mirkovitch, J., Ambs, S. *et al.* (1995) Nitric oxide and ethylnitrosurea: relative mutagenicity in the p53 tumor suppressor and hypoxanthine-phosphoribosyltransferase genes. *Carcinogenesis* **16:** 2069–2074
133. Trottier, Y., Walthe, W. I. and Anderson, A. (1992) Kinds of mutations induced by aflatoxin B_1 in a shuttle vector replicating in human cells transiently expressing cytochrome P4501A2 cDNA. *Mol. Carcinog.* **6:** 140–147.
134. Harris, C. C. (1993) p53: at the crossroads of molecular carcinogenesis and risk assessment. *Science* **262:** 1980–1981.
135. Aguilar, F., Hussain, S. P. and Cerutti, P. (1993) Aflatoxin B_1 induces the transversion of GT in codon 249 of the p53 tumor suppressor gene in human hepatocytes. *Proc. Natl Acad. Sci. U.S.A.* **90:** 8586–8590.
136. Hsu, I. C., Metcalf, R. A., Sun, T., Welsh, J. A., Wang, N. J. and Harris, C. C. (1991) Mutational hotspot in the p53 gene in human hepatocellular carcinomas. *Nature* **350:** 427–428.

137. Crespi, C. L., Gonzalez, F. J., Steimel, D. T. *et al.* (1991) A metabolically competent human cell line expressing five cDNAs encoding procarcinogen-activating enzymes: application to mutagenicity testing. *Chem. Res. Toxicol.* **4:** 566–572.
138. Pfeifer, A. M. A., Cole, K. E., Smoot, D. T. *et al.* (1993) Simian virus 40 large tumor antigen-immortalized normal human liver epithelial cells express hepatocyte characteristics and metabolize chemical carcinogens. *Proc. Natl Acad. Sci. U.S.A.* **90:** 5123–5127.
139. Pfeifer, A. M. A., Macé, K., Tromvoukis, Y. and Lipsky, M. M. (1995) Highly efficient establishment of immortalized cells from adult human liver. *Methods Cell Sci.* **17:** 83–89.
140. Sack, G. H. (1981) Human cell transformation by simian virus 40: a review. *In vitro* **17:** 1–19.
141. Woodworth, C. D., Kreider, J. W., Mengel, L., Miller, T., Meng, Y. L. and Isom, H. C. (1988) Tumoriginicity of simian virus 40-hepatocyte cell lines: effect of *in vitro* an *in vivo* passage on expression of liver-specific genes and oncogenes. *Mol. Cell. Biol.* **8:** 4492–4501.
142. Ke, Y., Reddel, R. R., Gerwin, B. I. *et al.* (1988) Human bronchial epithelial cells with integrated SV40 virus T antigen genes retain the ability to undergo sqamous differentiation. *Differentiation* **38:** 60–66.
143. Stoner, G. D., Kaighn, M. E., Reddel, R. R. *et al.* (1991) Establishment and characterization of SV40 T-antigen immortalized human esophageal epithelial cells. *Cancer Res.* **51:** 365–371.
144. Woodworth, C., Secott, T. and Isom, H. C. (1986) Transformation of rat hepatocytes by transfection with simian virus 40 DNA to yield proliferating differentiated cells. *Cancer Res.* **46:** 4018–4026.
145. Wyllie, F. S., Bond, J. A., Dawson, T., White, D., Davies, R. and Wynford-Thomas, D. (1992) A phenotypically and karyotypically stable human thyroid epithelial line conditionally immortalized by SV40 large T antigen. *Cancer Res.* **52:** 2938–2945.
146. Kulkarni, P. S., Sundqvist, K., Belshotltz, C. *et al.* (1995) Characteristics of human buccal epithelial cells transfected with SV40 large T-antigen gene. *Carcinogenesis* **16:** 2515–2521.
147. Burchell, B., Ebner, T., Baird, S. *et al.* (1994) Use of cloned and expressed human liver UDP-glucuronyltransferases for analysis of drug glucuronide formation and assessment of drug toxicity. *Environ. Health Perspect.* **102 (supplement 9):** 19–23.
148. Otterness, D. M., Wieben, E. D., Wood, T. C. *et al.* (1992) Human liver dehydroepiandosterone sulfotransferase: molecular cloning and expression of cDNA. *Mol. Pharmacol.* **41:** 865–872.

Index

A431 cells, 311
acetaminophen
  metabolism by hepatocytes, 418
  nephrotoxicity, 69
2-acetyl-aminofluorene, 120
N-acetyl-m-aminophenol, hepatotoxicity, 393
N-acetyl-β-glucosaminidase, in isolated perfused kidney, 69
N-acetyltransferase (NAT), expression in mammalian cells, 438
acrylamide, 164
Alamar blue test, cytotoxicity testing, 69
albumin
  metabolic parameter of toxicity, 397
  synthesis by cultured hepatocytes, 146
alcohol, see ethanol, 69
alginate culture matrix
  in chondrocytes, 188
  in hepatocytes, 414
allergic hepatitis, 396
allyl alcohol, 117
Alzheimer's diseases, 166
Ames test, genotoxicity testing, 325
4-aminobiphenyl, 120
p-aminohippurate, transport, renal slices, 70
amino-3-hydroxy-5-methyl-4-isoxazole, neurotoxicity, 161
aminoglycosides, nephrotoxicity, 82
aminonicotinamide, teratogenicity, 362
amphetamine
  metabolism, 423
  neurotoxicity, 169
β-amyloid protein, association with neurotoxicity, 169
Anchorin CII, extracellular matrix, in cartilage, 184
Anthracyclins
  hepatotoxicity, 119
  metabolism, 423
α1-antichymotrypsin, synthesis by hepatocytes, 146
antimicrobial agents, *in vitro* screening guidelines, 10–11
α1-antitrypsin, synthesis by hepatocytes, 146
apoptosis
  bcl-2 protein expression, 174
  hepatotoxicity, 377
  neurotoxicity, 17, 157, 174
    measurement, 174
  of neural cells, 16, 157
  and oxidative stress in neural cells, 162
arachidonic acid, in cutaneous models, 258
Aroclor 1254, 118
arylhydrocarbon hydroxylase, biotransformation enzyme, 140
2-arylpopionic acids, photosensitization by, 304
arylsulphatase, 141
astrocytes
  culture, 167
  membrane potential, 167
ATP measurement, luciferin–luciferase assay, 381
ATPase, neurotoxicity, 167
ATPase (Ca^2+), hepatotoxicity, 387
axonal transport, 170

bacterial gene mutation test, in genotoxicity testing, 33, 324
Balb/C 3T3 cells, use in phototoxicity testing, 34, 310
BAPTA, (1,2-bis(O-aminophenoxy)ethane-N, N,N′,N′tetraacetic acid tetra-[acetoxymethyl]-ester), 169
B-cell lymphocytes, 227
bcl-2 protein, 174
BEAS-2B cells, 434, 440–442
benoxaprofen
  effects on cartilage cultures, 198
  phototoxicity, 305
bile acids, nephrotoxicity, 85
Biotransformation activities, 139–144
  alkoxyresorufin-O-dealkylase, 140
  arylhydrocarbon hydroxylase, 147
  coumarin 7-hydroxylase, 141
  CYP450, 143, 147
  epoxide hydrolase, 143
  ethoxyresorufin-O-de-ethylase, 418, 420, 422
  7-ethoxycoumarin-*O*-de-ethylase, 143
  glutathione S-transferase, 142, 143
  7-methoxycoumarin-O-demethylase, 147
  NADPH-cytochrome c reductase, 143–144
  p-nitrophenol hydroxylase, 141
  testosterone hydroxylation, 141
  UDP-glucuronyl transferase, 142, 143
bovine cornea opacity test (BCOP), 274–275
brain cell aggregates, use in teratogenicity testing, 355
brain slices, 169
brain-derived neurotrophic factor (BDNF), 158
bromobenzene
  covalent binding, 383
  hepatotoxicity, 117
t-butyl hydroperoxide, lipid peroxidation induction, 384

C3H/10T1/2 cells, 435
cadherin, 158
cadmium, teratogenicity, 362
caffeine, teratogenicity, 362
calcein, cytotoxicity testing, 215
calcium, 387–392
  cellular homeostasis, 388
  channels, 388
    ligand-operated, 389
    voltage-dependent, 389
  hepatotoxicity, 391
  intracellular increase, 386
  measurement, 390
    fluo-3, 390
    fluo-3-AM, 390
    fura-2, 390
    indo-1, 390
    quin-2, 390
  pumps, 39, 17
CAMVA test, *see also* HET-CAM test, 272–274
Candida albicans, in phototoxicity testing, 301, 310
carbonylcyanid-p-trifluoromethoxyphenyl-hydrazone, 160
Carboxyseminapthorhodofluor-1 (SNARF), assessment of intracellular pH changes, in myocytes, 220
Carboxyseminapthorhodofluor-1 (SNARF), in neurones, 172
cardiac myocytes, 210–222, 215–221
  calcium homeostasis, 221
  cell viability, 215
  cellular energy capacity, 218
  contractile activity, 217
  cultures, 213–215
    adult rabbit, 214
    rat neonatal, 211–213
  mitochondrial function, membrane potential, 218
    proton motive force, 220
  reactive oxygen species, 217
  succinate dehydrogenase activity, 218
cartilage oligomeric matrix protein (COMP), 184
CAT-Tox assay, cytotoxicity testing, 446
cell adhesion molecules (CAM's), 158
  cadherin, 158
  collagen, 183, 244
  fibronectin, 146, 184
cell culture 35–42
  addition of chemicals to cultures, 49
    micronization, 49
    organic solvents, 49
    paraffin oil overlay, 50
    solubilization, 49
    sonication, 50
  cardiac myocytes, 22, 210
  chondrocytes, 184–195
  culture monitoring, 35, 36
    contact inhibition, 37
    growth, 36–38
    karyotyping, 36
    population doubling level, 36
    viability, 37
  fibroblasts, 3, 31
  finite cell lines, 35
  hepatocytes, 107–111, 131–148, 414
  keratinocytes, 245–249
  neuronal cells, 159–170
  perfused cell systems, 36
  renal cells, 62–64, 74–78
  skin cells, 242–250
cell lines in irritation testing, 46–48
  use in target organ toxicity, 40, 44–48
cephaloride, 70
cephalosporin, 71–72
c-*fos* expression, in hepatotoxicity, 412
c-*fos* expression, in neurotoxicity, 173
chaperonins, 173
chicken embryo teratogenicity testing, 356, 358–362
    advantages, 360
    culture, 359
    special studies, 360
chicken enucleated eye test (CEET), ocular irritation testing, 276–277
CHL cells, use in genotoxicity, 328
1-chloro-2,4-dinitrobenzene, 142, 418
chloroform, hepatotoxicity, 81
chlorpromazine hepatotoxicity, 106
  phototoxicity, 296
chlorzoxazone 6-hydroxylation, metabolism, 419
CHO cells, use in genotoxicity, 328
cholestasis, 395
chondrocytes, 184–195
  cartilage slices, 186
  immortalized, 189
  pharmacotoxicological effects, 196–198
    of anti-osteoarthritic drugs, 198
    of cytokines, 197
    of growth factors, 196
    of hormones, 196
    of non-steroidal anti-inflammatory drugs, 198
    of vitamins, 190–195, 197
    alkaline phosphatase, 196
    collagen, 192–195
      chains analysis, 193
      gene expression, 195
      global synthesis, 193
      immunological methods, 194
    proteoglycans, 191
      Alcian blue staining, 191
      prostaglandins synthesis, 191
  types of culture aggregate suspension, 189
    alginate beds, 188
    monolayer, 186
    suspension, 188
    three-dimensional, 188
chondronectin, 184
chorion allantoic membrane test (CAMVA), *see also* HET-CAM test, 274

chromosome aberrations, genotoxicity testing, 331
ciliary neurotrophic factor (CNTF), neutotoxicity, 158
cisplatin, 71–72
c-*jun* expression, neurotoxicity, 173
Clara cells, in lung toxicity testing, 46
clofibric acid, enzyme induction, 419
c-*myc* expression, hepatocytes, 412
cocaine, hepatotoxicity, 116, 119
co-cultures hepatocytes, 414, 417, 422, 423
  keratinocytes, 246
  neuronal cells, 17, 167
COLIPA, 300
collagen binding protein, 184
collagen solution, preparation from rat tail, 244
comet assay, genotoxicity testing, 446
computer-aided drug selection and design (CADD), 4
confocal microscopy, 219, 220, 221
COS cells, 435
coumarin 7-hydroxylase, biotransformation activity, 141
covalent binding, 392–395
  drug-protein adducts, 392
  hepatotoxicity, 393
  immunological detection of drug adducts, 394
  measurement, 393
cryopreservation, hepatocytes, 42, 160, 412, 415
cutaneous metabolism, 254–255
  models, 242–250
    dermal equivalents 242–244
    dermis, 244
    epidermis, 244–249
    excised skin, 250
    keratinocytes, 245–249
    metabolism by CYP450, 254
    metabolism by phase II enzymes, 254
    reconstructed skin, 249
  pharmacotoxicology, 250–260
    drug metabolism, 253–255
    tests for inflammatory processes, 258
    percutaneous absorption, 250–253
  toxicology, 255–260
    cytotoxicity tests, 256
    effects on differentiated functions, 257
cyclic AMP, 163
cyclosporin A, 78, 424
Cyp1a1/2, 392
Cyp1a2, 44, 140, 145, 416, 421, 434
Cyp2a6, 140, 437
Cyp2b1/2, 414, 416
Cyp2b6, 44, 140, 141, 145, 434
Cyp2c, 44, 393, 421, 434
Cyp2c11, 416
Cyp2c13, 416
Cyp2c8-9, 140
Cyp2c9, 437
Cyp2d6, 44, 434
Cyp2e1, 44, 140, 141, 415, 421, 434
Cyp2f1, 434–444
Cyp3a, 44, 421, 424, 434
Cyp3a1-3, 416
Cyp3a1/2, 416
Cyp3a3-5, 140, 142, 145
Cyp cutaneous models, 254
  distribution in human tissues, 436
  expression vectors, 442
  expression in mammalian cells, 437–445
    use in genotoxicity, 446
    use in metabolism studies, 445
  hepatocytes, 115, 416–419
  human hepatocytes, 139–144
  liver slices 115
Cyp4b1 44, 434
cytochrome b5 438
cytochrome P450, *see corresponding* CYP450s, 254
cytogenetic damage, 328–331
cytokines, 145, 229–231
  G-CSF, 231
  GM-CSF, 231
  interleukin 1, 228
  interleukin 2, 230
  interleukin 3, 230
  interleukin 4, 230
  interleukin 5, 230
  interleukin 6, 145, 146, 230
  interleukin 7, 230
  interleukin 8, 230
  interleukin 9, 230
  interleukin 10, 230
  interleukin 11, 230
  interleukin 12, 230
  interleukin 13, 230
  interleukin 14, 230
cytotoxicity testing, hepatocytes, 397–401
  Alamar blue, 69
  ATP levels hepatotoxicity, 379
    neurotoxicity, 171
  ATP production by mitochondria, 381
  Balb/C 3T3 cells, 42
  BCECF test, 215
  cardiomyocytes, 215–221
  CAT-Tox, 446
  cell division, 38
  cell growth, 38
  cell lines, 41
  cell metabolism, 38
  cell morphology, 38
  cell proliferation, 257
  cell staining, 38
  cutaneous models, 255–260
  DNA synthesis, 257, 305
  fluorescein leakage, 42
  hexosaminidase, 446
  Kenacid blue, 42
  lactate dehydrogenase, in cutaneous toxicity, 256
    in hepatotoxicity, 398

CAT-Tox *cont.*
in myocytes, 215
in neuronal cells, 168
in phototoxicity, 31, 304
LS-L929 cells, 42
membrane damage, 38
mitochondrial function, membrane potential, 380, 381
MTT, 42–43, 64, 109, 170, 218, 304, 398, 446
neuronal models, 170–175
neutral red, 31, 41, 42, 171, 256, 277, 304, 398, 446
pollen tube growth assay, 42
propidium iodide, 215, 446
renal models, 59–66
rhodamine-123, 446
sodium fluorescein, 446
lysosome function, neutral red assay, 38
V79 cells, 42
XTT 43

dermal equivalents, 242–244, 280
Bell's model, 244
Naughton model, 244
dermatitis, 256
dermis enzymatic dissociation, 243
isolation of fibroblasts, 242
dexamethasone enzyme inducer, 362
in culture medium, 134
dextrometorphan, metabolism, 418
diazepam, hepatotoxicity, 423
diclofenac protein adducts, 394
hepatotoxicity, 392–394
dihydralazine, 419
diisopropyl phosphorofluoridate, neurotoxicity, 163
2,4-dinitrophenyl-glutathione, 142
2′,7′-dichlorofluorescin, 217
DNA adduct formation genotoxicity, 332
phototoxicity, 446
damage, 331–334
mutagenesis, use of shuttle vectors, 447
photocleavage, 304
repair, genotoxicity, 333
Draize's eye test, ocular irritation, 265–271
Drosophila embryo, teratogenicity testing, 356
Drosophila embryonic cell, teratogenicity testing, 354
drug bioactivation, 377
drug metabolism, first-pass effect, 401
drug-metabolizing enzymes, 417–422
drug-metabolizing enzymes, inducers and inhibitors, 417–422
drug-metabolizing enzymes, metabolic rates, 422
drug-metabolizing enzymes, profiles, 422

ECVAM, (European Centre for the Validation of Alternative Methods), 26
elutriation, cardiac myocytes, 212
embryonic stem cell, teratogenicity testing, 355
engineered cells, *see also* Genetically engineered cells
expression vectors, 441
expression of human CYPs, 444
liposome-transfection, 442
mammalian cells used for cDNA expression of human CYPs, 435
enzyme inducers, clofibric acid, 419
dihydralazine, 419
ethanol, 419
isosafrole, 419
lovastatin, 419
methylcholantrene, 419
omeprazole, 419
phenobarbital, 118
rifampicin, 419
β-naftoflavone, 118
epidermal growth factor (EGF), 145
epoxides, covalent binding, 392
epoxide hydrolase, biotransformation enzyme, 143
erythromycin, hepatotoxicity, 396
Escherichia coli, genotoxicity testing, 324
ethanol, enzyme inducer, 419
7-ethoxycoumarin-*O*-de-ethylase (ECOD), biotransformation enzyme, 255
ethoxyresorufin-*O*-de-ethylase (EROD), biotransformation enzyme, 418, 420, 422
ethylene bromide, covalent binding, 121
Euro–Collins, 412
extracellular matrix cartilage matric glycoprotein (CMGP), 184
cartilage matrix protein (CMP), 184
cartilage oligomeric matrix protein (COMP), 184
collagen, 183
collagen binding protein, 184
fibronectin, 46–184
in neuronal models, 158
laminin, 158
proteoglycans, 183
EYTEX test, ocular irritation testing, 42, 47

fenfluramine, 169
fibroblast growth factor (FGF), 161
fibroblasts cell culture, 245–249
in cytotoxicity testing, 31, 304
fish embryo, teratogenicity testing, 356
flash photolysis, 295
flavin adenine dinucleotide mono-oxygenase (FMN), 391
fluo-3, 390
fluo-3-AM, 390
fluorescein leakage test, ocular irritation, 279
fluoroquinolones, chondrocytes, 198
fluperlapine, hepatotoxicity, 423
forskolin, neurotoxicity, 163

FRAME (Fund for the Replacement of Animals in Medical Experiments), 1
frog embryo, teratogenicity testing, 356
fructose, hepatotoxicity, 380
fura-2, 390
furosemide, nephrotoxicity, 72

GABA, neurotoxicity, 174
galactosamine, hepatotoxicity, 379
G-CSF, 231
gene mutation, tests, 326–331
genetically engineered cells, 437–445
applications, 445
bronchial cells, 440–445
human lymphoblast cell system, 438
limitations, 447
mutational studies in CYP450-expressing cells, 439
organ specificity, 448
toxicological testing, 446
genetically engineered cells, Vaccinia virus expression systems, 437–438
genotoxicity, DNA repair, 333
genotoxicity testing, 324–339, 318–339
bacterial gene mutation tests, Ames, 325
Escherichia coli 324
bacterial gene mutation tests, *Salmonella typhimurium*, 324
chromosomal fragments, 335
chromosome aberrations, 331
comet assay, 446
DNA damage, 331–334
mammalian cell tests, cell transformation, 336–337
chromosome aberrations, 331
cytogenetic damage, 328–331
gene mutation, 326–331
micronucleus, 335
structure–activity relationships, 331
use of inmortal cell lines, 337–339
yeast gene mutation tests, 335–336
mitochondrial mutation, 336
glia, 157
glia-derived neurotrophic factor (GDNF), 159
glial fibrillary acidic protein (GFAP), 162
glucagon glycogen depletion, hepatocytes, 400
in culture medium, hepatocytes, 135
glucocorticoids, 413
gluconeogenesis, hepatocytes, 398
β-glucuronidase, use in deconjugation of drug metabolites, 141
glutamate, neurotoxicity, 168
glutathione fluorimetric quantification, 386
hepatocytes, 142
glutathione peroxidase, determination of lipid hydroperoxides, 384
glutathione reductase, 379
glutathione *S*-transferase, isoform α, 420
in hepatocytes, 417
oxidative stress, 385
glycogen depletion by glucagon, 400
measurement in hepatocytes, 400
GM-CSF, 231
GQ ganglioside, 170
growth associated proteins, neurotoxicity, 158
GSH, *see* Glutathione,
GSH-enzymes *see corresponding* Glutathione enzyme(s)

haloalkene, nephrotoxicity, 82
halothane
covalent binding, 392
hepatotoxicity, 106
haptoglobin, synthesis by hepatocytes, 146
Harber–Weiss Fenton reaction, 384
heat shock protein, hsp-70, 173
hepatic models, 107–121
adult human hepatocytes, *see also* human hepatocytes, 131–148
adult rat hepatocytes, 107–109
liver slices, 111–118
use in drug development, 107, 144
hepatocyte growth factor (HGF), DNA synthesis in human hepatocytes, 145, 415–417
hepatocytes, culture systems, alginate, 414
capillary membranes, 414
co-culture, 414
collagen, 414
matrigel, 109, 414
monolayer, 414
three-dimensional, 415
dog, 424
fetal, 109–111
fetal human, isolation, 110
fetal rat, characterization, 110
fetal rat, isolation, 110
growth in vitro, 415–416
human, 131–148, 424
monkey, 424
rat, 424
adduct formation, 120
comparative transport, 119
DNA synthesis, 120
mechanistic studies, 119
functional characterization, 108
isolation, 107
multicellular agreggates, 109
survival in culture, 413
hepatocytoma, 147
hepatomas HepG2 cells, 434, 437
use in hepatotoxicity testing, 397
hepatotoxicity, 104–106, 144, 397–401
allergic hepatitis, 396
antibodies against CYPs, 396
autoantibodies, 396
drug antibodies, 396

hepatotoxicity *cont.*
immunological mechanisms, 395–397
lytic necrosis, 377
mechanisms, 105
mechanistic studies, use of human tissue
types of, 376
Hepatotoxicity testing, cytotoxicity parameters, 398
interpretation of results, 400
maximal non-cytotoxic concentration, 399
metabolic parameter, 398
predictive value, 400
reversibility, 401
reversibility of *in vitro* effects, 401
toxicity risk assessment, 401
HepG2 cells, 434, 437
HETC (Human Equivalent Toxic Concentration in Plasma), 50
HET-CAM test, ocular irritation testing, 42, 47, 272–274
HET-CAM test, *see also* CAMVA test
n-hexane, neurotoxicity, 167
2,5-hexanedione, 167
2-hexanol, 167
2-hexanone, 167
hexosaminidase, cytotoxicity testing, 446
HFL1 cells, for general cytotoxicity testing, 45
HGF (hepatic growth factor), 145
hippocampal slice culture, for neurotoxicity testing, 168, 169
histidine photo-oxidation test, 302–304, 310
human embryonic palatal mesenchymal cells, teratogenicity testing, 355
human hepatocytes, biochemical functionality, 138–139
human hepatocytes, biotransformation activities, 139–144
alkoxyresorufin-*O*-de-alkylase, 140
arylhydrocarbon hydroxylase, 147
coumarin 7-hydroxylase, 141
CYP450, 143, 147
epoxide hydrolase, 143
7-ethoxycoumarin-*O*-de-ethylase, 143
glutathione *S*-transferase, 142, 143
7-methoxycoumarin-*O*-demethylase, 147
NADPH-cytochrome c reductase, 143–144
p-nitrophenol hyroxylase, 141
testosterone hydroxylation, 141
UDP-glucuronyl transferase, 142, 143
culture systems, biomatrix, 135–136
co-culture, 137, 144
collagen gels, 135–136
fibronectin, 134
medium, 134
DNA synthesis, 145
drug metabolism enzymes, *see* human hepatocytes, biotransformation activities
immortalization, 147
isolation, cell viability, 134
collagenase, 131, 133
perfusion, 131, 133
isolation and culture techniques, 131–139
use in drug metabolism studies, 144, 422–425
use in pharmacotoxicology, 425
hydra, teratogenicity testing, 354

idiosyncratic, hepatoxicity, 376
IGF-2 (insulin-like growth factor), 158
immortalization, of human hepatocytes, 147
immortalized cell lines, 162
immunotoxicity, antigen-presenting cells, 227–229
dendritic cells, 227
macrophages, 228
monocytes, 228
immunotoxicology, 232–238
drug-induced immunosupression, 238
in vitro tests, 235
lymph node assay, 234
in vitro models extent and use by pharmaceutical industry, 3–6
present limitations, 5
in vitro skin corrosivity test, 18
in vitro tests, and QSAR modelling, 26
indo-1, calcium measurement, 390
indomethacin, chondriocytes, 197
inflammatory mediators, *see also* cytokines
arachidonic acid release in cutaneous models, 258
inhibitory concentration (IC50), 51
insulin, in culture medium, hepatocytes, 41, 14
interferon, 421
effects on CYP450 expression, 42, 15
interleukin 1, 173
interleukin 1β, 228
interleukin 2, 230
interleukin 3, 230
interleukin 4, 230
interleukin 5, 230
interleukin 6, 145, 146, 230
interleukin 7, 230
interleukin 8, 230
interleukin 9, 230
interleukin 10, 230
interleukin 11, 230
interleukin 12, 230
interleukin 13, 230
interleukin 14, 230
interleukin and cutaneous inflammatory processes, 258
effects in CYP450 expression, 421
intersystem crossing, 293
intrinsic, hepatoxicity, 376
irritation testing, *see* Ocular irritation, cutaneous toxicity
use of cell lines, 46–48
isolated rabbit eye test (IRE), ocular irritation testing, 275
isosafrole, enzyme inducer, 419

keratinocytes co-culture, 246
commercial models, 248–249
conventional cultures, 245–247
high-density culture, 245
isolation, 245
low-density culture, 246
three dimensional cultures, 247
ketoconazol, teratogenicity, 362
ketoprofen chondriocytes, 197
phototoxicity, 297, 298, 303
ketotifen, metabolism, 423
Krumdieck slicer, 113

L-929 cells, in biocompatibility assays, 46
lactate dehydrogenase cutaneous toxicity, 256
hepatotoxicity, 398
myocytes, 215
neuronal cells, 168
phototoxicity, 31, 3
laminin, extracellular matrix, 158
lauric acid, metabolism, 418
ligand-operated Ca^{2+} channels, 388
limb-bud cell culture, teratogenicity testing, 355
lipid hydroperoxides, determination with glutathione peroxidase, 384
lipid peroxidation hepatotoxicity, 381–384, 398
nephrotoxicity, 84
phototoxicity, 301–302
quantification methods, 382–384
quantification, with glutathione peroxidase, 383
with thiobarbituric acid, 382
lipid peroxides, fluorimetric determination, with thiobarbituric acid, 382
liposome-transfection, 442
liver perfusion, collagenase, 131–133
digitonin-collagenase, 419
liver slices, 116–119
cytochrome P450 levels, 115
drug toxic interactions, 116
incubation system, 114
mechanistic studies, 117
methodology, 111
peroxisome proliferation, 118
toxicity parameters, 118
liver-specific functions in cultured hepatocytes, 412–416
in isolated hepatocytes, 412
role in medium composition, 413
LLC-PK1 cells, in renal toxicity, 45
lovastatin, enzyme inducer, 419
LPS (bacterial lipopolysaccharide), 228
luciferin–luciferase assay, ATP measurement, 381
lymph node assay, immunotoxicology testing, 234
lymphocytes, 226

α2-macroglobulin, synthesis, by hepatocytes, 146
malondialdehyde determination, with thiobarbituric acid, 393
formation during lipid peroxidation, 383
mast cell degranulation, phototoxicity testing, 305
maximal non-cytotoxic concentration, 399
M-CSF, 231
MDCK cells, in renal toxicity, 45, 46
mephenytoin, metabolism, 418
mercuric chloride, nephrotoxicity, 71–72, 83
metamphetamine, neurotoxicity, 169
methotrexate, teratogenicity, 362
methoxyethanol, teratogenicity, 362
N-methyl-D-aspartate, neurotoxicity, 160
methyl-4-phenylpyridinium, neurotoxicity, 159
methylene dioxyamphetamine, neurotoxicity, 169
methyltetrahydrofolate, nephrotoxicity, 69
4-methylumbelliferone, 142
metronidazol, teratogenicity, 362
micromass culture, neuronal models, 170
micronucleus assay, genotoxicity testing, 446
microtubule-associated proteins (MAPs), 170
minaprine, metabolism, 423
mitomycin, use to inhibit fibroblast proliferation, 246
mitochondrial function, membrane potential, 171, 218, 380, 381
proton motility force, 220
in neurotoxicity testing, 170
mitotic index, 330
molecular chaperonin ubiquitin, 169
monkey hepatocytes, 424
monoaminergic neurones, 169
monochlorobimane, fluorimetric determination of glutathione, 387
mouse ovary tumour cells, teratogenicity testing, 355
MRC-5 cells in general cytotoxicity testing, 45
in phototoxicity, 311
MTT cytotoxicity testing in, cell lines, 39, 42
fibroblasts, 304, 31
hepatocytes, 398
myocytes, 218
neuronal cells, 170
myocytes, *see* Cardiac myocytes

NADPH-P450 oxidoreductase, 438
NADPH-cytochrome c reductase, bitranformation activity, 143–144
β-naftoflavone, enzyme inducer, 118
naproxen chondrocytes, 197
phototoxicity, 301
NCTC 2544 cells, in skin irritation, 46
necrosis, hepatocyte, 377
nephrotoxicity antibiotics, 82
bile acid, 85
chloroform, 81
cultured kidney cells, 64–69
glomerular injury, 83
haloalkenes, 82
heavy metals, 83

nephrotoxicity antibiotics *cont.*
  hydroperoxidase mediated, 84
  mechanistic studies, 8, 79, 81–85
    lipid peroxidation, 84
    role of hydroperoxidase, 84
    use of human tissue, 80–81
  renal models, cell-free systems, 78–79
    cultured kidney cells, 73, 78
    slices, 60
  testing, choice of the *in vitro* system, 59–62
    marker enzymes, 65
    micromethods, 66
    fluorescent probes, 66
    MTT, 65
    non-invasive methods, 68
    Alamar blue, 69
    epithelial barrier function test, 68
    selection of end-points, 64–66
nerve growth factor (NGF), neurotoxicity, 158
neural cell adhesion molecule, 170
neural differentiation, neurospores, 158
neural models, dissection of specific brain regions, 160
neural reaggregate cultures, 169
neural tissue cells, teratogenicity testing, 355
neurite growth, 16, 163
  neurofilament proteins, 164
neuroblastoma cell lines, 162
  teratogenicity testing, 355
neuronal differentiation, 157
neuronal models, 159–170
  co-cultures, 167–168
  complex primary cultures, 168–170
    cultured spinal neurones, 169
    hippocampal slice culture, 168, 169
    micromass culture, 170
    organotypic cultures, 169
    reaggregate cultures, 169
  hybrid cells, 167
  neuronal cell lines, 162–165
    human neuroblastoma (LA-N-2) 163
    human SKNSH neuroblastoma, 164
    mouse NB41A3 neuroblastoma, 164
    murine motor neurone (NSC19), 163
    murine septal (SN56), 163
    SHSY5Y neuroblastoma, 163
  neuronal differentiation, 164
  primary cultures, cerebral cortical neurones, 159, 16
    cerebral granule cells, 161
    chick embryo neurones, 161
    rat embryonic cortical neurones, 162
    rat embryonic septal neurones, 161
    rat hippocampal neurones, 160, 161
  transfected cells, use in genetic neural disease studies, 166
  transformed cells, use in genetic neural disease studies, 166
neuropathy target esterase (NTE), 163
neurotoxicity, 156–159, 170–175
  and apoptosis, 17, 157, 174
  assessment parameters, 170–175
  oxidative stress, 162
neurotoxicity testing, cellular ATP, 171
  intracellular calcium, 172
  intracellular pH, 172
  mitochondrial function, 170
  mitochondrial potential, 171
  neurotransmitter release, 174
  nitric oxide production, 172
  nitric oxide synthetase induction, 172
  pinocytosis, 171
  plasma membrane integrity, 171
  proto-oncogene expression, 173
  receptor binging, 174
  stress gene expression, 173
  synaptogenesis, 172
  transcellular traffic of solutes, 171
  transcription factors, 173
neurotrophic factors, 158
neurotrophins, 158, 16
neutral red test cell lines, 39, 41
  chondriocytes, 171
  cutaneous models, 256
  hepatocytes, 398
  ocular irritation, 277
  phototoxicity, 304, 31
NHEK cells, cytotoxicity testing, 46
nicotinamide, in culture medium, of hepatocytes, 413
nifedipine, metabolism, by hepatocytes, 418
nitric oxide CYP inhibition, in hepatocytes, 145
  neurotoxicity testing, 172
nitric oxide synthetase (NOS), 162
nitroblue tetrazolium, reactive oxygen species determination, in myocytes, 217
4-nitrophenol hydroxylase induction by ethanol, 420
  biotransformation enzyme, 141
non-steroidal anti-inflammatory drugs, phototoxicity, 119

Ochratoxin A, nephrotoxicity, 71–72
ocular irritation, 271–282
  cellular models, red blood cell haemolysis (RBC), 278
  isolated rabbit eye test (IRE), 275
  models, 272–281
  cellular models, 277–281
  organotypic cultures, 272–277
    BCOP, 274–275
    chicken enucleated eye (CEET), 276–277
    chorion allantoic membrane (CAMVA test), 274
    dermal tissue equivalent, 280
    EYTEX, 281
    HET-CAM test, 272–274

isolated rabbit eye (IRE), 275
test validation, 282–284
tests, *see also* Ocular irritation testing, 272–282
ocular irritation testing chicken enucleated eye (CEET test), 276
Draize's eye test, limitations, 266–267
refinement, 268–271
use, 266–267
fluorescein leakage test, 279
silicon microphysiometer test, 280
omeprazole, enzyme inducer, 419
organophosphates, neurotoxicity, 16, 161
organotypic models neurotoxicity, 169
ocular irritation, 272–277
oxidative stress glutathione, hepatocytes, 285
hepatocytes, 384–387
in neurotoxicity, 162
redox cycling, hepatocytes, 384
oxygen reactive species determination with nibroblue tetrazolium, in myocytes, 217
hepatotoxicity, 381–383
phototoxicity, 305

P450, *see* CYP
p53 gene, 447
palatal shelves, teratogenicity, 355
paraoxon, neurotoxicity, 163
parathyroid hormone, in culture medium, chondrocyte cultures, 196
pentoxyresorufin, CYP1A1/2 substrate, hepatocytes
pentoxyresorufin-O-depenthylation, hepatocytes, 418
Percoll, hepatocyte isolation, 109
percutaneous absorption, 250–253
drug concentration in skin structures, 252
interpretation of results, 252
kinetics, 252
phenacetin, metabolism, hepatocytes, 418
phenobarbital, enzyme inducer, 118
phenolsulphotransferases, expression in HepG2 cells, 438
phenytoin, hepatotoxicity, 106
phorbal esters, neuronal differentiation, 164
photoallergy, 291–293
photo–basophil–histamine release, in phototoxicity testing, 305
photodegranulation of mast cells, in phototoxicity testing, 305
photohaemolysis, in phototoxicity testing, 31, 300
photomutagenicity, in hototoxicity testing, 304
photosensitization mechanisms, 293–295
see Phototoxicity, Photoallergy, 290–291
phototoxicity, 291, 306, 311
phototoxicity testing, 299–306, 306–311
Candida albicans, 301, 310
DNA photocleavage, 304
fibroblasts, 304, 310–311
histidine photo-oxidation, 302–304, 310–311
lipid peroxidation, 301–302
lymphocytes, DNA synthesis, 305
measurement of reactive oxygen species formation, 305
peroxides determination, 308
photo–basophil–histamine release, 305
photodegranulation of mast cells, 305
photohaemolysis, 300, 309
side effects of drugs, 291–293
spectrophotometric tests, 300
physiologically based pharmacokinetic models (PBPK), 17
piroxicam, effects of chondrocytes, 197
Planaria, use in teratogenicity testing, 354
plasma protein synthesis, by hepatocytes, 398
poly-L-lysine, 160
pox virus, in teratogenicity, 354
predictive value, hepatotoxicity testing, 400
procainamide, metabolism, by hepatocytes, 418
proliferating cell nuclear antigen (PCNA), 17, 164
promethazine, prevention of lipid peroxidation, 383
propidium iodine, cytotoxicity testing, 215
proteoglycans, extracellular matrix, in cartilage, 183

QSARs (Quantitative Structure–Activity Relationships), 15–17
selection of chemicals, 23
development of predictive models, 18
relation to the dose applied, 18
in validation studies, 24–29
in *in vitro* studies, 23
limitations, 23
model development, 17
parameter selection, 17, 20–22
for *in vitro* studies, 23
dipole moment, 20, 21
octanol/water partition coefficient, 17
in predictive skin corrosivity, 18
quin-2, calcium measurement, 390
quinolones, phototoxicity, 292
quinones, hepatotoxicity, 385

rat hepatocytes (adult), 107–109, 119–121, 424
rat hepatocytes (fetal), 110
reactive oxygen species, *see* Oxygen reactive species
reconstructed skin Bell's model, 249
Boyce's model, 249
Naughton model, 249
red blood cell haemolysis test, phototoxicity testing, 278
renal, toxicity, *see also* Nephrotoxicity, 56–59
renal injury, mechanisms, 58
renal models, cell-free, 78–79
cellular models, cell organelles, 78
cytosolic systems, 62–64, 74–78, 79

renal models *cont.*
cell lines, 75–78
LLC-PK1 cells, 62
MDCK cells, 62
NRK cells, 62
OK cells, 62–63
PTC cells, 63
culture media, 62
distal tubular cells, 74
freshly isolated cells, 74
glomeruli cells, 75
medullary intersticial cells, 75
proximal tubular cells, 62, 74
complex culture systems, 69–73
glomeruli, 72
isolated nephron segments, 70, 71
enzymic dispersion, 72
mechanical shearing, 72
proximal tubular fragments, 72
renal cortical slices, conventional renal cortical slices, 70
precision-cut, 71
renal perfused kidney, 69
intact renal cellular systems, 69–73
renal toxicity, *see* nephrotoxicity
retinoic acid, neuronal differentiation, 164
neurotoxicity, 163
rhodamine-123
assessment mitochondrial potential
hepatocytes, 381
myocytes, 219
neurones, 171
labelling of mitochondria, 170
rifampicin, enzyme inducer, 419
rodent embryo culture, teratogenicity testing, 356
ruthenium red, blocking of mitochondrial Ca^{2+} sequestration, 161

S-9 fraction, preparation, 142
Saccharomyces cerevesiae genotoxicity testing, 335
Salmonella typhimurium genotoxicity testing, 324
sea urchin embryo, teratogenicity testing, 356
shrimp embryo, teratogenicity testing, 356
skin models, *see* Cutaneous models, dermal equivalents and reconstructed skin
toxicity, *see* Cutaneous toxicity
silicon microphysiometer test, ocular irritation testing, 280
sister chromatid exchange, genotoxicity testing, 333–334, 446
SKF525-A, CYP inhibitor, 117, 120
SNARF, *see* Carboxyseminapthorhodofluor-1, 172
spinal neurones, 169
S-thiolation of proteins, 386
suprofen, phototoxicity, 302

3T3 cells, in biocompatibility assays, 46–47

Taxol, neurotoxicity, 159
T-cell lymphocytes, 227
tenascin, extracellular matrix, 184
testosterone metabolism, for specific CYP measurement, in hepatocytes, 141
teratogenicity testing, 354–356
chicken embryo, 356
embryo cultures, 354, 356
FETAX test in frog, 356
human embryonic palatal mesenchymal cells, 355
in hydra, 354
in vitro potency, 357
sensitivity, 357
validation, 358
invertebrates, 354
limb-bud culture, 355
limb-bud cell, 355
mammalian cells, 354, 355
mammalian embryo, 363–368
advantages, 365
culture, 364
end-points, 365
mammalian organ cultures, 354, 355
mouse ovary tumour cells, 355
palatal shelves, 355
pharmaceutical applications, 356
viruses, 354
tetramethylrhodamine methyl ester, mitochondrial membrane potential, 219
TGF β, *see* Transforming growth factor β
theophylline, teratogenicity, 362
thioacetamide, hepatotoxicity, 378
thiobarbituric acid, fluorimetric measurement of lipid peroxidation products, 383
thiolation of proteins, 386
thioredoxin, dethiolation mechanisms, 386
three-dimensional cultures hepatocytes, capillary membranes, 415
keratinocytes, 247
tiaprofenic acid, phototoxicity, 3, 302
tienilic acid, hepatotoxicity, 106
TNF α, *see* Tumor necrosis factor α
tosufloxacin, metabolism, 423, 424
toxicity risk index (Tr), 401
transfected cells
see also Engineered cells, as neuronal models, 17, 166
transferrin, synthesis in culture, by hepatocytes, 146
transformed cells, in neuronal models, 166
transforming growth factor β BEAS-2B cells, 440
chondrocytes, 196
hepatocytes, 145, 421
trypan blue exclusion test, assessment of cell viability, 108, 134, 215
tumor necrosis factor α effects on human hepatocytes, 16, 145, 421
immunotoxicity, 23, 23
neurotoxicity, 173

TUNEL (translation of uridine end-labelling) assay, for assessment of apoptosis, 174

ubiquitin in hepatocytes, 142–143
  in neurones, 173
UDP-glucuronyl transferases, expression in mammalian cells, 438
unscheduled DNA synthesis, genotoxicity testing, 333
ureogenesis, hepatotoxicity, 398

V79 cells cytotoxicity testing, 42
  genotoxicity testing, 328
  teratogenicity testing, 355
vaccinia virus, expression systems for biotransformation enzymes, 437–438
validation of ocular irritation tests, 282–284
  of cellular *in vitro* tests, 24–25
    maximum average score, 28
  European Union/Home Office, Draize's test, 24, 25
  Quantitative Structure–Activity Relationships (QSAR), 24–29
valproic acid, chondrocytes, 198
voltage-dependent Ca^{2+} channels, 388

WI38 cells, in general cytotoxicity testing, 45

yeast gene mutation test, genotoxicity testing, 335–336